SCIENCE
FICTIONS

ALSO BY JOHN CREWDSON

By Silence Betrayed:
The Sexual Abuse of Children in America

The Tarnished Door:
The New Immigrants and the Transformation of America

SCIENCE FICTIONS

A Scientific Mystery, a Massive Coverup,
and the Dark Legacy of Robert Gallo

JOHN CREWDSON

LITTLE, BROWN AND COMPANY
BOSTON   NEW YORK   LONDON

First Edition

Library of Congress Cataloging-in-Publication Data
Crewdson, John.
    Science fictions : A Scientific Mystery, a Massive Coverup,
and the Dark Legacy of Robert Gallo / John Crewdson — 1st ed.
      p. cm.
    Includes index.
    ISBN 0-316-13476-7
    1. HIV (Viruses) — Research — History.   2. Gallo, Robert C.
3. Institut Pasteur (Paris, France) 4. Fraud in science.   I. Title.

QR414.6.H58 .C74 2002
616.97'92'009 — dc21   200103445

10 9 8 7 6 5 4 3 2 1

Designed by Paula Russell Szafranski
Q-FF

Printed in the United States of America

For Prudence

"We've learned from experience that the truth will come out. Other experimenters will repeat your experiment and find out whether you were wrong or right. Nature's phenomena will agree or they'll disagree with your theory. And, although you may gain some temporary fame and excitement, you will not gain a good reputation as a scientist if you haven't tried to be very careful in this kind of work."

— Richard P. Feynman,
in his 1974 commencement address
to the graduating class of Caltech

CONTENTS

Preface   xi

Timeline   xiii

Prologue *"This* Is What We're Going to Work On"   3

1. "Too Lucky to Be True"   13

2. "These Guys Have Found Something Important"   38

3. "We Were Wrong, and Barré-Sinoussi Was Right"   65

4. "This Looks Like It Could Be the Cause"   95

5. "Our Eminent Dr. Robert Gallo"   120

6. "We Assumed That Was *Your* Job"   141

7. "Only Because There Are So Many"   160

8. "Let Them Bark in the Wind"   177

9. "I Don't Want to Go to Jail"   200

10. "French Virus in the Picture"   226

11. "Bingo. We Win"   246

12. "A Small Guy Who Stumbled"   268

13. "Just Show Us the Proof"   279

14. "We Were Going to Get Killed"   293

15. "The Whole Thing Was Sordid"   311

16.	"Einstein, Freud — I'd Put Him on a List Like That"	330
17.	"I Have Probably Talked Too Much"	346
18.	"Of Course We *Did* Grow LAV"	369
19.	"If Chance Will Have Me King"	393
20.	"I Know I Don't Lie"	414
21.	"Intellectual Recklessness of a High Degree"	428
22.	"It Can't Be the Money"	442
23.	"Slander Is the Worst Crime"	458
24.	"The Steaks Are Not Done"	475
25.	"We Did It to Ourselves"	488
26.	"Dr. Gallo Is No Longer Here"	506
	Epilogue "Rather Does the Truth Ennoble All"	525
	Notes	541
	Dramatis Personae	621
	Glossary	629
	Index	643

PREFACE

This is not a book about AIDS. Nor is it really about science. It is a book about how scientists behave when the stakes are high, and the stakes were never higher than in the search for the cause of AIDS. The story of that search is drawn from thousands of pages of correspondence, memorandums, laboratory notes, transcripts, and other documents compiled during several years of official investigations. Despite the current fashion, none of the dialogue in this book is reconstructed. Words between quotation marks are those that I myself heard spoken, or which are contained in documents in my possession. If scientific-minded readers find the science oversimple, I ask them to remember that this book is not only for them. In this spirit I have presented technical terms in a consistent style, even though some of those terms may appear differently in articles and documents that are quoted. Thus, the human T-cell line HUT-78 is always referred to that way, even in a direct quotation from a document in which it may have been called HUT78 or Hut78 or HuT-78. So too with the human retroviruses, which Robert Gallo designated HTLV-I, HTLV-II, and HTLV-III (later renamed by others HIV). Because no other system of virological nomenclature uses Roman numerals, and to make such terms easier to read, I have called these viruses HTLV-1, HTLV-2, and HTLV-3 throughout. For the freedom to pursue this story in the face of what sometimes seemed inordinate pressure I owe a considerable debt to Jack Fuller, who edited the *Chicago Tribune's*

50,000-word account of the discovery of HIV, and also to Howard Tyner, who edited most of the subsequent *Tribune* reporting on the investigations inspired by the original article. Thanks also to my agent, Kathy Robbins, and my editors, Bill Phillips and Geoff Shandler, for their extraordinary patience and continuing conviction that the story of HIV is a story worth telling.

Bethesda, Maryland
August 2001

TIMELINE

December 1980: Bernard Poiesz and Francis Ruscetti discover HTLV in a patient with lymphoma.

January 29, 1983: At the Institut Pasteur in Paris, Françoise Barré detects a new human retrovirus, later called LAV, in cultured blood cells from Frédéric Brugière.

May 20, 1983: In *Science,* Robert Gallo reports isolating HTLV from one AIDS patient and detecting the virus in three others, including Claude Chardon. In the same issue, Barré, Luc Montagnier, and Jean-Claude Chermann report the isolation from Frédéric Brugière of a retrovirus different from HTLV.

May 30, 1983: Montagnier obtains second isolate of the AIDS virus, *Loi,* from Eric Loiseau, a French hemophiliac.

June 9, 1983: Montagnier obtains third AIDS virus isolate, *Lai,* from Christophe Lailler, a French homosexual with AIDS.

June 25, 1983: Pasteur obtains fourth AIDS virus isolate, LAV/Pri, from a Haitian patient.

July 14, 1983: Françoise Brun-Vézinet and Christine Rouzioux begin testing AIDS patients' blood samples for LAV antibodies in Paris.

July 17, 1983: Montagnier delivers the first sample of LAV from Frédéric Brugière to Gallo's house ("July LAV").

September 3, 1983: Montagnier obtains fifth AIDS virus isolate, *Eli,* from a Zairian woman with AIDS.

September 15, 1983: At Cold Spring Harbor, Montagnier reports LAV antibodies have been detected in 63 percent of patients with pre-AIDS and 20 percent of those with AIDS. Gallo proposes HTLV as "the almost-certain" cause of AIDS. Same day, Pasteur applies for a European patent on its blood test for LAV antibodies.

September 20, 1983: Mikulas Popovic uses July LAV to infect two T-cell cultures. One is sent to Matt Gonda, who photographs retrovirus particles in the cells.

September 22, 1983: A second shipment of LAV is received by Gallo's lab ("September LAV").

October 6, 1983: Popovic discovers that AIDS patients infected with HTLV are also infected with LAV, while others are infected with LAV alone. No AIDS patients are infected only with HTLV. He concludes that "we were wrong and Barré-Sinoussi was right."

October 24, 1983: Betsy Read uses LAV to infect five continuous T-cell lines; the virus grows best in Ti7.4 and HUT-78.

November 15, 1983: According to his later testimony, Popovic initiates the "Popovic pool" with material from three AIDS patients.

November 22, 1983: Popovic adds more material from the same three patients to the pool. His notes contain the notation "HUT78/V; Ti7.4/V = MOV."

November 29, 1983: Popovic uses MOV to infect a continuous T-cell line, H-4, cloned from the HUT-78 cell line.

December 5, 1983: Pasteur applies for a U.S. patent on its LAV blood antibody test.

December 14, 1983: Gonda informs Popovic he has photographed retrovirus particles in the Ti7.4/LAV and HUT-78/LAV cell lines. Montagnier obtains Pasteur's twelfth AIDS virus isolate, LAV/Rab.

December 23, 1983: In a telephone call, Popovic tells Montagnier that "we learned how to handle" LAV — but not that LAV is growing in continuous cultures in Bethesda.

December 29, 1983: Betsy Read infects HUT-78 with virus from Haitian AIDS patient R.F., the Gallo lab's first successful AIDS virus isolate.

January 2, 1984: Popovic adds material from seven new patients to the "Popovic pool" in hopes of saving the culture. Four of the seven samples are later found to contain no AIDS virus.

January 6, 1984: First blood antibody testing is performed in Bethesda by M. G. Sarngadharan, using the AIDS virus Popovic calls MOV.

January 19, 1984: Popovic clones the H-9 cell line from HUT-78.

February 7, 1984: At Park City, Utah, Gallo says his "only candidate" for the AIDS virus is HTLV or a close genetic variant. Chermann's presentation of the latest LAV antibody testing data from Paris persuades many of those present that LAV is the cause of AIDS.

February 8, 1984: Montagnier begins growing LAV in the FR-8 cell line, which he created by transforming normal B-cells into leukemic B-cells.

February 25, 1984: Popovic begins growing HTLV-3B in the H-9 cell line.

February 27, 1984: Françoise Brun-Vézinet finds LAV antibodies in 90 percent of Zairian AIDS patients.

February 29, 1984: Sarngadharan finds antibodies to MOV in 85 percent of pre-AIDS patients and 90 percent of AIDS patients.

March 9, 1984: After testing CDC blood samples, Pasteur reports LAV antibodies in 91 percent of pre-AIDS patients and 79 percent of those with AIDS, convincing the CDC that LAV is "the proximal cause of AIDS."

March 12, 1984: Testing many of the same CDC blood samples sent to France, Sarngadharan finds antibodies to HTLV-3B in 87 percent of pre-AIDS patients but only 48 percent of AIDS patients. Gallo's marginal results are later changed to positive.

April 1, 1984: Simon Wain-Hobson and Marc Alizon obtain the first partial genetic clone of LAV.

April 6, 1984: Meeting at Pasteur, the CDC's Don Francis shows Gallo and Montagnier the "remarkably similar" results of the comparative blood testing with LAV and HTLV-3B.

April 9, 1984: Gallo chooses HTLV-3B over R.F. as the AIDS virus to be used in commercial production of the Gallo blood antibody test.

April 23, 1984: Margaret Heckler announces that "our eminent Dr. Robert Gallo" has discovered the virus that causes AIDS and invented a blood antibody test for that virus.

May 4, 1984: Gallo reports in *Science* the isolation of HTLV-3 from forty-eight patients and the discovery of a continuous T-cell line, "HT," in which the virus can be grown. He suggests that "HTLV-3 and LAV may be different" viruses, although LAV "has not yet been transmitted to a permanently growing cell line for true isolation and therefore has been difficult to obtain in quantity."

May 15, 1984: Sarngadharan visits Institut Pasteur, bringing a frozen sample of live HTLV-3B, Gallo's principal AIDS virus isolate.

June 8, 1984: Gallo's lab obtains first partial clone of HTLV-3B, BH-5.

July 12, 1984: Montagnier sends LAV growing in a B-cell line to Bethesda.

August 16, 1984: Wain-Hobson and Alizon obtain first full-length clone of LAV, J-19.

August 23, 1984: Gallo tells Montagnier that LAV sent by Montagnier the previous month is highly similar genetically to HTLV-3B; he suggests that the HTLV-3B taken to Paris by Sarngadharan in May contaminated Montagnier's B-cell LAV cultures.

August 31, 1984: Gallo reveals that the source of HTLV-3B was a pool of material from several AIDS patients.

December 6, 1984: At the National Cancer Institute, Simon Wain-Hobson presents the first gene map of the AIDS virus. Gallo's group does not present a map of HTLV-3.

January 21, 1985: Pasteur publishes the DNA sequence and gene map of LAV.

January 23, 1985: Gallo publishes the DNA sequence of HTLV-3B, which is genetically indistinguishable from that of LAV. Gallo's misinterpretation of the sequence is reflected in his erroneous gene map of HTLV-3B.

March 2, 1985: The U.S. Food and Drug Administration licenses the Gallo blood antibody test for manufacture by Abbott Laboratories.

May 28, 1985: Gallo and HHS are awarded the American patent on their AIDS antibody test.

August 6, 1985: Raymond Dedonder leads a delegation from Pasteur to Washington to protest the administration's failure to grant Pasteur a patent on its LAV antibody test.

December 12, 1985: Pasteur sues HHS, alleging that HTLV-3B is LAV, that the French discovered the AIDS virus and developed the blood antibody test first, and that the Gallo test is therefore being manufactured with a virus discovered in France. Gallo insists that the LAV samples sent from Paris were "too small to be of practical use," and were "physically impossible" to grow.

February 19, 1986: Ten months after the application was submitted, the FDA licenses the Pasteur AIDS test for sale in the United States.

April 18, 1986: Gallo acknowledges that the pictures of "HTLV-3" he published in *Science* in May 1984 are actually the National Cancer Institute's pictures of LAV.

May 8, 1986: Gallo claims in *Nature* to have isolated the AIDS virus in late 1982, three months before Pasteur reported the isolation of LAV from Frédéric Brugière.

November 8, 1986: Gallo signs sworn declaration attesting that he "saw no evidence" LAV was the cause of AIDS "up through the allowance of the Gallo patent" in May of 1985.

March 31, 1987: President Reagan and French Prime Minister Chirac agree that HHS and Pasteur will share the American patent for the AIDS blood test.

August 1989: Gallo acknowledges that the H-9 cell line and its parent line, "HT," are actually HUT-78.

January 11, 1990: The NIH's Office of Scientific Integrity opens an inquiry into Gallo's AIDS research.

May 17, 1991: Pasteur reports that what was thought to be LAV_{Bru} is actually LAV_{Lai} from Christophe Lailler.

May 30, 1991: Gallo acknowledges in *Nature* that HTLV-3B is not an independent discovery but rather LAV_{Lai}, which Gallo claims accidentally contaminated virus cultures in his laboratory.

June 30, 1991: The Office of Scientific Integrity finds Mikulas Popovic guilty of scientific misconduct, and concludes that Gallo's actions "warrant significant censure."

January 30, 1992: A review panel of the National Academy of Sciences accuses Gallo of "intellectual recklessness of a high degree" and "essentially immoral" behavior by impeding the free release of HTLV-3B and the H-9 cell line to all requesting laboratories.

December 29, 1992: The NIH's Office of Research Integrity finds Gallo guilty of scientific misconduct for "falsely reporting [in *Science*] that LAV had not been transmitted to a permanently growing cell line."

June 3, 1993: The results of the ORI investigation, reported in *Nature*, show that both HTLV-3B and MOV are LAV_{Lai}.

November 5, 1993: Following Popovic's appeal, the Research Integrity Adjudications Panel reverses the ORI's finding that Popovic is guilty of scientific misconduct.

November 12, 1993: ORI declares that "recent decisions" by the Adjudications Panel make it "extraordinarily difficult for ORI to defend its legal determination of scientific misconduct regarding Dr. Gallo," and the finding is withdrawn.

July 11, 1994: Agreeing to cede the French some $6 million in future patent royalties, HHS acknowledges for the first time that "a virus provided by Institut Pasteur was used by National Institutes of Health scientists who invented the American HIV test kit in 1984."

SCIENCE
FICTIONS

PROLOGUE

"*This* Is What We're Going to Work On"

The virus. The Great White Shark of the microbiological kingdom, a relentless invader whose single-minded mission is to attack the cells of its unwilling host — a person, an animal, a plant — and do as much damage as possible. A million times smaller than the cells they infect, viruses are among the tiniest entities on earth — bare shards of genetic information wrapped in protein-covered packages, fifty thousand of which could fit on the head of a pin.

To call a virus microscopic is too generous. Because they are smaller than the wavelength of visible light, viruses can't be seen even with the most powerful microscopes. The answer to the question of whether viruses are alive, a late-night favorite among undergraduates, is "yes and no." Yes, because like people, animals, and plants, viruses can reproduce themselves, thus ensuring their continued survival. No, because viruses, which have no reproductive machinery of their own, must commandeer the genetic tools they find lying around the cells of their host.

Once a virus begins to reproduce, hundreds of thousands of copies issue forth each hour in search of new cells to infect. In as long as it takes to go from "I think I'm coming down with something" to a fever of 101, the unfortunate host is awash with virus. Depending on the nature of the virus and the cell under attack, the host either goes on living or not. If the invader is this year's strain of influenza A, the patient probably will survive an uncomfortable week of fever and aching muscles. If the virus is one that causes hemorrhagic fever, the host would do well to have his affairs in order. Between those extremes lie viruses that cause serious, but usually nonfatal, diseases like measles, mumps, and chickenpox, and some that appear to do nothing at all. But there are also a small number of very rare viruses, known as oncoviruses, that actually cause cancer.

The first cancer-causing virus was discovered early in the last century by Francis Peyton Rous at Rockefeller University in Manhattan. Following a visit from a farmer carrying an ailing Plymouth Rock hen, Rous noticed the fowl was afflicted with a kind of cancer called sarcoma. Rous cut the sarcoma out, ground it up, and inoculated it into healthy chickens. When some of the infected chickens developed sarcomas of their own, Rous concluded that the chicken cancer cells possessed a transmissible cancer-causing agent.[1] Years would pass before Rous's hypothesis — that the agent was a virus — would be taken seriously. But Rous had made his discovery as a relatively young man, and he lived to see other researchers discover tumor-causing viruses in birds, hamsters, pigs, cats, mice, cows, horses, sheep, and even snakes — and, near the end of his life, to receive the Nobel Prize for medicine.

As the number of animal cancer viruses mounted, it became evident that they possessed a curious distinction. In every case, it seemed, their genetic codes were inscribed not in DNA, but its more mysterious cousin, RNA. The significance of that distinction was only dimly understood when Howard Temin arrived at Caltech in the fall of 1955. At Swarthmore, where Temin had just finished his undergraduate degree, biology meant the study of cells, which were big enough to see beneath a microscope. The mystery of the structure of DNA, which would open the door to the submicroscopic world of molecular biology, had only been solved toward the end of Temin's sophomore year, with a letter that will forever rank among the most important pieces of scientific correspondence in history.

A mere nine hundred words in length, that letter, signed by Francis Crick and James Watson, would never be published today without reams of supporting laboratory data. When it appeared in *Nature*, in April 1953, Crick was thirty-five and Watson only twenty-four.[2] Because their hypothesis had been worked out in their heads and transferred to a crude wooden model in a Cambridge University lab, Crick and Watson's letter contained no experimental results or anything of substance beyond a drawing of what DNA must look like: two mirror-image strands of nucleic acids, wound one around the other in what is universally recognized today as the double helix.

Not addressed by Crick and Watson were the questions of *how* DNA encodes hereditary information in the form of genes, or of how that information is transcribed into proteins by RNA, problems whose full solution would require another twenty years. The letter does, however, suggest an answer to the mystery of how genetic information is passed from cell to cell, and ultimately from parent to offspring. "It has not escaped our notice," the authors wrote, in what may be the understatement of all time, "that the specific pairing we have postulated immediately suggests a possible copying mechanism for the genetic material."

The mechanism suggested has often been compared to a molecular copying machine. When a single cell divides to form two new cells, an event which occurs somewhere or another in the human body uncounted times each day, the double helix at the center of the cell unwinds. With the help of various enzymes, each of the complementary DNA strands manufactures a copy of itself. After each of the "parent" strands recombines with the complementary "daughter" strand, each of the new cells has an identical double helix of its own. "The whole business was like a child's toy that you could buy at the dime store," remarked the German physicist Max Delbrück. "All built in this wonderful way that you could explain in *Life* magazine so that really a five-year-old can understand what's going on. That there was so simple a trick behind it. This was the greatest surprise for everyone."[3]

Crick and Watson garnered celebrity, Nobel Prizes, bestselling memoirs, the envy and jealousy of their scientific colleagues, and near-veneration by the public as the men who had "solved the mystery of life." In fact, much more remained to be done.

By the time Temin reached Caltech, that institution had come to rival Cambridge as a world center for what was being called "the new biology." Walking across the Pasadena campus, it was possible to come upon the likes of Delbrück, Renato Dulbecco, François Jacob, Gunther Stent, and Sydney Brenner, now remembered among the giants of molecular biology, sitting under a tree and talking about how DNA encoded hereditary information in the form of genes, or how information is transcribed into proteins by RNA. Temin, working late into the night in Dulbecco's lab, found himself drawn to the RNA viruses. "I was always a virologist," Temin said later, "so I was interested in how viruses replicated, particularly the Rous Sarcoma Virus. My interest came out of the question of how viruses could cause cancer."

From Caltech, Temin landed at the University of Wisconsin, in those years a relative academic backwater where a young researcher had time to work and think without inordinate pressure to publish scientific papers. Temin's first important article, three years after his arrival in Madison, reported that an antibiotic, actinomycin B, already known to interfere with the copying of old DNA into new DNA, seemed also to inhibit the reproduction of Rous's chicken virus. The question was how. When ordinary viruses reproduce, the genes encoded in their DNA are transcribed, by RNA, into the functional and structural proteins of which those viruses are composed. But how did transcription occur with the Rous Sarcoma Virus (RSV), or any other virus whose genetic code was written in RNA?

The way Temin saw it, the RNA viruses must be translating their genetic codes into DNA, then splicing that DNA into the genome of the infected cell, where it would be available as a template for the production of more RNA viruses. Like Crick and Watson's letter to *Nature,* Temin's paper on actinomycin B contained a prescient sentence. "It is suggested," Temin wrote, "that the template responsible for synthesis of viral nucleic acid, either is DNA or is located on DNA."[4] That observation ultimately would bring Howard Temin his own Nobel Prize and enough honorary degrees, appointments, positions, and distinctions to fill a quarter page in *Who's Who.* But recognition was years in coming. At the time, Temin's idea threatened the fundamental doctrine of molecular biology — that all genetic information flowed in one direction only, from DNA to RNA — and it was flatly rejected by many of his colleagues. "Essentially ignored," Temin said later, "if not derided."

Temin concluded that RSV must manufacture an enzyme of its own that produced a DNA transcript of its RNA. "Once you had the idea that there was an enzyme, and that it had to be *in* the virus," Temin recalled, "it immediately clicked." With his postdoctoral fellow, Satoshi Mizutani, Temin began the search for the transcribing enzyme. But biochemistry was not Temin's forte, and the search lasted for four months. "If we had been competent biochemists,"

Temin said, "it would have taken an afternoon." Because Temin and Mizutani's enzyme reversed the direction in which genetic information was ordinarily transcribed, it would become known as reverse transcriptase.

In the hypercompetitive arena of the new biology, no discovery was safe from cooptation. Submitting a paper to *Nature* or another major journal posed certain dangers, since most journals first send promising manuscripts to other scientists, inviting their anonymous comments on whether to publish the work at hand. The practice, known as "peer review," doubtless prevents a good deal of misinformation from finding its way into print, though a fair amount still slips past the screen. But peer reviewers usually work in the same fields as those on whose research they are passing judgment, and reviewers have been known to reject or delay a competitor's manuscript, only to quickly reproduce the experiments it contains and submit a paper of their own to a rival publication.[5]

For Temin and Mizutani the threat of preemption was particularly acute, since finding reverse transcriptase wasn't that difficult, once one knew how to look. "If you send the paper to some journal," Mizutani recalled, "then somebody will pick it up very quickly. So we thought that to make it public was the best thing to do." As it happened, the Tenth International Cancer Congress was about to convene in Houston, with an opening declaration by Vice President Spiro Agnew that the 1970s would be remembered as "the decade against disease." Leaving Mizutani behind to perform some final experiments, Temin caught a plane from Madison to Chicago, where he connected with a flight arriving in Houston late on the evening of Tuesday, May 26, 1970.

The title of Temin's talk, "The Role of DNA in the Replication of RNA Viruses," provided no clue that his audience was about to learn of the discovery of reverse transcriptase. But before Temin had finished speaking, his listeners had begun rising from their seats and hastening from the room. "You could see certain people on the telephone," Temin recalled. "People called people in their laboratories, and had people immediately repeat the experiment." Temin remembered his particular amusement at seeing Columbia University's Sol Spiegelman juggling hastily scribbled notes in one hand and a telephone in the other. He was even more gratified when, over lunch, Rockefeller's Hidesaburo Hanafusa confessed that Temin's discovery explained things that had puzzled Hanafusa for years. "I had been following what was, to me, a solid line of argument," Temin said later. "I was completely convinced. I was waiting for the world to be convinced. And when that happened, I felt that this was the proper order of things."

On the evening of the most important day of his career, Temin celebrated by eating supper in his hotel room and going to bed early. The next morning, a Friday, he caught an early plane to Chicago. Before noon he was back in Madison, where Mizutani reported that the phone had been ringing nonstop. Several callers, Mizutani said, warned that already other labs had reproduced the reverse transcriptase experiment and advised Temin to publish quickly. Temin and Mizutani both recalled being unconcerned. If others followed their footsteps and achieved the same result, it only proved they were right.

Their unconcern lasted until Monday morning, when the telephone rang again. Mizutani remembered the caller, David Baltimore from the Massachusetts Institute of Technology, saying he had heard about Temin's talk in Houston and had "an important message for Howard." The message was that he, David Baltimore, had discovered reverse transcriptase. When Temin returned Baltimore's call, he got the same story. "He said, 'Rous Sarcoma Virus has a DNA polymerase,'" Temin recalled. "And I said, 'I know, and we found it.' And he said, 'We found it also.'"[a]

For seven years Temin had preached his heretical doctrine and suffered a certain amount of collegial abuse. Now, as he approached the finish line, David Baltimore had emerged from nowhere and beaten him to the tape. Worse, Baltimore already had mailed a manuscript to *Nature,* which meant Temin's talk in Houston no longer conferred priority for the discovery of reverse transcriptase. Temin, who hadn't imagined that he was facing any competition and hadn't finished writing his own manuscript, suggested to Baltimore that they ask the editor of *Nature,* John Maddox, to publish both articles in the same issue, an offer Baltimore declined. "He said that he would not like to do that," Temin recalled, "because he had previously been burned, or had some other negative consequence." Temin didn't think it seemly to call Maddox himself, so he took his case to a Madison colleague, Waclaw Szybalski, who agreed to intercede with *Nature* on Temin's behalf. According to Szybalski, Maddox replied that he would be delighted to publish both papers together.

In the pub-crawling that attends most scientific convocations, suspicions are still heard that David Baltimore, having somehow learned the details of Temin's talk in Houston, had quickly repeated Temin's experiment, written up his results, and sent them off to *Nature*, all within the space of a few days. Over the intervening years, the story has been embellished to include Polaroid photographs of Temin's presentation and late-night flights by Baltimore's postdocs from Houston to Boston. But Ken Manley, then a postdoc in Baltimore's lab, remembers that Baltimore had begun looking for reverse transcriptase before the Houston conference opened. "The entire series of experiments he did himself, with his own hands," Manley said. "It took him about two weeks. All his actions are consistent with the fact that he discovered it independently."

Baltimore's paper reporting the discovery of a "Viral RNA-dependent DNA Polymerase" in a mouse leukemia virus was received by *Nature* on Tuesday, June 2, one day *after* Baltimore's Monday morning telephone conversations with Temin and Mizutani. In an era before faxes and FedEx, the manuscript would have been mailed from Boston sometime during the week of the Houston conference, which meant the experiments it described could only have preceded Temin's talk. The two articles appeared, back-to-back, in *Nature*'s issue of June 27, 1970, Baltimore's first because it had been first to arrive in London.[b] In one of the more civilized gestures known to science, Temin's article acknowledged that "David Baltimore has independently discovered a similar enzyme in virions of Rauscher leukaemia virus."[6]

The discovery made front-page news in the *New York Times*,[7] which predicted, correctly, that the search for human cancer viruses would "accelerate rapidly." *Newsweek,* noting that Temin had long been ridiculed by his colleagues, viewed the discovery of reverse transcriptase as a "Triumph for a Heretic."[8] Five years later, Temin and Baltimore were awarded the Nobel Prize for medicine — and with it, induction into the high priesthood of the few scientists who have discovered something truly worth discovering.

With the missing piece supplied by Temin and Baltimore, it was at last possible to comprehend the workings of the animal *retroviruses,* as they were soon to become known — retroviruses, because they reproduced themselves in reverse, from RNA to DNA then back to RNA. Scientists now could search for retroviruses simply by testing laboratory cultures of cancer cells for reverse transcriptase, a certain clue to the presence of a retrovirus.

The discovery of reverse transcriptase coincided with the declaration, by President Richard Nixon, of what would come to be called the War on Cancer. In the months that followed, Congress, the White House, and the cancer research establishment each did what it could to advance the exciting idea that the discovery of a human, cancer-causing retrovirus was just around the corner — and with it a cancer vaccine. The American Cancer Society began running magazine ads showing a kindly doctor giving a shot to an apprehensive child. "One day," the caption read, "the scariest thing about cancer may be the needle that makes you immune to it."

Not a few scientists, Howard Temin among them, feared that such a day was far away, and that a Manhattan Project–style pursuit of human cancer viruses would ultimately fail, if only by raising expectations that could never be fulfilled. Scientists had known, in theory, how to make a polio vaccine or an atom bomb before those efforts were attempted. But not nearly enough was known about cancer or retroviruses to say how a cancer vaccine might be produced once a cancer-causing virus was discovered, assuming that one ever was. In the end, the public relations benefits of a cancer war, and the undreamed-of research funding, proved too compelling. When Nixon signed the Cancer Act of 1971 in a ceremony in the State Dining Room of the White House, it authorized $1.6 billion for cancer research — in those years a truly enormous sum. It was his hope, the president said, that history would "look back on this as being the most significant action taken during this administration."[9]

On paper, the National Cancer Institute, from which the War on Cancer would be waged, remained a part of the National Institutes of Health, a loose collection of federally funded medical research agencies that occupy a tree-shaded three-hundred-acre campus in the Washington, D.C., suburb of Bethesda, Maryland. But the cancer act had made the NCI virtually an independent agency, headed by a presidential appointee and governed by its own private group of overseers, the National Cancer Advisory Board. Most of the cancer board members were lined up to cheer the virus hunters on. One of the few exceptions was Jim Watson, now running a lab at Harvard, who worried that the Gold Rush mentality was likely to "scare off the sensible and leave the field to a combination of charlatans and fools."[10]

A Boston University researcher, Paul Black, pointed out that scientists still had no idea whether viruses caused cancer or whether cancer caused viruses.[11] But the virus hunters were determined to find the virus first and let the answers follow. In the spring of 1970, when David Baltimore descended on Bethesda to give a talk about reverse transcriptase, a junior NCI researcher named Robert Charles Gallo was in the audience. "He came right back upstairs," recalled Gallo's supervisor, Ted Breitman, "and he said, *'This* is what we're going to work on!'"[12]

"Too Lucky to Be True"

In the spring of 1981, a handful of young men began turning up in the emergency room at the UCLA hospital in West Los Angeles with the same mysterious complaint: a prolonged fever and swollen lymph glands, followed by a rare type of pneumonia previously seen only in the elderly or in malnourished children.

The most puzzling feature of their illnesses was what Michael Gottlieb, the UCLA clinician who examined them, described as an "acquired T-cell defect."[1] Something was causing the men to lose large numbers of T-cells, the class of white blood cells that orchestrate the immune system's response to infections. Presumably, it was this T-cell depletion that had allowed the pneumonia-causing protozoan *Pneumocystis carinii* to take hold in the lining of their lungs. But Gottlieb's patients weren't elderly or malnourished. The thing they seemed to have in common was that they were all homosexuals.

Within months, the same immune-system disorder was being reported in gay men in New York, San Francisco, Miami, and Washington, D.C., as well as in a few hemophiliacs and recent immigrants from Haiti. By the summer of 1982, 500 cases of what would come to be called *acquired immune deficiency syndrome* had been recorded in the United States.[a]

Few events capture the attention of doctors more readily than a new disease, and in August 1982 several hundred specialists in cancer, immunology, and infectious diseases convened at Mount Sinai Medical

Center in New York to share their ideas about its origins. It seemed that everybody had a different theory. Perhaps AIDS was the result of stress imposed on the immune system by an overload of different viruses, a syndrome often seen in developing countries. Perhaps it was the immune-suppressing properties of semen, or the chemical stimulants some gay men inhaled during sex. One researcher, noting that no cases were being reported in populous countries like China or India, suggested that AIDS might have a genetic component. The more realistic proposals included some kind of transmissible agent, probably a virus. Many viruses were on the suspect list, most of them known to be blood-borne or sexually transmitted. According to the National Cancer Institute's Dr. Robert Gallo, the most "reasonable candidate" was his own laboratory's recent discovery, a human retrovirus called HTLV.[2]

Gallo's quest for HTLV had begun a dozen years before, with what had appeared to be the first detection of reverse transcriptase in human leukemia cells.[3] Gallo wasn't claiming to have found a leukemia-causing human virus, only to have seen its biochemical footprints. But *Time* heralded Gallo's discovery as "a crucial clue" to the eventual isolation of the first human cancer virus.[4]

When another NCI laboratory, headed by a virus hunter named George Todaro, tried to reproduce Gallo's data, it failed.[5] Using Gallo's methods, Todaro's lab found it was possible to detect what *appeared* to be reverse transcriptase in normal human cells as well as leukemic cells. Since healthy cells weren't infected by retroviruses, Todaro reasoned that Gallo's test for reverse transcriptase must be detecting some other kind of enzyme.[b]

For the virus hunters, it was the first false start of many. Six months later, a team at the M. D. Anderson Cancer Center in Houston announced the isolation of the first human cancer virus. Named ESP-1, after Elizabeth S. Priori, the virologist who discovered it, the new virus had come from a five-year-old boy with a blood-cell cancer called lymphoma.[6] According to the *New York Times*, ESP-1 looked like the real thing. Experts in Houston and New York, the *Times* said, had "proved to their satisfaction that it is not a contaminating animal virus and that it is not any virus hitherto discovered."[7] Soon Gallo had confirmed the presence of reverse transcriptase in the cultures where ESP-1 was growing.[8]

It was George Todaro's lab that proved Priori was wrong. ESP-1 wasn't a new human virus, merely the same mouse leukemia virus in which David Baltimore had found reverse transcriptase, and which had somehow contaminated Priori's cultures.[9] Scarcely had the ink dried on Todaro's paper than Columbia's Sol Spiegelman announced the detection of a retrovirus in breast cancer cells.[10] But there wasn't any breast cancer virus in Spiegelman's lab, only another animal virus contamination.[11] More unfounded virus sightings followed, but rather than provoke a reassessment of the cancer virus program the false alarms seemed only to spur the cancer virus hunters on.

It was a rare weekend that didn't find Todaro or Gallo in their labs, but Gallo seemed to have a determination that even the other virus hunters lacked. "Gallo's a student of Roman history," recalled Dave Gillespie, who had left Spiegelman to become Gallo's chief molecular biologist, "and he ran his lab like a battlefield. Sometimes he would put two people on the same subject independently, knowing that one of them was going to get screwed and the other one would publish." On a visit to India, Gallo had even taken the trouble to seek out the briefly famous fifteen-year-old guru, Maharaj Ji, to ask where he might find the origin of cancer. "Look deep within the mysteries of life itself," the Perfect Master had replied, not a bad piece of advice.[12]

In newspaper and magazine articles, Gallo's single-mindedness was frequently attributed to the death of his five-year-old sister Judith from childhood leukemia, an event Gallo recalled as the most traumatic of his young life, and which had transformed the Gallo household into a grim and joyless place without music or laughter, where Thanksgiving and Christmas were no longer observed.[13] For all the grief it had doubtless caused, his sister's tragic illness brought the teenaged Gallo into contact with a succession of doctors and hospitals, ultimately including Boston's famed Children's Hospital and Sidney Farber, who pioneered the treatment of childhood leukemia with the chemotherapeutic drugs. What followed was an adolescent fascination with biology, then medicine and cancer — and, according to Gallo, an abiding resolve to track down and vanquish his sister's killer.

As spurious detections of reverse transcriptase continued to mount, those researchers who were *not* finding reverse transcriptase in every cancer cell were beginning to ask the obvious question: Where's the virus? RT, as reverse transcriptase was called for short, was unarguably the product of a retrovirus. But finding RT in a succession of human cancer cells without finding the virus was like following a trail of peanut shells without finding an elephant.

Gallo explained that testing for RT was easy, requiring a relatively small number of malignant cells, whereas actually isolating the virus that was producing the enzyme required many more cells than could be grown in the laboratory with existing methods. Leukemic blood cells multiplied ferociously in the human body, but not so well in a laboratory flask, where they seemed to be missing some stimulus the body provided. If the mysterious growth-enhancer could be identified, perhaps enough cells could be grown in a flask to isolate a leukemia-causing virus.

To search for the elusive "growth factor" Gallo teamed a talented virologist named Bob Gallagher with a Pakistani technician, Zaki Salahuddin, who had been visiting friends in Washington when war broke out between his country and India. After the first few days of fighting, news arrived that Salahuddin's father had been killed and one of his brothers thrown in jail. Salahuddin, who had already concluded that serious biological research was impossible in a country where issues of *Nature* arrived six months late, promptly answered Gallo's ad for a laboratory technician in the *Washington Post*.

Gallagher and Salahuddin began by screening white blood cells extracted from fetal tissue. If a cellular "growth factor" existed, Gallagher reasoned, it would be most plentiful during the fetal period, when many kinds of cells grow prodigiously. In what seemed a surprisingly short time, the pair had isolated a substance that seemed to keep one type of leukemic blood cells alive in the test tube. The cells, designated HL-23, had come from a Texas woman with myeloid leukemia, and they had previously tested positive for reverse transcriptase. With the addition of the new growth factor, the cells continued to multiply until there were enough to put beneath an electron microscope, which uses beams of electrons rather than rays of light to illuminate objects too small to be seen with an optical lens.

At the edge of one cell, magnified thousands of times, was a small, round object that vaguely resembled a weather balloon on the distant horizon of a pockmarked planet. Upon closer examination, the balloon became a particle with a dinnerplate-shaped core resembling a retrovirus. All Gallo needed to nail down the discovery was a demonstration that the particles could transform normal blood cells into leukemic ones, the *sine qua non* of cancer virology. But before that crucial experiment could be attempted, the freezer containing the laboratory's minuscule supply of growth factor somehow became unplugged.

It happened over a long holiday weekend, and by the time Gallagher and Salahuddin returned to work everything inside the freezer had thawed. Perhaps a janitor had knocked the plug from its socket. Perhaps a child had done it; people often brought their children to the lab on weekends. But neither possibility would explain why the controls on Salahuddin's incubator, a table-top oven that holds cultured cells at the approximate temperature of the human body, had been turned up to roasting levels. "Around that time a lot of weird things were happening," recalled a technician in Gallo's lab. "You'd go in on the weekends and somebody had changed all the dials on the counters. People were unplugging incubators. You'd come back on a Monday morning, and clearly something weird was going on. Because always, an attempt had been made to destroy something."

However the freezer had come unplugged, without new infusions of growth factor the HL-23 cells were soon dead, and with them whatever cancer-causing virus they might have harbored. Not only was the critical transmission experiment no longer possible, there wouldn't be any growth factor to supply other researchers who wished to confirm Gallo's results. But the original HL-23 cells remained, and Gallo could put things on hold while Gallagher and Salahuddin searched for a new source of growth factor. Or he could publish the data they already had collected, suggesting the presence of a virus that no longer existed.

Gallo chose to publish, not in *Nature* but in its American counterpart, the journal *Science*.[14] Even before the HL-23 paper appeared in print, Gallo's discovery was in the news. The *New York Times*, chastened by too many false virus sightings, was no longer reporting cancer-virus discoveries, but the *Washington Post* still thought they were front-page material.[15] While a half-dozen other human cancer virus claims hadn't panned out, said the *Post*, Gallo's newest virus had passed all the scientific hurdles. "I got up one morning and read the headlines with no forewarning whatsoever," Bob Gallagher recalled. "I was shocked to find that he'd been talking to the press. The paper was not out yet."[16]

Behind the scenes, Gallo was mounting a frantic effort to re-isolate the HL-23 virus, enlisting the help of a respected British retrovirologist,

Robin Weiss from the Chester Beatty Laboratories in London. Weiss, who had first encountered Gallo at a cancer meeting a few years before, had initially been put off. "He was so loud," Weiss recalled. "He was charismatic, and yet he was loud. He was complaining about others, and bragging that he was doing the greatest work. And I thought, 'Here's a guy to avoid.' I just didn't like his manner." By the time he arrived in Bethesda, Weiss had come to know Gallo better. "I saw that his aggressiveness and vanity was partly because he wore his emotions on his sleeve," Weiss recalled. "To my mind he wasn't covering things up. He was a raw, ambitious person. You knew where you were."

Like most European biologists, Weiss had been disdainful of the American virus hunters. "There was a certain amount of snobbishness about them taking the easy route," he said. "We real molecular biologists were working things out with chicken and mouse viruses. Sure there may be human viruses, but that became tainted with the excessive number of papers that never hardened up the claims. There was a monthly paper from Spiegelman's lab, bimonthly from Gallo."

Once he had seen it close up, Weiss was agog at the scope of the American cancer-virus program. Although British science has been spectacularly successful, it has traditionally been done with big intellects and small laboratories. But even Gallo's sprawling setup in Bethesda seemed modest compared to George Todaro's lab, recalled by Weiss as "a huge factory with a dozen postdocs and twenty-four technicians."

It took Weiss and Natalie Teich, a close colleague who accompanied him from London, only a few attempts before they hit pay dirt. Weiss and Teich hadn't found the missing growth factor, but they had somehow managed to re-culture the HL-23 cells without it, and to isolate once again what looked like a human retrovirus. Indeed, the virus that emerged from the new culture — Weiss named it HL23V, for HL-23 *variant* — grew even better than the original.

Carrying a supply of HL-23V-infected cells packed in dry ice, Weiss and Teich flew home to write up their dramatic rescue for *Nature*.[17] Samples of HL-23V had begun making the rounds of the other cancer-virus labs, where they were put to every conceivable test. Once again, it was George Todaro's lab from which the bad news emerged: HL-23V wasn't a human virus after all, but a mélange of three animal viruses — a woolly monkey virus, a gibbon ape virus, and a baboon virus — jumbled together in a retroviral cocktail.

Gallo and Todaro shared some common roots. Both had grown up in Italian-American families within a few dozen miles of one another, Todaro in New York City and Gallo in Waterbury, Connecticut, the Brass Capital of the World. Both had graduated from medical school in the spring of 1963, Todaro from New York University and Gallo from the Jefferson Medical College in Philadelphia. Both wanted nothing more than to find the first human cancer virus, but there the commonalities ended. Todaro's deceptively laid-back style and faintly melancholy demeanor contrasted sharply with Gallo's own hyperkinesis. When Todaro spoke, it sometimes seemed as if his brain was struggling to catch up with his mouth. Gallo's conversations often sounded as though a tape recording were being played back at faster than normal speed, and his syntax frequently lent the impression of someone whose first language was not English.

By all accounts, Todaro's seeming befuddlement disguised a Machiavellian brilliance. "Todaro totally intimidated Gallo," Dave Gillespie said. "If he had a meeting with Todaro, Gallo would be petrified going into the room." On this occasion it was Todaro who delivered the verdict that, once again, something had gone terribly wrong in Gallo's lab. "There was, ah, a meeting," Todaro recalled, "where some of us, uh, did try to talk to Bob and tell him, 'You have a contaminant.' He, er, resisted for quite a while, but the evidence became overwhelming." Gallo's capitulation came during a day-long cancer-virus symposium in Hershey, Pennsylvania, where one speaker after another presented data showing that HL-23V was not a human virus. "I certainly took a lot of punches," Gallo said, years later. "It wasn't one, it wasn't two — how about *three* primate retroviruses mixed together?"

Within a few months, *Nature* had published a retraction of HL-23V.[18] "You could look for faults and say someone should have been more cautious," said Robin Weiss, who regretted having gotten involved at all. "But I don't remember thinking that it didn't hold up, or that it didn't feel right at the time we got the paper submitted. I may have been over-influenced by Gallo as a pushy, charismatic fellow. I think we should have started wondering earlier. Gallo never quite forgave Natalie and myself for growing up that virus to the stage where it could be shown to be a contamination."

Nobody who worked with viruses, including Weiss, believed Gallo's lab had been the victim of an accidental contamination. "What else could it have been but deliberate," Weiss said, "if it was three viruses instead of one? Or at least two? If it was a rival group at NIH looking for human retroviruses, one could certainly make an enormous fool of Gallo." As Weiss thought back over his time in Bethesda, he remembered the weekend that George Todaro turned up unexpectedly at Gallo's lab. "He got me to let him in," Weiss said, "and he chose a time when Gallo and Gallagher and everyone else was out of town. He marched in and opened every incubator and looked at the cultures. He said, 'What are you growing there?' I distinctly remember this over-curiosity about details, that one quiet afternoon or evening."

"Totally untrue," Todaro says. "Absolutely not true. Never happened. I distinctly remember never having gone there on a weekend. You can get three viruses into a virus preparation easily just by being sloppy, and Gallo had plenty of sloppy people."

Courtesy of the War on Cancer, the National Cancer Institute's budget had more than doubled in four years, from $377 million in 1972 to $815 million in 1976, an extraordinary increase for any federal agency in peacetime. But even before HL-23, many of the cancer virus labs had been closed down in the face of protests from university scientists, who viewed the spectacularly unsuccessful cancer-virus program as a waste of precious research dollars that should have been flowing to other laboratories, preferably their own.

The debacle of HL-23 represented the final straw. What remained of the cancer-virus program was placed in serious jeopardy, and Gallo's career as well. "When the virus disappeared, the NIH would have preferred Gallo to disappear along with it," recalled Vincent DeVita, who then headed the NCI's Division of Cancer Treatment. "The only reason he didn't was me. He's a handful. He cost me a lot of time. I spent hours sometimes to calm him down. But there are two kinds of investigators in this world. There are people who discover things, and there are people who build a brick at a time. You need both. Discoverers are rarer, and I think Gallo, frankly, is one of those. That's how I saw him, his personality problems notwithstanding."

It would be said later that Doris Morgan was a technician who got lucky. But that would have been unfair. After years of culturing cells, it occurred to Morgan that she was at least as bright as some of the scientists who were designing the experiments she was carrying out. A divorce propelled Morgan into graduate school, from which she emerged with a Ph.D. in hematology and a postdoctoral fellowship at M. D. Anderson, followed by a job offer from Gallo as the HL-23 affair was coming to a head. Morgan leapt at the chance to work at the National Cancer Institute, but she was a bit apprehensive about her new boss. "A lot of the new people coming in had difficulty," she recalled. "It was not an atmosphere that really generated a lot of confidence for a young scientist."

Morgan's first assignment was to join the search for the erstwhile growth factor that could reignite the HL-23 culture. "My directive from Gallo," Morgan recalled, "was 'We have to grow myeloid leukemic cells, so we can reproduce HL-23.'" After many months in cold storage, the HL-23 cells were not in good shape. Morgan thawed them anyway, rinsed them with water, and put them in a bath of nutrients and amino acids, the molecules from which proteins are constructed. When the cells failed to grow, Morgan concluded that HL-23 was history, and turned her attention to culturing cells from other cancer patients.

With one group of cells Morgan had better luck. "If you kept these cells too far apart they didn't do well," she recalled. "They appeared to need contact and interaction with each other." Each morning Morgan went to her incubator, took out her test tubes, and studied the visible clumps of cells at the bottom. When the microscope confirmed that one batch was indeed multiplying, Morgan split it in two, feeding half the cells with a bean-plant extract called PHA. "I wasn't sure which way they would be happiest," she said. Eventually Morgan concluded that the PHA-stimulated cells were producing some kind of biochemical that encouraged them to grow. Moreover, the fact that the surviving cells were all of the same kind suggested that the growth factor was specific for one type of cell. But what kind of cell that was, Morgan had no idea.

Once a week, usually on Monday afternoons, Gallo summoned his staff to join in a roundtable critique of each other's work. A few researchers would be designated to speak about their current experiments, then subjected to questions that were not always polite. When Morgan's turn came to talk, she reported that she might have found a factor that induced white blood cells to grow in culture. When someone asked what kind of white blood cells, Morgan admitted she hadn't a clue. The response was far from enthusiastic. "There was a total indifference," Morgan recalled. "'This is not what we were after. This is a failure.'" The only encouragement came as the meeting was breaking up. "Bob Gallagher came up to me and said, 'I think you've got something really interesting. Take it to the immunologists and find out what it is.'"

The mid-1970s were the Dark Ages of cell biology, a time when it was barely possible to distinguish one type of blood cell from another. The immunologists told Morgan what she already suspected, that she hadn't been growing myeloid cells. They were, nevertheless, white blood cells, which meant they were probably lymphoid cells, or lymphocytes, then considered the dross of hematology. Myeloid cells were complex, while lymphocytes were simplistic. Myeloid cells were involved in interesting leukemic diseases. When lymphocytes became malignant, they caused uninteresting lymphomas. Soon a new joke was circulating at NIH: the good news is that Gallo has finally found a cellular growth factor. The bad news is that it's for growing lymphocytes.

In those years, lymphocytes were classified into two broad categories: B-lymphocytes, thought to come from the bone marrow, and T-lymphocytes, believed to originate in the thymus. According to the immunologists, Morgan's cells appeared to be mostly T-cells — not leukemic T-cells, but *normal* T-cells. Discovering something that induced healthy T-cells to grow was like finding a better way to grow weeds. "I was on the fringe," Morgan said, "and no one was paying that much attention to what I was doing. Gallo had no interest in this. It almost got discarded."

Morgan's self-appointed savior was Frank Ruscetti, who had joined the lab after encountering Gallo at a reception during a medical meeting in Atlanta. "I was hired at a cocktail party," recalled Ruscetti. "Gallo said, 'Don't you want to come to the lab that's going to win the Nobel Prize?'" Ruscetti accepted Gallo's invitation, only to discover that he, like Doris Morgan, was expected to find the erstwhile HL-23 growth factor.

Ruscetti had begun by searching established cell lines one at a time, but without any luck. When he sensed that Doris Morgan had found something interesting, his antennae began to shift in her direction. "Doris basically didn't know what to do with it," Ruscetti recalled. "So we sort of pooled our resources and our energies and did it together. She was constantly in trouble with Gallo, because she would only do things her own way. She could only grow these cells in test tubes, and not in flasks. I was basically trying to help her, because it was obvious that if she didn't change her ways she'd get fired."

It was help Morgan thought later she might have done without. When her discovery of what Gallo dubbed T-Cell Growth Factor was published in *Science,* in the fall of 1976, the authors of the article were Morgan, Ruscetti, and Gallo.[19] A follow-up paper a few months later was by Ruscetti, Morgan, and Gallo.[20] Not long after that, Doris Morgan was gone from Gallo's lab. "I was, I think the expression is, canned," Morgan said. "When I got fired, someone in the lab drew a silhouette of a person rejected, with a tear dropping. And under it he wrote, 'Don't cry, Doris. There's more to T-cell biology than any of us realizes.'"

The laboratory Doris Morgan left behind was no longer so close to the center of the scientific universe. Still, a postdoc with an interest in T-cell leukemias could find a less interesting place to work. Bernie Poiesz had spent the first year of a three-year NIH fellowship at the Veterans Administration Hospital in Washington, where he had seen a number of patients with relatively rare T-cell skin cancers. Poiesz had become curious about the origins of those cancers, and he wanted to use the remaining two years of his fellowship to do some laboratory research. He had chosen Gallo's lab, Poiesz said later, mainly because "I liked Ruscetti's spiel."

When Poiesz and Ruscetti drew up a proposal to study malignant T-cells, they decided, almost as an afterthought, to test the cells for reverse transcriptase as well. But the proposal hadn't met with much enthusiasm from Gallo and his staff, who were no longer looking for human cancer viruses. "They had kind of given up on it," Poiesz recalled, "but we told Bob that this was our project, and he told us to work on it for a few months." When Doris Morgan, who had found a new job in Daniel Zagury's lab at the University of Paris, heard that Frank Ruscetti was again growing T-cells, she was surprised. "After I left Gallo I thought the whole thing would be abandoned," Morgan said. "I said to myself, 'Why is Frank growing T-cells?'"

Some of the T-cells in Poiesz and Ruscetti's incubators had come from Charles Robinson, a twenty-seven-year-old patient at the VA hospital diagnosed with a T-cell skin cancer called mycosis fungoides. When one of Robinson's lymph nodes was biopsied, it had been Poiesz who authorized the surgery. He hadn't thought more about the man until he got a call from Adi Gazdar, an NCI pathologist who was interested in Robinson's case. Using a variety of laboratory tricks and a dash of T-Cell Growth Factor supplied by Ruscetti, Gazdar had succeeded in growing Robinson's leukemic T-cells in a flask. As long as the cells were fed with nutrients, they went on reproducing, transforming themselves into a self-perpetuating culture known as continuous cell line that produced an endless quantity of malignant blood cells to study.

In return for the T-Cell Growth Factor Gazdar promised to share with Ruscetti any continuous T-cell lines he was able to establish. In addition to the Robinson line, which Gazdar named HUT-102 (for *Hu*man *T*-cell line number 102), Gazdar had thrown in another line, HUT-78, established without T-Cell Growth Factor from the cells of a patient suffering from another kind of T-cell cancer called Sezary's syndrome.[21] When HUT-78 proved negative for reverse transcriptase — an indication that it didn't contain a retrovirus — Ruscetti stuck the cells in his freezer and forgot about them.

It was nearly Christmas of 1978 by the time Bernie Poiesz got around to testing Charlie Robinson's T-cells for RT. The cells were positive, but at such a low level that, according to the protocol previously established by Gallo's lab, further testing would have been pointless. "In order for something to be considered interesting," Poiesz said, "there had to be an extraordinary amount of reverse transcriptase. That would have required that the cell line be spewing out retrovirus. But I had done enough reverse transcriptase assays on normal T-cells to recognize that if there was a little bit of production, that's all you needed."[22]

When Robinson's cells were compressed into a pellet, thinly sliced and put beneath the electron microscope, Poiesz could see what Gallagher and Salahuddin thought they had seen five years before — retrovirus-like particles escaping from the surface of a cell. But plenty of people claimed to have detected "virus-like particles" in human cancer cells without ever isolating a virus.

After a decade of animal virus contaminations HUT-102 would have to be checked against every available animal retrovirus. Poiesz and Ruscetti agreed to keep Gallo in the dark until they were certain of what they had found. "Gallo wasn't even aware of its existence for something like six months," recalled Ruscetti's postdoc, Tina Eastment. "Because of the previous faux pas, they wanted to make sure to do all the right tests and everything. They knew that Bob would go and make a big deal out of it right away, and they wanted to make sure that neither they nor he were going to be made fools of."

Gallo, who had been on a visit to Europe when the cross-checking was finished, learned about the discovery of the first human retrovirus over cocktails in his backyard. "Gallo came back and gave a party," Poiesz recalled, "to which he invited John Minna, who was Adi Gazdar's boss and lived down the street," and who had known about the discovery for two or three weeks. "The last word I said to him," Poiesz recalled, "was 'Please don't tell Bob until after we're sure. And second of all, we should tell him, you shouldn't.'" Minna evidently hadn't been able to resist. "Gallo called me up in the middle of the night," Ruscetti said, "and gave me hell."

Even then, Gallo was skeptical that Poiesz and Ruscetti had succeeded where he had so often failed. "Gallo basically didn't believe it," recalled Ruscetti's technician, Andrea Woods. "He didn't believe Bernie's work, but Bernie pursued it." Once the importance of the discovery had registered, Gallo "was a bit astounded that this had happened," Poiesz recalled. "Because they had tried so long to find a retrovirus. Some very skilled people had tried it, and here was a junior member of the team coming in, and in the first months of working he finds the first human retrovirus. That seemed too lucky to be true."[23]

To make sure he and Ruscetti were really first, Poiesz began a search of the scientific literature. In an obscure European journal, he found what looked like a close call.[24] The year before, a group in the Netherlands had reported observing virus-like particles and detecting reverse transcriptase in cells from seven patients with mycosis fungoides and two more with Sezary's syndrome. The article contained several pictures, electron micrographs of particles that looked very much like those around Charlie Robinson's T-cells.

Most of the Dutch data was the work of a twenty-four-year-old graduate student, Elizabeth van der Loo, who had been finishing a degree in dermatology when she stumbled across what looked like a retrovirus in a mycosis patient. "It was like a hobby, you know, to look everywhere for retroviruses," van der Loo recalled. "I found them after searching a very, very long time." Not being a virologist, and not knowing how to isolate the virus she had seen, van der Loo had simply published her findings and continued her dermatology studies.

Poiesz made a copy of the van der Loo paper and gave it to Ruscetti, along with another article he had stumbled across, a three-year-old report from Japan of a previously unrecognized disease called Adult T-Cell Leukemia.[25] As Poiesz read about the Japanese leukemia patients, he thought the article could have been describing Charlie Robinson. The new disease involved T-cells. Once people began to exhibit symptoms, they didn't live very long. The Japanese patients had extraordinarily high levels of calcium in their blood. So had Robinson, and there were other similarities.

The one thing that set Robinson apart from the Japanese patients was that he had been diagnosed with mycosis fungoides. Nearly all the Japanese leukemia patients resided in the same area, Kyushu province on the southwestern tip of Japan, which implied that ATL might be caused by a transmissible agent. The Japanese doctors who had discovered the disease weren't ready to rule out genetic factors, but they urged that the possibility of a cancer-causing virus also be explored.

The tradition of naming viruses after their discoverers ended with Tony Barr and Yvonne Epstein, discoverers of the Epstein-Barr virus, a member of the herpesvirus family that causes infectious mononucleosis and may play some role in Burkitt's lymphoma. As the number of virus discoveries mounted it seemed less confusing to identify new viruses according to what they did or where they had been discovered, rather than who had found them. The name Gallo proposed for Poiesz and Ruscetti's discovery was Human T-Cell Leukemia Virus, or HTLV. Poiesz objected that Robinson had died of lymphoma, not leukemia. "Gallo wasn't real happy," recalled Andrea Woods. "He wanted a leukemia virus. He kept saying, 'Couldn't we call it a T-cell leukemia virus?' But the people around him said no."

Gallo's next suggestion, Human T-Cell Lymphoma Virus, still overstated the case. Poiesz had found the virus in a single patient — proof of nothing, certainly not that the virus had been the cause of Robinson's lymphoma. Nor did Poiesz have any conclusive evidence that the virus was human, only that it wasn't one of the animal retroviruses against which it had been compared. "We hadn't proven that it had caused disease," Poiesz said, "nor did we have any idea about where it was in the world. But HTLV is the name that Gallo wanted it to be."[26]

Only the year before, human cancer viruses had been dismissed as heresy by no less than the University of California's J. Michael Bishop, who declared in a widely reprinted lecture that "few investigators would now argue that infection with a retrovirus is the sole cause of any malignant process in human beings." The only justification for putting so much time and money into the futile search for human cancer viruses, Bishop said, was that the virus hunt had aided science's understanding of human cancer genes, "not the vague hope that human cancer will turn out to be a virus disease."[27]

With the scientific winds blowing so strongly against him, Gallo's chances of announcing the discovery of the first human retrovirus in *Nature* or *Science* were nil. But there was one journal where the paper might have a chance — the *Proceedings of the National Academy of Sciences*, to which prospective articles are "communicated" by a member of that august body, who thereby attaches his or her reputation to the significance of the data therein. If *PNAS* had more lenient standards than *Nature* and *Science*, it also had less prestige and visibility,[c] but what mattered was getting HTLV into print.

In search of sponsors, Gallo approached David Baltimore and Henry Kaplan, the Stanford radiologist whose pioneering treatment had made Hodgkin's disease a survivable cancer. Kaplan had gotten to know Gallo after being appointed by Vince DeVita, in the wake of HL-23, to provide an independent assessment of Gallo's research. Initially skeptical, Kaplan had come away impressed by Gallo's persistence. But Kaplan, like Baltimore, was wary of Gallo's latest claim. To allay their concerns, Gallo invited the two to meet with Poiesz and Ruscetti. "We presented our data to them," Poiesz recalled, "so they could tell us if they saw any flaws in it. And they couldn't find any flaws."

Scientific convention holds that first authorship of a scientific article be reserved for the person who has done the most to produce the data, with the second author having made the next-most-important contribution, and so on down to the last author, a slot traditionally reserved for the principal investigator of the study that produced the discovery or the chief of the laboratory in which it occurred. Shortly before the HTLV article was submitted to *PNAS*, Gallo took Frank Ruscetti aside to suggest that he, Gallo, should be the paper's first author. "He told me, 'You know, there's no reason that the person who did most of the work should be first author,'" Ruscetti said. When Poiesz learned what Gallo had planned, "I advised him that it would probably be best that he be the last author," Poiesz recalled. "I told him I felt fairly strongly about that."

When "Detection and Isolation of Type C Retrovirus Particles from Fresh and Cultured Lymphocytes of a Patient with Cutaneous T-cell Lymphoma,"[d] communicated by Henry Kaplan, appeared in December 1980, the first author was Bernie Poiesz, followed by Frank Ruscetti and Adi Gazdar, with Gallo bringing up the rear. Five years before, the discovery of HTLV would have caused a scientific sensation. But with memories of HL-23 still fresh, HTLV was ignored by the scientific journals and the popular press. A follow-up article, communicated to *PNAS* by David Baltimore, also sank without a trace.[28] The only interest in Gallo's new virus seemed to be in Japan.

Three months after the publication of Poiesz and Ruscetti's first paper, Gallo found himself at a former Buddhist monastery on Lake Biwa, in the mountains outside Kyoto, a place remembered by the French virologist Guy de Thé as "very beautiful and quiet, with lots of grass." The ostensible reason for the Lake Biwa symposium was to discuss recent advances in human tumor virology. The real topic of the meeting was the mystery of what caused Adult T-Cell Leukemia.

At first the Japanese thought ATL might be an aftereffect of the atomic bombing of Nagasaki, the capital of Kyushu prefecture, where the disease was most prevalent. That theory was discarded when ATL patients began showing up who were born after the bomb was dropped. Southwestern Japan is warm and humid, a place where insects thrive, and insects are responsible for the transmission of many exotic diseases. But if ATL were caused by an insect-borne microbe, why was it being seen only in adults and not children?[29] As the possibilities were considered and eliminated, the explanation that made the most sense was a slow-acting virus.

At the time of Lake Biwa, HTLV was a virus in search of a disease. Despite Charlie Robinson's diagnosis, when Poiesz and Ruscetti had tested blood cells from other mycosis patients they yielded no trace of HTLV.[e] Nor did HTLV seem to be present in people with ordinary T-cell lymphomas.[30] Indeed, the only other patients in whom Poiesz and Ruscetti reported any evidence of HTLV were a sixty-four-year-old Trinidad woman, M.B., and a merchant seaman from Boston, M.J.,[31] both of whom suffered from Sezary's syndrome. But when fifty other Sezary patients were screened for HTLV, every last one was negative. "We were striking out," Poiesz said.[32]

If HTLV didn't cause mycosis fungoides or Sezary's syndrome, Poiesz reasoned, perhaps it caused this new disease from Japan, and he recalled suggesting to Gallo that the Adult T-Cell Leukemia patients be tested for HTLV. The summer before Lake Biwa, Gallo had gotten in touch with the chairman of the microbiology department at Kyoto University, Yohei Ito, to ask if Ito could spare a few blood samples from his ATL patients.

The subject of Gallo's own talk at Lake Biwa was T-Cell Growth Factor, which Gallo now counted as a historic breakthrough in the annals of virology.[f] But the presentation most vividly recalled by Guy de Thé had come from one of Gallo's assistants, Marjorie Guroff, who reported that some of the ATL samples had indeed contained antibodies that reacted with HTLV — an indication that the patients from which they had come were infected with HTLV, or a virus very much like it.[g]

As Guroff spoke, Japan's most prominent virologist, Yorio Hinuma, the director of Kyoto University's virological institute, listened in imperious silence. Hinuma had intended to speak about his work with the Epstein-Barr virus. But as he recognized that the Americans were trying to link HTLV to ATL, and thereby gain the credit for discovering the cause of a Japanese disease, Hinuma informed Ito that he was changing the topic of his talk.

Like Marjorie Guroff, Hinuma had been testing ATL blood samples for evidence of a human retrovirus, and he had found a positive reaction in twenty-five cases out of twenty-five. The Japanese hadn't yet isolated the virus in question, which put them behind the Americans, but they had one crucial thing that Gallo lacked: incontrovertible evidence of virus-like transmission from one patient to another.

Around the time Bernie Poiesz was joining Gallo's lab, a young Japanese virologist, Isao Miyoshi, had drawn ten milliliters of blood from a farmer with ATL. When the farmer's cells were cultured in Miyoshi's lab they continued to grow, leading Miyoshi to suspect, correctly, that they must be making their own growth factor. Miyoshi named the cells MT-1, thereby christening the world's first human leukemic T-cell line.[33]

Miyoshi's most inspired experiment came with a second cell line, MT-2, established by mixing the cells of a forty-five-year-old female ATL patient with those from a healthy newborn baby.[34] It was Miyoshi's choice of a male baby which allowed him to distinguish, via chromosomes, the baby's previously normal blood cells from the woman's leukemic ones. When the baby's cells became leukemic, the only explanation was that the woman's cells contained a transmissible cancer-causing agent.

Judging from Hinuma's electron micrographs, that agent was a retrovirus. But the Japanese hadn't been able to fish their virus out, and over dinner Gallo offered to help, proposing that the Japanese provide him with more blood samples from ATL patients as well as from healthy Japanese living in the region where ATL was endemic. If Gallo could isolate a virus from the Japanese patients using the methods that had produced HTLV, that virus could be compared with HTLV. Perhaps the virus Hinuma and Miyoshi were chasing had already been discovered by Poiesz and Ruscetti.

Yohei Ito welcomed Gallo's proposal. But Guy de Thé remembered Hinuma declaring that no collaboration with the Americans would be necessary, that Japanese science could solve the riddle of ATL without the National Cancer Institute. What had begun as a collegial dinner in a celestial setting ended with what Guy de Thé recalled as "a silence that I will never forget."

"Gallo was far enough ahead on the virology that he thought he could scare the Japanese into being docile collaborators," said Frank Ruscetti, whose attendance at Lake Biwa had been canceled by Gallo at the last minute. "But he was stunned, because the Japanese had been working with typical Japanese enthusiasm and already had some data and some epidemiology themselves."

In the end, it was the Japanese who convinced the National Cancer Institute that HTLV was the genuine article. Because Miyoshi's report of MT-2 had appeared in a Japanese-language journal, Bernie Poiesz's library search had missed it. As punishment for Miyoshi's collaboration with Hinuma, Yohei Ito hadn't invited Miyoshi to present his data at Lake Biwa. For most Western scientists, the first chance to see the Japanese data came ten months after HTLV, in the autumn of 1981, when Hinuma's pictures of a "Type-C retrovirus" appeared in

PNAS, followed a few months later by Miyoshi's MT-2 data in *Nature.*[h]

Gallo rushed to tell Vince DeVita, now the NCI's director, about the reports from Japan, according to Gallo the first "clear-cut unambiguous and noncontroversial" association between a retrovirus and a human cancer, albeit a rare and exotic cancer. "The story," Gallo assured DeVita, "is really breaking very nicely."[35] DeVita's memories of HL-23 were too recent to permit much enthusiasm over Gallo's initial accounts of HTLV. Now that the Japanese had weighed in, DeVita allowed himself to believe that Gallo might have finally snared a human cancer virus. "This time it looks real!" DeVita wrote across the margin of Gallo's note.

It had been a decade since David Baltimore's NIH lecture had launched Gallo on his quest, five years since Gallo's public evisceration at Hershey. At last he seemed to have prevailed, and some of his colleagues applauded his perseverance.

"We stopped looking, but he didn't," said Stu Aaronson, one of George Todaro's postdocs. "I have a lot of admiration for that kind of constant drive. Rather than sort of going and hiding in a corner and giving up, he kept persisting. And that drive, it's unbelievable to me, the degree of that drive to find something. He's a very, very determined guy, and he finally found one. I've never seen a fighter like him, in terms of being willing to take on almost anybody."

Vince DeVita was persuaded that HTLV was real, but many of the questions raised by Bernie Poiesz's discovery had yet to be resolved. In addition to causing T-cell leukemia, was HTLV also the cause of Charlie Robinson's mycosis fungoides? What about M.B.'s Sezary syndrome? Three different diseases seemed a lot to ask of one virus. To answer such questions, the Japanese were eager to compare their Adult T-Cell Leukemia virus[36] with Gallo's HTLV. All they needed was some of Gallo's virus. Most major scientific journals require that, once an author publishes the discovery of a virus or a cell line, he is obliged to share it with other researchers. The NIH has a similar rule of its own.[37] But Gallo's seeming reluctance to allow HTLV to leave his lab led to what George Todaro recalled as "a feeling around NIH that there was something, ah, *wrong* with HTLV."

With Vince DeVita's ascendancy to the NCI director's office Gallo's future was assured, but Todaro's days were numbered. "They were constantly at war with each other," DeVita recalled. "The tension they created was very negative, and clearly they both couldn't stay. Todaro is the Mozart of schemers. He was absolutely brilliant at it. Very, very smart guy. He certainly had a capability of doing good science, and he did good science. He also had far-flung facilities, unbelievable money squirreled away, I think $13 million a year. We cut him back to about $3 million, at which point he decided to leave. Basically, we opted for Gallo, and Todaro left. They hate each other."

"Gallo was like a son to DeVita," Todaro said later. "At least I was Mozart, not Salieri."

Any comparisons between HTLV and ATLV would have to be done in Bethesda, and Miyoshi agreed to send Gallo the ATLV-infected cell line. To perform the comparison Gallo chose a forty-year-old Czechoslovakian virologist, Mikulas Popovic, whom he had met over a drink at a conference in Norway and invited to spend a year in his lab.[38] After Popovic reported in *Nature* that ATLV from Japan appeared identical to HTLV[39] Gallo began distributing HTLV to a few laboratories[i] — although not before changing its name from Human T-Cell *Lymphoma* virus to Human T-Cell *Leukemia* virus.[j] At last Gallo had his human cancer virus.

Only a supremely suspicious person — in Gallo's view, only a paranoid person — could seriously imagine that Gallo, having belatedly discovered HTLV to be yet another animal virus contamination, had induced the Japanese to send him *their* virus, then switched test tubes and passed the Japanese virus off to the outside world as the virus discovered by Poiesz and Ruscetti.

It was an impossible proposition to prove — or disprove. But that mattered not to Abraham Karpas, a Lithuanian émigré who had begun his career as a veterinarian tending Swiss milk cows. Karpas claimed an impressive succession of jobs: the Pasteur Institute in Paris, the Boston Children's Hospital lab of the legendary virologist John Enders, and with Albert Sabin, the co-inventor of the polio vaccine. "I must tell you," Karpas said of Sabin, "he's a terrible man. He treated his people terribly. That's one of the reasons he never got the Nobel Prize."

Abe Karpas presided over a small lab at the Molecular Biology Laboratory in Cambridge, England, the successor to the hallowed Cavendish Laboratory where Crick and Watson had started it all.

Karpas was a talented grower of cells, although not quite the sort of scientist one might have expected to find sharing a table at lunch with Sir Max Perutz or Professor Sir Aaron Klug, and there was some truth in the suggestions that Karpas's career owed much to his rapier wit and his talent for ingratiating himself with the mandarins of molecular biology.

Karpas considered Robin Weiss his archrival, and Weiss was convinced that Karpas had been carrying on a whispering campaign with the high priests of Cambridge to deny Weiss the thing he wanted most: the three initials after his name, "F.R.S.," that denote membership in the Royal Society, the British equivalent of the American National Academy of Sciences.

Karpas cheerfully acknowledged Weiss's suspicions. "I haven't exactly been whispering," he said, and Weiss was only slightly more charitable toward Karpas. "Abe was claiming he had viruses in this and that leukemia," Weiss said, "and he wouldn't collaborate with any molecular biologists. In the floors above him, in the same building, there were bunches of them. There were Nobel prizes sort of hanging off the windows."

But Weiss thought anyone who wrote Karpas off as a poseur was making a mistake. "Although he's difficult and truculent," Weiss said, and "does half-a-dozen half-baked things instead of one thing decently, he actually has some flashes of intuition which most of us don't get. I've always thought he's remarkably similar to Gallo, and that's why they hate each other. They think everyone else is out to get them, so it ends up that people are. They claim things in retrospect that never happened that way. They're very similar personalities, a mixture of paranoia and ambition, but with some real scientific imagination."

Like Gallo, Karpas had spent years looking for a human cancer virus, and he had watched with glee as Gallo's various discoveries turned to dust. "His level of biological intuition is very low," Karpas said, nevertheless insisting that his feud with Gallo wasn't personal. "He sets a very bad example for young people," Karpas said. To anyone who would listen, Karpas pointed out what seemed to him telling discrepancies in the HTLV story, including the absence of any evidence that HTLV was a human retrovirus, and the genetic differences between different isolates of HTLV.

Karpas, who thought two isolations of the same virus from different patients should be much more alike than not, was particularly fond of observing that the virus from Charlie Robinson bore only a superficial resemblance to the one from the Trinidadian woman, M.B.[k] Karpas seized on these and other disparities, such as the statement in one of Gallo's articles that an upcoming article by Poiesz would report the detection of HTLV DNA in leukemic cells from two new patients.[40] If true, that would make it far more likely that HTLV was indeed a human virus and not an animal contaminant. The fact that one of the two infected patients was described as "a child with acute lymphatic leukemia" was even more interesting, since HTLV-induced leukemia typically takes decades to show up. But when Poiesz's article appeared, it hadn't contained the promised data.[l]

In Yorio Hinuma, Abraham Karpas found a kindred spirit. Convinced that Gallo hadn't discovered what the Japanese had found, Karpas and Hinuma launched a search for ATLV in patients with mycosis fungoides and Sezary's syndrome. When no virus materialized from either group, Karpas and Hinuma declared that HTLV couldn't possibly be the same as ATLV,[41] and they weren't alone in suspecting something amiss with HTLV.

"When the American papers are closely scrutinized," another Cambridge scientist wrote to the British medical journal *The Lancet*, "they turn out to depend a great deal on cross linking and sometimes it is well nigh impossible to extract the evidence, but in order to disentangle them one has to spend many hours trying to unravel the threads. Conversely the Japanese work is impeccable, straightforward and highly regarded. . . . Quite a number of workers, including myself, are beginning to wonder what the situation really is."[42]

The principal interest in HTLV was not among clinicians, who except for those in Japan had never seen a case of Adult T-Cell Leukemia, but among molecular biologists, who wanted to know what made the first human retrovirus tick. Did it resemble the animal tumor viruses? Or was there some genetic oddity that distinguished HTLV from its animal counterparts?

The answers hadn't been forthcoming from Bethesda, because nobody in Gallo's lab was capable of cracking HTLV's genetic code. But the Japanese had the capability, and they were literally taking ATLV apart. Using a technique invented by the legendary Cambridge scientist, Fred Sanger, that made it possible to "see" DNA as smudges on a piece of X-ray film,[m] the Japanese had assembled the complete DNA sequence of ATLV, a string of 9,032 nucleic acids, or *nucleotides* — adenine, thymine, guanine, and cytosine — laid end-to-end.[43] "The Japanese worked very fast and very hard," conceded Bernie Poiesz. "They beat us to the punch."[n]

Not all the Japanese had accepted Mika Popovic's conclusion that ATLV and HTLV were the same virus by different names, and in their publications many Japanese had continued to use the term ATLV. Now that Gallo at last was willing to share HTLV, the Japanese could perform the same comparison on their own turf. Although there were some minor genetic differences, the Japanese agreed that ATLV and HTLV represented "the same species of retrovirus," and, therefore, that both were the cause of Adult T-Cell Leukemia.[44] Because Poiesz and Ruscetti had published first, with the exception of Yorio Hinuma the Japanese agreed to drop the term ATLV in favor of HTLV.

In public, Gallo repaid their deference. Addressing the biggest Japanese cancer meeting of the year, the Princess Takamatsu symposium in Tokyo, Gallo remarked how honored he was to be in Japan, "where so much of the important ground-breaking research in this field has been conducted." In the scientific literature, where it counted, it seemed to pain Gallo to give the Japanese any credit at all. In one article recapping the discovery of HTLV, Gallo accorded the Japanese two footnotes out of eighty-five.[45] When a colleague asked Gallo for a complete list of published papers on HTLV, he got back the titles of Gallo's own publications and the caveat that "much of the additional work, most of it from Japan, is really not terribly relevant."[46]

When *Science* returned a Gallo manuscript on HTLV with the suggestion that Gallo might include some reference to "other workers in the field," Gallo replied that he was "astonished by this request in view of the history of the field, the novelty of this work, and the incredible failure of the most obvious other laboratory in Japan to reference anything."[47] On a few occasions Gallo went so far as to declare that his lab, not Hinuma's, had forged the causal link between HTLV and Adult T-Cell Leukemia, including the first detection of HTLV antibodies in healthy Kyushu residents.[o] Only later, Gallo said, were "subsequent results obtained by investigators in several laboratories in Japan."[p]

As an editor of the definitive textbook on RNA viruses Robin Weiss tried to present a more balanced view, noting that HTLV had first been observed by Elizabeth van der Loo, and that the cell line in which HTLV was found had been established by Adi Gazdar. Weiss also accorded Hinuma the credit for linking Adult T-Cell Leukemia with HTLV.[48] "Hinuma did some very nice work, once the penny dropped," Weiss said. "I think he deserves real credit for that. The Japanese work, never mind who deserves most of the credit within Japan, was driven by studying the disease and the curious pattern of the disease. Gallo's work was driven by coming across this virus and being unaware of Japanese ATL."[49]

Gallo didn't think the lack of awareness was his fault. "The Japanese epidemiologists never knew there was an increase in leukemia in the southern part of Japan," Gallo said years later. "They missed it totally. If I lived in Japan, I would have discovered HTLV in the early seventies. It wouldn't have taken until the end of the seventies."

HTLV was interesting to virologists, but its discovery hadn't done much to advance the National Cancer Institute's primary mission, the treatment of cancer. Indeed, the link between HTLV and cancer was tenuous at best. Not only was Adult T-Cell Leukemia among the rarest of cancers, hardly seen in the Western Hemisphere, of every 200 Japanese infected with HTLV only one ever actually *got* Adult T-Cell Leukemia.[50]

Pushing such details aside, the NCI ranked the discovery of HTLV as "one of the most exciting stories of 20th Century biology," which put it on roughly the same plane as antibiotics and the double helix. When the NIH nominated Gallo for the National Science Medal, it lauded him not only for the "discovery and isolation of the first human retrovirus," but for "obtaining evidence that this virus, HTLV, is specifically associated with Adult T-cell Leukemia."[51] When they were mentioned at all, the Japanese were viewed as "adding weight to Gallo's new evidence."[52]

The Lasker Prize is American medicine's highest honor, often described as the "American Nobel," although much of its prestige has resulted from the careful selection of recipients who are only a few years away from winning the Nobel itself. When the Lasker jury met to choose the winners for 1982, there was general agreement that the list should be headed by Mike Bishop and his University of California colleague Harold Varmus, whose work with the Rous Sarcoma Virus had changed the course of cancer research.[q]

Vince DeVita was among that year's Lasker jurors, and DeVita didn't see how the jury could give the prize to Bishop and Varmus without including the discoverer of the first human cancer virus. "Gallo was tagged on at the last minute," Robin Weiss said. "They said, 'Oh, let's have the human as well.'" Gallo had missed the plane that carried Temin and Baltimore to Stockholm five years before. But as the recipient of the Lasker Prize for the "revolutionary discovery of the first retrovirus known to be associated with a human malignancy," he might make the trip with Bishop and Varmus.[53]

Not included in the Lasker citation was Frank Ruscetti, whose run-ins with Gallo had put him on the endangered list. "You don't actually get fired at NIH," explained Ruscetti's technician, Andrea Woods. "You lose your space and lose your technical help. When blood samples come in you aren't on the list to get them, you aren't invited to staff meetings. You basically dry up and blow away." Ted Breitman, Gallo's old boss, remembered a Saturday afternoon in the lab when "Gallo came back from Europe, and he was seething. Someone had approached him and asked him if he was 'still collaborating with Ruscetti.' I don't know whether it was coincidence or not, but Frank was out not long after that."

Bernie Poiesz, his cancer institute fellowship having come to an end, had departed Bethesda to set up a small research lab at the VA hospital in Syracuse, taking with him the rare satisfaction of having made a significant biological discovery. Poiesz needed more than memories to fund his research, but after arriving in Syracuse unsettling things began to happen. Applying for a grant to continue his work with HTLV, Poiesz asked Gallo for a letter of recommendation. What he got in return was far from an enthusiastic endorsement. "He basically wanted to make sure that he was the major player as the theme of HTLV worked its way out into the world," Poiesz said. "I think his competitive nature was such that, for some reason, there was a false sense of concern that I might do well with it."

Poiesz thought that calling Gallo the discoverer of HTLV was "like saying that Queen Isabella discovered America after Columbus came home and told her about it. *I'm* the discoverer of HTLV," Poiesz said, "working in Bob Gallo's laboratory. The moment of discovery was mine."[54]

"I think I've forgotten more than Poiesz and Ruscetti ever knew," Gallo says. "Times ten."[55]

"These Guys Have Found Something Important"

At the beginning of 1982, the National Cancer Institute's best source of information on AIDS was the chief of its pediatrics branch, Arthur Levine. "I probably knew more about AIDS than anybody else at NIH at that point in time," Levine recalled. "I had a very close colleague named John Zeigler, who had been in Africa before he joined the NCI. John went to San Francisco, and he was asked to consult on the first AIDS patients. When he saw these patients he called me and asked what I thought about this bizarre syndrome. That's what got me intrigued."

Levine had worked with a number of viruses, including retroviruses, and "as soon as I heard about the hemophiliacs and the Haitians, things began to fall into place. At that point we knew this probably was a blood-borne disease. Number two, it probably was slow-acting. So if this were going to be blood-borne and if it were going to be very slow-acting, it had to be a virus. If it were a virus, it had to be immuno-suppressive. So I went through the known viruses, eliminating each class that could *not* be the agent. And what I came up with, essentially, were retroviruses. So putting all this information together, I concluded that this was going to be a retrovirus related to HTLV."

Having worked out his hypothesis, Levine decided to tell Robert Gallo. "I'd known Bob a long time," Levine said. "His lab was next to mine at one time. I called him and I said, 'Have you heard of this bizarre syndrome that's happening in San Francisco and New York?' He hadn't heard of it. I described it to him. He agreed that it was very intriguing. And then I said, 'The most intriguing thing is that I think the cause of this syndrome is going to be a retrovirus related to HTLV,' and I told him why. He said 'That's very interesting,' and got off the phone."[a]

At the time of Levine's call, Gallo's attention was focused on a second human retrovirus, HTLV-2, which had emerged unexpectedly from a new T-cell culture in Gallo's lab and was even rarer than what was now known as HTLV-1.[b] "For Gallo, AIDS was 'Oh, God, yet another thing,'" recalled Doug Blayney, an NCI epidemiologist working on HTLV-2. "He had a lot of irons in the fire. It took direction from the top to get him to do it." That direction came from Vince DeVita. "When the whole AIDS business broke," DeVita said, "we went to Bob Gallo and said, 'Ratchet yourself fifteen degrees or so in the direction of AIDS. Commit some resources to it.' He resisted at first, then he recognized the opportunity."

Michael Lange, a physician at St. Luke's Hospital in Manhattan who was seeing increasing numbers of AIDS patients, had also concluded there might be a connection between HTLV and AIDS. Like Levine, the first person Lange called was Gallo, only to discover that Gallo "didn't seem to know much about AIDS." When Lange reminded Gallo that HTLV had begun showing up in the Caribbean, and that AIDS seemed to be prevalent among Haitian refugees in Miami, Gallo agreed to test blood from Lange's patients for antibodies to HTLV.[c] But when only one patient out of 140 was positive, Lange put aside the notion that Gallo's virus had anything to do with AIDS.

What Art Levine called "this bizarre syndrome" was being watched most closely by the Centers for Disease Control in Atlanta, the federal agency charged with protecting the public health. A few months before Levine's call to Gallo, a CDC epidemiologist named Don Francis had been the first to suggest that AIDS might be caused by HTLV.[d] The Japanese had shown that HTLV was transmitted by sexual intercourse as well as through mother's milk and transfusions of blood,[1] and considering the number of gay men with AIDS a sexually transmitted virus made sense. But HTLV was so rare in Europe and the United States that it had been dismissed by the CDC in favor of more common viruses.

"We were looking at every virus we could get our hands on," recalled Cirilo Cabradilla, one of Francis's CDC colleagues. None of those had panned out, and Cabradilla recalled that by the summer of 1982 "the only one we hadn't really looked at was the human retrovirus." Cabradilla, who had gotten to know Gallo slightly during his tenure as an NIH postdoc, made an appointment to talk about testing AIDS patients' blood samples for HTLV. "He didn't seem that interested," Cabradilla said later. "I don't think he wanted to get involved with a gay disease. What turned him around was Max."[2]

Myron T. "Max" Essex, a researcher at the Harvard School of Public Health in Boston, had worked out what he believed was a new way to determine whether individuals were infected with HTLV-1. Rather than searching blood samples for antibodies that reacted with the proteins of the virus itself, as Marjorie Guroff had done with the Japanese ATL patients, the "Essex test" looked for antibodies to a protein Essex had discovered on the outer surface, or membrane, of HTLV-infected T-cells.

Essex called the protein HTLV-MA, for HTLV membrane antigen — "antigen" being a catch-all term for any foreign substance capable of stimulating the production of antibodies — and he had concluded that HTLV-MA on the surface of a cell meant there was HTLV-1 inside. When Essex exposed AIDS patients' blood samples to HUT-102 and MT-2, two cell lines known to be infected with HTLV-1, a sizable percentage contained antibodies to HTLV-MA — evidence, in Essex's opinion, that the AIDS patients from whom the samples had come were also infected with HTLV-1.[3]

The concept of a cell-surface "marker" for retroviral infection had grown out of the notion, conceived by Essex as a postdoc, that white blood cells from cats infected with the feline leukemia virus also exhibited a unique protein on their surface. Essex dubbed that protein FOCMA, for "feline oncornavirus membrane antigen." The intriguing thing about FOCMA was that cats who had high levels of FOCMA antibodies seemed resistant to the ill effects of the feline leukemia virus itself.[4] If FOCMA were a by-product of the cell's infection with feline leukemia virus, it might represent confirmation of a cellular defense against cancer, at least in cats — "exciting stuff," one of Essex's colleagues recalled.

Essex's FOCMA research had been financed with hundreds of thousands of dollars in grants from the National Cancer Institute.

When Wolf Prensky, a precocious junior researcher at the Memorial Sloan-Kettering Cancer Center, dared to suggest on the basis of his own experiments that FOCMA was just a viral protein and not a cellular antigen, Vince DeVita selected Gallo, despite his co-authorship of a FOCMA article with Essex two years before,[5] to head an investigation of Prensky's claims. The investigating committee's verdict was equivocal: It was possible that Essex was right, and also that he wasn't. Considering the "scientific complexities" of FOCMA, the panel couldn't say which.[6] "I didn't understand FOCMA," Gallo admitted later.[7]

Neither did Murray Gardner, a widely respected animal virologist at the University of California at Davis, where Essex, a veterinarian, had gotten his degree. It wasn't that Gardner didn't understand the science behind FOCMA. "I couldn't confirm what Essex was saying," Gardner recalled. In collaboration with Prensky and Frank Ruscetti's wife, Sandy, Gardner published a definitive demonstration that the FOCMA protein was encoded by the feline leukemia virus itself, not a cellular by-product of infection.[8]

"Max was half right, in that if cats have this antibody they are protected," observed Jim Mullins, a junior member of Essex's department at Harvard. "He thought it was a cell-encoded protein, but he was wrong." The idea that cat blood cells had some built-in defense against cancer evaporated overnight. But rather than withdrawing or correcting his FOCMA articles, Essex simply stopped referring to them in his subsequent publications. "FOCMA just sort of died," Gardner said. "Time moves on. FOCMA's forgotten."

Without missing many beats, Essex had gone on to embrace FOCMA's successor, HTLV-MA. Depending on his choice of subjects, roughly a quarter of the AIDS patients' blood samples Essex tested were positive for antibodies to HTLV-MA — hardly conclusive evidence that HTLV caused AIDS, but too provocative to be ignored. Still, the Essex test was only circumstantial, fingerprints left on the windowsill after the burglar has fled.

Gallo wanted to catch the burglar in the act, a pursuit he assigned to Ed Gelmann, a Stanford postdoc whose temperamental brilliance matched the recently departed Frank Ruscetti's. Using a short piece of DNA from $HTLV_{CR}$, the Charlie Robinson isolate, Gelmann went fishing for complementary DNA fragments in T-cells extracted from patients with AIDS. After probing the cells of thirty-three AIDS patients — "basically everything we could get our hands on," Gelmann said later — only two appeared to be infected with HTLV. From only one of those, a thirty-two-year-old New York City resident named E.P., Mika Popovic had been able to isolate the virus itself.

Two HTLV-infected AIDS patients out of thirty-three was a fraction of the twenty-five percent in whom Essex was finding HTLV-MA antibodies. But HTLV in the United States is surpassingly rare, and Gelmann's results couldn't be dismissed until an equal number of healthy gay men had been screened for the virus.[9]

While Gelmann was arranging the necessary control experiments, a taxi bearing a virologist from the Hôpital Claude Bernard in Paris pulled up to the tall wrought-iron gates of the venerable Institut Pasteur. The plastic container Françoise Brun-Vézinet carried under her arm was filled with dry ice, and buried in the ice was a glass tube. Inside the tube, swimming in antibiotics, was the lymph node of a thirty-three-year-old fashion designer named Frédéric Brugière. A note from Willy Rozenbaum attached to the tube provided the patient's diagnosis: "persistent lymphadenopathy in a homosexual man."

An hour earlier on the morning of January 3, 1983, Brun had looked on as surgeons at the sprawling Hôpital Pitié-Salpêtrière, one of the largest in Europe, extracted the node through an incision under Brugière's left arm. When the operation was finished, Brun had taken twenty milliliters of Brugière's blood. For Brun and her colleague, Willy Rozenbaum, the brief procedure marked the culmination of a months-long struggle to focus the attention of the French research establishment on AIDS.

Rozenbaum, a specialist in infectious diseases, was one of the few French physicians who subscribed to the CDC's weekly *Morbidity and Mortality Weekly Report*, a pamphlet-sized chronicle of trends in death and disease across the United States. On the day the issue of *MMWR* arrived that contained Mike Gottlieb's report of the first American AIDS cases, Rozenbaum examined his first French AIDS patient. "I received it in the morning," Rozenbaum said, "and in the afternoon I had in my consultation room an Air France steward with cough and fever and lymphadenopathy."

By the end of 1981 Rozenbaum was taking care of three or four such patients, and he had been joined by a handful of Paris physicians in puzzling over a new disease for which there was no known cause or cure. With Brun and Jacques Leibowitch, a doctor from the Hôpital Necker, Rozenbaum had set up an informal AIDS working group. "We had contacts with the gay community, and with the Haitian community," Rozenbaum said. "The center was in the Hospital Claude Bernard," the main facility in Paris for treating infectious diseases. "But it was a center without any resources," Rozenbaum said. "We just had a meeting every month or so."

One of those invited to attend was David Klatzmann, a young French doctor who had abandoned the clinic for laboratory research and had been quickly drawn to AIDS. "People here in France had no interest in working on a disease affecting a bunch of gay guys," Klatzmann recalled. "At that time, the study group on AIDS was probably ten persons, and eight of us were Jewish — Leibowitch, Klatzmann, Rozenbaum, like that. There aren't that many Jewish physicians in Paris. It's not like New York. Maybe it was minorities taking care of minorities."

The most impetuous member proved to be Jacques Leibowitch, whose manic energy annoyed his more deliberate colleagues. "He had a lot of ideas," Rozenbaum said. "Sometimes they were on the ball. Sometimes. Several times he wanted to leave the group, and then he came back. It's his personality. Few people can work with him." But it was the Harvard-trained Leibowitch, whose English was the best of anyone in the group, who noticed an article in an American medical magazine quoting Gallo's suggestion at the Mt. Sinai conference that a retrovirus called HTLV might be the cause of AIDS.[10]

When Willy Rozenbaum was invited to lecture on AIDS at the Institut Pasteur, he used the occasion to press Leibowitch's point. "Everybody was there," Rozenbaum said, "all the heads of the laboratories. When I finished my talk I asked if there was a retrovirologist in the room. *'Y-a-t'il un retrovirologist dans la salle?'* It was my last question. Everybody smiled and nobody answered. Afterwards, I saw Françoise Brun. I told her, 'I can't understand why nobody at the Pasteur Institute is working on retroviruses. How can you explain that?' And she asked me, 'Was Jean-Claude Chermann there?' I said, 'I don't know him.' She said, 'Well, he taught the course on retroviruses at Pasteur.' So I told her, 'Why don't you try to call him?'"

Brun rang Chermann's office, but he wasn't in. Perhaps, Chermann's secretary said, Brun should speak with Chermann's boss, Luc

Montagnier. Although Montagnier had spent the better part of his career working with animal retroviruses, he confessed to Brun that he knew next to nothing about AIDS, beyond the fact that an American named Gallo had said it might be caused by HTLV.

He only knew that much, Montagnier said, because Institut Pasteur Production, the subsidiary that marketed vaccines and other products developed in Pasteur's labs, was using American blood plasma to make its vaccine for hepatitis B. To be sure the vaccine wasn't contaminated with HTLV, Montagnier had been asked to test a few of the imported plasma samples for reverse transcriptase. Two had been positive, suggesting that their donors were infected with a retrovirus. Montagnier assumed the retrovirus must be HTLV, and the tests had started him thinking about retroviruses and AIDS. "Probably I would have been less receptive to the group of Rozenbaum," Montagnier said later "if I had not had that request from Pasteur."

Brun explained that a hallmark of AIDS seemed to be a decline in the number of T-cells, and that her group thought AIDS might be caused by a retrovirus that infected and killed those cells. To Montagnier, that didn't sound like HTLV, which quite apart from killing T-cells transformed them into leukemic cells. "I told Montagnier we need to look for the virus in patients who don't yet have AIDS," Brun recalled, and offered to bring Pasteur a lymph node from someone in the early stage of the disease.

In Frédéric Brugière, Brun and Rozenbaum had found what seemed the ideal patient. A couturier employed by one of the top Paris fashion houses, Brugière had first consulted Rozenbaum in March 1982, after returning from a vacation in India.* Three months later he developed lymphadenopathy, the enlarged lymph nodes Rozenbaum now recognized as a precursor of AIDS. Brugière didn't yet have full-fledged AIDS but his lymphadenopathy had persisted, suggesting to Rozenbaum that the lymph nodes played an important role in the progression of the disease.

"I thought that the virus could kill T-cells," Rozenbaum said later, "and that if the T-cells are killed it could be difficult to find the virus in the cells that disappeared. So that was the reason I wanted to take somebody at an early stage of the disease."

---

*Although Rozenbaum discussed some of the published details of Brugière's case, he never violated his patient's confidentiality by disclosing Brugière's identity.

It was a little past noon when Brugière's lymph node arrived at the Pasteur, a jumble of modern and ancient buildings that line the rue du Dr. Roux, a short street named for the nineteenth-century Pasteur physician who discovered the cause of diphtheria and formulated the first treatment for that disease. On the top floor of the oldest building is the well-preserved apartment of Louis Pasteur himself, who gave the world the germ theory of disease, pasteurization, and a vaccine for rabies, and whose successors followed with sulfa drugs and a vaccine for tetanus.

For much of a century the Institut Pasteur had led the world in vanquishing infectious diseases, and its distinctive green-and-white medicine boxes bearing a cameo of Louis Pasteur remain a staple of hospitals and clinics throughout the developing world. Once, the Institut Pasteur was also at the forefront of molecular biology, having achieved its finest hour in 1965, when Jacques Monod, acknowledged as one of the two or three greatest minds in the history of modern biology, shared a Nobel Prize with two other Pasteurians, André Lwoff and François Jacob, for the fundamental discovery of how genes control the growth of cells.

In the twenty years since then, molecular biology in France had been overtaken by huge American laboratories at Harvard, Berkeley, Caltech, and M.I.T., veritable factories outfitted with vast arrays of high-tech equipment and manned by squadrons of postdocs and technicians on a scale unmatchable in Europe. Jacques Monod was dead, and André Lwoff, his faculties dimmed, had retired to a village on the Mediterranean. François Jacob was still in residence at Pasteur, but as a figurehead and fund-raiser who no longer spent much time in the lab.

It had been a while since the Institut Pasteur had discovered anything of earth-shattering importance, and Luc Montagnier was unquestionably overdue. Montagnier was viewed as an outsider by his Pasteur colleagues, having been raised and educated not in Paris, the center of all culture and learning, but in the precincts of the Loire Valley. His father, an accountant with an amateur's interest in science, had wished his son to become a doctor, and Montagnier had been admitted to study medicine at the University of Poitiers. "But I knew from the beginning that I would not be a doctor," Montagnier said. "Because I was more interested in science. I was fascinated by science, physics and biology. I was interested especially in the origin of the universe, how the stars were formed, astrophysics and nuclear energy."

Montagnier's natural shyness was magnified by his relatively short stature, barely five feet eight inches, for which he blamed the Second World War. At the age of twelve, his family's house had been partly destroyed by an American bomb intended for a nearby rail yard. "We were not hurt," Montagnier recalled, "but all the furniture and everything was in very bad shape. During the next four years I didn't eat well. The first years, in nineteen-forty and forty-one, we had nothing to eat but potatoes and bread. As a kid, I suffered. It affected my height. I was too young to be soldier, but I was a victim of the war."

Montagnier did study medicine, first in Poitiers and then at the Sorbonne, but halfheartedly. At twenty-three, rather than setting up a practice, he had taken a job as a junior researcher in a cell biology lab at the Curie Institute in Paris. A postdoctoral fellowship followed in the London laboratory of Kingsley Sanders, where Montagnier had developed a technique for growing malignant tumor cells in seaweed gel that remains in use today.[11]

When the cancer virus craze reached France, Montagnier had pioneered the culturing of viruses by using antibodies to interferon, a natural biochemical that impedes their growth.[12] A long dry spell had followed, during which Montagnier enlisted his tiny lab in the futile search for human viruses that might cause breast cancer. No breast cancer viruses had materialized on either side of the Atlantic, and Montagnier, approaching fifty, had resigned himself to a comfortable if undistinguished career as the Pasteur's chief of viral oncology.

The title sounded impressive, but the field of viral oncology was passé and the Viral Oncology Unit was one of the Pasteur's smallest, so small that Montagnier's domain extended only to his own lab, the laboratory of another researcher named Ara Hovanessian, and a third tiny lab occupied by Jean-Claude Chermann and his assistant, Françoise Barré-Sinoussi, whom Montagnier had reluctantly inherited from a Pasteur subsidiary.

"There was some conflict with Jacques Monod," Montagnier said, "so they had to leave and came back to the Foundation," as the main Pasteur complex on the Left Bank is informally known. Under Montagnier's tutelage, Chermann and Barré had begun working with mouse interferon antibodies, demonstrating that their use significantly enhanced the growth of mouse retroviruses by blocking the production of interferon. But after several years Montagnier had concluded that the pair were spinning their wheels and encouraged them to move on to something new.

Françoise Brun had expected to hand Brugière's lymph node to Jean-Claude Chermann. Told Chermann was at lunch, she took the box to Montagnier's lab on the second floor of the Bâtiment Henri Darré, named for a French doctor whose widow reputedly left his fortune to the Pasteur as penance for a wartime collaboration with the Nazis. But Montagnier had afternoon classes to teach, and it was after six when he removed the node from its antibiotic broth.

Working at the laboratory bench, Montagnier cut the tissue into small slices with a pair of scissors and placed the slices in a solution that made it easier to separate Brugière's T-cells from his other blood cells. Some of the T-cells Montagnier froze at minus 80 degrees Centigrade, the standard laboratory temperature for preserving cells and viruses. The rest he added to a solution containing a protein known to activate T-cells and induce them to replicate.

The solution was divided between two flasks, which Montagnier placed in an incubator set at thirty-seven degrees centigrade — the equivalent of 98.6 degrees Fahrenheit, the temperature of the human body. If the T-cells were infected by a virus and they remained alive, the virus should begin to reproduce. If the virus was a retrovirus, the first hint of its presence would be reverse transcriptase. After three days of no activity Montagnier added interferon antibody, followed by T-Cell Growth Factor from a Paris colleague, Didier Fradellizi at the Hôpital Saint-Louis. Still nothing. When it became necessary for Montagnier to leave Paris for a few days, he decided to transfer the Brugière cultures to a disused laundry room near where Jean-Claude Chermann had his lab.

Apart from their shared interest in retroviruses, Chermann and Montagnier were about as unalike as two Frenchmen could be. Where Montagnier was reserved, Chermann was demonstrative, and not infrequently emotional. Where Montagnier was short and slightly rotund, Chermann was tall, with movie-star good looks. Montagnier was self-effacing, sometimes painfully so. Chermann, the son of a seamstress who had worked his way through school, took himself quite seriously, insisting on being introduced at scientific meetings as *le chef du service du retrovirologie de l'Institut Pasteur,* without mentioning that his *service* consisted of himself and Françoise Barré.

Montagnier thought Chermann a bumbler, but he was comfortable leaving the cultures with Barré. "She had good techniques," he said. The only child of a middle-class Parisian family, who as a young girl had preferred microscopes to dolls, in high school Barré had become interested in "the mechanisms involved in human life." But she remained uncertain about a career in science until, while an undergraduate at the University of Paris, a friend had introduced her to Chermann. It was under his supervision that Barré had earned her doctorate, which had been followed by a postdoctoral fellowship in an NCI lab one floor below Gallo's, where she had gotten to know a few of Gallo's people.

Her time in Bethesda over, Barré had returned to the Pasteur and Jean-Claude Chermann, and if she hadn't proven to be a particularly creative or imaginative scientist, at least she was ultra-meticulous. Like a gardener tending a new plant, Barré nursed the Brugière culture along, adding the nutrients the T-cells needed to survive and checking for telltale signs of reverse transcriptase. Before leaving, Montagnier had emphasized that Barré should look for a retrovirus, but not necessarily HTLV, which produced no measurable reverse transcriptase during its first several weeks in culture. In order not to miss another kind of retrovirus, Barré siphoned culture fluid every three days and ran it through a machine that uses radioactivity to measure the level of RT — and, indirectly, the rate of viral replication.

For the first eleven days there was nothing. On the twelfth day, January 15, the meter showed 3,000 counts a minute.[13] "It could be something," Barré recalled, "but you are not sure. So we continued." By day twenty-three, the numbers on the digital readout had climbed to 22,000 for one flask and to 24,000 for the other[e] — clear evidence, unless the machine was malfunctioning, that a retrovirus was reproducing in the flasks. Worried that it might be a leftover mouse retrovirus, of which there had been many in her lab, Barré ran a series of experiments designed to rule out a murine virus contamination. When no trace of mouse virus was detected, Barré recalled, "I began to think we have found something important."

Upon returning to Paris, Montagnier sent a tiny pellet of Brugière's T-cells to Charles Dauguet, the scientist who presided over one of the Pasteur's electron microscopes. The photographs Dauguet returned were indistinct, but Barré thought they were good enough.[14] "We were sure that it was a retrovirus," she said. "The particles were exactly the same size as a retrovirus. For us there was no doubt. The thing we were surprised about was that it did not look exactly like HTLV."

To definitively eliminate HTLV, it would be necessary to probe Brugière's cells with the same kind of HTLV probes — short fragments of HTLV DNA — that Ed Gelmann was using in Bethesda. Under the right conditions, if the probes adhered to something in the cells it could only be HTLV DNA — proof that Brugière was infected with that virus. If the probes didn't react, it would mean the virus was something else.

Only two labs in the world had the necessary probes, Gallo's and one in Japan. Montagnier had no contacts with the Japanese. But he and Gallo had once shared a room at a scientific meeting in Sicily, and not long after the isolation of HTLV Montagnier had attended a Gallo lecture at the French national cancer institute in Villejuif, outside Paris, where he mentioned to Gallo his work with interferon antibody. Shortly afterward, Gallo had invited Françoise Barré to bring some anti-interferon to his lab and teach his people how to use it.

The following year Gallo had reciprocated with T-Cell Growth Factor to aid Montagnier's search for a breast cancer virus, and given their previous exchanges Montagnier had assumed that obtaining Gallo's HTLV probes would be no problem.[15] But when Montagnier called Bethesda, he couldn't get past Gallo's secretary. "I tried to get you on the phone," he wrote Gallo the next day. "Françoise Barré, Jean-Claude Chermann and I have detected some reverse transcriptase activity in cultures of T-lymphocytes from a French patient with an immunoproliferative syndrome. We would like to know whether this isolate has something to do with your HTLV."

Besides the probes, Montagnier asked Gallo to send some blood serum containing antibodies to the HTLV proteins, another means of testing for the presence of the virus. "If you agree," Montagnier said, "it would be very convenient for us if you could eventually give these reagents to Dr. Leibowitch who will shortly visit you."[16]

Once Montagnier's letter was in the mail the reverse transcriptase levels in the Brugière culture began to decline, a sign that virus production was falling.[17] Barré's first thought was that there must be a problem with the culture, and she summoned Chermann and Montagnier for an emergency consultation.

"We were finding the virus at the same time we were losing it," Chermann recalled. "We have a virus, and the cells are dying. What can we do now, other than discard the culture?" Barré suggested transferring the remaining live virus from the dying culture to a continuous T-cell line, which would provide the virus with an unending supply of T-cells to infect. But all Chermann's cell lines were frozen. They would have to be carefully thawed, and there wasn't time for that.

The next idea came from Montagnier: Why not keep the culture alive by feeding the virus *fresh* T-cells? The cells would have to be continually replenished as they became infected and died, but adding more would keep the virus alive. From the Pasteur's transfusion center Montagnier obtained the T-cells of a visiting Spaniard who had just earned a few extra francs by donating a pint of blood. Montagnier knew nothing about the man, including what other viruses he might have picked up in the Place Pigalle, but he was in a hurry. "The first donor who came was the right one," he said. With the addition of the Spaniard's T-cells to the flagging culture the reverse transcriptase levels fluttered and again headed upward, a signal that the Brugière virus was still alive and infecting fresh targets.[18] In addition to saving the culture, the experiment confirmed that Brugière's cells contained something capable of infecting uninfected cells — the hallmark of a viral isolation.

Montagnier, Barré, and Chermann remembered having had the same thought at approximately the same moment: Brugière's T-cells had been dying because the virus was killing them. The definition of AIDS was T-cell depletion, and a T-cell-killing virus could explain why AIDS patients had so few T-cells. Montagnier arranged with a nearby maternity hospital to supply him with blood from discarded umbilical cords, whose virgin T-cells are most susceptible to infection. When the culture dwindled again, an infusion of "cord blood" cells brought it back.[19]

As the Brugière culture was being rescued in Paris, Jacques Leibowitch was stepping off an airplane in America. Leibowitch's first stop was the Cold Spring Harbor Laboratory, the venerable Long Island research institution now headed by Jim Watson, to hear Gallo speak about HTLV.[20]

Despite what Ted Breitman described as Gallo's "Russian Army approach to research," according to Gallo's talk his methodical search for HTLV in AIDS patients wasn't going well. Blood and tissue samples arriving in Gallo's lab were put in culture, then tested for reverse transcriptase. Any culture exhibiting RT above a certain level was examined for the presence of HTLV. But the only culture from which HTLV had been isolated was still the New York AIDS patient E.P.[f] Just before Christmas, some promising cells had arrived from an M. D. Anderson physician, Jordan Gutterman, who suspected that an AIDS patient Gutterman called G.W. might be infected with HTLV.[21] The cells had been slightly positive for reverse transcriptase. But when they proved negative for any trace of HTLV, they, too, were discarded.[22]

Thanks to France's colonial links with Africa and the Caribbean, French physicians had access to a wider range of AIDS sufferers than their American colleagues, whose patients were mostly white homosexuals. Arriving in Bethesda from Cold Spring Harbor, Leibowitch handed Gallo a present from Paris, a number of blood samples packed in dry ice, including one from a Haitian woman who had recently died of AIDS and another from a Zairian named Elomata.[23]

Suspecting that Elomata might somehow provide the link between AIDS and HTLV, Leibowitch had gone to considerable trouble to obtain the man's cells. "We had information from cases that we had seen in Paris as early as 1979 that AIDS was in Africa," Leibowitch recalled. "I called my sister, who's a dermatology professor, and I told her to watch for an African that showed a lymphoma associated with HTLV. Three days later she calls me and she said, 'I have one.'"

Another Leibowitch sample had come from a French geologist who suffered a motorcycle accident in Haiti that cost him his left arm. During surgery in Port-au-Prince, the geologist, Claude Chardon, had been transfused with eight pints of Haitian blood. Four years after returning to his family in Paris, Chardon had become ill with AIDS. "He realized he had a very serious disease," recalled his physician, Robert Modigliani. "But as we had no treatment, we didn't tell him he had AIDS."

Claude Chardon was dead, but his T-cells had remained in Modigliani's freezer at the Hôpital Saint-Lazare. When Leibowitch attended a Modigliani lecture on the curious case of Claude Chardon, he immediately recognized its significance. "It was a clear case of AIDS," Leibowitch said, "and it was a *transfusion* case of AIDS. I was strongly motivated to get the cells of this guy, because I thought this guy was clean in terms of homosexual complications. It could serve the political purpose of demonstrating that the cause of AIDS was not homosexually related."[g]

When the nine Leibowitch samples were logged in Gallo's register, Claude Chardon became number 3731, Elomata 3734, and M.A., the Haitian woman, 3735.[h] Frank Ruscetti's former technician, Andrea Woods, remembered "something funny about those samples that came from France. Maybe the person who came wasn't supposed to bring them. Or maybe it was what Gallo was supposed to do with them when he got them. I have some recollection that Gallo would have preferred they weren't French samples."

As it turned out, several of the Leibowitch samples had been taken from the serum collection painstakingly assembled by Françoise Brun — according to Brun, without her knowledge or permission.[24] "The week after he learned that we found something in Pasteur, he went right to Gallo," Willy Rozenbaum said.

In Bethesda, Leibowitch discovered just how far Gallo was from linking HTLV with AIDS. After probing blood samples from nearly a hundred AIDS patients, including sixty provided by the CDC, an increasingly skeptical Ed Gelmann hadn't found any HTLV-infected patients beyond the original two. While Gelmann continued to probe, Marjorie Guroff and Doug Blayney had begun testing blood from the same patients for antibodies to HTLV. But fewer than 10 percent of those samples were proving positive, well below the 25 percent Max Essex was reporting with antibodies to HTLV-MA. Unless more evidence turned up soon, Leibowitch glumly informed his colleagues in Paris, "it is evident that Dr. Gallo's team will lose interest in this story."[25]

The cells Leibowitch carried across the Atlantic seemed at first to offer no help. Elomata, the Zairian man whom Leibowitch had thought held such promise, proved to be a case of HTLV-induced lymphoma, which had nothing to do with AIDS. Another sample, from a French journalist, B.U., had been slightly positive for reverse transcriptase. When B.U.'s cells tested negative for HTLV, they too were put aside.

With two of the Leibowitch samples, however, the story was different. Not only were the cells from the Haitian, M.A., slightly positive for reverse transcriptase, they reacted with an antibody to one of the main HTLV proteins — an indication the woman had been infected with HTLV. So, apparently, had Claude Chardon, whose cells were strongly positive for both reverse transcriptase and HTLV antibodies.[26] An article by Modigliani and his Paris colleagues, recounting Chardon's death from AIDS, was already in press at *The Lancet*.[27] The article said nothing about the cause of Chardon's disease. But when an excited Jacques Leibowitch passed the news from Bethesda, Modigliani added a last-minute paragraph noting that Chardon had been infected with the human retrovirus HTLV.[i]

The provenance of the virus that infected Frédéric Brugière was still unclear, mainly because Leibowitch had returned to Paris without the HTLV probes and antibodies urgently requested by Montagnier. When Montagnier called to stress the importance of his request, Gallo again was unavailable. "I am very sorry you didn't reach me by telephone," Gallo wrote Montagnier the next day. "I tried to return the call twice, but I did not get an answer. We too have evidence for HTLV in some immune abnormality diseases, and I am very pleased to have your interest and Jean-Claude's in this problem. Your results sound very interesting."

Gallo agreed to send the HTLV antibody, but not the DNA probe. Although Harvard's Jim Mullins already had the probe, Gallo informed Montagnier that he wasn't able to release it to other laboratories until its existence had been reported in a scientific journal.[28]

Gallo's attention was distracted by the two manuscripts he was preparing for *Science,* one reporting Ed Gelmann's detection of HTLV in the two homosexuals with AIDS, the second describing Mika Popovic's isolation of HTLV from E.P. *Science* was also keen to publish Max Essex's latest results with HTLV-MA, and Gallo wanted all three articles to appear in the same issue. But Ruth Kulstad, *Science*'s biology editor, thought two HTLV-positive cases out of thirty-three AIDS patients was weak evidence at best.[29] To strengthen the manuscript, Gallo added the news that HTLV had been detected in two additional AIDS patients from France.[j]

Gallo had recently been invited to join the company, founded by Max Essex and one of Essex's Harvard colleagues, William Haseltine, that owned the rights to Essex's test for HTLV-MA. Cambridge

BioScience originally had been set up to market Essex's blood test for the feline leukemia virus, which the company's advertisements described as "a leading killer of cats." But if HTLV was indeed the cause of AIDS, Essex's test for HTLV-MA looked like a much bigger money-maker.

Gallo's detection of HTLV in four patients with AIDS could only help the company's prospects, and Essex and Haseltine offered Gallo a position as a "scientific associate," with an option to buy 10,000 shares of the company's stock at $1 a share — a small stake compared to the 600,000 shares controlled by Essex and Haseltine, but enough to send Gallo to the NCI's associate director, Peter Fischinger, to inquire about the legality of the arrangement.

Fischinger thought the deal was fine, as long as Cambridge Bio-Science didn't do business with NIH. Just the same, Fischinger said, NCI would prefer that the company kept quiet about Gallo's participation. Fischinger especially didn't want to see any mention of the company's relationship with Gallo in the prospectus announcing the sale of its stock.[30]

Scarcely had the ink on the Cambridge BioScience prospectus dried when Fischinger began receiving phone calls from other scientists, asking whether Gallo's arrangement with a company whose potential value was enhanced by his research represented a conflict of interest. Incensed that Cambridge BioScience had made its relationship with Gallo public, Fischinger ordered Gallo to sever his ties.

"It was certainly thoughtful of you to set aside for me some of the future potential of Cambridge BioScience," Gallo wrote the company's president, Gerald Buck. "I think that the future of Cambridge BioScience is not linked to me but more broadly to the scientific community. Therefore, it is my decision to return to you . . . all the options for the stock you set aside for me."[k]

Once Gallo's HTLV-specific antibody reached Paris, it hadn't taken long to determine that, as Barré and Montagnier had suspected, the virus growing in Brugière's T-cells wasn't HTLV.[31] To make sure nothing was amiss, Barré tested Brugière's own blood with antibodies designed to react with his virus-infected T-cells. The reaction was positive — no surprise, since Brugière was bound to have antibodies to his own virus. But the positive reaction showed Barré's test was working, and that the negative result for HTLV hadn't been a mistake.[32] "For us," Barré recalled, "it was the first proof that the virus was different."

More sophisticated experiments confirmed the initial results, and other tests added compelling evidence: The virus's genetic material indeed was RNA, and the particles emerging from Brugière's T-cells were the correct size and density for a retrovirus. No matter how Montagnier, Chermann, and Barré looked at their accumulating data, they arrived at the same conclusion. Whether or not it was the cause of AIDS, they had discovered a new human retrovirus.

On the Monday before Easter 1983, Gallo rang Montagnier to inquire about the state of research in Paris. When Montagnier remarked that he was writing a paper for *Nature* reporting the Pasteur's discovery of the third known human retrovirus, Gallo suggested the French submit their manuscript to *Science,* along with those from his lab and Max Essex's. Montagnier quickly agreed, since joining a Gallo-Essex package virtually guaranteed publication for a paper that might not have been accepted by *Nature.* "Gallo said you have to hurry," Montagnier recalled, "so I rushed to write the paper."[33]

Over a frantic weekend, Montagnier and Barré summarized the data generated in their respective labs. In recognition of Barré's initial detections of reverse transcriptase, Montagnier agreed that she should be the paper's first author. As chief of the department where the discovery occurred, Montagnier put his own name last. In between were Jean-Claude Chermann, Françoise Brun, Willy Rozenbaum, and nine other Pasteur researchers and technicians.

The article described Brugière, not identified by name, as a homosexual with "more than fifty partners per year and travels in many countries," including North Africa, Greece, India, and New York City, which he had visited on one occasion four years before. In the interim, Gallo's HTLV probe had finally arrived in Paris. But the experiments with the probe, which verified that Brugière wasn't infected with HTLV, had been done too late to be included in the paper.[1]

Even so, the article contained a surfeit of evidence that the virus afflicting Brugière was something quite different from HTLV. It couldn't be a leukemia virus like HTLV, because it hadn't transformed the Spaniard's uninfected cells into leukemic cells; nor, for that matter, did Brugière have T-cell leukemia. Moreover, Brugière's blood contained antibodies to the core protein of the French virus, but not to the core protein of HTLV — a further, and compelling, indication that the French had discovered a new virus.

The only caveat was an experiment by Jean-Claude Chermann purporting to show that antibodies in Brugière's blood had reacted "strongly" with two HTLV-producing cell lines. Although not wishing to wound Chermann's considerable pride, Montagnier and Barré suspected, correctly as it turned out, that the experiment had been mishandled. The reactive proteins in the cell lines belonged to the cells themselves, rather than the virus.[m]

To Montagnier's eye, the particles in the electron micrograph that accompanied the paper resembled HTLV.[n] When Barré pointed to all the evidence suggesting the French virus *wasn't* HTLV, Montagnier concurred. But there wasn't any reason another kind of retrovirus shouldn't *look* like HTLV, and the description would remain. As for the most important question — whether the new virus caused AIDS — the manuscript noted that the relationship between virus and disease "remains to be determined."[34]

One of Montagnier's technicians had a daughter married to a scientist at the National Cancer Institute who worked in the same building as Gallo. By happenstance, the woman, Jacqueline Gruest, had plans to visit her daughter in Bethesda over Easter weekend. Rather than entrust the manuscript to the mail, Montagnier asked Gruest to deliver it to Gallo in person, along with a sample of DNA extracted from the Brugière virus. Although the normal method of submitting a paper is to send it to the journal in question, Montagnier reasoned that Gallo would have been chosen by *Science* to review the paper anyway. Why not save a few days?

As Gallo scanned the manuscript he noticed the French had neglected to write an abstract, the crucial paragraph at the beginning of scientific articles that summarizes the results and conclusions to follow, the only portion of most articles that goes into computer databases and which many increasingly busy scientists have time to read. To wait while the French composed and mailed an abstract to *Science's* office in Washington would delay by a week or more the publication of what had now become a four-paper package. "Then Gallo called," Montagnier said, "and he said, 'I could write for you the abstract.'"

To his everlasting regret, Montagnier agreed. Gallo's abstract seemed to describe a different paper from the one Montagnier and

Barré had written. Genetically, the French had found nothing in common between HTLV and the Brugière virus. As summarized by Gallo, however, the French manuscript appeared to be reporting, if not the isolation of HTLV itself, then of a very closely related virus. "Gallo called when he was writing this abstract," Barré said, "and on the phone he was reading what he wrote to us. Montagnier asked me to come to his office when Gallo called, to check together. It was very difficult by phone in fact to object. Gallo was speaking very fast. You cannot read, you just hear. I don't think we really objected at that time. It's our fault, because we forgot to write the summary."[35]

Montagnier later expressed his dismay at the abstract's description of the core proteins of HTLV and the French virus as "similar." "I would not ever agree on that," he said, "because we showed no cross-reaction. The core proteins did not cross-react. We had evidence that the virus was different."[36] Nor had Montagnier noticed, until it was too late, that Gallo had also changed the text of the article, describing the French virus as a member of the "Human T-Cell *Leukemia* Virus" family, and the latest in a series of *"previous* HTLV isolates."

"It was *not* a leukemia virus," said Montagnier, who had used the term Human T-Cell *Lymphotropic* Virus, meaning a virus attracted to lymphocytes. "We called it lymphotropic *deliberately,*" Montagnier said. "He thought my paper would support his own paper on HTLV, because he thought my virus was HTLV. Gallo didn't believe there could be more than one kind of human retrovirus. He was fully convinced that HTLV was the right one, that there was only one human retrovirus involved in AIDS. I believed myself this was wrong, but I could not really say this is wrong to Gallo. Because I have too little evidence at that time."[37]

An impartial peer reviewer might have noticed that the virus described by the French had a number of important differences from HTLV. But the reviewers for the Pasteur paper were Gallo and two of his assistants, and when Gallo sent the manuscript to *Science* he gave it his enthusiastic endorsement.

"This paper is of obvious immediate great importance and relevance," Gallo wrote Ruth Kulstad. "It will be of *very* great interest to virtually all scientists and clinicians. The work is careful. The discussion is clear and well thought out. It should be published as rapidly as possible." His changes to the text, Gallo assured Kulstad, were "mainly stylistic and grammatical," and Montagnier "agrees with all."[o]

Science published Essex-Gallo-Pasteur papers in an extraordinarily short time, twenty-four days from submission to publication.[38] When they appeared, in May 1983, the National Cancer Institute trumpeted the discovery by "scientists from the National Cancer Institute and Harvard University" that some AIDS patients were infected with HTLV, "a virus associated with an unusual form of adult leukemia and lymphoma." In what seemed an afterthought, the NCI noted that "a fourth paper, from the Pasteur Institute in Paris," reported an isolation of the same virus "in a homosexual patient with a series of infections and persistent lymph node enlargement, who may be at risk of developing AIDS."[39]

The significance of Max Essex's report, that between a quarter and a third of the AIDS patients he tested had antibodies to HTLV-MA, wasn't lost on the stock market. A few weeks before the *Science* articles were published, Cambridge BioScience had gone public at $7.25 a share. The day Essex's paper appeared, the stock passed $11 on its way to $16. By sundown, Essex was nearly $2 million richer than when he awakened that morning. Had Gallo retained his stock options, they would have been worth more than $100,000.

Ignoring Vince DeVita's caution that HTLV might be a "passenger" virus that had nothing to do with AIDS, the newspapers and networks followed the NCI's lead. "Detection of cancer virus is called a strong clue to the cause of AIDS," proclaimed the *Washington Post*, which mentioned the Pasteur Institute, incorrectly, as one of the laboratories where "signs of human T-cell leukemia viruses" had been detected in AIDS patients.[40] *Newsweek* reported, also incorrectly, that "three separate laboratories," including one in Paris, had found "elevated levels of antibodies to HTLV in a third of the blood samples from AIDS victims."[P] Even *Nature* mischaracterized the work by Pasteur as confirming "that HTLV is indeed somehow linked with AIDS."[41]

By the spring of 1983 1,200 Americans had been diagnosed with AIDS, and physicians in San Francisco, New York, and Los Angeles were seeing more AIDS patients each week. For nearly two years they had been desperate for some clue about the cause of the disease they were confronting, and how it might be treated. Now they were being told AIDS might be caused by a leukemia virus. According to the *Philadelphia Inquirer,* "dozens of laboratories here and abroad" were already working to take advantage of "this possible breakthrough in understanding the disease."[42]

Within days, other researchers were volunteering to help Gallo confirm HTLV as the cause of AIDS — and, in the bargain, to play a role in what looked like a historic discovery. From Montreal and Brussels, from London and Tel Aviv, researchers implored Gallo to send them HTLV antibodies and DNA probes so they, too, might search for his virus in their AIDS patients.[43]

If the idea that a leukemia virus might be responsible for a fatal immune deficiency didn't make immediate sense, most of those who read the *Science* articles put their confusion down to lapses in their own knowledge. "I didn't consider myself capable of questioning Max Essex," one researcher recalled. "Max Essex was a person at Harvard. That meant that Max Essex would probably be right. The likelihood that he needed me to re-evaluate his data was zero."

For the scientists who did have questions, Gallo and Essex had answers. Asked why, if HTLV was the cause of AIDS, he had found antibodies to HTLV-MA in fewer than half the AIDS patients he tested, Essex replied that his test probably wasn't yet sensitive enough. To those who wondered why Gallo had been able to detect HTLV in only four AIDS patients out of nearly three dozen, Gallo suggested that the virus was difficult to find when the number of remaining T-cells was small. As for how a virus that transformed T-cells into wildly proliferating leukemic T-cells could also kill those same T-cells, Gallo proposed that a "subtle change" in the genetic structure of HTLV might account for the difference.[44]

Of all the anomalies in Gallo's HTLV hypothesis, the most perplexing was the virtual absence of AIDS in Japan, where there were far more people infected with HTLV than anywhere on the planet. If HTLV caused AIDS, Gallo was asked, shouldn't that disease have been seen in Kyushu long before it was recognized in Africa, Haiti, or the United States? Gallo replied that maybe AIDS simply hadn't yet been noticed in Japan, or that perhaps the Japanese responded differently to HTLV than Africans or Americans. Or maybe the Japanese were more resistant to the immune-suppressing effects of HTLV.

A few days after the *Science* articles appeared, Gallo wrote Yohei Ito to ask whether AIDS had been seen in Kyoto. "Despite my apparent successes," he added, "I don't feel very happy." He was feeling "unusually severe" pressure, Gallo said, after accepting Vince DeVita's offer to head the cancer institute's new task force on AIDS.[q] On top of that, "I still get terribly stressed and distressed by Hinuma. He has teamed with a sick, paranoid man, A. Karpas in England, and Karpas in particular is doing many bad things like sending out insane letters to all journal editors that I took [HTLV] away from Hinuma!"[45]

Gallo wasn't alone in his distress. Though a publication in *Science* wasn't an everyday event for French researchers, the paper from Montagnier, Barré, and Chermann hadn't been received well at the Pasteur — partly because of Montagnier's outsider status, partly because some of his colleagues feared that "working on a homosexual disease" might threaten the substantial private donations on which the institute depended.[46]

The paper fared no better in America. As Montagnier read the news from the States, he recognized that the work at the Pasteur was being viewed not as an important and original discovery, as Montagnier had expected, but merely as a confirmation of Gallo and Essex. Recognizing the urgent need to get across the message that the Brugière virus was *not* HTLV, Montagnier, Barré, and Chermann resolved to present their data at any scientific conference that would have them.

First up was Barré, who flew to New York at the end of May for a major tumor virus meeting at Cold Spring Harbor. The topic of the meeting was animal cancer viruses, and the program's cover sported sketches of prominent scientists depicted as the animals in whose viruses they specialized: Harold Varmus and Mike Bishop as chickens, David Baltimore and George Todaro as mice, and so on. The French virus wasn't a cancer virus, but it was still a retrovirus, and Barré hoped she might be allowed a few minutes to speak. Barré's request arrived too late for her name to be added to the program, but the session chairman, an NIH lab chief named Malcolm Martin, allotted her five minutes anyway.

In her heavily accented English, Barré struggled to recap the data in the Pasteur's *Science* article, emphasizing the ways in which the virus the French now called *Bru* was different from HTLV.[47] One member of the audience, sitting behind Gallo and Essex, recalled the two men "talking very loudly to one another, and pretending to ignore what was happening on the podium." But as he listened to Barré, the scientist remembered thinking, "Gee, maybe they've got it."[48] Also impressed were Mal Martin, who invited Barré to present a seminar in his lab, and Ci Cabradilla, who asked whether she had time to stop at the CDC in Atlanta on the way back to Paris.

Less impressed was Gallo, who told Barré over dinner that if the French virus wasn't HTLV, the Pasteur ought to move on to other things. "He was completely convinced," Barré recalled, "that the AIDS virus was an HTLV leukemia-like virus. It was not even possible to engage him in a conversation about any other possibility."[49]

Arriving at the CDC in Atlanta, Barré had some fresh news from Paris. In her absence, Montagnier had isolated a *Bru*-like retrovirus from a second patient, a teenage hemophiliac named Eric Loiseau. Like most hemophiliacs, Loiseau received regular infusions of clotting factors, and whatever was causing AIDS was transmitted via the blood as well as through sex. Most important, antibodies to the *Loi* virus, like antibodies to *Bru*, had been detected in a number of AIDS patients.[50]

The experiment that would forge the irrevocable link between virus and disease — inoculating a healthy individual and waiting to see whether he or she got AIDS — was impossible on ethical grounds. Such an experiment, however, could be attempted in animals, and Barré offered to send the CDC's Don Francis enough virus to infect a few rhesus monkeys. Francis, who taken his doctorate in Max Essex's lab and was leaning toward the Essex view of HTLV as the probable cause of AIDS, agreed to try the monkey experiment anyway. In return, Francis promised Barré a few AIDS patient blood samples from the CDC's growing collection.[51]

Following a final presentation at Sloan-Kettering in New York, Barré headed for Paris, where Montagnier had isolated a third virus from the lymph node of a French student named Christophe Lailler.[52] When Barré returned to the lab she was astonished by the virulence of the *Lai* virus. It had taken only five days for the level of reverse transcriptase in the *Lai* culture to reach 43,000 counts per minute, twice that achieved by the *Bru* virus after twenty-five days.[53]

The *"Bru* room," as Barré and Chermann had begun calling their tiny retrovirus lab, was becoming dangerously crowded, with flasks of virus-infected T-cells from Brugière, Loiseau, and Lailler kept in the same incubator and cultured under a single "hood," a metal chimney designed to waft airborne virus particles away from the laboratory workbench. But there was no place else to work, and Barré lived with the constant worry that a virus from one of her cultures might contaminate the others.

Next to travel was Montagnier, who upon Barré's return headed for Frankfurt and the first European roundtable conference on AIDS. In addition to describing the Pasteur's three virus isolations, Montagnier reported that antibodies to *Bru* had been found in blood from six of nine AIDS patients — evidence that the virus was common, if not ubiquitous, among people with AIDS.

Then Montagnier dropped a bomb. David Klatzmann, Montagnier said, had discovered that *Bru* preferentially infected a special subset of T-cells, known as T-4 cells, that control the immune system's response to infection — further evidence that the French virus played a key role in a disease characterized by multiple "opportunistic" infections like Pneumocystis carinii.[54]

Klatzmann's discovery was especially impressive in that it marked his first foray into laboratory science. The Pasteur Institute had plenty of immunologists, but they weren't interested in putting aside their ongoing research to work on AIDS. Klatzmann, having no other research to put aside, had told Montagnier that, rather than studying the virus, he wanted to focus on the T-cells that were being infected by the virus. "He said, 'Fine,'" Klatzmann recalled, "even though at that time I had very little knowledge about viruses." There wasn't room for Klatzmann in Montagnier's lab so he moved in with Chermann, whom Klatzmann found not very helpful. "I never got a single idea or one valuable comment from discussing anything with Chermann," Klatzmann said later.

JAMA, as the *Journal of the American Medical Association* now prefers to be known, is not as highly regarded as its principal competitors, the *New England Journal of Medicine* and *The Lancet*. A kind of "Doctor's Home Companion," *JAMA* regularly publishes poetry and photography from its readers, and among its most popular features is a weekly tally of physicians who have passed away. But *JAMA* tries to keep abreast of the medical news, and in June 1983 a *JAMA* reporter sought Gallo out to ask why he was looking for HTLV in patients with AIDS.[55]

A number of reasons, Gallo replied. AIDS was a new disease, and HTLV was a newly discovered virus. The feline leukemia virus caused immune suppression in cats; so might HTLV cause immune suppression in humans. HTLV was endemic in the Caribbean and there appeared to be a fair amount of AIDS in Haiti.[r] HTLV was transmitted sexually and through blood. So was whatever caused AIDS.

Last but not least, HTLV wasn't a ubiquitous virus, "very uncommon in our environment. So its detection in patients with a particular disease is certainly suggestive." In Gallo's view, a key piece of evidence was "the finding of HTLV or a virus similar to HTLV by the Pasteur group."

What Gallo didn't say was that, before the *Science* papers were published, his lab had compared the *Bru* virus DNA delivered by Jacqueline Gruest with DNA from HTLV — and discovered the French were right: Genetically, *Bru* had nothing in common with HTLV.[s] Even Gallo's own staff had begun to doubt they were chasing the right virus.[t] Whatever Gallo was saying in public, in private he agreed with his staff. "The evidence for an HTLV or a related retrovirus role in AIDS," Gallo confided to a Swedish virologist, George Klein, "is far less than the T-cell leukemias where I think we have virtually established a causative role."[56]

With Montagnier back in France, it was Jean-Claude Chermann's turn to convince the scientific world that the French virus wasn't HTLV. But despite the pleasures of Italy in the spring, Chermann wasn't looking forward to the conference in Naples. "In every meeting where we talk about *Bru*," Chermann complained, "there has been a big fight. Because the Americans are saying that our virus is not true."

Naples was no exception, but at least one American at the meeting didn't think the French had found the wrong virus. "I was sitting in about the tenth row, on the right-hand side of the auditorium," recalled UCLA's Mike Gottlieb. "It was a very sparsely attended meeting. Chermann was at the lectern, and David Klatzmann as well. They presented this data on reverse transcriptase activity associated with a retrovirus isolated from a lymph node.

"And I was — the words that come to mind are amazed, astonished," Gottlieb said. "I was sitting there hearing something that clicked, saying 'These guys have found something important. These guys are on the right track.' These guys were on the trail of a human retrovirus that destroyed the cells it initially lived in."[57] Over breakfast the next morning, Gottlieb mentioned that he was helping to organize the first general-session AIDS conference in the United States, to be held at a Utah ski resort the following February. Would Chermann be willing to come to Utah to speak about *Bru*?

At the end of June 1983 Gallo dropped Montagnier a note. "I believe in fairly short order it would be reasonable to make available your cell lines if they are established and producing virus," Gallo wrote. If nothing else, Gallo said, sending the French virus to Bethesda would show Montagnier's "good faith to members of my laboratory. . . . Both your laboratory and ours have shown the interest, have put our necks out first, and have shown that we can work together."[58]

The Fourth of July found Gallo in Cambridge, delivering a special lecture to the *illuminati* of the Molecular Biology Laboratory on the historic discovery of the first human retrovirus. Following what Abraham Karpas thought an unnecessarily effusive introduction by Robin Weiss, Gallo spoke for more than an hour about HTLV. When at last he called for questions, Karpas was the first to rise. Waving one of Poiesz and Ruscetti's articles in the air, Karpas demanded to know why Gallo hadn't searched for genetic evidence of HTLV in fresh leukemic T-cells from Charlie Robinson.

Struggling to remain calm, Gallo explained that Poiesz and Ruscetti hadn't been able to purify enough HTLV DNA to perform that particular experiment. Karpas retorted that, according to the paper he held in his hand, they had had enough DNA to perform a number of less significant experiments. When Karpas persisted in asking why precious DNA had been wasted on comparisons with tissue from Robinson's kidneys, Gallo took a question from someone else — only to find Karpas lying in wait as he emerged from the lecture hall. "He walked over to me," Karpas recalled, "and he indicated in no uncertain terms that I should see a psychiatrist. I haven't seen one yet."[59]

• 3 •

"We Were Wrong, and Barré-Sinoussi Was Right"

By the summer of 1983 Frédéric Brugière still didn't have full-fledged AIDS. But Brugière's lymph glands were still swollen, and Luc Montagnier suggested renaming the *Bru* virus LAV, for lymphadenopathy-associated virus. The viruses from Christophe Lailler and Eric Loiseau, both of whom did have AIDS, were christened IDAV, for immune deficiency associated virus. Montagnier had no doubt that LAV and IDAV were the same kind of virus, although the unusual virulence of the Lailler virus left open a question about whether it possessed some important genetic difference from the other two.[1]

Montagnier, Françoise Barré, and Jean-Claude Chermann were virologists, and their approach to demonstrating that LAV/IDAV caused AIDS had been to isolate the virus from as many different groups of AIDS patients as possible. Their evidence was encouraging, but an airtight case for the cause of AIDS still hadn't been made. Virus isolations took time — growing up T-cells in primary culture, transmitting whatever the cells contained to fresh, uninfected T-cells, then waiting to see what *those* cells produced — and they weren't always successful. The French had found the virus in four AIDS patients, but there were several others from whom they had failed to isolate any virus at all. That might mean the level of circulating virus in those patients was too low. Or it might mean something else was killing them.

Diagnostic blood testing in France for herpes and hepatitis viruses had been established by Françoise Brun, and for more than a year

(65)

Brun had been storing blood from AIDS patients in her lab at Claude Bernard Hospital. To Brun, testing those samples for antibodies to LAV seemed an easier way to forge the link between the virus and the disease. With Christine Rouzioux, a graduate student from the University of Paris she recruited as an assistant, Brun approached Montagnier with a proposal. "We said to Montagnier, 'We know how to do an ELISA,'" Rouzioux recalled.

The ELISA, short for enzyme-linked immunosorbent assay, is a relatively simple test, employing a tiny shard of virus as a lure for blood-borne antibodies specific to that virus. When virus and antibody form a cohesive unit, called an antigen-antibody complex, an enzyme added to the ELISA changes color, visual evidence that the donor of the blood either is, or once was, infected with that virus.

Marjorie Guroff had used the ELISA to test the blood samples from Japan, and Christine Rouzioux thought it "a very nice and a very easy approach to look for antibodies. With the ELISA, you can show that the virus is not in healthy patients, but only in those who are sick." Not entirely convinced, Montagnier nevertheless asked Brun's superiors at Claude Bernard to lend her to the Pasteur. "Why they agreed, I don't know," Brun said later. "I think the main reason was that nobody was very interested at this time in LAV."

At the beginning of July 1983 Brun moved her base of operations to Chermann's lab. Before experimenting with LAV, she used the ELISA to test serum from AIDS patients from Europe, Haiti, and Africa for antibodies to HTLV.[2] When fewer than fifteen percent were positive, Brun's superiors, who had been reading Robert Gallo's declarations about HTLV in the scientific journals and the newspapers, thought something must be the matter with her test.[3] "The people in France did not believe us," Rouzioux said. "We received samples from physicians and they wrote, 'We want to have serology for HTLV.' We said, 'That's not the right virus.'"

There was an upside to being ignored. "They did not believe us, so they did not disturb us," Rouzioux said. "It was quiet, very easy to work." Convinced that HTLV had nothing to do with AIDS, Brun and Rouzioux moved on to LAV, calibrating their ELISA by first testing Frédéric Brugière's blood for antibodies to his own virus.[4] The second blood sample was from Rouzioux herself, to see whether the ELISA could tell the difference between someone who was infected with LAV and someone who wasn't. To her relief, Rouzioux was negative.

The blood testing began in earnest on July 14, 1983, Bastille Day, the most important holiday in France. Ignoring the festivities outside, Brun and Rouzioux spent the morning coating plastic plates with microscopic quantities of inactivated LAV. Rouzioux, three months pregnant at the time, remembered Chermann fussing about the way she was handling the virus. "He was telling us, 'Change your clothes, change your shoes,'" Rouzioux said. "We told him, 'Don't worry, Jean-Claude, it's OK.'"

The pair tested blood from five AIDS patients that day, including an Englishman who had lived for several years in Angola.[5] All five carried antibodies to LAV. In the days that followed, Brun and Rouzioux continued to adjust the ELISA, altering the concentration of virus and the incubation time to achieve the optimum binding of virus and antibody. "We worked very hard," Brun said, "Saturday and Sunday and in the night. You have a lot of things to standardize, because if you play with the ELISA you can have a lot of very different results."

By the end of August the ELISA was finding LAV antibodies in more than 60 percent of patients with enlarged lymph nodes and other symptoms of pre-AIDS.[6] What puzzled Brun and Rouzioux was the presence of antibodies in only 20 percent of those patients with full-fledged AIDS. Was it possible that LAV caused lymphadenopathy but not AIDS? That seemed unlikely, since nearly everyone who got AIDS got lymphadenopathy first. A better explanation might be that AIDS patients lost antibodies to the virus as their immune systems deteriorated. Or perhaps the ELISA was less precise than it needed to be.

Still, it wasn't likely to be a coincidence that substantial numbers of AIDS and pre-AIDS patients — but hardly any healthy individuals — had antibodies to a virus that infected T-4 cells. In the summer of 1983, such a finding by an American laboratory would have been submitted to the *New England Journal of Medicine;* already Max Essex had made headlines by reporting half that number of AIDS patients with antibodies to HTLV-MA. But Brun and Rouzioux continued to test. "Nobody was saying to stop and write a paper," Brun said. "I was excited by the results, but I was completely inside the work. I did not think to publish. We were thinking about making a test."

The invitation list for the premiere meeting of the National Cancer Institute's AIDS Task Force included three dozen researchers, among them Max Essex and Bill Haseltine from Harvard, Wade Parks from the University of Miami, and a Duke University virologist, Dani Bolognesi, whom many of Gallo's colleagues considered his closest friend — "like brothers," recalled one of Gallo's technicians.

In hopes of improving relations with the CDC, Gallo had added Don Francis and Francis's boss, Jim Curran, to the list. Also invited was Montagnier, to whom Gallo had again complained a few days before about still not having received a sample of the French virus.[7] On the plane to Washington, Montagnier carried three tiny plastic tubes packed in dry ice — one filled with Frédéric Brugière's blood, another containing thirty-nine micrograms of LAV DNA, and a third that held ten milliliters of LAV-infected culture fluid.[8]

In what would prove a prescient move, before Montagnier left Paris, the Pasteur's patent coordinator, Danielle Bernemann, deposited a dated, certified reference sample of LAV in the freezers of the French National Collection of Micro-organisms, a kind of national germ-bank.[9] As a further safeguard, the Pasteur lawyers had drawn up an agreement, to be signed by Gallo, specifying that the NIH could use LAV for basic scientific research as long as no commercial purpose was involved. The sole exception was the cloning, or copying, of the viral genes, which would have to be done by Pasteur scientists in Bethesda "under the direction of Dr. Montagnier."[10]

As Montagnier's plane approached Washington's Dulles Airport on the afternoon of Sunday, July 17, his immediate problem was what to do with the package. The task force meeting wasn't until the next day, and after a night in the Bethesda Holiday Inn the virus would thaw and die. Montagnier telephoned Gallo, who suggested Montagnier jump in a taxi and deliver the box to his house.[11] When Montagnier pulled up, Gallo was in the midst of a backyard volleyball game. "Was I so excited to get the thing?" Gallo asked later. "No, I really wasn't. I put it in my freezer and I went out and played volleyball."[12]

Gallo began the next day's meeting by reciting the now familiar litany of reasons that HTLV made a "very attractive" candidate for the cause of AIDS.[13] Montagnier had heard the same spiel a month earlier, during a conversation with Gallo in Guy de Thé's fifteenth-century apartment on the Île Saint-Louis in Paris, where Montagnier recalled presenting "one argument after another" in favor of LAV and against HTLV. Gallo, Montagnier said later, "would have none of them," insisting, as he had with Françoise Barré, "that LAV was a variant of HTLV."

Gallo's arguments were bolstered by Wade Parks, a former Todaro postdoc, who reported that a third of the Haitian refugees flowing into South Florida, including all Haitian women who had given birth to children with AIDS, had antibodies to HTLV. But not everyone at the meeting was in the HTLV boat. A researcher from George Washington University thought AIDS might be caused by a defective thymus. Sloan-Kettering was looking at an adenovirus isolated from the urine of several AIDS patients. An NCI scientist, Gene Shearer, reminded everyone that sperm and semen could be immune-suppressing. The Food and Drug Administration thought AIDS might be due to a herpesvirus infection.[14]

When Montagnier's turn came to talk, he described the virus isolations from Brugière, Loiseau, and Lailler. In every instance, he said, what had emerged was a human retrovirus genetically distinct from HTLV, and Montagnier had brought a set of electron micrographs that were clearer than the ones published in *Science*. To Matthew Gonda, the chief of the electron microscope lab at the NCI's satellite campus in Frederick, Maryland, the particles they showed appeared to have a bar-like core quite different from the dinner-plate-shaped core of HTLV.

Gonda thought the French virus most resembled a horse virus, the Equine Infectious Anemia Virus, discovered around the beginning of the last century. EIAV, which causes an autoimmune disease in horses, belongs to a special class of slow-acting retroviruses, called lentiviruses, that infect larger animals like cows, goats, and sheep and that can take several years to cause disease.[15]

A few decades before, one lentivirus, the visna virus, had nearly destroyed the sheep population of Iceland. But lentiviruses didn't cause cancer, and they were something most NCI researchers knew little about. Matt Gonda was one of the few who had published on animal lentiviruses; when Gonda said he thought LAV looked like a lentivirus, the CDC's Jim Curran wrote the word on his notepad and drew a circle around it.[16]

Montagnier recalled having the same insight a month before, following a luncheon conversation with a Pasteur virologist, Ewald Edlinger.[a] The excited Montagnier had gone so far as to obtain a sample of EIAV from the veterinary school at Maisons-Alfort, as well as serum from EIAV-infected horses, which to his surprise contained antibodies that cross-reacted with the core protein of LAV — more evidence that LAV was a lentivirus, unrelated to HTLV.

The task force meeting marked the first time since the Mt. Sinai conference that so many researchers and clinicians had gathered in one place to discuss the current state of knowledge about AIDS, but the official accounts of the meeting did nothing to cast doubt on the link to HTLV.[17] Marjorie Guroff's presentation showing HTLV antibodies in fewer than 10 percent of AIDS patients wasn't mentioned in the Public Health Service's report of the meeting.[18]

Neither was Matt Gonda's suggestion that LAV belonged to an entirely different class of retroviruses than HTLV. The NCI's account referred only to "a single isolate by the French group from an AIDS patient," which the NCI described — over Montagnier's objections — as "HTLV type 3."[b] Under the circumstances, a Franco-American collaboration hardly seemed auspicious. "Overcome with exasperation," Montagnier returned to Paris with the unsigned agreement in his pocket.[19]

One of the few in Bethesda who wasn't discounting the Pasteur's research was Mikulas Popovic, the Czech virologist who had arrived in Gallo's lab on a fellowship the year before. Popovic's title was Visiting Associate, the lowest rung on the NIH ladder, but he was no junior researcher. After a stint as a doctor in the Czechoslovakian air force, Popovic had trained under the famed virologist Jan Svoboda and later headed a ten-person virus laboratory at the Slovak Academy of Science in Bratislava.

Popovic's first paper from America, the comparison of HTLV and ATLV, had appeared in *Nature*,[20] a nice change from years of publishing in obscure Eastern Bloc journals. Popovic had decided to stay in America, telling the U.S. Immigration and Naturalization Service he was afraid to return home because his brother, a Czech government official, had defected to Switzerland. Other high-profile articles followed, including Popovic's transmission of $HTLV_{CR}$ to uninfected cells — a demonstration, three years after Isao Miyoshi had done the same with ATLV, that HTLV was indeed a virus.[21]

Satisfied that Popovic had learned how to work with HTLV, Gallo assigned him to search for that virus in AIDS patients. Popovic and his technician, Ersell Richardson, had been deluged with blood and tissue samples, but except for isolating HTLV from Claude Chardon and E.P., they hadn't had any luck. During the spring and summer of 1983, Richardson's logbook recorded one failure after another: "Cells died." "Cells could not be grown for testing." "Cells died; not tested;

no growth." Only the cells from Chardon had continued to grow, eventually producing enough virus to photograph.[22] But by the time of the task force meeting, the last Chardon culture was dead as well — a strange dénouement for HTLV-1, which was supposed to make T-cells immortal.[23]

Zaki Salahuddin had pleaded with Gallo for a chance to work on AIDS, to no avail. "Bob would always say, 'No, Mika's going to do it,'" Salahuddin recalled. Salahuddin had grown to detest Popovic, and he thought the feeling was mutual. "He would come into my lab and curse my mother," Salahuddin said. "If I didn't have the balance of nature within me, I would have killed him. But as time passed and Mika got no results, Bob got worried."

In May, Gallo abruptly told Salahuddin to go ahead. But Salahuddin, like Popovic, was following the protocol for isolating HTLV, and he was getting the same results: occasional borderline levels of reverse transcriptase with no trace of virus, followed by a flask of dead cells.[24] Still, Salahuddin had seen something interesting. In a few instances when he mixed fluid from his sputtering cultures with uninfected T-cells, the new cultures would produce reverse transcriptase. Then *those* cells would die. The only explanation was that a retrovirus had been passed from the first culture to the second. But if there was a virus in any of his cultures, Salahuddin couldn't get it out.

In the hands of a talented virologist like Zaki Salahuddin, so many dead T-cell cultures wouldn't be expected if the cells harbored a leukemia-causing virus. Popovic was becoming troubled by what he later called Gallo's HTLV "mindset,"[25] and he had more respect for European science than did some of his American colleagues. As he listened at the task force meeting to Montagnier's description of how LAV behaved in the laboratory, Popovic thought the French virus sounded like a better candidate for the cause of AIDS.

Waiting on Montagnier's desk when he returned from Bethesda was the finished manuscript marshaling David Klatzmann's evidence that LAV infected T-4 cells and killed them.[26] "Very important," Montagnier said later, "one of the critical proofs that the virus was the cause of AIDS." The Pasteur had gotten its first paper into *Science* because it carried Gallo's imprimatur, but Montagnier understood that Gallo, to whom such a paper would surely be sent for review, could close the pipeline to *Science* as well as open it. Instead, Montagnier decided to submit Klatzmann's manuscript to *Nature,* which was more receptive to research from Europe and which hadn't yet published a major paper on AIDS.

The Times of London has called *Nature* the bible of the church of science, and its cantankerous editor, John Royden Maddox, the high priest.[27] With a better haircut and a three-piece suit, Maddox might have been mistaken for an English public school headmaster or a retired British Army colonel. But Maddox's taste ran to faded khakis and madras shirts, his passions to old Jaguars and older Bordeaux, and his eccentricities were legendary. Scientists often joked that because Maddox, who had been trained as a chemist, determined what appeared in *Nature* and what did not, he was the most important scientist in the world. To which Maddox replied in all earnestness, "Well, I am."[28]

Maddox also had a taste for glitz, and it was said that while articles published in *Science* were more likely to be right, those in *Nature* were more likely to be interesting. Of the two hundred lengthy research manuscripts that arrived each week at *Nature's* threadbare offices in London's Little Essex Street, only two or three were printed, which made "a *Nature* paper" worth ten or even twenty in nearly any other journal. Montagnier knew he was taking a chance, but he also knew that publishing Klatzmann's paper in *Nature* would do more than bring an urgent piece of information to the attention of other AIDS researchers. It would amount to John Maddox's ratification of the Pasteur's discovery of LAV.

As a CDC field officer, Don Francis had worked in Africa and India as part of the World Health Organization's program, eventually successful, to eradicate smallpox from the planet. Upon returning home, Francis had taken a sabbatical to earn a doctorate in Max Essex's lab at Harvard, with a brief time-out for a visit to the Sudan, where he had been dispatched to investigate the first outbreak of Ebola fever.

"When I joined Max's lab," Francis recalled, "it was at the end of this incredible war about there being such a thing as retroviruses that cause disease. Max and Bob were part of the minority fighting against all those at NCI. I think there's a long-term affection there, because they were on the side of a winning battle." When Max Essex proposed that HTLV might be the cause of AIDS, Francis had paid attention. "Those studies of Max's were very enticing," Francis said.

Francis had been conducting trials of a vaccine for hepatitis B in Phoenix when AIDS was first recognized, and he returned to Atlanta to organize the collecting and storing of blood from AIDS patients across the country. Cy Cabradilla had sent sixty of those blood samples to Gallo at the beginning of 1983,[c] but the NCI complained that they hadn't been "the specimens of greatest interest."[29]

Gallo was convinced the CDC was reserving its best blood samples for Max Essex, and he couldn't understand why Jim Curran was warning reporters that the Gallo-Essex research on HTLV shouldn't be "prematurely overinterpreted" as evidence that HTLV caused AIDS.[30] "It is obvious," Gallo wrote Curran, "that neither we nor anyone else claims to have proven that a member of the HTLV family causes AIDS. On the other hand, it is just as clearly the best published lead to date."[31]

Much of the friction between Gallo and the CDC stemmed from the difference between the CDC's mission and that of the National Cancer Institute, where scientists engaged in basic research that often took years to bear fruit. The CDC's job was more urgent: to monitor the public health and respond, often within hours, to outbreaks of infectious disease. With the advent of AIDS, the CDC found itself faced with the most serious threat since polio, and it was in a hurry to find the cause. When Gallo appealed for more blood samples, Cy Cabradilla suggested that Gallo send his HTLV antibodies and DNA probes to Atlanta and let the CDC test its *own* samples for HTLV.[32]

The CDC samples Gallo wanted most were the so-called matched pairs, taken from donors who had previously given pints of blood and hospital patients who received transfusions of that blood and later got AIDS.[33] Those transfusion recipients who had no other risk for AIDS must have been infected by an agent in the blood of their donor. Isolating the same virus from donor and recipient would amount to a virtual guarantee that the virus caused AIDS.

Max Essex had gotten some of the matched pairs, and Gallo demanded that the CDC send the same samples "as rapidly as possible to the laboratory with the best chance of isolating the suspect virus, namely to me." There was, Gallo assured Jim Curran, "no higher priority in AIDS research."[34] When Francis reminded Gallo that he had refused to send his HTLV probes to Atlanta, Gallo replied that what might look like his own lack of collaboration was "more disorganization than running away." But Gallo admitted his concern that, once he began sharing his HTLV probes, the CDC would "go off independently" in search of the AIDS virus. "Keep away from the origin of AIDS independently," Gallo warned Francis. "CDC can do it with my help or I do it alone."[35]

While the National Cancer Institute pressured the CDC to cooperate with Gallo, at the end of July 1983 Francis invited Gallo, Essex, and Jim Mullins, a virologist from Essex's department at Harvard, to talk things out at the CDC's redbrick headquarters on the periphery of Atlanta's Emory University.[36] "There was a big fight," Mullins recalled, "between the CDC and Gallo over who was supposed to be doing research and who was supposed to be gathering data for the research. Gallo felt they should be gathering data, and he should be doing the science."

Mullins had been looking for a retrovirus in AIDS patients almost from the day he arrived at Harvard in the summer of 1982. He hadn't found any HTLV. But in a CDC blood sample from a homosexual AIDS patient, Mullins had stumbled across a retrovirus that didn't react with Gallo's HTLV probes. Now, face-to-face with the CDC, Gallo demanded the same sample Mullins had been given. "We retired to a closed meeting with about eight people," Mullins recalled, "and Gallo turned off his smile and started screaming at me for taking his probes and doing these experiments without his permission. He pointed out that I had grants through his good graces from the Leukemia Society. He tried to bring it up as 'Look at what I've done for you, and you turn around and do this to me.'

"He knew very well we were using the probes for AIDS diagnosis. He supported it and he encouraged it. But at this meeting, he chose to lambaste me in front of a congressional appointee and Jim Curran and Max Essex and everybody else — the most important people at that time in the field. In the middle of the meeting, Cy Cabradilla got up and walked out. He said, 'I refuse to submit to this, I quit the CDC.' He relented later, but all I could do through this entire harangue was to say, 'This just isn't true, you're not telling the truth.'"

In the end Gallo got the blood sample, and he hand-carried it to the airport packed in dry ice. "When we were walking to the cars after the meeting," Mullins said, "Bob said to me, 'You're trying to solve the AIDS epidemic by yourself. You can't do it, you won't do it, so don't try.'" When Gallo reached Bethesda, the cells were dead.[37] "There wasn't enough dry ice, and they warmed up," Mullins said. "He accused the CDC of doing that on purpose."[d] But before September was over Gallo had what he wanted from the CDC: matched sets of blood samples from more than a hundred transfusion-AIDS patients and donors.[38]

A few weeks earlier, a manuscript from the University of Nebraska had arrived at the Chicago offices of *JAMA.* The sender, a virologist named David Purtilo, had been testing blood samples from AIDS patients for antibodies to HTLV. Unlike Max Essex, Purtilo was looking for antibodies to an entire virus, not just a protein on the surface of T-4 cells. But in more than a hundred attempts Purtilo's lab hadn't found a single AIDS patient who was positive for HTLV.

Purtilo's curiosity about HTLV had been piqued by one of his postdocs, Shinji Harada, who had trained under Yorio Hinuma and who had been growing ATLV, the Japanese version of HTLV, in Purtilo's Omaha lab. What Max Essex was saying about HTLV and AIDS hadn't made sense to Harada, who began a fruitless search for HTLV in some of the AIDS patients' blood samples Purtilo had assembled for another study. When Purtilo saw the Gallo-Essex papers in *Science,* he thought the time had come to make Harada's data public. But *Science* wasn't interested in publishing anything that undercut its high-visibility articles, and Purtilo hoped *JAMA* would be more receptive.

"The undocumented implication that this virus causes AIDS," Purtilo wrote *JAMA*'s editor, George Lundberg, "has grave consequences to all of the individuals at risk for AIDS."[39] *JAMA* wasn't interested either. But Shinji Harada had stayed in touch with Hinuma, who was now in touch with Abraham Karpas, and Karpas had a plan. Hinuma and Karpas would independently confirm Harada's results, and the combined data from Cambridge, Kyoto, and Omaha would be published in a single article.

When Karpas suggested asking Hinuma's old professor, Werner Henle at the University of Chicago, to sponsor their paper for *PNAS,* Purtilo replied that Henle didn't want his name on a paper that was likely to annoy Gallo, as Henle had previously received "a bombastic telephone call from Dr. Gallo" for having sponsored Hinuma's paper on ATLV. Henle suggested Robert Good, the former head of Sloan-

Kettering, and although Good thought the manuscript worthwhile he didn't want to put his name on it either.[40]

Most of Purtilo's blood samples had been provided by a Manhattan physician, Joseph Sonnabend, whose Greenwich Village practice included a large number of AIDS patients. Sonnabend also edited a small journal called *AIDS Research,* and as a last resort he agreed to publish Purtilo's manuscript there.[41] "It was pretty strong," Sonnabend recalled. "I toned it down somewhat, which I sort of regret now. I even added a sentence at the end, to the effect that maybe the difference between our results and Max Essex's could be attributed to the different geographical origin. But I was just being polite." Not long after the article appeared, the publisher of *AIDS Research* replaced Sonnabend with Dani Bolognesi, who promptly installed Gallo on the journal's editorial board.

By the end of August 1983, Jean-Claude Chermann and Françoise Barré had stockpiled ten liters of LAV-containing fluid, enough for many ELISAs.[42] Montagnier, his skepticism overcome by Brun's initial results, felt the time had come to inform the French government that the Pasteur had developed a rudimentary blood test for the virus that almost certainly caused AIDS.

Already two dozen AIDS cases had been reported in the United States among men and women who had received hospital transfusions, and Montagnier fired off letters to the director general of the National Center for Scientific Research, the director general of INSERM, the French equivalent of the NIH, and the chief of the Ministry of Research, arguing that it was imperative to begin testing French blood donors for LAV.[43]

The French government didn't agree. There were only about a hundred confirmed cases of AIDS in all of France, most of those in homosexuals — in the government's opinion, hardly a public health emergency that warranted wholesale vetting of the national blood supply. Moreover, Gallo, Max Essex, the NCI, and the CDC were all pointing to HTLV as the most likely cause of AIDS. In the government's opinion, testing the blood supply for LAV would be a waste of time and money.

Montagnier got an extra 500,000 francs, then about $50,000, in research funding and "a nice answer" to his letters. "But nothing was done," he said. "We had the test by the summer of 1983. It was for research studies, but it could have been used for blood supplies. Some time, perhaps a few months, could have been gained, if people had believed what we said. Some lives could have been saved. The test was not as sensitive, so we missed more than half of the AIDS patients. But for people who were just healthy carriers"— the people for whom such a test would be most useful — "it was OK. We could detect a very high proportion."[44]

Having rejected Montagnier's offer, the French national transfusion center turned to Gallo for advice about how to test the French blood supply for HTLV.[45] Mika Popovic had failed to isolate HTLV from nearly every AIDS patient whose cells Ersell Richardson had cultured, and Marjorie Guroff had failed to detect HTLV antibodies in all but a tiny fraction of those patients. Yohei Ito had managed to locate only a single Japanese AIDS patient who was infected with HTLV.[46] But rather than discard his HTLV hypothesis, Gallo struggled to salvage it.

As it happened, the HTLV isolated by Popovic from the New York AIDS patient, E.P., was a bit different from the Charlie Robinson prototype, $HTLV_{CR}$. The two were mostly the same, but the DNA for E.P.'s viral envelope contained a slightly different genetic twist.[47] Such a minor difference, Gallo thought, might explain how HTLV could cause both leukemia and AIDS. The original HTLV, which Gallo now dubbed "Type A," was clearly a leukemia virus. Perhaps the E.P. variant, which Gallo named "Type B," caused immune suppression and AIDS.[48]

That would explain Marjorie Guroff's failure to find Type A antibodies in many AIDS patients, and why the Japanese, who were infected with HTLV Type A, didn't have AIDS. But Gallo's theory depended on a high prevalence of HTLV Type B in Central Africa, where there was so much AIDS that many researchers believed the disease had originated there.

Most of the African countries where AIDS was most prevalent were former European colonies, and several European universities still maintained African research stations to study tropical diseases. To his European colleagues, Gallo appealed for more blood from African AIDS patients. The quest for HTLV in Africa, Gallo said, had become the "current focus" of his lab.[49]

Max Essex was still looking for HTLV in American AIDS patients, and in early September 1983 Essex reported that two out of three hemophiliacs with AIDS had antibodies to HTLV-MA — "new evidence," according to the *Philadelphia Inquirer*, "that AIDS may be caused by a rare cancer virus."[50] Even his newest numbers, Essex explained, were probably lower than the actual levels of infection, since the test still might not be sensitive enough.[51]

No one seemed interested in LAV, including the editors of *Nature*. "Your manuscript has now been seen by two referees whose comments are attached," one of John Maddox's assistants informed Montagnier and Klatzmann a week after Essex's latest paper appeared. "In view of their criticisms I am afraid we are unable to offer to publish your manuscript in *Nature* and I am therefore regretfully returning it. I hope you find our referees' comments useful."[52]

"One referee was not very critical," Montagnier recalled, "a few minor points which could have been corrected. The second referee was a little more nasty." On one point, both of the anonymous reviewers agreed: If Klatzmann's findings were true, they would be "of considerable importance." The only problem, according to the second reviewer, was that LAV might not be a human virus. He wouldn't be surprised, the reviewer said, if the Pasteur's "putative human virus" was really one of the mouse viruses with which Barré and Chermann had been working before AIDS, and which had contaminated their cultures.[e]

"Gallo's laboratory," the reviewer reminded Montagnier, "spent almost 2 years carefully characterizing HTLV before they first ventured into print. Had the data been as rudimentary as for the Paris virus, no-one would have taken the findings seriously. The potential importance of an AIDS virus is too great to rush into print with one item papers." To Montagnier, the reviewer didn't seem to be commenting on the manuscript he had submitted to *Nature*. "He is questioning the work previously published in *Science*," Montagnier complained to Maddox, "on the isolation of a new retrovirus, the 'Paris Virus' as he calls it with a touch of contempt. We agree with the referee that this virus is not HTLV."

As for the possibility of a laboratory contamination, Montagnier observed that "we are not that naive to the stage of not having considered it before submitting our work to *Science*. We are tempted to conclude that the referee has not carefully read our *Science* paper, and that he has some difficulties in admitting that a new virus possibly involved in AIDS [could] be discovered in places other than Bethesda or Boston."

For the rejection, Maddox later would blame his deputy, Peter Newmark, whom Maddox described as having been "very much in charge" of *Nature*'s AIDS coverage. "Frankly," Maddox said, "at that time, in 1983, I would have published anything that purported to be an explanation of AIDS. As Peter would be the first to admit, I think he's too cautious and too conservative."

"There's no doubt I'm more cautious than John Maddox," Newmark replied. "So is everyone else at *Nature*. It's easy in retrospect to say you've been too cautious. Faced at the time with decisions that have to be made and with referees' comments, you act in a different way. But I certainly don't remember him saying 'Publish everything we can get our hands on.'"

Dejected, Klatzmann and Montagnier rewrote the paper for submission to *PNAS*. André Lwoff, one of the few French members of the National Academy, agreed to act as communicator. When Lwoff asked Montagnier for the names of two prospective reviewers, Montagnier suggested one French scientist and one American. "In order to be fair," Montagnier said, "I put the American first. The French reviewer immediately answered and said, 'That's fine, it's perfect, you can publish it,'" Klatzmann recalled. "The other reviewer, the American, never, ever reviewed it."

Still feeling the sting of *Nature*'s rejection, Montagnier arrived at Cold Spring Harbor on an unseasonably chilly day in mid-September of 1983 for what must have been the largest scientific meeting ever devoted to a single virus.

The topic was HTLV, and the meeting's organizers, Gallo and Max Essex, had invited more than a hundred researchers, seemingly everyone who had ever worked on HTLV except Frank Ruscetti, Yorio Hinuma, and Abraham Karpas.[53] Gallo, just back from Brussels, would give the opening address,[54] followed by sessions on the molecular structure of HTLV, the effect of HTLV on T-cells, and the epidemiology of HTLV-related diseases. The title of the meeting's final session was "Possible role of HTLV in AIDS."[f]

A contingent of Japanese were present at Cold Spring Harbor, including Isao Miyoshi and Yohei Ito, and in Hinuma's absence they agreed with Gallo that the time was propitious to sign a multilateral accord stipulating "an internationally agreed nomenclature for these human retroviruses and their associated diseases."[55] Henceforth, the virus that caused Adult T-Cell Leukemia would be referred to as *HTLV-1*, or as HTLV "when no other related virus is under discussion."

As other human retroviruses were discovered that were "related to" HTLV-1, they would be numbered in sequence. Since there was already an *HTLV-2*, the next such virus would be called *"HTLV-3"*—perhaps not coincidentally, the term the NCI had already used to describe the Pasteur's new virus.

The Cold Spring Harbor convocation represented a celebration of sorts for the dozens of retrovirologists whose scientific stature had been lifted immeasurably by Bernie Poiesz's discovery of HTLV. Murray Gardner recalled having "stood up at meetings since 1968 as an advocate for the study of retroviruses, defending why I, an M.D., would be working with wild mice, parakeets, cats, monkeys and whatnot. I always had to explain why we could not find these viruses in man, and promise that they were going to be there, even if they were lurking in the deep. I have had to explain to my mother, kids and friends why I was studying things that apparently did not have anything to do with humans."

Thanks to Gallo and Essex, in the space of a few months HTLV had risen from virological obscurity to become the leading candidate for cause of the most visible disease in decades, a candidacy now bolstered by the latest finding from Essex that 70 percent of some groups of AIDS patients had antibodies to HTLV-MA.[56] "A strange and dangerous new cancer virus," observed the *Boston Globe* reporter who covered the Cold Spring Harbor meeting, "has been identified by scientists as the almost-certain cause of the disease called AIDS."[57]

For the French, Cold Spring Harbor represented the best chance so far to convince their American colleagues that the likely cause of AIDS was LAV. "I was the only one at the meeting," Montagnier said later, "who was not talking about HTLV." In accepting Gallo's invitation, Montagnier had asked for more time to speak, explaining that "I find it very hard to report in fifteen minutes all our new data on LAV."[58] Gallo gave Montagnier an extra five minutes, but left him at the end of the program. "I could present some data," Montagnier said later, "but not all, because I had no time."[59]

Montagnier had new and even better pictures of LAV, but by the time he stepped to the microphone many of the conferees had departed. Viruses immunologically identical to LAV, he told the half-empty room, had now been isolated from five patients with AIDS or pre-AIDS — two homosexuals, a hemophiliac, a Haitian, and now an African woman from Zaire[60] — and none of those patients had had antibodies to HTLV. Montagnier once again pointed out the similarities between LAV and the Equine Infectious Anemia Virus — "because it showed again that this virus has nothing to do with HTLV"— and summarized David Klatzmann's discovery that LAV infected T-4 cells. But the highlight of his talk was the first public presentation of the ELISA testing by Françoise Brun and Christine Rouzioux.

LAV antibodies, Montagnier said, had been found in 63 percent of pre-AIDS patients and 20 percent of those with AIDS, but less than 2 percent of the general population — a strong suggestion that the presence of LAV in patients was more than coincidental. Brun's most recent data was even better, 75 percent positives in pre-AIDS patients and 37.5 percent in AIDS patients, but she hadn't given Montagnier an update before he left Paris. "We were happy with the first results," she explained later.

When Montagnier's twenty minutes were up, the session chairman, Don Francis, cut him off and called for questions from the floor.[g] "There were all kinds of nasty questions," Montagnier recalled, mainly those from Gallo. "Because Gallo could not understand a cell-killing retrovirus in man. He was questioning the reality of the reverse transcriptase activity. Was it really a retrovirus? Could it be an animal contaminant? Guy de Thé said, 'Well you are right. You have a new retrovirus, but why do you have to involve that retrovirus in AIDS? AIDS is caused by HTLV.'"

"That was the first time Gallo had ever heard of any of this stuff," one onlooker recalled, "and he insulted Montagnier. It was a disgusting display, absolutely disgusting. He told him it was terrible science, that there was no way it could be true. He ranted and raved for eight or ten minutes. I said to one of the guys in Gallo's lab, 'This is it.' I went up to poor Montagnier afterwards. He was sitting in the corner. He looked like he'd been beaten over the head with a sledgehammer. I said, 'The data looks good, I'm sure you've probably got it, don't take to heart what these guys have said to you.'"[61]

During the proceedings, Gallo slipped Montagnier a scribbled note asking for *more* LAV.[h] "Gallo had two positions," Montagnier recalled. "The public position he took was very aggressive, saying 'Well, you are not sure of anything.' I mentioned in my talk that this data would be applied to testing blood donations. I said, 'the Pasteur Institute is interested, and they will be producing soon a test.' Gallo stood up and said it would be very dangerous for the Pasteur Institute to take that position, that it was premature, there was no evidence that this virus is the cause of AIDS. And privately he was saying, 'I need more material, I want to test my own sera, and so on.'" When Montagnier asked Gallo later why he had launched such a vitriolic attack, Gallo's reply was "You punched me out."[62]

Bernie Poiesz, the discoverer of HTLV, had joined the search for HTLV in AIDS, but Poiesz recalled thinking that Montagnier's presentation on LAV had "seemed pretty reasonable." Like Mika Popovic, Poiesz had found reverse transcriptase in some AIDS patients' T-cells, and he figured that "if anybody could make a T-cell grow with a virus, I could." But Poiesz couldn't. "I kept growing these cultures from these guys," Poiesz said, "getting reverse transcriptase . . . and the cell lines kept dying."

Perhaps because Poiesz had written the HTLV protocol, he was the first to recognize that Gallo's lab had been following the wrong recipe for finding the AIDS virus. "They were doing pretty much what I had set up as a way to find HTLV," Poiesz said. "People were trying to hang in there, growing their cultures a little bit too long. It was Barré who finally said 'This virus kills cells, you can't get it immortal, you just gotta add cells to it.'"

By the time Poiesz heard Montagnier speak, he was wide open to the possibility that LAV was the cause of AIDS. "He obviously didn't have it fully developed," Poiesz said later, "and he certainly didn't have a lot of proof, and he couldn't find antibodies in every patient. But he had gone a substantial way, and it was plausible to me that they had found something that was different."[63]

Robin Weiss was among those who left Cold Spring Harbor early, to catch a plane back to London with *Nature*'s Peter Newmark. Based on the Pasteur's *Science* paper, Weiss had had serious doubts that the French really had found a new human virus — an opinion much like that of the anonymous *Nature* reviewer who had rejected Klatzmann's T-4 cell manuscript. But when Weiss heard about Montagnier's Cold Spring Harbor data, "it made me take that first paper much more seriously."[64]

From Cold Spring Harbor Gallo was off to a virology symposium in Vienna, where he discovered that European scientists who had been following his comments in the medical journals thought he still believed that classical HTLV, the virus Gallo now called Type A, was the most likely cause of AIDS. Upon returning to Bethesda, Gallo appealed to several German researchers for help in dispelling that impression.

"In my opinion," Gallo wrote the Germans at the end of September, "an HTLV *variant* is the *most likely* candidate, and if it isn't this, it is an as yet unknown virus"— meaning something other than LAV. Gallo's lab had isolated HTLV from ten AIDS patients out of forty,[i] but he wasn't sure what those numbers meant. Of one thing, however, Gallo was sure. His laboratory had "never seen the virus that Luc Montagnier has described."[65]

Mika Popovic couldn't say the same. Most of those at Cold Spring Harbor had left the meeting still leaning toward HTLV as the progenitor of AIDS, but Popovic had paid close attention to Montagnier's presentation. "He had excellent data," Popovic said later. "He was most advanced, there is no question about that. He picked out the correct virus, but the conclusion, of course, does not follow that this is the cause of AIDS."[66]

The death of Claude Chardon's HTLV-infected T-cells had reinforced Popovic's own conviction that HTLV, which didn't kill T-cells, couldn't be the virus he was looking for.[j] There had to be something else in Chardon's cells, most likely a second, cell-killing virus. Popovic thought the second virus was probably the one the French called LAV; before leaving for Cold Spring Harbor, Popovic had unthawed the LAV delivered by Montagnier to Gallo's house and cultured it, Pasteur style, with cord blood T-cells.

Upon his return, Popovic sent two flasks of LAV-infected cord blood cells to Prem Sarin, Gallo's deputy lab chief, whose duties included the lab's testing for reverse transcriptase.[k] One of the LAV cultures was positive for RT, but at levels far below those reported by the French.[l] "I couldn't reproduce Barré's data," Popovic said later. "I used the same LAV, the same protocol as they used, [but] they had 22,000, and we got only 741." When Popovic called Montagnier for advice, "he told me to be patient, that the virus will come up after a while."[67]

Suspecting the problem lay in Prem Sarin's RT testing, which Popovic now considered "erroneous to the point of being misleading,"[68] Popovic collected a tiny amount of LAV culture fluid and sent it to Matt Gonda in Frederick.[69] Under Gonda's electron microscope, the particles that emerged were "quite distinct" from HTLV: tiny viruses with a dark, bar-like core of DNA magnified eighty thousand times, surrounded by a translucent envelope — not at all like HTLV, but exactly like the pictures of LAV Montagnier had taken to Bethesda in July.

Gonda had thought in July that LAV looked like a lentivirus. As Gonda examined his electron micrographs, he still thought so.[70] Berge Hampar, the general manager of the NCI's Frederick facility, remembered Peter Fischinger, then the NCI's associate director, storming into his office "and going into a tirade because Gonda had identified LAV as a lentivirus."[71] But Fischinger's outburst was nothing like what Gonda experienced when he took an unexpected phone call from Gallo.

"The guy is calling me from Japan or Germany or wherever it is," Gonda recalled. "He was very upset. So he yelled and screamed and I sat there and listened to the first fifteen minutes of his argument. And I said, 'Now you have to listen to mine.' I said, 'Something looks like a duck, I don't care if its feathers are black and white, it looks like a duck, it's still a duck. I'm not going to call it something different.'"[72]

Gonda had played tennis with Gallo, "and he hits the ball real hard the first time. Then after that, you got him. It's the same way he plays science. He plays rough right up front, and then once you can convince him, his name is on the paper. He had Bill Haseltine telling him, 'We want to reclassify these. We are going to call them type-T viruses.' I said, 'Why do you guys have to change the world? I mean, they got a name for these things.'"[73]

On the sixth day of October 1983, Mika Popovic lined up cells from Frédéric Brugière and nine other AIDS and pre-AIDS patients, including a half-dozen patients known to be infected with HTLV-1. The cells were tested in turn, first with antibodies to HTLV, then with Brugière serum containing antibodies to LAV. That Brugière's own LAV-infected cells reacted with LAV antibodies in his blood was no surprise. Nor was it surprising when the HTLV-1-infected AIDS patients were positive for HTLV-1 antibodies. When three of the HTLV-1 patients tested positive for LAV, the bulb over Popovic's head glowed brightly: None of the AIDS patients were infected *only* with HTLV-1, but *all of them* were infected with LAV.[m]

For more than a year Gallo had been chasing down the wrong road, dragging Popovic, Ed Gelmann, Marjorie Guroff, Doug Blayney, Zaki Salahuddin, and much of the retrovirological community behind him. A half-dozen AIDS patients, among them the Haitian woman M.A. and Claude Chardon, had indeed been infected with HTLV-1. Now Popovic understood that those infections were coincidental: both M. A. and Chardon must also have been *infected with LAV*. At that moment, Popovic said later, "I came to the conclusion that we were wrong, and Barré-Sinoussi was right."[74]

It was a classic case of confounding. Gallo had been sent blood and tissue samples from AIDS patients who tested positive for HTLV-1 because he, and by extension his collaborators, thought HTLV-1 might cause AIDS. Gallo's people had isolated HTLV from a few of those AIDS patients, because they knew *how* to isolate HTLV. They detected it in others because they had the monoclonal antibodies and DNA probes they needed to look for HTLV.

They hadn't isolated or detected LAV because they had no LAV reagents, and because the protocol for isolating HTLV didn't work for LAV. But LAV had been there all along, in uncounted billions of T-cells stored in Gallo's freezers. Too late Popovic realized "that we probably had this type of retroviruses in the lab for one and a half years."[75]

The day after Popovic's Eureka! experiment, the National Cancer Institute nominated Gallo for the prestigious General Motors Cancer Research Award, in prestige right behind the Lasker and the Nobel itself. In explaining why Gallo deserved the $100,000 GM prize, the NCI cited his research implicating HTLV as the possible cause of AIDS.[76]

Hours before Montagnier spoke at Cold Spring Harbor, the Pasteur's lawyers applied for a European patent on Françoise Brun's LAV ELISA. What made the French ELISA patentable wasn't the technique it used, which already had been patented by the Dutch company Organon. What made it unique, and therefore patentable, was the virus it employed.

Three years before, the United States Supreme Court had ruled for the first time that the patent laws applied to the products of genetic engineering and molecular biology. At issue in that case was a petroleum-ingesting microbe that might be useful in cleaning up oil spills. The General Electric scientist who developed the microbe initially had been denied a patent on the grounds that nature's handiwork couldn't be patented, but the Supreme Court had sided with the scientist.[77]

Until then, the prevailing wisdom had been that nature was unpatentable. When Edward R. Murrow had asked Jonas Salk who owned his polio vaccine, Salk replied, "Well, the people, I would say. There is no patent. Could you patent the sun?"[78] It still wasn't possible to patent the sun, or anything else simply found in nature — a rock, a tree, even a virus. The inventor of the oil-eating microbe was entitled to a patent because he had *improved* on nature, by altering the DNA of an existing bacterial strain to make it more useful than nature had. Like any other inventor, said the Court, the scientist should be entitled to reap the rewards of his "human ingenuity and research."

LAV, being a product of nature, couldn't be patented either. But Brun and Rouzioux had been first to use the ELISA technique to search for antibodies to LAV. A LAV-based ELISA therefore represented a novel invention, and when Danielle Bernemann learned Montagnier was going to include the ELISA results in his Cold Spring Harbor talk, she scurried to assemble a patent application. Under the patent laws of most countries, but not the United States, an application must be on file before the existence of an invention is publicly disclosed. Without such an application on record, the moment Montagnier began to speak at Cold Spring Harbor the Pasteur would have been barred from patenting the ELISA in France and nearly everywhere else in the world.

Alongside the LAV sample from Frédéric Brugière, Bernemann now deposited the viruses from Loiseau and Lailler in the National Collection of Micro-organisms. The language in the patent application she copied from a draft of Montagnier's Cold Spring Harbor presentation. Since the manuscript was in English, Bernemann found it easier to write the application in that language than translate the technical terms into French. The application had been registered at the British Patent Office in London, a cavernous Victorian pile that still has James Watt's patent on the steam engine in its files.[79] Under international patent treaties, the Pasteur would get credit almost everywhere in the world for its disclosure, on September 15, 1983, of the invention of a blood test for LAV.[n]

A month after their confrontation at Cold Spring Harbor, Montagnier and Gallo met again, at a chateau near the Loire river in Seillac, a popular venue for scientific conferences in France. The Pasteur's blood-testing data, Montagnier told his audience, had improved significantly. "At Cold Spring Harbor I mentioned twenty percent of AIDS patients had antibodies against LAV," Montagnier said. "At Seillac it was forty percent." But neither that news, nor Montagnier's report that Pasteur now had a sixth isolate of LAV, made a ripple.°

The only reaction at Seillac came from Françoise Haguenau, a French electron microscopist, who informed Montagnier, according to Gallo's recollection, that "This is all bullshit, you have no retrovirus." Montagnier recoiled, but Chermann was incensed.

"We know that we have the virus," Chermann said later. "But everybody was saying that we were wrong. But it was not a joke, and I tried to convince Gallo. We took a bicycle ride, Gallo, Guy de Thé, Françoise Haguenau and myself. I said to Gallo, 'You know me for a long time. I can tell you we have the virus. I will not fight anymore with you. You don't want to be convinced. Just take the virus that we sent to you. Because you told me that you put it in the fridge. Make a pellet and look for the virus. Make an electron microscope.'"[80]

Unbeknownst to Chermann, those things had already been done in Bethesda. Chermann recalled that when the foursome returned to Seillac, "Gallo pushed me in the swimming pool with my suit on. Everybody was very surprised. He said later he mistook me for somebody else."

Montagnier fared no better the following month at the Palais des Congrès in Paris, at a meeting of the French Association for Cancer Research, which had just awarded Gallo its Griffuel Prize (and whose president, Jacques Crozemarie, would later go to prison for conspiring to steal $50 million in cancer research funds).[81] The Paris conference was a replay of Cold Spring Harbor, Gallo pushing HTLV and Montagnier arguing for LAV. If Gallo knew about the Eureka! experiment six days earlier, he hadn't mentioned it. Claudine Escoffier-Lambiotte, the medical editor of *Le Monde,* accorded victory to the Americans, on the basis of Gallo's failure to find the French virus in any AIDS patients.[82]

"Gallo and Montagnier had a big fight," Escoffier recalled. "And during that fight one really had the impression Montagnier was a little boy and Gallo was a genius. Because Montagnier didn't argue well.

He presented a few cases. His test result was positive only one time out of three or four. Gallo was extremely tough and rough in the discussion. So coming out of the meeting one really had the impression that Montagnier's case was not a solid one."

Jacques Leibowitch, who still believed fervently that HTLV was the agent of AIDS, was at the meeting, and according to Escoffier "he talked all the time. He was definitely on the side of Bob Gallo, and that contributed to the fact that Montagnier's arguments seemed so weak." The day the meeting ended, Françoise Barré obtained the Pasteur's seventh and eighth isolates of LAV from two more AIDS patients.[83] The day after that, she isolated two more.[84]

Having established in his own laboratory that LAV was probably the cause of AIDS, Mika Popovic's next task was to find a better way to grow the French virus. At Cold Spring Harbor, Montagnier and Popovic had discussed the difficulties of growing a virus that killed the cells it infected, but Popovic thought there must be an easier way to keep the cultures alive than by continuously adding fresh T-cells.[85]

"Mika eventually came up with the idea that it was too much of a pain in the tail to keep adding tons of T-cells," Bernie Poiesz said. "And if you wanted to get a hundred liters of virus, you had to have something that grew without T-Cell Growth Factor. So he started to look for some T-4 cell line that could accept the virus and propagate it without dying."

Chermann and Barré had had the same idea, and they had asked Daniel Zagury at the University of Paris, Gallo's closest French friend, to lend them some continuous T-cell lines. But neither of the cell lines offered by Zagury had been the right ones for growing LAV. The first, HSB-2, didn't contain any T-4 cells. The second, CEM, established in Boston twenty years earlier from a four-year-old girl with leukemia, was a genuine T-4 cell line. But when Chermann put LAV into CEM he only got very low levels of reverse transcriptase, and after two weeks he abandoned the project.

There were several T-cell lines in Gallo's freezers, including the HUT-78 line that had been sitting there since Adi Gazdar gave it to Frank Ruscetti five years before. But before Popovic could begin infecting cell lines with LAV, a family crisis arose in Czechoslovakia that required an emergency visit to Switzerland.[86] Gallo didn't want to delay the work with LAV until Popovic's return, and he asked Prem Sarin's technician, Betsy Read, if she were willing to help with LAV. "I remember Dr. Gallo saying to Mika and me, 'We really need to get this done,'" Read said, "'because Luc wants to know an answer. Do we get the same results that he does?'"[87]

Read had some concerns about working with Popovic, whose Eastern European mannerisms his American colleagues found disconcerting. Popovic had retained an Old World gentility — upon being introduced to a woman he would bow slightly from the waist — but life in the Czech police state had also left him slightly paranoid. "The windows of his lab facing the corridor were taped over with newspapers," Zaki Salahuddin said. "If you walked in while he was reading something, very quickly he would close the book so nobody could see what he was working on." Read put aside her concerns and agreed to Gallo's request. "When I first went in the lab everyone said, 'Oh, watch out for Mika,'" she recalled. "Then I got to know him, and I really found him a very interesting sort, and very knowledgeable about virology and science."[88]

As Popovic was leaving for Switzerland, he scribbled out a set of instructions for how Read should go about infecting HUT-78 and four other cell lines with LAV.[89] When Read copied Popovic's instructions in her notebook she added one of her own: "Test at 9 days against *Bru* sera,"[90] a reminder to check the cell lines for virus growth by exposing the cells to the LAV antibodies in Brugière's blood.

The July LAV delivered by Montagnier to Gallo's house had been used up by Popovic's Eureka! experiment. But at Cold Spring Harbor Gallo had asked Montagnier for more virus, and in late September Françoise Barré had sent a new LAV shipment to Bethesda, along with more of Brugière's blood and the interferon antibody Gallo seemed so eager to obtain.[91] Accompanying the package was an agreement promising that the materials it contained would be used by NIH only for research, and "not for any industrial purpose without the prior written consent of the director of the Pasteur Institute." Gallo was still in Vienna when the shipment arrived, and Popovic scribbled his own signature on the document and thought no more about what would become a fateful moment.[P]

On October 24, 1983, a Wednesday, Betsy Read used the newly thawed LAV to infect five T-cell lines selected by Popovic. When he returned from Basel, the French virus was still growing in four of the five, which suggested that those four cell lines were able to generate new T-cells at a faster rate than LAV was able to kill them. When the cultures were tested for reverse transcriptase, the two in which LAV seemed to be growing best were a cell line from M. D. Anderson bearing the cryptic designation Ti7.4, and Adi Gazdar's HUT-78.[q]

The continuous growth of LAV represented an advance, a source of virus that, in the months to come, would make possible a number of further experiments. But when Gallo's AIDS task force met in early November, Popovic said nothing about a breakthrough. The theme of the meeting once again was HTLV, with Max Essex now reporting that 16 percent of people living in the Kyushu prefecture of Japan were positive for HTLV-MA.[92] But what Essex's test was measuring still wasn't clear, because the genesis of HTLV-MA wasn't clear. Did the protein belong to the T-cell? Or to the virus itself? Was its presence a sure sign the cell was infected with HTLV-1? The "unequivocal determination that [HTLV-MA] is a viral protein is of utmost importance," the task force concluded.[93]

The French hadn't published anything with international visibility since their initial *Science* article the previous May, and the AIDS researchers and clinicians who hadn't heard Montagnier speak at Cold Spring Harbor or in Seillac or Paris, which was most of them, remained unaware of the accumulating data at the Pasteur.

That included Jay Levy, a retrovirologist from the University of California in San Francisco, who had flown to Paris in October to attend his brother's wedding. Levy, who spoke fluent French, had taken advantage of the visit to stop by the Pasteur. Not until then, Levy recalled, had he realized the French were *not* working with HTLV. "Everyone thought they had HTLV," Levy said, "because they had published in *Science* with Gallo."

There were more AIDS cases in San Francisco than anywhere except New York City, and Levy had been pursuing the AIDS virus in his own lab. Long before arriving in Paris, Levy had become convinced Gallo was on the wrong track, and he had assumed the French were mistakenly following in Gallo's footsteps. "We had already worked out that this couldn't be HTLV," Levy recalled. "It just didn't make sense." Among other things, Levy reasoned, hemophiliacs were coming down with AIDS, and hemophiliacs received blood-clotting factors that were free of cells, whereas HTLV needed T-cells to survive.[94]

At the Pasteur, Jay Levy had an epiphany. "By visiting their lab," Levy said, "it was the first I knew that it might be a lentivirus. It was almost too good to be true: It grew in T-4 cells, it killed the cells. I came back to the hotel room and I told my wife, 'Sharon, I've been looking for this virus, and I think they've found it.' But if I hadn't gone to see them, I would have never known."[95] Levy encouraged the French to keep going, but he declined Montagnier's offer of a LAV sample to take home. "One of the things I've learned in virology," Levy said, "if you want to confirm somebody, don't bring their virus into your lab. Because you never know."

Instead, Levy set out to isolate the French virus from the blood of a San Francisco man with AIDS. Using Françoise Barré's protocol for LAV, it took him two weeks. "At the end of October we got our first RT activity," Levy said, "and then in early November we had our first isolate. We asked Françoise for serum against her virus, and they sent us *Bru* serum. It reacted with the viruses we isolated. In retrospect, I regret that we didn't immediately publish at the end of 1983."

Word that Levy had isolated LAV from an American AIDS patient was the first good news to reach the Pasteur in many months. Françoise Barré learned about it on the way to a retrovirus conference in Tokyo, where she planned to present the latest ELISA results, and to announce that Pasteur now had ten isolates of LAV, including viruses from a hemophiliac, two Zairians, two homosexuals, a Haitian, and a Caucasian living in Africa.[96] At Narita airport Barré encountered Gallo, who was headed for the same conference, and they agreed to split the expensive cab ride to their downtown hotel. According to Barré, Gallo mentioned during the ride that *his* lab had just isolated a virus that appeared to be identical to LAV. The new virus killed T-cells, Gallo said, and AIDS patients had antibodies to it. Barré recalled Gallo saying the pictures of his new virus looked just like LAV.[97]

The only LAV-like pictures in Gallo's lab were Matt Gonda's pictures of LAV. Two days after the cab ride, Popovic sent more cells from his LAV-infected cultures to Gonda — who, once again, was able to photograph the same lentivirus-like particles he had seen in Popovic's first LAV cultures in early October. Of the two dozen other AIDS cultures Popovic sent Gonda that day, none had contained any visible virus.[98] Besides LAV, the only non-HTLV virus Popovic had been able to culture from an AIDS patient had come from a North Carolina hemophiliac code-named S.N. But S.N.'s cells had died, and Gonda hadn't been able to see any virus there either.[99]

Mika Popovic was no longer looking for HTLV, but Gallo was telling colleagues the HTLV story had become "much more interesting now."[100] In mid-December Gallo sent *Science* a paper that appeared to validate Max Essex's results by concluding that HTLV-MA protein was almost certainly a viral protein, a product of HTLV itself.[r] The only effective test for HTLV, Gallo declared, was the Essex test, which was now finding HTLV-MA antibodies in 90 percent of some groups of AIDS patients.[101]

The still-unpublished data in Gallo's own lab told a very different story. According to Gallo, the reason Marjorie Guroff and her co-investigator, Doug Blayney, had detected HTLV in fewer than 10 percent of AIDS patients was probably the inaccuracy of the ELISA Guroff had used. But Guroff and Blayney thought their data was rock-solid, and Blayney had been fretting for months over Gallo's reluctance to publish. "It was my interpretation," Blayney said later, "that Essex was picking up something else that had to do with God knows what. I thought this thing was important, and we ought to get our data out. But it was delayed by Gallo."

Months before, Guroff had sent Blayney a copy of the finished manuscript. "Gave a copy to Dr. Gallo today," she wrote. "Not sure he will want to publish on AIDS at this time, but we'll see."[102] Gallo didn't. When he finally submitted the Guroff-Blayney manuscript to *The Lancet,* at the end of December 1983, the manuscript was careful to note "possible explanations" for the yawning disparity between Guroff's 7 percent positives and Essex's 90 percent.[s] One possibility was that AIDS might be caused by a "minor variant" of HTLV that Guroff's blood test didn't pick up — Gallo's Type A/Type B hypothesis.[103]

Not by coincidence, such a minor variant had just been discovered by a Gallo postdoc, Beatrice Hahn, in the process of comparing the genetic makeup of several HTLV isolates. Using a technique called restriction mapping, which employs a handful of enzymes that digest certain DNA molecules, Hahn had taken the DNA fingerprints of a number of HTLVs and compared them to the Charlie Robinson original. The Claude Chardon virus was a carbon copy of $HTLV_{CR}$. But another HTLV, isolated by Mika Popovic from a Houston AIDS patient, was different. The Houston virus mapped like $HTLV_{CR}$, but only up to a point.[104] After that the fingerprints diverged — just like the "Type B" mutant Gallo had predicted a few months before as the possible cause of AIDS.

Gallo named the new virus HTLV-1B.[105] When his chief molecular biologist, the Chinese-born, UCLA-trained Flossie Wong-Staal, sent the HTLV-1B manuscript to *Science,* she made sure the editors understood that HTLV-1B represented a significant discovery. "We are excited about this work," Wong-Staal wrote *Science.*[106] Only after the manuscript was in the mail had Beatrice Hahn gotten around to comparing the DNA fingerprint of the Houston virus with the HTLV isolated from Elomata, the Zairian man who had died of T-cell lymphoma.[107]

The two were a dead match, which meant HTLV-1B hadn't come from an AIDS patient after all. As Hahn sorted through her DNA samples, she discovered the source of the mistake. Ersell Richardson had assigned the Houston patient the code number 3774. Elomata's number was 3734. Somehow the two samples had gotten mixed up. Hahn blamed Richardson's dyslexia, but how the mix-up happened hardly mattered.[t] What mattered was that Gallo's "new variant" of HTLV had nothing to do with AIDS, and the HTLV-1B paper never appeared in print.[u]

Nineteen eighty-three had begun at the Institut Pasteur with the discovery of a new human retrovirus. For the balance of the year, new isolates of that virus had emerged from the labs of Montagnier and Françoise Barré at the rate of better than one a month; the twelfth isolate, LAV/*Rab,* had been obtained on December 14.[v] But as 1983 drew to a close, the French had lost the battle to convince the world.

Through some logic it never made clear, the National Cancer Institute concluded that LAV was really the Equine Infectious Anemia Virus.[108] Its highest priority, the NCI told Congress in December 1983, remained "the elucidation of the role of human T-cell leukemia virus (HTLV) in AIDS."[109] Over Montagnier's objections, the World Health Organization followed the NCI's lead, concluding that the best candidate for the cause of AIDS was HTLV.[110] On the same December day Matt Gonda made his latest pictures of the LAV growing in Popovic's lab, Gallo assured other scientists that "we still have not seen the Montagnier group's type of virus in a patient here."[111]

Since the previous April, the French had sent Gallo three shipments of LAV DNA, two of the LAV virus itself, several vials of blood from Frédéric Brugière, and several more of anti-interferon. Beatrice

Hahn had confirmed that LAV was genetically distinct from HTLV.[w] Mika Popovic had succeeded in growing the French virus in continuous culture, and discovered that it infected the other AIDS patients' blood cells in his inventory. Matt Gonda had sent Popovic enough pictures of LAV to paper the walls of Gallo's lab.

But there hadn't been a word from Gallo about what his lab had done with the Pasteur's virus. A few days before Christmas, an exasperated Montagnier received an urgent telex asking for still more material. "Regarding antibody to alpha interferon," Gallo wired, "you agreed to send this to Dr. Popovic a few weeks ago. Need definite answer. Can we depend on this being shipped or not?"

When there was no reply from Paris, Popovic called Montagnier at home. An angry Montagnier demanded to know whether Popovic had made any progress with LAV before sending yet more material. Popovic replied that "we learned how to handle the virus. What I didn't tell him," Popovic said later, "that it grows very well in permanent T-cell line . . . I thought, it is our discovery so we should first publish it and later inform them. I didn't consider that it was my duty to inform him in detail that we have a breakthrough."[112]

• 4 •

"This Looks Like It Could Be the Cause"

The first person Jean-Claude Chermann saw when he walked off the plane in Salt Lake City was Robert Gallo. During the forty-minute bus ride to Park City, high in the Wasatch Mountains, the two resumed the dispute that had been interrupted the previous October by Gallo's dunking of Chermann.

"He say, 'Jean-Claude, nobody believes your virus,'" Chermann recalled. "'You have to prove that you have a reverse transcriptase and a true retrovirus. You cannot speak about LAV as a retrovirus. You don't know if it is a retrovirus.' I say, 'Bob, you know that I am working with retrovirus for twenty years. I have fifteen minutes to speak, I don't want to lose any minutes to speak about what is a retrovirus. I have much more to say.'"[1]

Gallo, whose "best candidate" for the cause of AIDS was a version of HTLV,[2] had been tapped to present the keynote address, and the meeting's co-organizer, Jerome Groopman of Harvard, assured Gallo that he could "speak for 45 minutes, 90 minutes, or two days if you would like."[3]

Groopman opened the conference by reminding his listeners why they had come to Utah in February.[a] "As I think everyone in this room knows," Groopman said, "AIDS is a devastating disease that spans a diversity of disciplines. AIDS has been designated the number one health priority in the United States. We're challenged to discover its etiology. We're pleased tonight to have Dr. Robert Gallo, chief of the

Laboratory of Tumor Biology at the National Cancer Institute, as the keynote speaker."

Gallo talked for over an hour about the history of his research on AIDS, somehow without mentioning Mika Popovic's confirmation that LAV was indeed a new human retrovirus that infected many AIDS patients.[4]

"When I came into this," Gallo said, "there were a lot of ideas discussed in the newspaper and in the literature as well — ideas such as amyl nitrate and other drugs. Ideas such as sperm. 'Antigens' I often heard described as the cause of the disease, which means there is no cause. And in the last six months or so a fungus was described as a possible etiologic agent with enthusiasm, cyclosporin."

The cyclosporin incident had unsettled Gallo, who was in San Francisco when he got a call from an unhappy Vince DeVita. As Gallo remembered the conversation, DeVita began by saying, "'I thought you told me it was going to be a new retrovirus that was the cause of AIDS.' I said, 'Well, tell me the data.' And he told me, 'On television they're claiming it's a fungus that releases cyclosporin.'

"I started to get palpitations. I said, 'Oh, my God.' I thought, 'Wait a minute — cyclosporin?' I remembered Einstein's statement that Mother Nature's not mean, but she's never that simple. And then I thought better than that. Hemophiliacs are now getting AIDS, and they had Factor VIII"— a blood-clotting agent — "and Factor VIII's filtered. It couldn't be a fungus. So we breathed easier."

Gallo's intuition had led him to HTLV as the likely cause. "When I speak of HTLV," Gallo said, "I want to cautiously state I mean the *family* of T-lymphotropic retroviruses. Because what we're isolating is not always Type 1. This is not published yet, and I don't know what to call it. Call it '1B.' It came from a patient from Africa. We were initially told this man had AIDS.[b] Later we were told he has an immune abnormality, and we don't know what. We have to find out. I can't tell you if this is the important virus in AIDS or not."

Anyone who might be tempted to interpret Marjorie Guroff's negative blood-testing data as evidence that HTLV couldn't be the cause of AIDS was reminded by Gallo that there were other diseases where the number of virus-infected patients was considerably higher than the number who had detectable antibodies to that virus. "The antibodies of people with hepatitis to core proteins, I've read, are around the same," Gallo said, "around ten percent.

"I see some scorn from the faces of one or two people," Gallo said. "Dr. Sachs? That's not true?"

"I just had an itch," Sachs replied.

"The best way to handle it," Gallo said, "is to scratch it. It's certainly not data from me. I've just read this in a review. I don't know if it's true."

Gallo admitted he hadn't proved that HTLV-1 was the cause of AIDS. "It *could* be," he said, "but it doesn't mean it *has* to be. It could be something else. It could be another member of the family. And that's exactly what we're trying to find out. It's not easy to isolate this class of virus from people with AIDS. We have a total now of about seventeen, I guess it is exactly seventeen isolates.

"And let me put 'isolates' in quotes," Gallo went on, "because it depends how you define an isolation. We like to define it when we've characterized what we have in detail and when we've been able to successfully transmit it, to be able to hand it out to somebody. So it's better for me to say we have seventeen samples from people with AIDS that we've cultured. In some cases the virus is in fact isolated, five or six. In others the process is just on the way."

At the following day's symposium on AIDS, chaired by Gallo, Max Essex remained convinced that HTLV was "a leading candidate" for the AIDS virus. Essex was followed on the program by Murray Gardner, the California researcher who had undone Essex in the FOCMA affair, then by Bill Haseltine and Jean-Claude Chermann. But Haseltine had continued to talk while Chermann's allotted time dwindled away.

"Groopman added Haseltine as a speaker because Groopman had Harvard connections," recalled Mike Gottlieb, the meeting's other co-organizer, who had invited Chermann to Park City. "I had been told by Groopman that Haseltine was only going to talk for ten minutes. Haseltine is still going at thirty minutes, and it looks like he's going for forty-five.

"At these ski meetings," Gottlieb said, "the pressure is to get the morning meeting done by noon, so we can get out onto the slopes. And I hunt down Groopman, because he's responsible. I said, 'Hey, Jerry, this is your guy, who we said could have ten minutes, and he's cutting into Chermann's time. What kind of behavior is this?' Jerry got the chair's attention, and Gallo said something to Haseltine. Groopman told me later that Haseltine was livid."[5]

"I'm sorry I had to rush Bill," Gallo told the audience, "but it is because we are late and I guess there has to be things on time. Bill's talk was going to be a short one, but there's a lot of data and a lot of information. I don't think there's really time for questions. The next speaker is Jean-Claude Chermann from the Pasteur Institute in Paris, and he's going to talk about the human retrovirus which they find associated with lymphadenopathy, and he's going to give us the latest on some characterizations and whatever other studies they have."

Since their *Science* paper nine months before, the French had been relegated to publishing in European journals that American and British scientists didn't read, and their best work hadn't been published at all. When Montagnier sent *Science* a manuscript reporting that LAV cross-reacted with the Equine Infectious Anemia Virus and was therefore most likely a lentivirus, the manuscript was returned.[6] Just before Christmas, Françoise Brun and Christine Rouzioux had written up their ELISA results and sent them to *The Lancet:* 75 percent of pre-AIDS patients, and 38 percent of those with AIDS, positive for antibodies to LAV.[c] By the time of Park City there hadn't been any word about when the paper might appear.

Park City was the last chance for the French to persuade the Americans that they had probably found the cause of AIDS. But Chermann was the Pasteur's least articulate spokesman, and as he reached for the microphone he fumbled with his notes. "I would like," he began, "to thank the organizers for the opportunity to convince you about this new retrovirus. I have heard three times in this conference that it looked like an *arenavirus*. I am sorry. I will show you that it is not an arenavirus but a retrovirus."

Flipping through his slides, Chermann provided an abbreviated summary of what the French had accomplished in less than a year and Françoise Brun's blood testing data, now showing 40 percent of AIDS patients and 88 percent of pre-AIDS patients positive for LAV.[d]

When the time came for questions, Gallo was first to speak. How, he asked, could the French be sure that each of the viruses they were calling LAV was really the selfsame virus? "How do you know the individual isolates are individual isolates?" Gallo asked. "How do you know they're the same exact strain?" Chermann explained that the French had tested their isolates for reactivity to blood antibodies from Brugière and several other patients with AIDS and pre-AIDS. All the patients, Chermann said, had antibodies that reacted with each of the viruses, the whole virus as well as the core protein.

After a few questions from others, Chermann returned to his seat. "It was very difficult for me to speak," Chermann said later, "and it was a very, very short time. And there was practically no discussion." But Chermann had gotten his message across. "He was a little flustered by the events," Mike Gottlieb said later, "and his English isn't that great anyway. Jean-Claude, I love him, he's a great guy, but his presentation was a little discombobulated. But people were sitting there ready to go skiing and all of a sudden there were people saying 'Hey, these guys have something.' These were people who hadn't read the *Science* paper, they hadn't heard the story."[7]

Chermann hadn't been able to gauge the audience's reaction, and when he got back to his room he was disconsolate. Soon there was a knock on his door, then another, and another: Donna Mildvan from Beth Israel in New York, Mike Lange from St. Luke's, even Murray Gardner. "Donna Mildvan said, 'You have the true virus,'" Chermann recalled. "Murray Gardner was also convinced." The clincher, Gardner said later, had been the LAV isolates from Africa. The only African viruses in Gallo's lab were HTLV.

Toward the end of the meeting someone approached Gallo with a question from Jay Levy, who hadn't been invited. Levy wanted to know why, if HTLV caused AIDS, AIDS patients didn't have T-cell leukemia. Gallo admitted it was a reasonable question, but when he answered Levy in writing he took issue with the premise. "I never said HTLV caused AIDS," Gallo replied. "From the beginning, I have said we are testing the *idea* that a human T-lymphotropic retrovirus is involved. In short, we are looking for HTLV 'relatives' and variants of which we now have several types isolated. All have common features, including the isolate from Paris." But Gallo wasn't about to knock on Chermann's door. "HTLV itself," he told Levy, "*could* still cause AIDS."[8]

From Utah, Françoise Brun flew to New York for a little shopping while Chermann went on to Bethesda, where he had been invited to give a seminar to the members of Gallo's lab. "Gallo was not there," Chermann said, "but a lot of people were there. I do my seminar, there are no questions, or few questions." Afterward, Chermann went in search of Mika Popovic. "I said to Mika, 'We send you twice or three times the virus,'" Chermann recalled. "'We need to know if you are replicating or not the virus.' And he told me, you know, with his pipe like this, 'I cannot speak. Only the boss can speak.' I mean, here I was just making a seminar, giving all I know about LAV at this time. This is not what I would consider to be collaboration."[9]

The day before Chermann's visit, Popovic's new technician, Betsy Read, arrived at work to find things not as she remembered leaving them the previous evening. The AIDS cultures in Read's incubator had been shuffled around, and next to the incubator sat an unfamiliar coffee cup. Read's experiments had been sabotaged before —"I have seen my CO_2 switched off," she said. "I have had freezer alarms turned off."

A few weeks earlier, Read and Popovic had transferred their AIDS cultures to a new workspace down the hall, and locks hadn't yet been installed on the door. The cultures hadn't been moved by Popovic, and no one else had any business in their lab. "I became rather paranoid," Read recalled, "because of the important cells I had in my incubator, and I went and told Dr. Gallo."[e]

Popovic was reluctant to say who he thought might have tampered with Read's cultures, if that was indeed what had happened. "It is difficult to imply anything," he said. "But obviously we were afraid that there was certain reshuffling, and God knows what could happen and things might be out of our control. I cannot tell whether somebody went in or not, or who, and what would be the reasons."[10]

Chermann's next stop was Atlanta, where Don Francis and his CDC colleagues had become thoroughly disenchanted with Max Essex's irreproducible HTLV data. As Essex's correlation between HTLV-MA and AIDS crept ever higher, Cy Cabradilla had used the Essex method to test blood samples from patients with autoimmune diseases like lupus. When Cabradilla got the same results Essex was reporting with AIDS patients, he began to get "really uncomfortable."

Don Francis, who had continued to promote HTLV as the "best lead" for the AIDS virus for longer than he would later care to remember,[11] now agreed with Cabradilla. By the time Chermann arrived in Atlanta, a CDC virologist named Paul Feorino had succeeded in growing the LAV sample Chermann had handed a CDC courier in New York while changing planes on the way to Utah.[12] "It had become clear," Francis said later, "that we had all made a very big mistake."

That included Francis's boss, the CDC's AIDS chief, Jim Curran, who hadn't heard Chermann speak at Park City. "But when he came to Atlanta, I heard him," Curran said. "I saw his data. A lot of people at CDC were very encouraged, because he had serologic data from a variety of different groups of people, not only from gay men. It may not have been perfect, but the unifying hypothesis about AIDS was that it was occurring in these disparate populations, hemophiliacs and others."

Curran's boss, Walter Dowdle, was also on board with the French. "We came away from there convinced that they had the agent," Dowdle said. "The lesson was brought home to CDC. We didn't know what was happening in Gallo's lab. We only knew he was working on something and we were providing sera. The French were speaking openly, and there wasn't this open discussion from Gallo's lab. There was no real way to compare what was going on in both labs, except what was being told to us."

Within the U.S. Department of Health and Human Services, word that the probable cause of AIDS had been found — not at NIH or CDC, but in France — moved quickly up the chain of command. The CDC's director, a rangy, sandy-haired doctor named James Mason,[13] informed the assistant secretary, Ed Brandt, who sent a confidential memo to Margaret Heckler, a doughty former Massachusetts congresswoman whom Ronald Reagan had chosen as his secretary of health and human services, and who had declared finding the cause of AIDS the nation's "most urgent health priority."[14]

"Scientists at L'Institut Pasteur in France," Brandt told Heckler, "have isolated a retrovirus known as the Lymphadenopathy Associated Virus (LAV) from some seven [sic] patients with AIDS. The apparent importance of this virus is that it is the first one that is consistent with a plausible theory for the development of AIDS. Since these findings must be tested further, we must not discuss them now. I will keep you informed."[15]

The mood at the Pasteur was considerably improved upon Françoise Brun's return to Paris. For months Jean-Claude Chermann had tried to persuade the Pasteur's molecular biologists to help with the genetic cloning of LAV, a critical step in determining exactly how the virus worked. "Because my lab was near the computer," Chermann said, "all the molecular biologists had to cross my corridor. I tried to stop some people to say, 'Could you help us to clone?' The molecular biologists said, 'Oh, it is not difficult, you take the RNA and so on.' But nobody believed us. If one had taken the bet to say 'maybe they're right,' in January '84, the virus would have been cloned."[16]

In desperation, Montagnier approached a senior Pasteur colleague, Pierre Tiollais, whose lab had cloned the hepatitis B virus from which Pasteur was making its vaccine. Tiollais was aware that other Pasteur labs were refusing to help Montagnier and his group, some because they didn't want to work with the AIDS virus, others because they didn't think LAV *was* the cause of AIDS. But Tiollais couldn't ignore a direct appeal from a fellow Pasteur professor, and he put the proposition to Simon Wain-Hobson, an Oxford-educated British expatriate who was teaching gene-cloning courses at the Pasteur.

"He told me, 'I've just seen Montagnier,'" Wain-Hobson recalled. "He said, 'Montagnier wants us to clone his virus. I can't ask you to do it, but if it interests you, why not?' We discussed a long time. I had heard noises about Montagnier's virus, but I didn't know much about it. Everyone saw the *Science* paper, but one didn't know what to say. It was simply 'Well, what can you say with one isolate?' Most people skip papers quickly. You don't read the details." In any case, Wain-Hobson told Tiollais, "I wanted to have a go. He said, 'Now look, Simon, I'll give you six months. Promise me if it hasn't worked after six months you'll come back to hepatitis-B.' I said, 'Well, I've got a few things to finish off, and I'll start as soon as I can.' Perhaps we should have got going earlier, but I must confess that I was terribly unimpressed at the time."[17]

The principal shortcoming of the Pasteur's ELISA, its inability to find LAV antibodies in a convincing percentage of AIDS patients, had persisted into early 1984. In January, thirty CDC blood samples had arrived from Don Francis, ten drawn from AIDS patients, ten from pre-AIDS patients, and ten from healthy controls.[18] All ten of the pre-AIDS patients had been positive for LAV antibodies, but only three of the ten with AIDS.[19] Such a discrepancy wasn't so important in the real world, where it was the people who didn't yet exhibit the symptoms of AIDS who needed to know whether they were infected with the virus. But for establishing a causative link between AIDS and LAV, the numbers were crucial.

The biggest surprise to greet Brun's return was a new and prolific source of LAV.[20] A couple of months before, frustrated by Chermann's failure to grow the virus in existing T-cell lines, Montagnier had created a new continuous cell line, not with T-cells but with B-cells, the other major component of the immune system.[f] While Chermann and Brun were in Park City, Montagnier had inoculated his new B-cell line with LAV. The virus had taken hold and grown, in significantly larger quantities than had been achieved by adding fresh T-cells.[21] Encouraged, Montagnier had switched to an established B-cell line, BJAB, which proved even more productive.[22]

With plenty of virus for their ELISA, Brun and Rouzioux no longer needed to be so selective in their blood testing. Their newfound ability to test many samples, and to test the same samples over and over, finally answered the question that had vexed them for months — why weren't more AIDS patients positive for LAV?

Brun and Rouzioux had designed their ELISA to yield the smallest possible number of "false positives," erroneous indications that LAV antibodies were present in a blood sample when there really were no antibodies. To rid the virus used for the ELISA of any nonviral proteins or other contaminating debris, Chermann had put LAV through not one, or two, but three purification cycles. "We were purifying the virus at the maximum," Brun recalled, "and when you purify the virus you lose the envelope, because the envelope protein is very fragile. At that time the main component of our virus preparation was the core protein, but some patients have antibodies only against the envelope of the virus. It was the reason we had in AIDS patients a not very high percentage of results."

The breakthrough with Montagnier's B-cell line couldn't have come at a more auspicious time. A large collection of blood samples, drawn from thirty-six Zairian AIDS patients and a number of healthy controls, had just arrived from the Institute of Tropical Medicine in Antwerp. "Montagnier said he had discovered the virus and developed a serological test," recalled Peter Piot, the Belgian AIDS researcher who shipped the coded samples to Paris. "So I sent him some serum samples to see if his tests agreed with our diagnoses."[23]

Piot's samples were the first to be tested with an ELISA made with LAV that had been purified only twice, and the difference was dramatic. Before, fewer than half of AIDS patients had detectable antibodies to LAV. With the new ELISA, *90 percent* of the Zairian AIDS patients were LAV positive.[24] "When Montagnier called me and gave me his results, I couldn't believe how well they fitted with ours," recalled Piot, who would later become chief of the World Health

Organization's program on AIDS. "That was one of the most thrilling phone calls of my life."[g]

Rather than pausing to publish the Zairian data, Brun and Montagnier told Don Francis they were eager to put their virus to the acid test. According to the plan, Francis would send the French dozens of coded CDC blood samples — not just any samples but the CDC's gold-standard "pedigreed sera," from homosexuals, blood donors, hemophiliacs, and transfusion recipients with confirmed diagnoses of AIDS and pre-AIDS. Mixed in among them would be blood taken from healthy homosexual men and heterosexual blood donors not at risk for AIDS. But none of the samples would be labeled. If the French blood test found LAV antibodies in the samples from people who had AIDS or were at risk for AIDS, and not in those who didn't have AIDS and weren't at risk, the case for LAV would be made.

A few days after Mika Popovic's late-night phone call to Montagnier, Popovic had sent a sizable quantity of virus to Litton Bionetics, one of the private companies in and around Bethesda that held multimillion-dollar NCI contracts to perform services for Gallo's lab.[25] Popovic's virus, dubbed MOV, was delivered to M. G. Sarngadharan, a Bionetics researcher who had worked closely with Gallo since the early cancer virus days.[h]

In early January 1984, six months behind Brun and Rouzioux, Sarngadharan used MOV to make the first antibody blood test in Bethesda. But Sarngadharan's initial ELISA couldn't tell the difference between antibodies to LAV and those to HTLV-1 and HTLV-2.[26] After a few weeks of adjustments during which many samples were tested, the ELISA was able to detect strong antibodies to MOV in the blood of a New Haven prostitute named Locklear, and also her newborn infant.[i] The child, who already had AIDS, had certainly gotten it from his mother, either in the womb, during birth, or through mother's milk.

When Sarngadharan saw that both Locklear mother and child were infected with MOV, his "gut feeling" was that Popovic's new virus "probably is going to be the virus involved in AIDS. So I went to Gallo and told him."[27]

Of the available T-cell lines in which to grow the AIDS virus, Popovic had settled on Adi Gazdar's HUT-78 as the most promising.

But Popovic thought he could improve the virus yield even more by cloning the line — selecting those individual HUT-78 cells that were most susceptible to infection with the MOV, then allowing each of the selected cells to reproduce in a flask of its own, thereby generating many new substrains of HUT-78.

Popovic had tried the single-cell cloning technique the previous November, and in one HUT-78 clone, called H-4, the virus had grown better than in the original HUT-78.[28] In mid-January he tried again, this time selecting fifty-one HUT-78 cells that, through the miracle of cell division, would become fifty-one brand-new HUT-78 clones.[29] When the newest clones were infected with virus, the best producer was clone number nine, which Popovic labeled H-9.[30]

Despite the promising work by Popovic and Sarngadharan with MOV, as February drew to a close Gallo still thought HTLV-1 "one of the best candidates" for the cause of AIDS.[31] With the H-9 cell line spewing virus, Sarngadharan had enough MOV to run through his ELISA sixty of the coded AIDS patients' blood samples Marjorie Guroff had found negative for antibodies to HTLV.[32]

At the end of February 1984, Guroff and Sarngadharan met in Gallo's office to break the code. More than 90 percent of the AIDS patients, and 85 percent of those with pre-AIDS, had antibodies to Popovic's MOV — nearly as good as the results the French had gotten with Peter Piot's Zairian samples two days earlier. At that moment, Sarngadharan recalled, Gallo became "convinced that we had a reliable test"— and that Popovic's new virus must be the cause of AIDS.[33]

The CDC blood samples, more than a hundred in all, arrived in Paris on February 28, 1984. Within a few days another consignment, including many of the samples sent to Pasteur, was shipped from Atlanta to Bethesda, in response to a request from Gallo following Sarngadharan's results with the Guroff sera. If the French intended to use the CDC to prove they had found the cause of AIDS, Gallo would do the same.

Christine Rouzioux remembered standing in Jean-Claude Chermann's office, listening on another line as Chermann read the ELISA results to Don Francis over the phone. "Chermann would say 'C43 — positive,'" Rouzioux recalled, "and Don Francis would say, 'That's a hemophiliac with AIDS.' 'C63 — positive.' 'That's another AIDS patient.' 'C93 — negative.' 'Oh, that's my technician.' 'C72 — negative.' 'Oh, that's me. Thank you very much.'"

When the score was tallied, 91 percent of the CDC's pre-AIDS patients had antibodies to LAV, and 79 percent of those with AIDS — not quite as good as the Pasteur's results with the Zairian sera, but in Françoise Brun's mind convincing beyond a doubt.[34] "Everything was corresponding very well," Brun said. "We were very happy."

Curran and Francis had continued to brief the CDC's director, Jim Mason, on developments with LAV, and Curran recalled that, the moment the ELISA results were tabulated, "we told Dr. Mason that this stuff the French are doing is really looking good. This really looks like it could be the cause."[35]

Under other circumstances, the French might have sent off an updated paper to The Lancet or one to the New England Journal, announcing that they had found the likely cause of AIDS and requesting expedited publication. But the blood testing had been done in collaboration with the CDC, and by sending many of the same samples to Gallo Don Francis had made it a three-way collaboration. "If you are collaborating with some people," Montagnier said later, "before you can publish all the collaborators have to agree."

Don Francis got the Pasteur's blood test results on March 9, 1984, a Friday. The following Monday, Jim Curran flew to Bethesda to break the code with Gallo and Sarngadharan, who five days before had finished testing the CDC samples with MOV.[36] Over lunch at a French restaurant, Sarngadharan read off the results for each sample while Curran scanned the computer printout he had carried from Atlanta. "Gallo was busy that day," Curran recalled. "He had a lecture to give. He was primarily interested in how well his test had done."

The answer was not as well as Pasteur's. Eighty-seven percent of the blood samples from pre-AIDS patients had been positive for antibodies to MOV, compared to 90 percent at the Pasteur — a wash. But only 48 percent of Gallo's AIDS patients' samples were positive, compared to the Pasteur's 72 percent.[37] Still, Gallo's numbers were persuasive enough to convince Curran that both Pasteur and Gallo had the AIDS virus.

"I told him I thought his serologic results were compatible with the cause of AIDS," recalled Curran, who didn't mention the parallel blood testing in Paris. "Gallo was aware that we were also collaborating with the French," Curran said later. "My purpose in meeting with him wasn't to compare his results to the French. I didn't have the French results with me. But part of the reason I was so pleased was because of the concordance of Gallo's results with Pasteur. Part of the reason I was convinced he was on the right track was that Pasteur was also on the right track. I was convinced that Gallo's virus was the same virus as the French. We all knew you couldn't get the same results with viruses that were not the same."

Leaving Curran and Sarngadharan to finish their lunch, Gallo confided that he had isolated the AIDS virus from *fifty* AIDS patients. More important, he had developed a "revolutionary" secret technique for viral isolations that would soon be revealed in *Science*. Curran remembered wondering whether CDC, which had collected the blood samples and arranged the competition that established LAV and MOV as the presumptive cause of AIDS, was going to share the credit in the days and weeks to come.

In addition to collaborating with Gallo and the French, the CDC had been using LAV to test its own blood samples, not with an ELISA but a more sophisticated test, a radioimmuno precipitation assay, and the CDC's results matched those from Paris. That made it a three-way confirmation. "We got the French isolate to grow," Cy Cabradilla said later. "We were the first ones to set up a competitive radioimmuno-assay for it. We beat Gallo at his own game. We were doing *tons* of serology. We were working twenty-four hours a day. We were able to confirm that other isolates were related to LAV. We had all that data. Gallo knew exactly what we had."

One thing CDC had, arguably more important than anything at NCI or the Pasteur, was an ironclad link between the virus and AIDS. The previous December, the CDC's chief virologist, Paul Feorino, had isolated a retrovirus from a thirty-six-year-old woman who developed AIDS after receiving a hospital transfusion. The woman was married, didn't use intravenous drugs, and wasn't a hemophiliac, which meant she could only have become infected via the transfusion. The CDC had tracked down her blood donor, a twenty-two-year-old homosexual who had gotten AIDS a month after making the donation. The donor's T-cells had also had yielded a retrovirus. When Feorino compared the two viruses, they were indistinguishable — from one another, and from LAV.[38]

Testing for blood antibodies with an ELISA, as Gallo and the French had done, was tantamount to a game of probability, to asking what the chances might be that a virus which infected AIDS patients, but not healthy subjects, was *not* the cause of AIDS. On that score the ELISA results, at least those from France, were conclusive. But Curran and Francis thought the virus isolations from the CDC's "transfusion pair" represented the nearest thing possible to a nonprobablistic proof that LAV was the cause of AIDS.

"We wanted to publish that manuscript simultaneously with Gallo's," Curran said. But the CDC couldn't answer the obvious question such a publication would raise — whether the viruses from the transfusion pair were also indistinguishable from Gallo's virus — because Gallo hadn't shared MOV with the CDC. "The only reagents we had to work with," Curran said, "were reagents that were given to us by the French."

Over the weekend Gallo pondered his ELISA results, and when Curran got back to his office in Atlanta Gallo gave him a call. Almost all Sarngadharan's equivocal blood-testing scores, recorded as "plus/minus," had come from AIDS patients' blood samples, and Gallo thought the CDC should allow him to change his borderline results to positive.[39] Pasteur hadn't asked to change any of its results after the fact, and Don Francis was against allowing Gallo that extra advantage. "The French felt more comfortable with their test and gave us an absolute number," Francis said later. "Whereas between the time of the initial report and the final telephone call, Bob was saying, 'We call all the plus-minuses positives.'"

Jim Curran agreed to Gallo's request, he said later, "because the plus-minuses were almost all people that should have been infected." But moving the cutoff between positive and negative gave the Gallo ELISA nearly equivalent accuracy with the Pasteur test. Of the ninety CDC blood samples tested jointly in Paris and Bethesda, now Gallo and the French each scored 92 percent of the pre-AIDS patients positive. Among AIDS patients, the French had gotten 80 percent right to Gallo's 78.

The most important difference between the ELISAs was told by the incorrect scores. The Gallo ELISA incorrectly identified two "healthy controls" as positive for MOV, whereas the French had scored a single control positive for LAV. More ominous, the Gallo ELISA had identified *three* blood samples from AIDS patients as negative, compared with only one for the French.

But the relative false-positive and false-negative rates of the two ELISAs didn't seem important in the spring of 1984. The mystery of

AIDS at last had been solved. Its cause was a previously unknown human retrovirus. The French called the virus LAV. Having abandoned the term MOV, Gallo called it HTLV-3. Jim Curran didn't care what it was called. "I just wanted somebody to find the cause of AIDS," he said.

The day after learning the CDC's verdict, Gallo began spreading word of his discovery and denigrating the work in Paris. To Jean-Paul Levy, the dean of Paris retrovirologists, Gallo confided that he had "many" isolates of HTLV-3. It wasn't clear whether HTLV-3 was related to the Pasteur's virus, Gallo said, because it was difficult to say "what is being measured in their seroepidemiological studies."[40] To Ian Munro, the editor of *The Lancet,* Gallo complained that "No one has been able to work with their particles," because LAV had never been grown in a continuous cell line.[41] On the other hand, Gallo's own "very very exciting" blood test results showed that more than 95 percent of AIDS patients had antibodies to the new virus, which he now had isolated from more than forty patients.

Marjorie Guroff's manuscript showing tiny percentages of AIDS patients infected with HTLV-1 was still awaiting publication at *The Lancet,* and Gallo told Munro he was worried "that other data we will submit for publication in the future might be misinterpreted if we published this paper now." Fearing the Guroff manuscript "will be construed as negative to *all* HTLV," Gallo asked that it be placed on hold. "I need some time," he said, "to think about the best way to present this to avoid confusion."

On French soil Gallo was more charitable. At a scientific conference in Marseille a few days after the code-breaking in Bethesda, Gallo spoke for the first time in public about "a virus that we call HTLV-3." Gallo described his new virus as "very similar to what Jean-Claude Chermann, Montagnier, and Sinoussi-Barré [*sic*] have reported in the literature earlier, identifying in a patient with AIDS and a few more." But Gallo claimed to be far ahead of the French. "We have many isolates of '3,'" he told his audience. "Their genes are being cloned, and being compared to 1 and 2.[j] These three form distinct groups, but they are all related to each other. They all belong to the HTLV family."

Montagnier wasn't in Marseille, but Gallo telephoned him from somewhere on the Côte d'Azur. "He said he had a virus growing to very high titer on a continuous cell line," Montagnier recalled, "and he believed it was the cause of AIDS." It was the first Montagnier had heard that Mika Popovic had infected a continuous cell line with the AIDS virus, and Montagnier recalled telling Gallo that he, too, had LAV growing in a continuous B-cell line. But when Montagnier asked whether Gallo had compared HTLV-3 to LAV, Gallo didn't reply.[42]

When word of Gallo's remarks in Marseille reached Bethesda, Vince DeVita began worrying — as it happened, with good reason — about the premature disclosure of what promised to be the most important discovery in the history of the National Cancer Institute.[43]

"Bob was wheeling and dealing," DeVita said. "People would call me up, tell me these sorts of things. I had never any doubt, quite frankly, that he had already told plenty of people. My real concern was Ed Brandt. Ed Brandt was a very good assistant secretary, maybe the best I've ever seen. He was always fair with us. I said to Bob Gallo, 'You're not going to blindside Ed Brandt. He's going to know what's going on. The minute you have something written on paper, you and I are going downtown.'"

In keeping with the historic occasion, Gallo hoped to publish not just one or two articles about his historic discovery, but a set of four articles in *Science*, the most from a single laboratory ever to appear simultaneously. The lead article would feature Mika Popovic's discovery that the AIDS virus could be grown in a continuous T-cell line. As a reward for his labors, Gallo had agreed to let Popovic attend one of the UCLA ski meetings, and after a long string of twelve-hour days Popovic was looking forward to "a nice vacation in the mind."

Before leaving for Park City, Popovic finished a draft of his *Science* paper, and when Gallo returned from Marseille he found it waiting on his desk. Popovic's manuscript began by noting that "a new variant of HTLV," called LAV, had recently been isolated from a patient with lymphadenopathy in Paris. Using LAV as a "reference virus," Popovic had begun searching for a T-cell line in which the AIDS virus could grow without killing the cells.

Two such lines had been found, one of which Popovic had cloned fifty-one times. The manuscript didn't identify the cell line, but it reported that the AIDS virus had grown best in three of its clones: H-4, H-6, and H-9. In fact, the H-4 cell line had been producing virus continuously since the previous November. But Popovic didn't say where the AIDS virus that infected those clones had come from.

Explaining that, in his paper, LAV would be called HTLV-3, Popovic's manuscript recounted his search for an AIDS virus of his own. He had found HTLV-3 in the cells of four AIDS patients, code-named R.F., B.K., L.S., and W.T., sent to Bethesda by a University of Pennsylvania clinician, James Hoxie.[44] When Popovic thawed Hoxie's cells and cultured them according to the methods he had used with LAV, there had been some reverse transcriptase activity. Before the cultures could die, Popovic had transmitted the viruses they contained to H-4 or H-9.[k] Antibody tests had confirmed that the cells were producing the AIDS virus, although with the exception of R.F. at very low levels.[45] A fifth culture, from the North Carolina hemophiliac, S.N., had briefly produced low levels of virus and it, too, was included in the *Science* paper.[l]

Popovic flew to Utah on March 18, 1984, a Sunday. The following Friday, he got a message to call Gallo at once.[46] When Popovic found a phone, he learned that Gallo had major problems with his manuscript, especially Popovic's description of his experiments with LAV. If LAV had to be mentioned at all, Gallo said, it should be at the very end of the article, and there were other complaints. Sensing that he was losing control over the presentation of his work, Popovic decided to cut his trip short.

The manuscript Popovic saw when he walked into the lab on Monday afternoon bore little resemblance to the one he had left behind. Entire sentences, even whole paragraphs, had been excised, replaced with Gallo's scrawled additions. Crossed out altogether was the paragraph in which Popovic acknowledged the Pasteur's discovery of LAV and explained that the French virus was "described here" as HTLV-3.

"I just don't believe it," Gallo had written in the margin. "You are absolutely incredible." Also gone was Popovic's description of his use of LAV as a "reference virus" in his search for a permissive T-cell line. Next to that strikeout, Gallo had scribbled "Mika you are crazy."

Gallo's original deadline for the completion of the *Science* manuscripts had been the end of April 1984. Now, Gallo said, the papers were going to be submitted by the end of March. If Popovic's manuscript wasn't finished in a few days, it wouldn't be published with the others.[47]

When Gallo asked Zaki Salahuddin to comment on Popovic's paper, Salahuddin pointed out what he considered a glaring omission: the manuscript said nothing about the patient who was the source of the AIDS virus Popovic had used to infect H-9 and the other clones. Nor did it describe the patient, or patients, from whom the H-4 and H-9 cell lines had been derived. "It is very important," Salahuddin advised Gallo, "for this paper to make the details of this unusual cell line available to the reader."[48]

Salahuddin had just finished drafting his own manuscript for the *Science* package, enumerating the AIDS patients in whom HTLV-3 had been found. Gallo thought Salahuddin's paper important enough that it should follow Popovic's — and also too important for Salahuddin to be the lead author.

"I walked into Gallo's office for something else," Salahuddin recalled, "and he said to me, 'Mika tells me that I should be the first author on your paper.' I said, 'Why doesn't he tell you to be first author on *his* paper?' He said, 'I don't know, but he wants me to be first author on your paper.'"

Salahuddin's paper — now Gallo's paper — made an impressive addition.[49] Titled "Frequent detection and isolation of cytopathic retroviruses (HTLV-3) from patients with AIDS and at risk for AIDS," it reported that HTLV-3 had been "isolated from a total of forty-eight subjects," a prodigious achievement, except that the paper didn't describe any of the forty-eight patients, or provide any information about the viruses their T-cells had supposedly yielded. From the fine print, it wasn't even clear that the forty-eight isolates were the same kind of virus.[m]

The third paper in the series, from a Swiss postdoc named Jorg Schupbach, concluded, on the basis of purported protein similarities with HTLV-1 and HTLV-2, that HTLV-3 was "a true member of the HTLV family." The fourth and last paper contained the results of Sarngadharan's ELISA testing, reporting antibodies to HTLV-3 in 88 percent of AIDS patients and 78 percent of those with pre-AIDS. It was those data, Sarngadharan had written, which "suggest that HTLV-3 is the primary cause of AIDS."[50]

Gallo's remarks in Marseille had caused consternation that continued to reverberate at the Pasteur. Was the virus Gallo called HTLV-3 the same as LAV? If so, had Gallo therefore simply confirmed Pasteur's discovery? Or was HTLV-3 somehow different from LAV, in which case either the French were wrong or AIDS patients were infected with two different viruses? "The CDC knows the results of Gallo," recalled Jean-Claude Chermann. "The CDC knows our results, but we were not knowing the results of Gallo."[51]

Chermann wanted a tripartite meeting in Paris, with Don Francis present, at which the data from the blood testing in both labs could be examined by everyone involved. When Francis called Gallo to set up the meeting, "I said, 'Look, you're going to be in Switzerland on such and such a day. Can we meet in Paris the next day?' Bob said, 'Sure, that'll be fine.' I said, "'Well, I'll fly over then and we'll all be there.'" Francis also remembered telling Gallo that his lab, the Pasteur, and the CDC had "all scored identically, all three labs," on the same group of blood samples.

When Gallo called Francis a few days later to confirm the meeting date, he took the opportunity to complain about the French. Montagnier was in the newspapers every day talking about LAV, Gallo said. But the French had better have what he, Gallo, had, or there was going to be "a major battle." Even if the French did have the same virus, Gallo had more isolates than Montagnier. Gallo intended to say more in public about his work soon, but he was concerned that his discoveries be kept confidential until then. If he made a premature announcement, his discovery might be stolen by other NIH scientists.[52]

The day the four manuscripts from Gallo's lab were delivered to *Science,* Gallo and Vince DeVita were ushered into Ed Brandt's office in the Hubert H. Humphrey Building, the labyrinthine headquarters of the Department of Health and Human Services at the foot of Capitol Hill. After Gallo offered a brief summary of his discoveries, Brandt said he'd like to keep copies of the manuscripts for later perusal. Gallo hesitated. Could Brandt be trusted? Gallo asked DeVita.[53]

By the time Ed Brandt saw Mika Popovic's manuscript, it had gone through at least eight drafts. According to the latest version, the source of Popovic's H-9 cell line was now identified: a previously unheard-of cell line, "HT," that had been established from the cells of "an adult with lymphoid leukemia." Any suggestion that Popovic had used LAV in his experiments, or that LAV might be the cause of AIDS, had vanished. The only reference to LAV was now in the next-to-last paragraph, and it sounded as though the French had the wrong virus:

A few T-lymphocyte retroviruses that differed from HTLV-1 and HTLV-2, but were associated with lymphadenopathy syndrome were detected earlier. One such virus, called LAV, was reported to be unrelated to HTLV-1 or -2. Moreover, serum samples from 37.5 percent of patients with AIDS were found to react with it. In contrast, HTLV-3 is related to HTLV-1 and -2 and, by all criteria, this new virus belongs to the HTLV family of retroviruses. In addition, more than 85 percent of serum samples from AIDS patients are reactive with proteins of HTLV-3. These findings suggest that HTLV-3 and LAV may be different. However, it is possible that this is due to insufficient characterization of LAV because the virus has not yet been transmitted to a permanently growing cell line for true isolation and therefore has been difficult to obtain in quantity.[54]

Popovic was distressed by what Gallo had done to his manuscript.[n] "I thought it would be better, far better," Popovic said later, "that we would refer to the LAV data and would be included in the paper. I mentioned it several times."[55]

Gallo's first destination in Europe was Zurich, for a conference sponsored by the pharmaceutical firm SmithKline Beecham.[56] The evening before, Gallo joined several of the other speakers, including Murray Gardner, for dinner at the Hotel Dolder. One of the diners, a Swiss physician named Michel Glauser, recalled the highlight of the meal as a "vivid discussion between Gardner and Gallo about the discovery of a new virus responsible for AIDS."

The subject had come up, Glauser said, after Gardner mentioned that he had just discovered a virus responsible for an AIDS-like disease in monkeys known as simian AIDS, or SAIDS. Not to be outdone, Gallo retorted that *he* had discovered the virus responsible for AIDS in *humans*. When pressed for details by his dinner companions Gallo had demurred, explaining that "he could not mention this discovery before a public announcement later in April or May."[57]

Gallo was more forthcoming during his talk the next day, illustrated with slides of HTLV-1, HTLV-2, and a picture of "the new one. We call it HTLV-3." Gallo had "a lot" of isolates of HTLV-1 from AIDS patients, one of HTLV-2, and "a lot" of HTLV-3. "We're focusing on this," he said, pointing to a micrograph of HTLV-3. "There is not time, nor is it yet proper for me to discuss this data with you. But if you're interested, I recommend following the literature over the next few months carefully, and the story will be told in some detail."

As Gallo finished talking, Professor Walter Siegenthaler, the head of the German Society of Internal Medicine, rose to his feet. Siegenthaler had been at dinner the night before, and he knew there was more to the story. "If you could just say a few words more," Siegenthaler implored, "about the HTLV-3?"

"I'll say what I can," Gallo replied. "The truth is, we know quite a bit about the virus. In fact, the genes are cloned of it. But it needs to go properly into the literature first. I can't discuss openly yet everything about it. I'll tell you what I feel comfortable about. We have now over fifty of this virus. The genes are fairly well characterized . . . when you analyze the genome, it clearly and conclusively is in the HTLV family."

The breakthrough, Gallo said, had occurred when Mika Popovic had learned to transmit the AIDS virus "to a particular cell line developed in our lab. That happens to be HT, a new line." For anyone wondering about reports of an AIDS virus from France, Gallo said, he was still trying to determine whether HTLV-3 was "related to what in the Pasteur Institute is called LAV."

Gallo, who had helped shepherd the Pasteur's first paper into *Science,* enthusiastically endorsing its publication and making changes along the way, now declared that the French paper hadn't been "up to snuff. I got some criticisms for its acceptance. But the virus that was published had morphology that was interesting and peculiar. The protein data was obscure at best. The serological data indicated 20 percent of normal homosexuals, 20 percent of AIDS — not so good."

The Pasteur paper hadn't contained any serological data, but Gallo continued his critique. "There was no further characterization of the virus," he said. "They had trouble doing things with it. They came to my lab first to learn the technology for T-cell growth. And the idea was, we would collaborate with them if they got an isolate. Dr. Montagnier wanted us to collaborate if it was in the HTLV family, because then we would have probes to get it. What he first sent to us had no relationship to HTLV. I frankly didn't believe very much, because I believe all human retroviruses are in that family. So I kind of dismissed it."

Gallo conceded that LAV "looks very similar" to HTLV-3. "And also," he added, "I have heard recently that their serological data has gotten very good, almost as good as I know we have with these. So the two may come together." But Gallo wondered whether the virus the

French had been using in their recent blood testing was the same virus they claimed to have discovered in 1983.

"Now what did they send us before?" Gallo asked. "Was it the same virus? I don't know. Did they have something else and get this now? Or was it that they just couldn't grow it? They never were able to grow it very well, they say. So they may have just not really had virus. They have a picture, then they go to give it out and they give out not very much of anything. That may have been the problem. What you need to do is convince the world. I think that is going to happen."

The morning after the Zurich conference found Gallo and Murray Gardner on the same Swissair flight to Paris. But Gardner recalled that there was no chance to talk, because Gallo was sitting in first class and Gardner in economy. The first item on Gallo's agenda when he arrived at Pasteur was yet another lecture, before what Simon Wain-Hobson recalled as an overflow audience in the Amphithéâtre Jacques Monod.

"I was told before the lecture by Montagnier and Chermann, and by others behind their back, that they had no credibility," Gallo said later. "No one believed their results. I was grabbed by Harvey Eisen, who told me, why did I allow Montagnier to introduce me? Nobody here believes anything he says. He said some things much worse than that, that I won't repeat."[58]

Gallo recalled closing his talk with a picture of HTLV-3 and stating that "I was sure it caused AIDS, and that almost surely it was the same as their isolate from a case of lymphadenopathy called LAV. The mood was jubilant. It was like the archangel came down and blessed them." But Simon Wain-Hobson remembered the occasion differently.[o] "Gallo was saying maybe HTLV-3 and LAV are two different viruses," Wain-Hobson recalled. "I remember sitting down and talking to Montagnier and saying, 'It's clearly the same thing.' We were all naive. We had never been in the big leagues. We didn't know how all this worked."

A week before Gallo's arrival in Paris, a young Pasteurian named Marc Alizon had obtained the first partial clone of LAV.[59] Barely out of medical school, and knowing next to nothing about molecular biology, Alizon had taken a chance by joining Wain-Hobson's group. "People were not sure that LAV was really a retrovirus," Alizon recalled. "But I had nothing to lose. I wanted to be at the Pasteur Institute."

From Pierre Tiollais's lab Wain-Hobson enlisted another fledgling doctor, Pierre Sonigo, a medical school classmate of Alizon's who shared his affinity for black leather jackets and large Japanese motor-cycles. The pair had struggled long into the night to master cloning technology, and they had finally succeeded in cloning a part of LAV's full complement of DNA. "It would have gone faster if a whole team had decided to put their arms into it," Wain-Hobson said later. "But we got no help."

Still, after months of frustration and obscurity, the French were on a comparative roll. Montagnier's paper linking LAV to the Equine Infectious Anemia Virus, a demonstration that LAV was a lentivirus and not a leukemia virus, at last had appeared in print, not in *Nature* or *Science* but in the *Annals of Virology*.[60] A second paper, a bio-chemical characterization of LAV's reverse transcriptase, had been accepted by another journal.[61] A week before Gallo's arrival, the French had published a major paper in *The Lancet,* reporting the iso-lation of the AIDS virus from Eric Loiseau and his brother, also a hemophiliac.

The *Lancet* paper, the most important publication on AIDS from any laboratory, opened the first window onto the epidemic to come.[62] While seventeen-year-old Eric Loiseau had AIDS, his thirteen-year-old brother was healthy. But there was no doubt the two had become infected at almost the same time, via the contaminated blood-clotting factor with which they were regularly injected.

That the younger Loiseau still hadn't developed any symptoms of AIDS could only mean that the virus took longer — in this case, years longer — to cause disease in some patients than others. That, in turn, could only mean there were uncounted gay men, intravenous drug users, hemophiliacs, and transfusion recipients who were unwittingly carrying, and spreading, the AIDS virus — the "asymptomatic carrier state" that would make the AIDS epidemic one of the most insidious in history.

The article also contained the first description of how the Pasteur ELISA was made and how it worked, and it reported that antibodies to LAV were "widely distributed in the population at risk of AIDS." With the *Lancet* article and Marc Alizon's success, Montagnier's group had been in something approaching a celebratory mood. But when Gallo, Murray Gardner, Don Francis, Barré, and Chermann retreated to Montagnier's office, the atmosphere immediately chilled.

Francis had brought an eleven-page, single-spaced computer printout showing the final results of the competition between the Pas-teur and Gallo ELISAs.[63] Murray Gardner, invited into the room as an arbiter, remembered the moment as "electrifying," proof beyond a doubt that the cause of AIDS had been found both in Paris and Bethesda.[64] For Montagnier and the French, "it was confirmation of what we already knew, that we had the virus first."

Gallo later denied having seen the CDC printout or learning anything about the French blood test data.[p] But Don Francis recalled "three or four fingers going down these columns, looking at the similarities and dissimilarities. Gallo was standing right there. He certainly was part of the conversation. We were going 'Look, Bob, here's one with a variation, here's one that's really different.' A couple of them were quite different. Most of them were remarkably similar."

Montagnier and Gardner remembered a heated discussion between Gallo and Francis over what the data meant, ending with Gallo's abrupt insistence that Don Francis leave the room. Murray Gardner recalled being told by Gallo, "You keep this guy away."[65] According to Montagnier, Gallo insisted that "'Don Francis is not a retrovirologist and he has to go out.' Don Francis told him that CDC has also this LAV-like virus in culture. And Gallo said, 'That's nothing. You have only one isolate. We have forty-eight isolates.'" Chermann's memory agreed with Montagnier's. "Gallo don't want to discuss with the CDC," Chermann said. "Don Francis has to leave, and we were discussing, Gallo, Montagnier, and myself, about the results directly. It was exactly the same results from the CDC, Pasteur, and NCI."[66]

Once alone with Montagnier, Chermann, and Barré, Gallo had a surprise. "He said he had several papers to be published shortly in *Science*," recalled Montagnier, "and he didn't know exactly how this would be announced, that perhaps a press conference would be done."[67] The way Gallo remembered the moment, "I said, 'Look, one thing. Don't panic if I get attention. And I'm going to get attention. Don't panic. A month later we'll come back and make a joint announcement. I'll analyze your virus and we'll go together.'"

When Montagnier asked Gallo, again, why he hadn't already compared HTLV-3 with LAV, in order to be able to say in *Science* whether the two viruses were one and the same or whether he had discovered something new, Gallo replied that Popovic hadn't been able to grow enough LAV to make any comparisons.[68] The day ended with a tour of the Pasteur's newly completed facility for growing large quantities of LAV, a prelude to the commercial production of the French ELISA by a new Pasteur subsidiary, Diagnostics Pasteur. Françoise Barré remembered everyone, including Gallo, drinking champagne to christen the lab.

As the visitors walked out through the Pasteur's front gate, Gallo caught up with Don Francis. "He told me, 'Well, I guess we've all got it now,'" Francis said. But during the long evening that ensued, Gallo apparently had second thoughts. Distressed by the contretemps in Montagnier's office, Chermann had tried to restore some comity by inviting everyone to join him in a night on the town, dinner followed by a lavish floor show at a tourist nightspot, the Paradis Latin. Montagnier, Barré, and Gardner declined, but Gallo, Don Francis, and David Klatzmann were game.

Much later, finding himself alone with Chermann in the *pissoir*, Gallo suggested cutting Francis and the CDC out of the forthcoming announcement. "We can do this together," Chermann remembered Gallo saying. "We don't need CDC."

Chermann let the remark pass, and when the Paradis Latin closed its doors Gallo and Francis retired to the Club Meditel, a small hotel for visiting physicians around the corner from the Pasteur. Over coffee and croissants the next morning, Gallo offered Francis the same proposition he had made to Chermann.

"He told me, 'You and I can do this together.'" Francis recalled. "'We don't need the French.'"[69]

"Our Eminent Dr. Robert Gallo"

Murray Gardner, convinced beyond a doubt that the French had been first to find the cause of AIDS,[1] remembered a nervous Robert Gallo rushing to catch the early-afternoon plane to Washington. "He was saying, 'I've got to get back home and get my lab working on this stuff,'" Gardner recalled.[2] The Institut Pasteur already was setting up commercial production of its LAV ELISA, and if the Americans didn't want to relinquish the AIDS blood-testing market to the French they would have to come up with a commercial AIDS test of their own.

The AIDS virus used for experiments in Gallo's lab was being grown in relatively small amounts by Gallo's contract laboratories. But commercial production of an ELISA would require much larger quantities of the virus Gallo called HTLV-3. Those could only be produced in the huge stainless-steel fermentation vats at the NCI facility in Frederick, Maryland, used by the army to develop its fearsome biological weapons before large portions of Fort Detrick had been ceded to the NCI by Richard Nixon as part of the War on Cancer.

The day after Gallo's return home, a Frederick researcher named Larry Arthur made the 75-mile round trip to Bethesda to bring back a sample of HTLV-3B, the AIDS virus strain with which Gallo's lab was performing its ELISAs and conducting other experiments.[a] But Mika Popovic didn't think 3B was the right choice for a commercial AIDS test.

"I, personally, as well as Betsy, told 'Let's take out the prototype, the R.F.,'" Popovic recalled. "Dr. Gallo told no, we have to rush because it is a blood bank assay. We have to give that one, HTLV-3B, because this one is the best one at this time."[3]

R.F. was Roland Ferdinand, a Haitian immigrant dying of AIDS in a Philadelphia hospital, whose cells had been sent to Gallo by Jim Hoxie the previous November.* None of the other four patient samples mentioned in *Science* had yielded more than transient amounts of virus. But after a month Betsy Read noticed that R.F. was producing "multinucleated giant cells," a precursor of T-cell death and something Read had observed before — virus-infected cells placed in culture, some reverse transcriptase, followed by giant cells, then dead cells.

With no way to "rescue" the viruses infecting those earlier cultures, Read had been forced to watch them die. By late December of 1983, however, she had a life-preserver: HUT-78, the T-cell line in which LAV was growing abundantly.[4] Figuring that if one AIDS virus could flourish in HUT-78 so might another, Read had used what live virus remained in the R.F. culture to infect a flask of HUT-78, "and nursed that along."[5] After an initial "crisis" R.F. had taken hold and continued to grow,[6] though not nearly as well as HTLV-3B. R.F., Read later concluded, was more "cytopathic," quicker to kill the T-cells it infected.

That was one reason Gallo wanted HTLV-3B, his best-growing virus, as the basis for the commercial blood test. But Gallo also favored 3B, he said later, because it was "American instead of Haitian."[7] Mika Popovic still preferred R.F., even though he conceded it wasn't the better candidate.

"Obviously production was lower," Popovic said later. "In order to be in a good position to go ahead with R.F., we needed at least four weeks of work to concentrate on that one, and that wasn't done. At that point still it was in our minds, if we transfer [R.F.] into the large-scale production, to Frederick and so on, would behave cells the same way as in the small scale? We didn't know."[b]

In the end, it was Matt Gonda's repeated failures to see any virus in R.F.'s cells that persuaded Popovic. "If we had to go ahead," Popovic admitted later, "the best was 3B."[8]

The day after HTLV-3B reached Frederick, a reporter from the BBC in London arrived in Gallo's lab. The topic of the interview was human leukemia viruses, but after a few minutes of conversation

---

*Hoxie never revealed his patient's identity, referring to the man only as "R.F."

about HTLV Gallo abruptly changed direction. "He said, 'You don't really want to hear about that, that's old hat,'" recalled the reporter, Martin Redfern. "'What's much more interesting is that we've just discovered the cause of AIDS.'"

Like most science reporters, Redfern had been under the illusion that Gallo believed the cause of AIDS was HTLV-1. "When my hair had flattened on my head again," Redfern said, "I asked him if he was prepared to talk about that. To which he said yes, certainly, the papers would be appearing within a couple of weeks in *Science*." As Redfern's tape recorder turned, Gallo reprised his remarks in Marseille, Zurich, and Paris, mentioning that "about eight or nine months ago, we developed a cell line in our laboratory which is susceptible to infection by these viruses. . . ."[c]

At Gallo's request, Redfern agreed to hold the HTLV-3 story until the *Science* articles were in print. "He then went on to say," Redfern recalled, "that he thought a number of papers in the States, and he mentioned the *New York Times* and the *Washington Post*, were onto the story and might well put it out in the next few days, possibly over the next weekend. He was waiting for someone to call him back — he didn't say who."

Redfern asked whether he was free to report Gallo's discovery if the story broke first somewhere else. "He agreed that if it did, I couldn't be expected to keep what I knew under wraps any longer," Redfern said. "When the interview had finished, and without prompting from me, he said, 'Would you like pre-prints of the papers?' To which I said, 'Dead right.' He went through to his main office and asked one of his colleagues to get them out. The chap's eyes opened rather wide and he said, 'Are you sure? All four of the AIDS papers?' And Gallo said 'Yes, I trust this man.' There were several people around who were a little surprised that he'd given me the story."[9]

Gallo also thought it prudent to outline his discovery for a few influential European scientists who might be miffed if they heard about it first on television. To Harald zur Hausen in Heidelberg, Gallo reported that "the AIDS situation is now very exciting. I can now tell you with some assurance that I believe we have it worked out. It is a variant of HTLV which we call HTLV-3."[10] To Fritz Deinhardt in Munich, Gallo confided that he had had the AIDS virus "isolated for almost two years but couldn't analyze it in a way I would have wanted my name attached to, until a breakthrough in growing it so that we could do the analyses correctly."[11]

Evidently unaware that Gallo already had talked about his discovery to three scientific audiences in Europe and a reporter from the BBC, the NCI's associate director, Peter Fischinger, alerted the NIH's patent attorneys that Gallo had made "a very important invention with world-wide significance." To preserve the government's foreign patent rights for the AIDS blood test, Fischinger said, a patent application would have to be on file before the *Science* papers were in print.[12]

While the NIH lawyers labored over the patent, the Department of Health and Human Services pondered how best to break the good news to an anxious nation. Ed Brandt, having decided the announcement was too important to be left to the Surgeon General, planned to hold a news conference himself once Gallo's four papers were accepted for publication. "I am very pleased to announce," Brandt's prepared statement began, "that intramural scientists at the National Cancer Institute have discovered that variants of a human cancer virus are the primary cause of Acquired Immune Deficiency Syndrome (AIDS)."[d]

Gallo's manuscripts were accepted by *Science* nineteen days after their submission, a process expedited by the journal's biology editor, Ruth Kulstad, who invited Mika Popovic, Prem Sarin, and Sarngadha-ran to her home on the Saturday before publication to go over the page proofs.[13] No other scientist could recall having been invited to a *Science* editor's home for a weekend working session, but for *Science* the Gallo papers represented a singular coup. When Kulstad had dared to suggest that four articles from the same laboratory might be too many, and suggested combining Jorge Schupbach's paper with one of the others, Gallo had reminded Kulstad "of the existence of other journals that would like the papers."[14]

To flesh out Schupbach's paper, Gallo proposed adding a collage of electron micrographs comparing HTLV-1, HTLV-2, and HTLV-3. "Gallo came to me," Zaki Salahuddin recalled, "and he said, 'Make a nice picture to go with the article by the Swiss guy.'" Gallo had plenty of pictures of HTLV-1 and HTLV-2, but pictures of HTLV-3 were harder to come by. Matt Gonda had one hazy micrograph of a virus Salahuddin had isolated from J.S., a soldier at Walter Reed Army Hospital with pre-AIDS, whose cells had survived only long enough to produce what Salahuddin described as "experimental amounts" of virus.[e]

Salahuddin admitted that the J.S. micrograph "wasn't a very good picture," but he insisted on using it to illustrate the paper of which he was now the second author. Gallo agreed, on the condition that Salahuddin come up with another picture of HTLV-3 for the collage. Salahuddin's first thought was the obvious one — use a picture of Popovic's R.F. But despite three tries over a three-month period, Matt Gonda had never seen any virus in R.F.'s cells — a result that sent Popovic into a fury.[15] "He was extremely antagonistic," Gonda recalled. "He kept muttering something about, you know, 'You guys are terrible, you are no good, you should be able to find a virus. I don't understand what is wrong with you guys.'"[16]

When Salahuddin, desperate, called Gonda's lab in search of *any* picture of HTLV-3, Gonda's technician took the call, then called Gonda at home. "He said, 'I don't really understand what they want,'" Gonda recalled. "'Maybe you can come in and pick them out.'"[17] Gonda, who was leaving for a European vacation the following day, recalled stopping by the lab on the way to the airport. "I selected the photographs," Gonda said later, "but I didn't know what the samples were. The pictures were brought out and I said, 'Take that one, and that one, and that one.'"

Whatever pictures were chosen that day, the Schupbach manuscript now contained an impressive collage: six electron micrographs comparing HTLV-1 and HTLV-2 with HTLV-3 in different stages of maturation. The pictures of HTLV-1 were identified as the Charlie Robinson isolate, $HTLV_{CR}$, and those of HTLV-2 as Mika Popovic's isolate from the New York cab driver, J.P. But the pictures of HTLV-3 were described only as having come from an unidentified "patient with pre-AIDS," which happened to be the diagnosis of Frédéric Brugière.

Kulstad declined to say who had reviewed and approved the four Gallo manuscripts in so short a time, except that they were "competent authorities." Whoever they were, it must have escaped their attention that none of the four papers contained a clue to the origin of the AIDS virus with which Popovic had infected H-9 and his other T-cell clones, or of the "HT" cell line from which the clones had come.

An astute reader might have noticed that Gallo's conditions for labeling a virus as HTLV-3 were so ambiguous that nearly any retrovirus, animal or human, would have qualified. In light of Popovic's acknowledgment that he had "not yet proved" all the HTLV-3 isolates were the same kind of virus, a perceptive reviewer might even have questioned Gallo's claim to have found the presumptive cause of AIDS. Anyone who attended the Park City meeting might have wondered why none of the 122 footnotes in the four articles referenced the presentation by Jean-Claude Chermann, much less the recent *Lancet* article on the Loiseau brothers. But such questions evidently hadn't been asked.

From Bethesda, Martin Redfern had flown to Boston for interviews at Harvard, the HTLV-3 story "burning a hole in my pocket." Redfern remembered sitting in his hotel room on a Friday morning and thinking that "this is the biggest story I've ever had and probably ever likely to have, and I don't want to be caught with it sitting in my suitcase. Let's have a go at writing it up."

"I knew it was a weekend coming up," Redfern said, "and I was traveling back to London on Sunday. So I thought, 'If it comes out, we don't want to miss the thing by a whole week.' And Gallo had said it might come out in the States over that weekend." BBC correspondents were permitted to write freelance articles for print, and in addition to his broadcast script Redfern typed out a short news story. That done, he telephoned Fred Pierce, the news editor at a London magazine, the *New Scientist*, "who put me onto a chap called Omar Sattaur, who at that time looked after their AIDS coverage."

"He said, 'Can you read us the story over?'" Redfern recalled. "I dictated it over the phone, from the office of the press person at the Harvard Medical Area. And I gave the same conditions: that Gallo had said it was coming out in *Science* in a couple of weeks and we're not to run it until then unless it breaks in the American newspapers." Redfern arrived back in London, jet-lagged, on Monday morning, April 16, "to the telephone ringing and Omar Sattaur saying, 'Do you want a byline? It's in this week.' To which I said, 'Has it broken, then?' And he said 'Well, there was a piece in the *Wall Street Journal* that sounds as if it's the same story.' And I said 'Well, if you're sure.'"

The *Journal*'s story was brief, reporting mounting speculation "that researchers soon will announce discovery of a new variation of human cancer virus that may cause acquired immune deficiency syndrome."[18] Gallo dismissed the speculation as "premature," but other American papers picked the story up for their Tuesday editions. According to the *Washington Post*, Gallo had found "very strong signs that a newly discovered form of the Human T-Cell Leukemia (HTLV) virus infects victims of AIDS."[19]

As readers in Washington, San Francisco, and several other cities were learning of Gallo's discovery over their Tuesday breakfasts, the first copies of the *New Scientist* containing Martin Redfern's no-longer exclusive story were arriving at news dealers in London.[20] Soon, Redfern's interview with Gallo was being heard around the world. "Next thing I knew," Redfern said, "I was coming in on Wednesday morning to discover my assistant editor in an anxious phone conversation with the director of the National Cancer Institute."

At three in the morning London time, Vince DeVita had awakened a prominent British scientist, Walter Bodmer, who had given DeVita the number of the BBC's science department and gone back to sleep. To Redfern's editor, DeVita was now protesting that Gallo's embargo had been broken, not by the *Wall Street Journal* or the *Washington Post*, but by Martin Redfern, whom Gallo accused of having stolen the four *Science* manuscripts from his office while his back was turned.[f]

The NCI's civilian overseers, the National Cancer Advisory Board, hadn't been officially informed of the triumph about which they were now reading in the papers, and Vince DeVita quickly assembled a package of material and shipped it to each board member by Federal Express for Saturday morning delivery. The *Post* story had mentioned that "promising work" with HTLV variants was also under way in Paris, and DeVita thought it prudent to address the inevitable question of whether Gallo had simply rediscovered what had already been discovered by the French.

"It is not yet clear," DeVita told the NCAB members, "whether the 50 isolates of HTLV-3 are related to the virus or viruses reported by the French scientists. Until more detailed studies of the biochemistry, immunology, and epidemiology of the French virus or viruses are completed, it is not possible to draw the conclusion that they are the same or that they are different." Even if they proved to be the same, DeVita said, Gallo had been "the first to report the ability to isolate the HTLV-3 viruses repeatedly from a large number of AIDS patients."[21]

It wasn't true, but the premature publicity had forced Ed Brandt to scrap plans for announcing Gallo's discovery himself, in favor of a formal news conference by the HHS secretary, Margaret Heckler, who was attending to official duties on the West Coast. While Brandt awaited her return, the press set about tracking Gallo down. They found him at a tumor virus meeting in Cremona, Italy, accompanied by the NIH director, James Wyngaarden, who remembered that Gallo "was up half the night with reporters on the phone." Before the meeting ended, the organizers presented Gallo with a special prize, a plastic telephone. "Cremonians like to brag that they are a city noted for their three t's," Gallo said later. "Their tower, their torte, and a female endowment. We can add a fourth, the telephone."

When Wyngaarden called Ed Brandt to tell Brandt what he already knew, that the Gallo story was leaking everywhere, Brandt replied that Wyngaarden and Gallo should be in Washington for Heckler's news conference the following Monday. Gallo later recalled that, before leaving Cremona, he had showed Robin Weiss his HTLV-3 data, and that Weiss had asked "'Is it the same thing Montagnier described last year?' I said, 'I bet it is. But we're going to publish this now.'"

Wyngaarden also remembered Weiss lecturing Gallo for trying to steal the spotlight from the French; Wyngaarden recalled the moment clearly, he said later, because it was the first he had heard of a French virus called LAV.[22] Robin Weiss didn't remember delivering such a lecture, or seeing Gallo's data, or for that matter learning of Gallo's impending publication in *Science*.[g] What Weiss did recall was telling Gallo about the achievement that was then "uppermost" in his mind — his own success in growing LAV in the CEM T-cell line.[h]

Weiss had gotten hold of LAV after Montagnier, at a meeting in Brussels, appealed to his audience for help in convincing the scientific world that LAV was the cause of AIDS. Anyone who wished to work with the French virus was welcome to it, Montagnier said, who offered to send a technician from the Pasteur along with the virus to demonstrate how it should be grown.[23]

Weiss wasn't at the meeting, but when he heard about the appeal he told Montagnier he wanted to try infecting some T-cell lines at his laboratory in London.[24] "I thought, 'OK, he claims it's a retrovirus,'" Weiss recalled. "'We're quite good with retroviruses. Let's have a go.'" By the time of Cremona, the LAV-infected CEM line in Weiss's London lab was throwing off two million counts of reverse transcriptase.[i]

As Gallo and Wyngaarden arranged their hasty return, a young attorney, Bill Bundren, was still sweating over the patent application for the Gallo AIDS test. "We got the *Science* manuscripts either Thursday evening or Friday morning," recalled Bundren, whose small patent-law firm worked under contract to NIH. "They were messengered over to us. We were told that a press conference would occur on Monday morning, and that it had to be on file by then."

HHS had asked Bundren to prepare a single patent application. But as he began to absorb the material in the *Science* articles, Bundren realized there would have to be two patents, one for the blood test and another for the HT cell line.[25] "I wrote those things over the Easter weekend," Bundren said. "Some people never get groundshaking patent applications during their career. You know that one's come in, and you only have a couple of days to do the best job you can. You know that something everybody's going to read could be better."

In return for the exclusive right to make, sell, and profit from an invention, prospective inventors are obliged to tell the United States Patent and Trademark Office whatever they know about previous work by others in the same field —"prior art," in the archaic terminology of the patent laws.[26] Bill Bundren hadn't been given time to do a search of the scientific literature, and although he spent much of the weekend in consultation with Sarngadharan, the Gallo applications didn't reference a single one of Pasteur's eleven presentations or publications on LAV.[j]

Neither did they mention the existence of the Pasteur blood test, although by the time Bundren drew up the blood-test patent the French had been testing blood for LAV antibodies for nearly nine months, and had described their ELISA in *The Lancet* only two weeks before. "We didn't know anybody was working on it, other than Gallo," Bundren said later.[k] Nor had Bundren been aware that the CDC, a branch of HHS, the agency in whose name the patents were being sought, had found the French ELISA to be more accurate than Gallo's. Or that Montagnier had begun growing LAV in a B-cell line at almost the same time Popovic had done the same with HUT-78. Or, as Jim Wyngaarden had learned in Cremona, that Robin Weiss's LAV-infected CEM line was already producing industrial quantities of virus in London and Paris.[27]

Vince DeVita had obtained Ed Brandt's assurance that Brandt wouldn't tell the CDC about Gallo's discovery, lest Curran, Don Francis, and Cy Cabradilla try to expedite publication of their own isolations from the transfusion pair. Despite Brandt's promise, a few days before Margaret Heckler's return to Washington word reached

Atlanta that something was up in Bethesda. When Jim Curran tried to call Gallo, a secretary said she had no idea where Gallo was.[28] The call was returned hours later by Prem Sarin, who mentioned that four papers on HTLV-3 would soon appear in *Science.*

Only when Curran called *Science* did the CDC learn about Secretary Heckler's impending news conference. "We had *no* idea," recalled Curran's boss, Walt Dowdle. "Gallo had given us no indication he was ready to come out with anything. The French had made their data available, they had talked about their data in the open. They came to CDC, and we had come away convinced that they had the AIDS agent. We were concerned that whatever was said at the press conference, it should be said that the French had similar data and had published similar data. And so we told [CDC director Jim] Mason."

Mason had an appointment that same afternoon with Lawrence K. Altman, the medical correspondent of the *New York Times,* that had been arranged a month or so before when Altman checked in with Mason to see what was new with the LAV story. Mason explained that the CDC's blood samples were being tested with LAV and HTLV-3, but that it was too early to say anything for sure. "He said, 'There's still a chance that this thing isn't real,'" Altman recalled. "He said, 'We have to compare these results, and if they don't compare it's not going to be the same thing.'" Mason suggested Altman drop by CDC sometime in the next few weeks, and Altman agreed. "I was going to be in Alabama anyway," Altman said, "and I said I would come by on the way back and talk over all of this stuff. Don Francis had been over in Paris talking to Montagnier, to iron out the results of what was done at CDC and what was done in Paris. Things heated up while I was in Alabama, and I came to Atlanta on a Friday."

Unlike most medical writers, Larry Altman was a physician, and before becoming a journalist he had spent three years as an epidemiologist at the CDC. The Pasteur's *Science* paper had caught his attention, and the progress of the work in Paris had remained on Altman's list of stories to pursue. "In the year since Montagnier's paper, I had gotten no one, but no one, to support his virus," Altman said. "So I couldn't write much about it. Everybody said, 'Oh, that's just one more paper, there's no belief in it.' I always thought there was something to it. Don Francis will tell you how, over and over again, I kept yelling at him, 'What about this virus?'"

Altman hadn't been at Park City for Chermann's talk, but he had sensed some movement in the story. "I began hearing things," Altman said. "But I didn't hear it as 'Oh, boy, this is it.' It moved from cold to simmer, it moved up in degrees. But it's clearly what I was nosing in on by the time of Mason's interview. What they were saying was what I had long suspected."

In Mason's office on the afternoon of Friday, April 20, Altman learned that the CDC's transatlantic blood testing had established both LAV and HTLV-3 as the presumptive cause of AIDS. As Altman walked out of Mason's door with the story in his notebook, Don Francis and Jim Curran were walking in with the news that Margaret Heckler was going to announce Gallo's discovery of the AIDS virus on Monday. What followed, Curran said, "were a lot of discussions about what the French did, what we did, who did what and what the impact of the articles would be."

Borrowing Mason's telephone, Curran and Francis warned Ed Brandt that Heckler was about to make a huge mistake: the French, not Gallo, had been first to find the cause of AIDS, and the CDC had confirmed the French discovery by isolating viruses from the transfusion pair that were identical to LAV. "The line I used," Francis recalled, "was that this is going to look really silly, for the United States government to describe that they have the cause of AIDS. And a few weeks later another agency, namely us, publishes in the same journal that they have evidence that a virus causes AIDS and it's identical to the French isolate." According to Francis, Brandt's response was, "'I understand what you're saying. I'll look into it.'"

Back in his hotel room, Larry Altman went over his notes. All the news stories appearing in the last few days had been about Gallo's impending announcement of an AIDS-causing variant of HTLV. Now Altman had been told that AIDS was caused by a virus that *wasn't* HTLV, and that had been discovered in France more than a year before. "I talked to the science desk that night," Altman said, "and there was no way we could get the story into the Saturday paper under any circumstances. They decided they wanted to go with it for the Sunday paper. At that time I knew nothing, and so far as I knew neither Mason nor anyone else there knew anything, about the press conference the following week."

Altman found out when he called Mason early on Saturday morning, at home. "I said, 'I just want to be sure, I want to repeat to you, so there's no misunderstanding, that this is what you're saying,'" Altman recalled. "At that point he had heard there was going to be something coming up the next week. I think he found out on Friday night. He asked me if I could hold the story and I said no, because the interview took place before." Mason remembered telling Altman that if the story appeared, "I'd probably get fired."[29]

Larry Altman wasn't the only reporter onto the LAV story, as Mal Martin learned when he got a call from Gallo that evening at home. "It was about 10:30 on Saturday night," Martin recalled. "He said, 'You're in big trouble with people downtown in the department. They're really upset with you. Who the hell are you to go to reporters and tell them about a retrovirus as the cause of AIDS?'"

Martin, the NIAID lab chief who had allowed Françoise Barré to speak at Cold Spring Harbor, had stopped at the Pasteur a few days before, on his way home from a lecture tour of India. "I had never met Montagnier," Martin recalled. "They showed me the results. I said, 'This sounds really interesting. Can you give me some virus?' They gave me all this material. When I came back to the United States I told some of my friends what I'd learned in France."[1]

Along with the sample of LAV, Martin had smuggled a substantial quantity of unpasteurized French cheese through customs, and he was hosting a wine-and-cheese party when the telephone rang. "I told Gallo, 'Look, I don't want to talk to you now,'" Martin recalled. "'I have a bunch of people in my house. If you want to, call me in the morning.'"

The source of Gallo's agitation wasn't Larry Altman's story, which was just beginning to hit the street in New York and didn't quote Martin anyway, but a shorter report that had moved on the Associated Press wire a few hours before. By the time the AP reporter called, Martin had read the reprints of the Pasteur's articles given him by Montagnier. "Gallo was as usual not around," Martin said. "He was out of the country or something. I didn't know anything about Gallo, and I told this guy, 'I don't know what he has.' Then he said he knew that I knew something about a retrovirus and AIDS. And I said, 'Well, yes I do.' And I proceeded to read him the abstracts of these various papers from Pasteur."

"Researchers in the United States and France," the AP story began, "have strong, new evidence that a type of virus first identified in AIDS patients in France last year might be the long-sought cause of the deadly disease." The story quoted Martin as calling LAV "the best game in town." Both the CDC and Gallo, the AP said, had "subsequently isolated from their AIDS patients viruses that they believe are identical to the French virus."[30]

At eight-thirty Sunday morning, Gallo phoned Martin again. "Every magazine, every newspaper is calling," Gallo said later. "What do I arrive and see? Headlines, Pasteur and CDC and quotes all over the place of Mal Martin. What the hell, is Mal Martin involved in this? What is going on? So, the tension level, the blood pressure, was way up. I didn't know what the heck to do. I had no collection of my thoughts."[31]

"He proceeded in his usual way," Martin recalled, "all the threats and all the other bullshit. I said, 'Look, if you want to talk that way I'll hang up.' So Gallo ranted and raved at me, and then *he* hung up. And then he called me back three minutes later. He said, 'Now I know who the real bad guys are.' I said, 'Who's that?' And he asked if I had seen the *New York Times*."

Larry Altman's story appeared at the bottom of page one, under a two-column headline: "Federal Official Says He Believes Cause of AIDS Has Been Found."[32] Mason was quoted as saying that "I believe we have the cause of AIDS, and it is an exciting discovery. The public needs to know that this is a breakthrough and that it is significant."

Mason couldn't explain why it had taken so long for the significance of the French work to be recognized, or why there had been "so little excitement in the scientific community when the French came up with their announcement last May." Not until Chermann's presentation at Park City, Mason said, had American scientists become enthusiastic about LAV.

The *Times* story didn't mention Gallo until the twentieth paragraph. "Federal health officials," it said, "have scheduled a news conference in Washington for 1 P.M. Monday, presumably to discuss findings made by an AIDS researcher, Dr. Robert Gallo, and his colleagues at the National Cancer Institute concerning a retrovirus they have reportedly called HTLV-3. It is believed to be different from another retrovirus called HTLV-1 that had been a focus of research into AIDS. A report by Dr. Gallo's group is scheduled to be published soon in the journal *Science*." Altman couldn't reach Gallo for comment. But his story quoted scientists "familiar with the research" as saying HTLV-3 and LAV were simply different names for the same virus.

Martin hadn't yet seen the *Times* story when Gallo called. Neither had Ed Brandt.[33] But the morning was still young when Brandt heard from Heckler's chief of staff, C. McLain Haddow. Brandt didn't like Haddow, and talked to him "as little as possible," but on this occasion he had no choice. Brandt remembered that Haddow had "turned the air blue," shouting that Mason's comments to Altman had been "a deliberate embarrassment" to the secretary and demanding that Mason be fired. When Brandt refused, Haddow told him the secretary wanted Mason in Washington the next day.

Mason flew from Atlanta to Washington on Sunday night, coincidentally on the same plane as Larry Altman. When he arrived at HHS headquarters on Monday morning, Mason said later, "I really got in the doghouse. They took me to the woodshed as soon as I got up there. It was not a very happy moment. When Altman interviewed me, I wouldn't have cared if it had been on the record, because I didn't know what was going on at NIH. But when it got to the weekend, I could see a real problem if he put out something that got in front of Margaret Heckler."

With him Mason brought a memo prepared by Fred Murphy, the legendary CDC officer who had identified the Ebola virus and who now ran the agency's Center for Infectious Diseases. "CONFIDEN-TIAL," the memo began. "For use only by Dr. Mason in his one-on-one meeting with Dr. Brandt, 4-23-84." The memo recounted the extensive blood testing done in collaboration with Pasteur and Gallo, and pointed out that "a high proportion" of people with AIDS or pre-AIDS had been found to be infected with LAV "or a related virus."

As recalled by Brandt, Mason described the comparative blood testing with the French and Gallo viruses and the ELISA with which the French had conducted their part of the study — the same invention on which HHS was shortly to apply for a patent.[34] When Mason finished running over Murphy's points, his job was safe. "I was convinced he believed the Pasteur scientists deserved the credit he gave them in the *New York Times*," Brandt said. "I learned from him that day that they both had the virus and a blood test."

As for LAV and HTLV-3, Brandt recalled that "after hearing the CDC, the only conclusion I could come to was just that the two were identical." By then it was "too late" to pull back the Gallo patent or to stop Margaret Heckler's press conference. "Whatever the French had done," Brandt said, "we had done certain things. No one said, 'Don't hold the press conference.'"

But Mason insisted that if the secretary were going ahead, she give credit to the Pasteur in her remarks. "I was upset when I saw the draft," Mason recalled. "Because it didn't mention the French. I felt it was in Heckler's best interest if she acknowledged their contribution. I just argued that it deserved to be in there."

While Bill Bundren hustled the patent documents across the Potomac River to the U.S. Patent Office in Virginia, Margaret Heckler, her voice hoarse from the effects of a lingering cold, accorded Gallo and DeVita a personal moment; "commending him for his work and that kind of stuff," Brandt recalled. As Gallo and DeVita were leaving, Heckler asked them to look over her prepared statement, which thanks to Mason had a new fifteenth paragraph.[35]

"And as is so often the case in scientific pursuit," it read, "other discoveries have occurred in different laboratories — even in different parts of the world — which will ultimately contribute to the goal we all seek: the conquest of AIDS. I especially want to cite the efforts of the Pasteur Institute in France, which has in part been working in collaboration with the National Cancer Institute. They have previously identified a virus which they have linked to AIDS patients, and within the next few weeks we will know with certainty whether that virus is the same one identified through the NCI's work. We believe it will prove to be the same."

According to Mac Haddow, the paragraph had been added over Gallo's "strenuous" objections. "Gallo called me," Haddow said later. "He was very specific: 'You can't give credit to the French.'" The offending paragraph, Haddow said, was deleted from Heckler's copy of her statement — but not from the copies that had already been prepared for distribution to the press. "It was at the last minute that that stuff was taken out," he said. "There wasn't time to make changes and Xerox new copies."[m]

The reporters who filed into HHS headquarters on the afternoon of April 23, 1984, were handed a four-page news release, headlined "NCI Isolates AIDS Virus," and preprints of Gallo's four *Science* articles.[36] At the podium stood Margaret Heckler in her trademark red suit, biting her lip. To Heckler's left were Gallo and Jim Mason. On her right sat Vince DeVita, Jim Wyngaarden, Peter Fischinger, and Ed Brandt, who remembered thinking that Heckler seemed more nervous than usual.[37]

"As I believe you anticipate," Heckler began, "this press conference will be devoted to the subject of AIDS, in which area there is, of course, important news. But unfortunately we have not made similar breakthroughs in the field of laryngitis, so I apologize for the state of my voice today." The important news, Heckler explained, was that "the probable cause of AIDS has been found, a variant of a known human cancer virus called HTLV-3." Not only had the AIDS virus been identified, "a new process has been developed to mass produce this virus."

> This discovery is crucial because it enables us for the first time to characterize the agent in detail and to understand its behavior. Thirdly, with discovery of both the virus and this new process, we now have a blood test for AIDS which we hope can be widely available within about six months. We have applied for the patent on this process today. With the blood test, we can identify AIDS victims with essentially 100 percent certainty. Thus, we should be able to ensure that blood for transfusion is free from AIDS. We should be able to prevent transfusion-related AIDS cases, as well as those which might appear in hemophiliacs. We'll also be able to promptly and easily diagnose people who may have been infected by the virus, and perhaps develop ways to prevent the full syndrome from occurring. Finally, we also believe that the new process will enable us to develop a vaccine to prevent AIDS. We hope to have such a vaccine ready for testing in about two years.

As Heckler's voice began to crack, Ed Brandt jumped to fetch the secretary a glass of water, which she ignored. "In particular," Heckler went on, "credit must go to our eminent Dr. Robert Gallo, chief of the National Cancer Institute Laboratory of Tumor Cell Biology, who directed the research that produced this discovery. And to Dr. Edward Brandt, the Assistant Secretary for Health, who has led the Public Health Service effort in the fight against AIDS since its inception. And Dr. Vincent DeVita, very eminent Director of the National

Cancer Institute. And Dr. James Mason and Dr. James Curran of the Centers for Disease Control, and their scientific teams."

It was there that Heckler's statement had contained the acknowledgment of Pasteur's work — and it was there that she stopped reading.[n] "I would like to turn now," Heckler said, "to the eminent scientist who has made the breakthrough which prompts the conference today, to call upon Dr. Robert Gallo, with the applause and appreciation of the Secretary of Health and Human Services and the appreciation of the American people."

"I had never been in a press conference in my life before," Gallo said later. "That was my first time. It was one of the largest press conferences you will ever want to see. It was a sea of reporters as far as you could see almost, with television cameras and lights on me. I was a nervous wreck. I was deadly worried about how this is going to be interpreted on the other side of the ocean."[38]

Gallo began by mentioning "someone who came to us from Czechoslovakia, who has been on a rather permanent stay with us — Dr. Mikulas Popovic, who played a very major role in some of the growth of cells that would be permissive for large-scale production of the virus." But Popovic wasn't there to take a bow on the most important day of his career, having been dispatched by Gallo at the last minute to attend an obscure medical conference in Tampa.

Gallo acknowledged someone else who wasn't present on the dais, "a technician who did a lot of work with, I think, a reasonable amount of risk, Betsy Read." There was also a backhanded mention for Max Essex, who "has had his neck out for some time, sometimes with criticisms, for using an assay for antibodies in the serum of patients with AIDS or pre-AIDS that was not always completely one hundred percent certain, but an assay that he believed was giving him important leads."

Gallo wanted to make sure nobody thought the Essex test for HTLV-MA was a commercial alternative to his own ELISA. "There might be some false positives," Gallo said. "It's not as specific. It certainly is not going to be as good as the assays that will come out of having mass-produced the exact right virus. But the fundamental data published by him and in collaboration with CDC in part, I believe to be correct."

That morning the *Washington Post* quoted Gallo as having been "astounded" on his return from Italy at the "hullabaloo" caused by "sour-grapes" comments from unnamed scientists who seemed "threatened" by his accomplishments.[39] But Gallo assured reporters covering the news conference that all was well between the NCI and the Pasteur. "Many of you," Gallo said, "or all of you, have seen discussions about work in Paris. There was — there is not — there has never been any fights or controversies between us and a group in France. The laboratory at the Pasteur Institute and my laboratory have been friends for about fifteen years."

Perhaps there had been some "miscommunications" while he was out of the country, Gallo said, "some misunderstandings" between himself and the French, but nothing more. "We have an active collaboration in the coming month," Gallo said. "If what they identified in *Science* a year ago is the same as what we have now produced more than fifty isolates of, and in mass production, and in detailed characterization — if it turns out to be the same I certainly will say so, and I will say so with them in the collaboration."

A reporter who had scanned the *Science* articles observed that the evidence that HTLV-3 caused AIDS was only circumstantial, and asked whether Gallo's virus had been shown to cause AIDS in animals. "That is the classic test," the reporter asked. "Is it not?"

"I think we have something potentially better than that," Gallo replied. "In collaboration with the CDC, Jim Curran and I, and other members of the CDC and members of my laboratory, have been doing prospective studies [of] people who donate blood in blood banks, who then are recipients, develop AIDS as a consequence of that blood transfusion."

"Excuse me," Heckler said, cutting Gallo off. "I'd like to have Dr. Curran respond as well."

Somebody whispered to Heckler that Curran hadn't been invited.

"He's not here?" Heckler said, looking puzzled. "Dr. Mason, how about you? Would you like to make a comment for CDC?"

It was Mason's chance to point out that the CDC had isolated viruses from the transfusion pair that were indistinguishable from LAV, and to mention the blood-test results from France. But Mason shook his head.

"How about letting Dr. Gallo complete his statement?" Mason suggested.

"I think what she wanted to do," Gallo went on, "is to show you that they have these blood donors, and they have the serum samples. And we have been testing them and broke the code with Jim Curran, who belongs to the CDC. In any case, it was appropriate for an interruption."

The press wanted to know how long it would be before there was a vaccine for AIDS. "We're estimating a minimum of two years," Brandt said, "probably more like three years."

"Excuse me," interjected another reporter. "The French told me this morning that they would predict at least five years. And Luc Montagnier said he thought it might be five to ten years. Why are you more optimistic than the French are?"

"I'm just more optimistic, I guess," Brandt said.

A reporter pointed out that no effective vaccine had ever been developed for any of the animal retroviruses.

"I can only say that we have the problem of mass production solved," Gallo replied. "I haven't seen anything published from France, or anywhere else, that if these two viruses are the same, that they even have it continually grown in the laboratory. I haven't seen any publication that says they have a line that's permissive, that mass produces. That's one of the significances of what we are telling you today. Therefore, we can develop reagents, and we will develop those reagents rapidly. And it will be less than two years that those reagents will be available."

Someone asked what it meant to have antibodies to HTLV-3 — whether "the presence of HTLV or the presence of antibodies to HTLV indicates that in nine months, or some period of time, this person is definitely going to have AIDS."

"Before you keep saying HTLV," Gallo interrupted, "say HTLV-3, and say that it may *in time* be the same as what has been called LAV in a couple of publications."

Brandt, who evidently hadn't read the Pasteur's *Lancet* paper, replied that he didn't know whether there was "a carrier state for this disease at the present time. So the answer is no, you can't be certain that the presence of the virus would indicate that full-blown AIDS would develop."

Someone else wanted to know when Gallo had discovered HTLV-3. The correct answer was on the day of Mika Popovic's Eureka! experiment with LAV. But Gallo replied that "There's no one day I can tell you, only that we have large numbers of isolates that were openly discussed at NCI in meetings that involved thirty or forty people in our lab, and many outside people, including members of CDC. We could not say what they were because we couldn't get them to grow, but we believed firmly for many reasons they were in the HTLV family. But because we couldn't get the cells to grow, we were stuck in saying what they were. And we didn't want to report on it because we didn't know the significance of it.

"But when we got — and I believe this is the only one that exists right now — a permissive cell, that is, a cell that will grow forever and not be hurt by infection with the virus, that will mass-produce the virus — when we can do that reproducibly, we now can characterize that virus in detail, make what we call reagents against the mass-produced virus, its proteins, get its nucleic acids, go back to all the earlier isolates and have the answer. The first time we saw what *wasn't* HTLV-1 and 2, I don't know exactly when. It was certainly over a year ago, a year and a half ago. I don't know."

The next question came from Cristine Russell, who had written that morning's story in the *Washington Post*. "Dr. Gallo," she said, "could you describe how you will work with the French to figure out if they have got the same virus? And also, why hasn't that been done already?"

Before Gallo could answer, Ed Brandt cut him off. "Well, Cris," Brandt said, "that's going to take a long time to describe that in any detail."

"We have been waiting," Russell shot back, "for the science to be presented, and this is the opportunity that many of us have."

"All right," Brandt said. "If Dr. Gallo wants to take a quick, easy shot at it, why that's fine."

"Our problem," Gallo said, "has been this. Originally, one of the French co-workers, Françoise Barré, came to our lab to learn the techniques to grow T-cells. That was two years ago. We provided them with reagents of HTLV-1 and HTLV-2. In other words, in fact, they started out by learning the techniques to grow T-cells in obtaining T-cell growth factor from our laboratory. There's been a collaboration from day one, in short."

The LAV he had been sent from Paris, Gallo said, hadn't reacted with HTLV-1, but no further comparisons had been possible because the French hadn't sent more virus. "It's probably because they really didn't have enough material," Gallo said. "They didn't have enough material to send us. That's what's been the delay. They don't have a mass producer. As of a few weeks ago, they didn't have it successful in a cell line."

"I talked with Chermann and Montagnier today and two weeks

ago," Gallo said. "They believe they're getting it into a cell line just now. When you see the papers published in *Science,* you will see that we've been mass-producing it for six months. Okay? So we've had it in the cell line for a long time. I was developing reagents over that period of time to go back and do the analyses."

If the French could send him more LAV, Gallo promised to compare it to HTLV-3. "In retrospect," he said, "if the viruses are the same as what we now have in numbers, we already know they clearly do belong to the HTLV family . . . and we will see if there is a relationship with the genes we are cloning now from HTLV-3. One of my co-workers, Dr. Sarngadharan, will go over there in the last week of April, which is very soon, I guess, or the beginning of May, and we will work on protein comparisons directly with them.

"I'm not sure they have enough quantity to do everything I'd like to do," Gallo went on. "But I feel confident that in a matter of a month's time or less, we should be able to have a more definitive answer. The problem before is there would not be a definitive answer from lack of amount of materials that was sent to us. And we think the two laboratories are very likely to come together, although I cannot say at this point whether the viruses are identical."

"Dr. Gallo," another reporter said, "I have sort of a political question. And that is if, in fact, your — the virus you discovered and the French are the same, it sounds like both you and the French believe, isn't this announcement sort of stealing a little bit of thunder from the French? I mean, it seems somewhere we're taking the credit where the French should share it."

"Well," said Brandt, "I think Dr. Gallo said in his opening statement that if this turns out to be the same virus, he's readily going to give them credit for reporting it first."

Gallo, who had already returned to his seat, rose abruptly and walked back to the podium. "I could have presented an electron micrograph and reverse transcriptase activity of a variant a long time ago," he said, looking annoyed. "What I'm telling you is there are fifty isolates. They are characterized. The test is available for blood banks. The reagents are available to characterize anything now and a method is available to isolate this virus routinely. If I held that back from you, you would be mad at me for other reasons."

• 6 •

"We Assumed That Was
Your Job"

To those who watched the evening news and read the next morning's papers, it must have seemed a historic and reassuring moment. Three years earlier, AIDS was unknown. Two years before, it didn't have a name. Now a government laboratory had found the cause, and developed a diagnostic blood test as well — a triumph for the National Cancer Institute, the National Institutes of Health, the Reagan administration, and American science.

Robert Gallo was flying high. "Getting one paper in *Science* is a lot," Gallo said later. "Getting two is fantastic. Getting three was a record. We had four at one time. This was really something."[1] Gallo wanted Margaret Heckler to know that he had been "deeply impressed" by her "graciousness, calm and dignity during the sometimes stressful press conference."[2] But Jim Mason was "devastated" by Heckler's failure to recognize the French. "There was no mention of Pasteur," Mason said later. "I think Margaret really wanted a big scoop. Everyone likes to get all the credit they can for their department and their country. I think she just wanted all the glory to go in the direction of the USA and the Department of Health and Human Services."

The tone of the media's coverage was set by *Time,* whose two-page article accorded Pasteur two paragraphs and made the French sound like late-comers to Gallo's party. Following the first reports of Gallo's discovery, *Time* said, "a scientific team in Paris rushed to call attention to their own work on an AIDS virus." A Nobel Prize was "possibly at stake."[3] Nearly every story about the news conference described HTLV-3 as a newly discovered variant of HTLV-1, and therefore the newest member of Gallo's HTLV family. According to *Science*, the turning point in Gallo's research had come "about 10 months ago," when Popovic discovered his new cell line and was "able to mass-produce the virus for the first time."[4] When Luc Montagnier saw *Science*, he shook his head. "If Gallo has been mass-producing HTLV-3 in June of 1983," Montagnier said, "why was he publishing in *Science* about HTLV-1?"

Only the *New York Times* seemed inclined to offer Pasteur's side of the affair, reminding its readers that Gallo had been promoting HTLV-1 for many months after the French reported the first isolation of LAV from Frédéric Brugière. "At the time of the first LAV report," Larry Altman wrote, "Federal and other researchers said they were not excited by the prospects of that retrovirus as the cause of AIDS."[5] Altman also noted that Pasteur had been "sending samples of the virus to any other scientific team that asked for it," including "about 10" laboratories in Europe and the United States — among them Gallo's lab.

Nature chose Robin Weiss to explain Gallo's discovery to its readers. Weiss's article managed to annoy both Gallo and Montagnier, Gallo by predicting that LAV and HTLV-3 "will turn out to be the same virus," Montagnier by asserting that Pasteur had "published first, but with skimpy data," while Gallo's group had "delayed submission until a thorough characterization of their virus and repeated isolations from different patients had been accomplished."[6]

Weiss observed that a year had passed since the first report of LAV appeared in print, and that a permanent cell line producing LAV was "not yet available" to other scientists — a curious comment from someone who had been growing LAV in a permanent cell line for more than two months. Asked later why he had failed to mention his own success, Weiss replied that "It's not good form to advertise your unpublished work."[7]

For comment, San Francisco reporters summoned their local AIDS expert, Jay Levy. "I remember being called down to 'Live at Five,'" Levy said, "and being asked, 'What do you think of this press conference?' And I must have looked like a fool, because I said 'Well, we've got the virus too.'"

Levy, whose own manuscript was about to be submitted to *Science*, had obtained the first isolates of the virus he called ARV, for AIDS-related virus, in November 1983, and the first electron micrographs the following January. But anyone watching Heckler's news conference would have been surprised to learn the AIDS virus had been growing for five months in a laboratory in San Francisco.

"We were probably the first group to isolate it in the United States," Levy said. "I think I'm the second person to find the virus, very frankly, after Françoise. When Gallo made his announcement, he stole the thunder. We're the first group to confirm the French. I think Bob all along thought it was an *arenavirus*. Bob never believed the French. He never thought LAV was real, he thought everything they wrote was wrong, that they aren't good. Then when he found that they were right, he tried to rewrite history."[8]

After the news conference, Gallo called Montagnier in Paris. "He said, 'It's over now,'" Montagnier recalled. "He said, 'I mentioned your contribution and I think everything is fine.'"[9] But when the French learned what Gallo had really said, there was more enmity at Pasteur.

Montagnier remembered what he said had been Gallo's promise, following Cold Spring Harbor, to spend six months determining whether the French were right about LAV. Now Gallo had mentioned LAV in "a single sentence at the end of one paper, suggesting that our virus was insufficiently characterized."[10] Montagnier was equally infuriated by Gallo's assertion that the French had used T-Cell Growth Factor from Bethesda to isolate LAV, and incensed at the suggestion that the French were just now getting their virus into a cell line. "His attitude toward our findings," fumed Montagnier, "was to minimize their importance or to demolish them."

Françoise Barré was angriest over Gallo's statement that she had been trained to grow T-cells and HTLV in his lab.[11] "I remember Gallo saying I learned the technology in his lab," Barré said later, "but he was not mentioning *why* I stayed in his lab"— teaching Gallo's people how to use Pasteur's anti-interferon to isolate primate retroviruses —"or that I stayed there only six weeks."[a]

Barré, who hadn't had any contact with Gallo's HTLV group during her brief sojourn in Bethesda,[12] also thought Gallo had been dishonest to announce that he "broke the code" with Jim Curran — but not that the French had done it first, and with more convincing results. "He knew that the CDC was giving the same samples to us and to him," Barré said. But she was most offended by Gallo's assertion that the French "essentially followed our HTLV-1 protocols for getting LAV."[13] If Gallo's HTLV protocol was the right one for discovering the AIDS virus, wondered Barré, why hadn't he done it himself?

If Barré was furious and Montagnier irate, Jean-Claude Chermann was apoplectic. "'The breakthrough of a new virus, HTLV-3, has been found,'" Chermann said, mimicking Heckler's words and waving his arms in the air. "We never heard about HTLV-3, you know. I was surprised by the new name. Till before, we were speaking all together of the AIDS virus, or the LAV. I mean, I don't know why this name change. I feel very angry. He was just saying, 'We don't know if it be the same.' And that scientifically for me, ethically and morally, was not acceptable. He can say what he wants. He knew it was the same virus."

Gallo professed to have been mystified by Chermann's reaction. "Here's a guy who used to treat me with kid gloves," Gallo recalled, "you know, with great respect all the time. And now I have this guy yelling at me from across the ocean."[14]

With the attention of the scientific world focused on HTLV-3, Gallo set about expunging the evidence that he had spent two years chasing the wrong virus. At the Cold Spring Harbor meeting, Gallo had promoted HTLV-1 as "the almost-certain cause of the disease called AIDS."[15] There hadn't been any mention of HTLV-3, because HTLV-3 hadn't existed in September of 1983. Now, in his capacity as coeditor of the proceedings of the Cold Spring Harbor conference, Gallo replaced his remarks about HTLV-1 with a paper reporting the isolation of HTLV-3 from more than fifty patients.[b] Montagnier's paper on LAV appeared exactly as it had been presented. "The organizers asked people who are speaking to give in their manuscripts at the time," said Montagnier, who could have updated his paper with many more isolates and near-perfect blood test results. "I was the only one to do that."

Jean-Claude Chermann's presentation at Park City also appeared in print exactly as it had been delivered. But after the four Gallo papers had gone to *Science,* one of Gallo's assistants sent Mike Gottlieb a revision of Gallo's Park City presentation reporting fifty isolations of HTLV-3. The same thing happened to David Klatzmann, who had given a paper on his T-4 cell data before the New York Academy of Sciences the previous November.[16]

Like Montagnier, Klatzmann had turned in his paper at the conference. "I made no single change," Klatzmann said, recalling that Phil Markham from Gallo's lab had presented data on HTLV-1 in AIDS patients at the same meeting. "Now I open the proceedings," Klatzmann said. "There is no more trace of HTLV-1. Instead, there is updated results on HTLV-3.[c] Mine are the results I wrote in November 1983. Theirs is the results they got in 1984."[d]

When Marjorie Guroff's paper reporting that fewer than 10 percent of AIDS patients were infected with HTLV-1 finally appeared in *The Lancet,* it no longer offered explanations for why HTLV-1 might still be the cause of AIDS.[17] Instead, the paper blamed Max Essex for having "compelled one to consider HTLV-1" as a prospective cause. "I don't know what Max was detecting," Gallo said later. "Truthfully, I don't know. I really don't know. I don't mean this critical of Max."

Whoever won the patent for the AIDS blood test, it wouldn't be Essex. Declaring that the test for HTLV-MA was "inoperative and therefore lacks utility," the patent office summarily rejected Harvard's application. Essex's data, the patent office observed, "leads one to the conclusion that the assay may result in a large number of false positive test results."[18]

"That's Max's history. That's FOCMA," said one of Essex's Harvard colleagues who spoke for many. "He knows the right people. He's very charming and effective. He's very reserved and never gets excited and comes on very sincere and open. He's very politically adept. At Harvard that counts for a lot. If you're politically adept you can succeed as well as if you do good science."

The discovery of HTLV-3 had brought the National Cancer Institute more visibility and acclaim than anything that had emerged during the entire War on Cancer. But Vince DeVita didn't want to see the National Cancer Institute transformed into the National AIDS Institute. "Cancer was still a big problem," DeVita said later. "Plenty of people were going to work on AIDS, and I had to pay attention to the cancer problem. Otherwise we'd be gobbled up." When some of Gallo's friends suggested that DeVita devote as much money to AIDS research as the NCI had spent chasing cancer viruses, DeVita threatened to "come out in public and tell everybody" how the cancer-virus program "almost destroyed NCI."[19]

Cancer still killed more Americans by far. But AIDS was the disease of the moment, and the Reagan administration's priority was putting Gallo's blood test into service. At least twenty-three million tests a year, the government estimated, would be needed to keep the blood supply virus-free. In case the blood banks and other prospective customers might be tempted to buy the Pasteur ELISA, Gallo offered a reminder that "no one else but our NCI laboratory has the cell line that produces this virus. Without the specific virus, they can't have a specific test."[e]

Gallo's professions of uncertainty about whether LAV and HTLV-3 were the same virus had dampened enthusiasm for the Pasteur ELISA, and within days of Heckler's news conference companies had begun lining up for licenses to manufacture the Gallo test. First to apply was Baxter-Travenol, which took the opportunity to praise Gallo for "the outstanding work you have just reported on the relationship between AIDS and HTLV."[20] Within a week, more than twenty other companies had requested applications, prompting the official in charge of licensing government patents to complain that "the phone is ringing off the hook regarding Dr. Gallo's inventions."[21]

The applicants ranged from pharmaceutical powerhouses like Becton Dickinson and Warner-Lambert, to biotech boutiques like Seragen, Chiron, and Cetus. Even Max Essex's Cambridge BioScience, apparently hoping to recoup its misbegotten investment in the test for HTLV-MA, had submitted an application.[22] Also on the list were the three Gallo contract companies that had helped grow the AIDS virus and perfect the blood test: Biotech Research Laboratories, run by Gallo's one-time postdoc, Bob Ting; Electronucleonics, which had been put in charge of culturing the Chardon virus; and Litton Bionetics, where Sarngadharan had developed the Gallo ELISA.

The most formidable competitor by far was Chicago's Abbott Laboratories, which had pioneered the field of diagnostic blood testing and dominated the worldwide market. Although Abbott's consumer items were household names, the bulk of Abbott's business was done with hospitals and laboratories, to many of which Abbott already was selling an ELISA for antibodies to the hepatitis B virus.

Racing to meet Heckler's six-month deadline, an HHS committee charged with evaluating the competing applications chose Abbott first and Baxter-Travenol second, followed by the three Gallo contractors — but only after Electronucleonics and Biotech had formed hasty commercial partnerships with Organon and DuPont to manufacture and distribute their tests.[23] Vince DeVita remembered being concerned that the three contractors, who had been working with HTLV-3 for months, had taken advantage of an inside edge in what was supposed to be an impartial government competition. "The companies who heard about it and tried to compete from scratch were at a competitive disadvantage," DeVita said.

For Margaret Heckler, who evidently didn't have similar concerns, the licensing agreements marked "an important milestone in our drive to conquer AIDS."[24] *Science* headlined its story "Five firms with the Right Stuff," but there wasn't anything magic about the number five.[25] The government had been free to issue as many licenses as it liked, or as few. "If all of the applications had met the criteria," declared the committee's chairman, a senior HHS executive named Lowell Harmison, "all would have been awarded a license." But Harmison didn't explain how three government contractors in the Maryland suburbs had rated ahead of Becton Dickinson, Warner-Lambert, Chiron, and Cetus.

The official reason for requiring government licenses at all was to ensure the quality of the AIDS test.[26] In fact, the licenses were royalty agreements that had nothing to do with the accuracy of the individual tests. No AIDS test could reach the market until its quality had been verified by the U.S. Food and Drug Administration, the agency charged with approving all medical devices. The real reason for the patent licenses, an HHS lawyer acknowledged, was to give the five chosen companies "the opportunity to develop a strong market position."[27]

In return for HTLV-3B and the H-9 cell line, Abbott and the four other companies agreed to pay HHS five percent of their gross sales. Assuming the companies sold twenty million tests a year at three dollars apiece, HHS would pick up an extra $3 million annually — a miniscule sum by government standards. The real benefit for the government, one HHS attorney admitted, was "scientific pride."[28]

The theology of the biotech industry held that small companies could move faster than large ones, and Abbott was a gargantuan bureaucracy. But the head of the company's diagnostics division, Jack Schuler, intended to beat the smaller companies at their own game by creating a small company inside a large one. To head Abbott's ELISA team, Schuler chose a twenty-eight-year-old researcher and gave him ten people. Schuler's only instructions were that Abbott must be first to win FDA approval. "I told them, nobody is going to remember who was second," Schuler said.

The HTLV-3B carried to Frederick by Larry Arthur in April as seed stock for the ELISA virus production had gotten off to a faltering start.[f] HHS had hoped to have enough virus to supply the five companies at the end of May, but two weeks before the deadline Arthur sent Gallo an urgent request for more virus.[29] It was mid-June when representatives of the five companies finally gathered in Frederick to pick up HTLV-3B, the Abbott contingent arriving in one of the company's fleet of corporate jets — a gesture, Schuler said later, that he hoped would send a message to the rest of the company that Abbott was serious about being first.

Although Gallo claimed to have more than fifty isolates of HTLV-3, Popovic's *Science* article had identified just five, including R.F. But scientists eager to begin work on a cure or a vaccine for AIDS were all being given the isolate Gallo called HTLV-3B. "We received the HTLV-3B isolate in May of '84," recalled Robin Weiss. "We got none of the ones listed in Popovic's paper. We asked for them and we never received them. And we kept asking and not getting them."

Gallo's research had been paid for with millions of taxpayer dollars, and Gallo had long been aware of the NIH policy that its cell lines and other discoveries be made available to any qualified scientist who requested them.[g] But Gallo treated HTLV-3B and the H-9 cell line in which it grew best like his personal property. Anyone who wanted either would first have to promise, in writing, not to provide them to another laboratory without Gallo's permission. Moreover, all experiments performed with 3B or H-9 would be done in collaboration with Gallo, who was to be kept informed of his competitors' research in progress, and who retained the option of appearing as a co-author on any resulting publications.[h]

To what was already an unprecedented collaboration agreement for a government laboratory, Peter Fischinger and Lowell Harmison added the admonition that recipients must "maintain in confidence" all information relating to HTLV-3B and H-9. Written confidentiality agreements would have to be obtained "from all employees to whom the proprietary materials or information will be made available."[30] The reason for the secrecy, Fischinger told Jim Wyngaarden, was to protect the possibility of "further patents by the Government"— particularly those involving H-9, which would be released only at Gallo's discretion, and only then after "a discussion of the resulting collaborative plan."[i]

Between May and December 1984, at least sixty-three laboratories received either HTLV-3B, H-9, or both.[j] The rules, however, were stricter for some than for others. Daniel Zagury got HTLV-3B more than a week before the Heckler news conference.[k] Before the *Science* articles were in print, several of Gallo's other friends had received private invitations to take HTLV-3B and H-9 into their labs.[31] Jerry Groopman, who had introduced Gallo at the Park City symposium, got H-9 three weeks after Margaret Heckler's news conference. When a request arrived from Mike Gottlieb, who had interceded for Chermann at Park City, it was turned down.[32]

For a few others, Gallo tried to impose conditions on which experiments they could perform and which they could not. The agreement drafted for Jim Mullins's signature provided that he could infect H-9 only with viruses that *didn't* cause AIDS — an absurd condition for an AIDS researcher. Disgusted, Mullins never bothered to sign the form.

Bill Haseltine, whom Flossie Wong-Staal considered her principal competitor, got H-9 with the caveat that it could be used only "for the specific purpose of studying expression of HTLV-LTR linked genes."[l] The only scientist explicitly exempted from the collaboration requirement was Robin Weiss. "Collaboration *at will* for Dr. Weiss," Gallo noted on Weiss's agreement, meaning that it was up to Weiss whether to include Gallo as a co-author on his own papers.[m]

"There were lots and lots of people who got reagents from Bob Gallo," Vince DeVita said later. "One of the issues, though, is whether or not there were people who were excluded by a mechanism we could not get a handle on. There were rules that you had to send out to everybody. Would Bob quietly prevent something from going out to a single individual? My guess is he would. If he doesn't like you, you could die of thirst before he'd give you a drink."

Gallo was generous with Murray Gardner, but he was worried about some of Gardner's California colleagues. "Please feel *free* to do any research you want with HTLV-3," Gallo told Gardner. "My colleagues and I would be pleased to collaborate with you at any time, but we should be involved only when we make real contributions. The cell line is *yours* now. I would appreciate if periodically you keep me informed of projects and collaborators. Obviously, there are some people in your part of the country one can only wonder about."[33]

Gallo didn't say whom he had in mind. But the day Gallo's *Science* articles were published, Jay Levy had written to request Gallo's reagents. "In our studies of AIDS in San Francisco," Levy explained, "we have also isolated retroviruses and now would like to know if any of them are related to the HTLV-3." Levy was growing his AIDS viruses from San Francisco patients in HUT-78, but he wanted Gallo's H-9 cell line as well. Gallo never replied to Levy's request.[n]

Mal Martin's boss, the head of the National Institute of Allergy and Infectious Disease, had underlined for Vince DeVita the urgent need to know whether HTLV-3 and LAV were different viruses — a comparison Martin could easily have performed in his lab with HTLV-3 and the LAV sample Martin obtained in Paris.[34] But the collaborative agreement Gallo prepared for Martin contained the provision that any work with HTLV-3B "not be published without prior approval by Dr. Gallo," and it required Martin's written agreement not to use HTLV-3 "in comparisons with other viruses."[35]

The uninfected H-9 cell line, especially useful to any researcher wanting to make his own isolations of the AIDS virus, had been shared with a half-dozen labs — but not the Pasteur, and Mal Martin wouldn't get it either. The reason, Gallo informed Martin, was that H-9 was "still being characterized." In the event it did become available, Gallo wanted to know what Martin intended to do with the cells. "For instance," Gallo wrote, "I do not think it would be appropriate for you to put the French isolate in them. That is for them to do in collaboration with me and my co-workers and is on-going."

Martin never got either HTLV-3B or H-9. The real reason, Gallo admitted later, was his reluctance to provide his virus or cell line to those he "could not trust," who might "stab me in the back" or "embarrass me or call me dishonest if there was something wrong."[36] Apparently, that description also fit the CDC, whose blood-testing program was expanding rapidly and which faced the same dilemma outlined by Martin's boss: which virus, LAV or HTLV-3B, should be the gold standard for AIDS testing?

That question couldn't be answered without comparing LAV to 3B. But when the CDC met Gallo to take delivery of his virus, the occasion was described by Fred Murphy as "a tense moment, fraught with the possibility of non-delivery."[37] Gallo began by insisting the CDC promise in writing not to compare 3B with LAV. "Our tack," Murphy reported later to Walt Dowdle, "stated in several different ways, was that public health purposes were paramount."

According to Murphy, "Dr. Gallo agreed" with the urgency of the situation. But when Murphy offered "to have certain comparative tests between his HTLV-3 and the French LAV done at CDC, Dr. Gallo declined each time, stating that such work would be done in his lab."

When Murphy pointed out that Max Essex and other collaborators had HTLV-3B in *their* labs, Gallo replied that he viewed the CDC not as a collaborator but a competitor. Only after the CDC complained to Ed Brandt did Gallo agree to release a small quantity of HTLV-3B.[38] But the CDC still couldn't make any comparisons with LAV, and it would have to *pay* the NCI for the virus, at a cost of $72 per liter.[39]

"Gallo's friends received tons of virus for free," recalled Berge Hampar, the manager of the NCI-Frederick facility. Every two weeks, Hampar said, Max Essex was sent the virus-rich cells left over from growing virus for others, including the CDC. When Jim Mason told Jim Wyngaarden that the H-9 cell line was also badly needed by the CDC, Wyngaarden replied that H-9 was being given only to those "who want to collaborate" with Gallo.[40]

Gallo had promised to send Sarngadharan to Paris "very soon" to take part in a formal comparison of HTLV-3B and LAV. But when Robin Weiss arrived in Bethesda on May 11 to pick up his sample of HTLV-3B, he found Gallo on the verge of canceling Sarngadharan's trip.

Weiss spent "much time persuading Gallo that Sarngadharan should indeed go," he told Montagnier later. "Much politics is going on at the moment in the USA," Weiss explained, and Montagnier's name was "being used by CDC to exacerbate difficulties that I believe you yourself have no part in whatsoever. I therefore persuaded Bob that it was imperative for your laboratories to co-operate. In that sense my weekend in Bethesda was probably more valuable than all the research we are pursuing in London."[41]

By the time Sarngadharan arrived in France it was the middle of May. The anger over Gallo's remarks at the news conference, and the Pasteur's treatment in his *Science* articles, was still palpable, and Sarngadharan remembered being greeted by "some animosity."[42] Gallo had initially agreed to let Sarngadharan carry only inactivated HTLV-3B to Paris, which would have been adequate for the comparative studies but wouldn't have been able to grow in the Pasteur labs. "But at the last minute he changed his mind," Montagnier said, "and Dr. Sarngadharan brought live HTLV-3B growing in H-9 cells to our lab."

The unexpected arrival of Gallo's live virus presented the unwelcome possibility of a cross-contamination with LAV, and a nervous Montagnier decided to keep HTLV-3B locked in his own lab, in a different building from where Chermann and Barré were working with LAV. "We both went to his lab," Sarngadharan recalled. "He took a key, opened the door. We walked in and the door automatically locked behind us. And then he took the sample and he gave it to his technician to put it in the hood."[43]

It took Sarngadharan and Chermann four days to agree that the proteins that comprised LAV and HTLV-3B were the same sizes and weights — and, more important, that the core protein Gallo called p24 and the French called p25 was the same molecule, despite their different designations.° The two viruses behaved the same way in culture, and AIDS patients had antibodies to both. It was Montagnier's idea to make a chart comparing their principal features —"to show that there were some points that he agreed on," Sarngadharan said later, "and there were some points that we needed to work out."[44]

The only real disagreement concerned a protein, gp41, that Sarngadharan thought was part of the viral envelope. The AIDS patients tested at Pasteur didn't appear to have gp41 antibodies, and Montagnier had reasoned that gp41 must be actin, a cellular protein found in muscles and other contracting tissues.[45] Sarngadharan had been wrong himself, in concluding that the AIDS virus RT had a molecular weight of 100,000 (nearly twice its actual size). But he thought Montagnier was wrong about gp41, and that HTLV-3B and LAV were the same kind of virus.ᴾ

Sarngadharan's conclusions were confirmed upon his return to Bethesda, when he repeated the experiments using a fresh sample of LAV. As they had been in Paris, the core proteins of the two viruses were a perfect match.[46] When another NIH researcher asked

Gallo whether he should use HTLV-3 or LAV in an upcoming series of experiments, he was advised that "LAV is identical."[47]

As Sarngadharan was leaving Paris, Montagnier asked whether he should destroy the live HTLV-3B culture. "It gave me a shock," Sarngadharan said. "I mean, I was really not expecting that kind of a question from him. I immediately said, 'No. I brought it for you to use. Please keep it. Don't destroy it.' For a second I was confused, but I knew right away if I said, 'Yes, destroy it,' absolutely no way would I know that he indeed destroyed it. The moment I walked out of the lab I stopped knowing anything about the culture."[48]

Don Francis heard about the Paris experiments from an excited Chermann, for whom they represented proof positive that the French had discovered the cause of AIDS.[q] Gallo didn't think it mattered. "I don't give a crap that they are the same or not," Gallo told Francis, who was taking his customary telephone notes.[49] "I'm honest," Gallo told Francis. "I am not trying to say that I was the first to isolate the cause of AIDS. We started the field. We predicted AIDS. We were the first to find cause. You created the problem. If anyone asks who first identified the virus I say the French."

That wasn't what Gallo had been saying in the weeks and months leading up to the Heckler news conference, or at the news conference itself. Gallo had planned a post–news conference visit to France, to attend a small convocation in the village of Talloires near lac d'Annecy. When he canceled at the last minute, Francis and Chermann approached the session chairman, Robin Weiss, who had just published a commentary in *Nature* suggesting that the similarities between 3B and LAV were more striking than the differences.

"We said, 'If you would like, we can update you on LAV and AIDS,'" Francis recalled. "There was a tremendous amount of pressure on Robin to cancel Jean-Claude and me, but Robin allowed us to speak. Robin's a straight guy." Chermann gave what Weiss described as "his usual disorganized talk, bringing the Institut Pasteur group's work up to date." When Francis's turn came, he talked about the CDC's transfusion pair, describing it as "a very tight natural experiment, very important for determining the natural course of AIDS."

"At that point we broke up," Francis said. "We were sitting around a table, and Bill Haseltine came up to me and said, 'Don, how could you possibly have given those specimens to Institute Pasteur and not given them to Bob? How can you justify that?' I turned to him and I said, 'Bill, we gave all those specimens to Bob. Don't stick your god-damn nose in something you don't know anything about.'"

His encounter with Haseltine still fresh in his mind, when Francis got home he composed an appeal to Gallo, reminding him of the tri-partite meeting in Montagnier's office three months before.[50] "I tried to tell you all," Francis said. "I opened our printouts on the serologic results and showed you my summaries. Unfortunately, I understand from you, I did not succeed since you still don't feel that those data have been shared. But I tried to show you that either isolate, when used as a target antigen, scored similarly."

> I tried to reinforce the fact that probably what you had, what we had and what the French had were the same. Jim Curran did the same and encouraged you to complete comparisons before making any broad announcement. On the Sunday before your press conference, I tried again to show you that the bugs were probably the same. The lack of pre-announcement comparison, the lack of substantial mention of the French work at the press conference, and the minimum of credit given the French at subsequent talks and interviews made it look like you wanted to be given credit for first identifying the cause of AIDS. Thus, the perception (and I agree, Bob, it is percep-tion) by me was that you did not want to give due credit to the French. My defense of the French has been because I per-ceived that they were not being given the credit that I knew they were due.

Due credit aside, in the United States the French were being por-trayed as sore losers. According to *Science Digest,* it was Gallo who had "solved the most compelling medical mystery of our time."[51] The *Baltimore Sun* thought Gallo had been victimized by the CDC, which "wanted to ride on the French coattails and share in the credit" for one of the most important medical discoveries in decades.[52] When the *Boston Globe* dispatched its chief science corre-spondent, Loretta McLaughlin, to find out why there was such bitter-ness at the Pasteur, Montagnier again blamed Gallo.[53] "He could have grown our virus and analyzed it when we sent it to him," Monta-gnier said. "But that is not his way. His way is not to confirm the work of others."

Chermann thought Gallo's behavior was explained by the fact that "they have been under more pressure in the States to come with some answers fast. They were very concerned with a molecular biology approach. We were looking for a virus. It was sort of like they were looking for a door with one or two keys — HTLV-1 and HTLV-2 — while we were also looking for a door, but telling ourselves that an entirely different type of key might open it."[54]

The correspondence flying between Bethesda and Paris was more embittered than the public statements. It wasn't "easy or pleasant" to revisit the past, Gallo told Chermann in a letter he copied to Jim Wyngaarden, Ed Brandt, Vince DeVita, and Peter Fischinger. But Gallo thought a proper accounting of recent history was necessary, "after the peculiar press treatment we have received . . . and the statements attributed to you, Luc Montagnier, and the 'unnamed' people at the Pasteur Institute."[55]

The package Montagnier delivered to Gallo's house in July, Gallo said, had contained "no detectable virus particles." The second shipment, sent by Françoise Barré in September, did contain LAV, but Popovic had only grown it in fresh T-cells, not HUT-78 or any other continuous cell line. Despite what the French obviously suspected, Gallo had never "mass-produced" the French virus. "We assumed that was your job," Gallo told Chermann. "We also did not want to cross contaminate our lines."

Gallo mainly wanted Chermann to know that the French hadn't been first to find the AIDS virus. "Our first identification of HTLV-3," Gallo declared, "was November 1982. We had several more isolates in February 1983, but did not choose to report on our electron microscopy or reverse transcriptase studies until we had further characterized the virus."[56]

"I am confused," an astonished Chermann replied, "by your statement that your first isolate of HTLV-3 was in November 1982. Is this a typographical error or did you really withhold this information from me for that long of a period?"[57]

Gallo and Montagnier found themselves face-to-face in mid-June, at a tumor virus meeting in Denver, whose organizers had arranged a joint news conference.[58] In the corridors at the Denver meeting, the consuming topic of conversation was the mounting tension over the relationship between HTLV-3B and LAV; Fred Murphy recalled being assured by a member of Gallo's lab that, whatever the CDC might think, 3B and LAV were different viruses.[59] At the news conference, Gallo was equivocal. "There is data now," he said, "that they *could* belong to the same virus group of the same virus family."

But Gallo cautioned that the data was only preliminary. A final determination would have to await the comparison of the two viruses at the DNA level.[60] Montagnier tried to point out that the comparisons by Chermann and Sarngadharan had established that the two viruses were the same, but his attempts to explain the subtleties of competitive radioimmunoassays hadn't succeeded. "I was not quite happy about that press conference," Montagnier said later. "Gallo speaks faster than me in English."

According to Gallo, one of those spreading "the plot and innuendo" in Denver "about HTLV-3 and LAV being the same" was George Todaro, who had landed in Seattle after leaving the NCI.[61] Besides running a lab at the University of Washington, Todaro was serving as scientific adviser to a small Seattle company, Genetic Systems, that had been among the losers in the competition to license the Gallo AIDS test.

The Harmison committee had credited Genetic Systems with superior scientific experience and technology. Its only shortcoming, the panel said, was the fact that the company had never marketed an ELISA. But Genetic Systems's CEO, a flamboyant thirty-six-year-old scientist named Robert Nowinski, was convinced the real reason for the rejection was the longstanding enmity between Gallo and Todaro. "George and I probably had more experience in retroviruses than all the applicants put together," Nowinski said.

Genetic Systems's only products, a set of monoclonal antibodies for the diagnosis of herpes, chlamydia, and other sexually transmitted diseases, had come on the market the year before. But most of the company's value had been created by Wall Street's fascination with biotech stocks, and that fascination wouldn't last forever without some earnings. Genetic Systems was looking for a score, and the AIDS test was a guaranteed moneymaker. If Nowinski and Todaro couldn't sell the Gallo ELISA, they would get around the Gallo patents by going to France.

Todaro remembered having been impressed by Montagnier's presentation at the scientific sessions in Denver. "His data were so much better than anyone else's," Todaro recalled, "and they were ignoring him. I convinced Montagnier to change his plans and come out to Seattle to meet with the executives at Genetic Systems."

The Pasteur had everything Genetic Systems needed: an AIDS virus and a cell line in which to grow it, and a patent application that had been filed months before Gallo's.[62] "We made our deal with the Pasteur in one day," Nowinski recalled. "We flew to Paris, we arrived at four o'clock and by eleven o'clock that night we had the arrangement made. The collaboration was really exceptional." "Let them bark in the wind," Gallo told the *Wall Street Journal*. "Genetic Systems is interested in money. I'm not."[r]

Once the discovery of HTLV-3 was in print, the appetites of the medical and scientific journals for articles about AIDS became insatiable. The French, whose efforts to publish their most important findings had been stymied for months, were quick to take advantage of the opening.

Montagnier sent *Science* an article on his successful transmission, the previous February, of LAV to a continuous B-cell line.[63] Françoise Brun submitted a report of her detection, also in February, of LAV antibodies in 90 percent of Peter Piot's Zairian AIDS patients.[64] Hoping the third time would be a charm, David Klatzmann included the manuscript on T-4 tropism that had been rejected by *Nature* and *PNAS*.[65] Appearing in the same issue of *Science* with Klatzmann's paper was the CDC's report on the transfusion pair.[66]

Had any of those papers appeared before Gallo's publication of HTLV-3, they would have created enormous excitement. But when the articles from Paris and Atlanta finally saw print, they were virtually ignored. Another long-overdue paper to appear was the manuscript Brun and Rouzioux had sent *The Lancet* the previous December, and which unaccountably had languished in the journal's offices for nearly six months.[s] The data in that article was from the fall of 1983, but the *Lancet* editors had permitted Brun to update her results with an addendum.

"Since submission of this paper," it read, "we have introduced . . . technical modifications to the ELISA [which have] increased the sensitivity of the test." With the new test, 75 percent of the AIDS patients and more than 90 percent of those with pre-AIDS were positive for antibodies to LAV. The last of the backlogged articles, Jay Levy's isolation of ARV from seven San Francisco AIDS patients, appeared in *Science* at the end of August.[67] "We published it third," Levy said, "but that doesn't mean we found it third. We've always been like, 'Oh, yes, there was Jay Levy,' when actually we were right there at the beginning."

In the world outside the laboratory, facts mattered less than perceptions. It appeared to be true, as Levy claimed, that he was the first American researcher to have isolated the AIDS virus.[t] But Levy was a long way from Harvard and the NIH. He wasn't a major player in the retrovirological establishment. He didn't chair major scientific meetings or edit their proceedings. He didn't command half a hundred scientists and technicians, and he didn't have any contract laboratories to call on for help. No editors were expediting the publication of his papers, and the secretary of health and human services wasn't announcing his discoveries. At a critical moment Jay Levy had done some outstanding science, but that mattered less than who Jay Levy was — or wasn't.

"It's all Hollywood," said Flossie Wong-Staal's husband, Steve Staal, on the verge of leaving the NCI to set up a private oncology practice. "The whole business has the ethics of a used-car lot. It's what you can get away with. The older-style scientists are falling by the wayside. To be a success in science these days, you need a big operation. You need a different sort of talent than just the ability to be a good experimenter or to ask the right questions or be good at the bench. It's become an entrepreneurial business, and Gallo's good at that. He enjoys most of all making contacts and wining and dining and traveling. He works the European connection very heavily."[68]

In the wake of the discovery of the cause of AIDS, the awards and honors flowed in Gallo's direction. From Detroit, the General Motors cancer prize, conferred in recognition of Gallo's "profound" influence on cancer research. From Bombay, the Second Triennial Rameshwardas Birla International Award. From Tokyo, an invitation to deliver the Henry Kaplan Memorial Lecture at the annual meeting of the Princess Takamatsu Cancer Research Fund. From the Italian-American Foundation, headed by frozen pizza magnate Jeno Paulucci, an award for scientific achievement that compared Gallo to Galileo.[69]

Mindful of how much the Nobel Prize had done to enhance Sweden's stature in the world, the Japanese had created their own scientific prize, richer even than the Nobel. Consisting of a gold medal and ten million yen, the Japan Prize was to be awarded each year "on an auspicious day in November."[70] When the National Cancer Institute nominated Gallo, it cited the discovery of HTLV-1 and HTLV-2. In the NCI's opinion, however, it was the discovery of the AIDS virus for which Gallo most deserved to be rewarded.[71]

The NCI's citation didn't mention the French. But Robin Weiss, who was among those asked by the Japanese to submit nominations, did. "They wanted an opinion from a non-French, non-American retrovirologist," Weiss said. "So I had to write a reasoned appraisal of who was prizeworthy. I pushed Françoise Barré. She's the one who did the work. I knew perfectly well they were never going to pick Françoise, because they don't pick women. Women are assistants."[72]

The judges ignored Barré's contribution and selected Montagnier to share the prize with Gallo. But half of the first Japan Prize was cold comfort for the French. To the rest of the world, Robert Gallo was the discoverer of the cause of AIDS, and the Institut Pasteur and Jay Levy among the also-rans.

"Only Because There Are So Many"

The Japan Prize found an honored place on Gallo's wall. But the honor for which he might have traded all the others continued to elude his grasp: election to the National Academy of Sciences, whose 1,700 members (and a handful of foreign "associates") are collectively the most distinguished scientists in the world. "He really wanted to be in the Academy," George Todaro recalled. "He would tell you himself that was one of the things that made him unhappy in life."

Although its annual elections are conducted amidst stringent secrecy and are reputed to be pristine, Gallo had begun lobbying selected Academy members not long after the discovery of HTLV.[a] That strategy hadn't worked, and a few months after Margaret Heckler's news conference Gallo implored Peter Fischinger that "it is almost vital to get in this year. I would appreciate it very much if you would remind Vince [DeVita] at the correct time to speak with Paul Marks," the influential head of the Memorial Sloan-Kettering Cancer Center in New York City. "Also, some comment, perhaps directly from you, to Jim Wyngaarden," an academy member, "would probably be very useful."[1]

Even the *New York Times* was now describing Gallo as the discoverer of the AIDS virus.[b] But once again Gallo failed to make the academy's cut, and behind the doors of his laboratory trouble was brewing. The source of the trouble was Roland Ferdinand, the Haitian AIDS patient from Philadelphia. The "R.F." isolate, which had only materialized months after Mika Popovic began working with LAV, represented Gallo's first independently discovered AIDS virus. Of the five isolates described in Popovic's *Science* paper, only the R.F. culture in the H-4 cell line had remained productive, although yielding virus at a rapidly diminishing rate.[c]

In hopes of establishing a more virulent culture that could produce enough virus to study and characterize, in late June of 1984 Betsy Read took the original R.F. cells from the freezer and re-isolated the virus in the H-9 cell line.[d] In the interim, a Southern blot from the original R.F. culture had delivered some troubling news. On a genetic level, HTLV-3$_{RF}$ differed substantially from HTLV-3B, by 10 percent or more. Worse, it also differed by the same 10 percent from the viruses isolated by Popovic from a half-dozen other AIDS patients after the *Science* papers were in press.

Unlike HTLV-3$_{RF}$, the other viruses appeared to be carbon copies of HTLV-3B.[e] At first, the recognition that Popovic's newest AIDS viruses were indistinguishable from HTLV-3B hadn't come as a shock. Isolates of HTLV-1 from Japan and the Caribbean had virtually the same DNA sequences, and there was no reason to think one AIDS virus would be different from any other AIDS virus.[2] When Montagnier's LAV-producing B-cell line arrived in Bethesda, LAV looked exactly like HTLV-3B and Popovic's other viruses.[3] "We said, 'Oh, gee, we got what they got,'" recalled Beatrice Hahn. "'We must all have the same thing.'"

But the genetic map of HTLV-3$_{RF}$ had thrown Gallo a curve. Genetically speaking, if LAV, HTLV-3B, and the other Popovic viruses were standing at home plate, R.F. was out in far left field.[f] "We started to wonder," Hahn recalled, "why is this one different and all these others the same?"[4] Mika Popovic also remembered it as "a big surprise, that one AIDS virus should be so different from all the others."[5]

The AIDS virus might be genetically stable, like HTLV-1. Or it might vary from region to region, like the influenza viruses. But no virus could be both stable *and* variable at the same time. "The dogma," said Hahn's husband, George Shaw, "was that retroviruses were similar, not divergent. It took a little bit of time to understand exactly what we were seeing."[6]

Mika Popovic understood. As Popovic, who hadn't seen his family since his brief visit to Basel the year before, boarded a plane to Vienna for another family reunion, he carried with him the fourth and fifth drafts of his *Science* article to leave with his sister for safekeeping — the versions in which Gallo had excised Popovic's references to his work with LAV.

On a late-summer evening in 1984, the telephone in Luc Montagnier's office chirped.[g] The caller was Robert Gallo, and Gallo began by remarking that HTLV-3B and LAV appeared to be "rather close" in their genetic composition. According to Gallo, Montagnier replied "'So what? They should be close. They're the same kind of virus.'"

No, Gallo explained. He had another AIDS virus, from the Haitian R.F, that was quite different from 3B and LAV.[7] That meant HTLV-3B and LAV were likely to have come from the same patient. "It's a contaminant," Gallo recalled telling Montagnier, "and *you* did it."[h]

According to Gallo, the live HTLV-3B culture Sarngadharan had taken to Paris in May had contaminated the Pasteur's cultures of LAV. The following month, when Gallo asked Montagnier for his LAV-producing B-cell line to facilitate more "comparative studies" of 3B and LAV,[8] Montagnier had unwittingly returned HTLV-3B to Bethesda, labeled as LAV. Or so Gallo said.[9]

Gallo didn't mention the half-dozen other AIDS virus isolates that were also identical to 3B and LAV, which would place the locus of contamination in Bethesda, not Paris. Nor did he tell Montagnier that Popovic had unthawed what was left of the LAV sample sent by Françoise Barré the previous September — months before HTLV-3B existed — and that it, too, was indistinguishable from 3B, which would absolutely rule out a contamination in Paris.

Montagnier, recalling his distress a few months before at learning that Sarngadharan hadn't brought inactivated HTLV-3B to Paris as planned, and realizing that he had perhaps been set up as the eventual culprit in Gallo's transatlantic contamination scenario, leaped "out of my chair, on the verge of apoplexy."[10]

Gallo's scenario was impossible, Montagnier shouted, because the French hadn't *had* any HTLV-3 in Paris at the time the B-cell line was infected with LAV.[i] Moreover, Mal Martin had been given a LAV sample in Paris in April, more than a month before Sarngadharan's arrival at Pasteur. The fact that Martin's LAV was also identical to HTLV-3B could only mean that any contamination had occurred in Gallo's lab.[11]

The National Cancer Institute preferred Gallo's version of events. When Peter Fischinger heard the Paris contamination story, he rushed to inform Vince DeVita that "what Montagnier is sending out to others as the LAV infected cell line is HTLV-3 and not LAV."[12] Fischinger, who thought the facts should come out, wondered what "degree of visibility" DeVita thought appropriate. "Allow Brandt to say it publicly," DeVita suggested. Appearing before a House subcommittee a couple of weeks later, Ed Brandt reported that "recently, scientists at the NCI have determined that LAV is an HTLV-3 virus."[13]

Brandt knew only what he was being told by the NCI, but there were signs he was losing patience with the NIH's star researcher. When Gallo speculated publicly on the risk of transmitting AIDS to women via heterosexual contact, Brandt tried to muzzle him, observing that "Dr. Gallo is not an epidemiologist."[14] But Gallo wouldn't stay quiet. After Jerry Groopman and Zaki Salahuddin reported detecting the AIDS virus in the saliva of nearly half of pre-AIDS patients,[15] Gallo warned the American people that "direct contact" with saliva "should be avoided," setting off alarms about the safety of oral sex, water fountains, restaurant cutlery, and cardiopulmonary resuscitation.[j]

Besides searching for the AIDS virus in bodily fluids, Gallo was battling the French over whether the virus was "a true member of the HTLV family."[16] In the summer of 1984 Gallo's position appeared to have been bolstered by a new paper from the CDC, declaring that LAV and HTLV-2 were similar "over most of their genomes."[17]

Because the CDC paper included studies with LAV, as a courtesy Montagnier, Françoise Barré, and Jean-Claude Chermann had been included as co-authors. But Montagnier, who had just published a paper demonstrating that LAV was a lentivirus *not* related to the HTLVs,[18] demanded that the CDC delete the paragraph about HTLV-2. "We knew it wasn't true," Montagnier said. "I called them on the telephone, but it was too late to change anything."[k]

The following month, Gallo published his own data purporting to make it official: the AIDS virus rightfully belonged to the HTLV family.[19] But when the similarities between HTLV-1 and HTLV-3 were added up, they were about the same as any retrovirus shared with any other retrovirus, animal or human.

Whatever Gallo was saying in print, in private he was far from certain that the AIDS virus had anything in common with the HTLVs.

Ten days after submitting his latest paper to *Science,* Gallo acknowledged to another scientist that HTLV-3 was "only distantly related" to HTLV-1 and HTLV-2, as demonstrated by Gallo's "own failure in numerous experiments."[1] But Gallo's *Science* article nonetheless contained something of considerable significance, buried in a single paragraph in the middle of the text.

HTLV-3B had been the only AIDS virus employed in nearly all the experiments reported in Gallo's four *Science* articles. It was the only AIDS virus allowed out of Gallo's lab for study by other scientists, and it was being used by Abbott and the other licensees to manufacture the American AIDS antibody test. But its origins remained unknown. When Bernie Poiesz and Frank Ruscetti described their discovery of HTLV-1, they had identified Charlie Robinson as "a 28-year-old black man . . . with a diagnosis of cutaneous T-cell leukemia or lymphoma." The Pasteur's first paper in *Science* had described Frédéric Brugière as "a 33-year-old homosexual male." But in the more than four months since HTLV-3B had come on the scene, Gallo hadn't said a word about the patient in whom Popovic had found it.

At last there was an answer: there *was* no such patient. HTLV-3B had been isolated from the T-cells of *several* AIDS patients, whose cultured cells Popovic had pooled together. Don Francis thought it curious that there hadn't been any mention of a patient pool in Popovic's *Science* paper three months before. "Why not say where the virus came from?" he asked. Francis thought it odder still that Popovic had pooled patient material in the first place, something Francis viewed as a certain way *not* to know which patient was the source. "Mixing doesn't make sense," he said. "Why do it?"

The French hadn't pooled blood samples from Brugière, Loiseau, Lailler, or their other AIDS patients. "If you have several isolates and you mix them," Montagnier said, "you will never know which isolate you will get at the end." Jean-Claude Chermann thought Popovic must have simply assumed the AIDS virus would be genetically stable, like HTLV-1, and therefore impossible to trace back to the patient from whom it had come. "At this time," Chermann said, "nobody could predict that LAV could be mutating, so variable."

Gallo dismissed such mutterings as uninformed. "To any virologist it's obvious," he said. "Anybody knows why we would mix. We weren't doing well with singles." But it was less than obvious even to some of Gallo's own people. "Not the cleanest scientific experiment," admitted Lee Ratner, one of Gallo's molecular biologists. "It confused things endlessly. I don't know why you'd ever mix things. All I know is Mika did it."[20] The revelation surprised even Sarngadharan, who had been working with HTLV-3B for months and hadn't heard anything until now about the virus having come from a patient pool.[21]

Ed Brandt was less concerned about how Popovic had found HTLV-3B than whether LAV was also the cause of AIDS, a question Brandt believed to be of critical importance to AIDS research. Although the CDC was still under orders not to compare LAV and HTLV-3B, its separate blood antibody tests of many AIDS patients with both viruses had left no doubt that LAV and HTLV-3B were two names for the same virus.[22] Robin Weiss had come to the same conclusion, based on his sequential testing of hundreds of blood samples in Britain with 3B and LAV.[23] But matters had been confused by a report from Copenhagen that 64 percent of Danish hemophiliacs were positive for antibodies LAV, while only 9 percent had antibodies HTLV-3B.[24]

Months had passed since Brandt had ordered Gallo to carry out a direct comparison of the French and American viruses and Sarngadharan had flown off to Paris. Now Peter Fischinger explained to Brandt that the final comparisons of LAV and HTLV-3B had been delayed — not by Gallo, but by the Pasteur.[25] To help "break the logjam," Brandt offered to intervene with his counterpart in Paris, and put an end to "the French foot-dragging."[26] But there wasn't any foot-dragging in Paris. The logjam was in Bethesda, where Gallo had too much data showing that HTLV-3B and LAV were indistinguishable.

The best evidence was from unpublished experiments by Flossie Wong-Staal comparing the restriction enzyme "maps" of HTLV-3B with Ti7.4/ LAV, the culture Betsy Read had started the previous October. It was impossible to tell 3B and LAV apart, leading Wong-Staal to conclude "that LAV and HTLV-3 are independent isolations of the same virus"— an acknowledgment, at last, that the French had found the AIDS virus first.

But there was something else. No other known isolate had a genetic fingerprint identical to one clone of HTLV-3B — except for one clone of LAV. HTLV-3B and LAV weren't just the same kind of virus. They had come from *the same patient.*[m] Nor had there been any cross-contamination in Paris. The September LAV used by Wong-Staal had arrived in Bethesda eight months before HTLV-3B crossed the Atlantic in the other direction.

Although Gallo later claimed Wong-Staal's data was never written up,[27] a manuscript had been prepared for *The Lancet*, intended for eventual publication as part of the joint comparisons with Pasteur.[28] But the secret that HTLV-3B was LAV wouldn't keep that long, because there was another laboratory where HTLV-3B and LAV were growing in the summer of 1984.

The University of California's Murray Gardner had brought home a sample of LAV from the tripartite meeting in Paris, packed in dry ice beneath his seat on the Air France flight to Los Angeles. Gardner also had Jay Levy's ARV, and Gallo had sent Gardner HTLV-3B "to do any research you want."[29] The UC-Davis hospital, eager to make its own ELISA for screening blood transfusions, had asked Gardner to develop a test for antibodies to the AIDS virus. Considering that LAV had been isolated in Europe, HTLV-3B on the East Coast, and ARV on the West Coast, the three strains seemed to represent the broadest possible spectrum of AIDS virus types.

"We wanted to make sure that of the known viruses, the ELISA wouldn't miss anything," recalled Marty Bryant, the graduate student Gardner assigned to the task. "And it did pick them all up. Then we decided to do some restriction analysis," the same kind of genetic fingerprinting done by Flossie Wong-Staal. When Bryant compared 3B and LAV, they were a dead match —"right down to a gnat's eyebrows," Gardner said later.[30] But ARV was about as different from both LAV and 3B as R.F. had been in Gallo's lab.

Like everyone else, Bryant had expected all the AIDS viruses to be more or less alike. Thinking he had fouled up the experiment, he repeated it several times. Each time it came out the same. "We were in the heat of the battle," recalled Paul Luciw, a researcher from Chiron Corporation who was collaborating with Bryant. "We couldn't really see what was on the next ridge. It didn't really hit us until we saw ARV."

Bryant had been working on a paper about the monkey virus, discovered by Gardner, that causes an AIDS-like disease in primates. To his manuscript he added a section showing that the human AIDS viruses and the monkey AIDS viruses were not genetically related. The new material included the DNA maps of HTLV-3B, LAV, and ARV. Although Bryant's paper left the reader to work out the significance, to anyone who could read a restriction map the conclusion was obvious: LAV and HTLV-3B were too different from ARV — and too much alike — to have come from different patients.

"When I gave the paper to Murray," Bryant recalled, "he said we should send it to Dr. Gallo as a courtesy." Gardner sent a copy to Jay Levy as well, with an anxious note attached. "This preprint describes our comparison of HTLV-3, LAV and ARV," Gardner wrote. "We would appreciate your critical review — anything short of jettisoning the whole project. Marty has worked too hard. I am sending this to Gallo and the French — and am holding my breath!"[31]

Mal Martin, who still hadn't received HTLV-3B from Gallo, was one of many who assumed that all AIDS viruses were the same. Martin's first clue to the contrary had come at an AIDS meeting in Montana in early November 1984, when Murray Gardner, in the midst of a talk about his monkey virus, mentioned Marty Bryant's data.[32]

Jay Levy was in the audience, and as soon as Gardner finished speaking Martin took Levy aside. "Mal said to me, 'Jay, your virus is so different from the Gallo-Montagnier virus,'" Levy recalled. "'You'd better be careful. It looks like a maverick.'"

"I said, 'Mal, we have two others, and they're different too,'" Levy said. "There was an 'Oh, my God.' And then I realized it as well: actually, they're *all* different."[33]

Gallo wasn't at the Montana meeting, but once he had seen Marty Bryant's manuscript he was on the phone to Murray Gardner.[n] "Bob browbeat me, in his way, for about an hour," Gardner recalled. "He questioned my patriotism. He asked me, 'Are you French or are you an American? Aren't you an American?' He asked me to hold off until he and Montagnier could sort it out. He said, 'We have the data, we're onto this, let us do the comparison.'"[34] Gallo's warning was reinforced a few days later by Peter Fischinger, who took Gardner aside during a meeting at NIH. "He told me, 'You would be wise not to get in the middle of this,'" Gardner said.[o] "He implied I would be smart not to touch the comparisons."

When Gardner told Marty Bryant the virus comparisons were being removed from his paper, Bryant was devastated. "I ended up rewriting it with the monkey comparison as the headline and leaving the other stuff out," Bryant said, "just showing that probes made from the human virus didn't pick up the monkey. I was real disappointed. It ended up months later in some obscure place no one ever saw."[35]

With the publication of Bryant's comparisons scuttled, Gallo's secret was safe for the moment, but the moment wouldn't last. In Paris, Marc Alizon and Simon Wain-Hobson had finally succeeded in obtaining a complete clone of LAV, the most important step toward cracking the virus's DNA code.

"Marc and I were in the wilderness until we got the clone," Wain-Hobson said. "No one was interested. It was the two of us against the whole world. Malcolm Martin was the only one who gave us any comfort. When he was in Paris he came to see us. He came by and went through our data, and he said, 'Keep going boys, keep going. You're doing a great job.' And then of course when we got the clone and we started showing it to people, people started showing interest in us — 'These kids have done it,' you know. We started getting encouragement. We realized we were in a race."

Wain-Hobson named the first LAV clone J-19, "J" in honor of his young son, Julien. The second clone of LAV to emerge from Wain-Hobson's lab was J-81. The LAV clones were unveiled during a Thanksgiving-weekend meeting at the Pasteur to which a number of Americans had been invited, including Mal Martin and one of Gallo's assistants, Beatrice Hahn, who by then had extracted two clones of HTLV-3B.ᴾ Hahn brought her restriction maps to Paris, and when Martin compared them to Wain-Hobson's, he discovered what Marty Bryant and Flossie Wong-Staal already knew.

Except for a few trivial differences, all four clones were virtual carbon copies. But it was one of the microscopic differences that caught Martin's attention. The restriction enzymes used by Wain-Hobson and Hahn included *Hind*III ("Hindy three"), a product of the bacteria *Haemophilus influenzae,* which digests only the nucleic acid sequence *AAGCTT. Hind*III had taken a bite out of one of Hahn's clones, and Martin saw that one of Wain-Hobson's clones had a *Hind*III bite in exactly the same place. But Hahn's second clone didn't have the *AAGCTT* sequence. Neither did Wain-Hobson's second clone.

To Martin, it seemed beyond the realm of probability that two AIDS viruses, isolated at different times and from different patients in laboratories 3,000 miles apart, should each have given birth to a clone with a maverick *Hind*III restriction site that existed in no other clone of HTLV-3B, LAV, or ARV. Indeed, Martin had seen the same *Hind*III "signature" in his own sample of LAV.[36] And, like Murray Gardner's LAV, Mal Martin's LAV couldn't have been contaminated by HTLV-3B in Paris, because there hadn't been any HTLV-3B in Paris at the time Martin brought his LAV sample home. "Before," observed George Todaro, "you had two thumbprints that were identical. Now it's like you also have two index fingers that are exactly the same. There aren't enough zeros in the universe to calculate the odds of that."

When Martin returned to Bethesda, he got a call from Jay Levy. "He was quite upset," Martin wrote later in a memo to the file, "because of pressure being put on Dr. Murray Gardner by the NCI staff not to publish data presented at the Montana workshop. He likened the situation to 'a Watergate cover-up' and stated that all data pointed to apparent theft of the French AIDS virus by Gallo."[37]

Convicted killers have been freed from prison upon the discovery that their DNA doesn't match DNA recovered from the scene of the crime. But in rare cases genetic fingerprints can be misleading. The only definitive way to match two pieces of DNA is a side-by-side comparison of their nucleotide sequences. Pasteur had begun "sequencing" the J-19 clone of LAV in September 1984. "We had to handle the sequencing quickly," Marc Alizon recalled, "because Gallo already had a full-length clone and we knew it."

The team of Wain-Hobson, Alizon, and Pierre Sonigo was temporarily expanded to five, with the loan of Olivier Danos and Stuart Cole from other Pasteur labs. For the young French researchers, cloning LAV had been the most difficult task. Sequencing the clones was merely drudgery, going over the same stretch of nucleic acids again and again to ensure as few errors as possible.

"We did it five times," Wain-Hobson said. "We sequenced fifty thousand nucleotides to get ten thousand. With the overlap you get a very good quality sequence. We worked in shifts."

By November the sequence was complete,[38] more than nine thousand "A"s, "T"s, "G"s, and "C"s strung together like so many beads. With the LAV sequence in hand, Wain-Hobson could scan for the three-nucleotide groups, called codons, that mark the beginning and end of each viral gene and, in between, dictate the sequence of amino acids in the particular protein produced by that gene.

The moment the gene map was finished, Wain-Hobson began drafting a paper. "It took us longer to write the paper than it took to do the sequence," Wain-Hobson said, "because we're terrible at writing. We tried to make a nice paper of it."[39]

For the sequencing of HTLV-3B Gallo had assembled a consortium of researchers headed by Lee Ratner, an M.D.–Ph.D. from Yale, that included another NCI lab, Bill Haseltine's lab at Harvard, and two companies, DuPont and Centocor.[40] "There were nineteen of us," Ratner recalled, "and we worked our tails off for three to four months."[41] Ratner's group finished the sequence of HTLV-3B on November 29, two weeks behind the French, and sent their paper to *Nature* the same day.[42]

Worried that Gallo's sequence would be the first to appear in print, Montagnier called Sam Broder, an NCI lab chief who was organizing a cancer institute symposium on HTLV, to lobby for a slot to present the Pasteur's findings. "Montagnier said, 'Could Wain-Hobson speak? He's got some interesting stuff on the genetics of the virus,'" Wain-Hobson recalled. "And Broder sort of hemmed and hawed and said, 'Well, maybe, perhaps.'" After a letter from Montagnier and another telephone call, Broder belatedly agreed to let Wain-Hobson have twenty minutes. "Then they pushed in Arsène Burney," one of Gallo's Belgian collaborators, "to give us less time."

The predicament for the French was how much of their data to present in Bethesda. If Wain-Hobson didn't show the gene map of LAV, and if Gallo or Wong-Staal presented a map of HTLV-3B, everyone would conclude the French had lost the race to decode the virus. But any data that appeared on an overhead screen at a scientific meeting was fair game. If Gallo's team hadn't completed its sequence, or had gotten part of it wrong, Wain-Hobson wasn't sure he wanted to show them the map of LAV.

On the morning of December 6, 1984, the largest auditorium on the NIH campus, Wilson Hall, was overflowing with retrovirologists from around the world. Gallo, who had just returned from a week in Vienna, used his opening lecture to reiterate the similarities between HTLV-3 and the other HTLVs. Next came Flossie Wong-Staal, whom Montagnier and Wain-Hobson had expected to show at least a partial gene map of HTLV-3B.

When Wong-Staal didn't present any genetic data on the AIDS virus, Montagnier thought he understood Broder's reluctance to allow Wain-Hobson to speak: Gallo's team hadn't finished its gene map. As Wain-Hobson walked to the dais, it dawned on him that he had a clear field, and as his twenty minutes drew to a close Wain-Hobson put up a slide of the LAV gene map.

For two human retroviruses, LAV and HTLV-1 could scarcely have been less alike. Where HTLV-1 had only four genes, LAV had at least five, and there were important differences in their sizes and placement.[q] Just before Wain-Hobson finished his talk there was a rustling sound, followed by a sudden exodus from the auditorium. "I remember Bill Haseltine stomping out of there with a contingent of people," said Cy Cabradilla. "I also remember him grabbing people and saying, 'No, no, his sequence is wrong. *We've* got the right sequence.' Bill Haseltine was very upset. Molecular biologist, cloner, sequencer, supposed to be a top gun, and here he got upstaged by the French."[43]

When the time came for questions, Haseltine and the others filed back to their seats. "Gallo walked to the microphone," recalled Paul Luciw, now running a lab at the University of California in Davis, "and he said, 'I have a question for Dr. Wain-Hobson.' But he didn't ask a question, he made a speech. He talked for more than ten minutes." When Gallo's soliloquy finally ended, it was with a question. "He asked me, 'Why do you stress the differences between HTLV-1 and HTLV-3?'" Wain-Hobson said, "I answered, 'Only because there are so many.' Everyone was taken by surprise."[44]

"The people from Gallo's camp couldn't believe it," Cabradilla said. "They were shocked. This small band of molecular biologists out of the Pasteur Institute had just beaten these guys from NCI and Harvard. Other groups, myself included, were saying, 'Hey, good job.'"[45]

Paul Luciw, whose paper containing the sequence of Jay Levy's ARV was already in the mail to *Science*,[46] accorded victory to the French. "Simon Wain-Hobson had the story," Luciw said, "and everyone else, including us, was close but behind. I talked to Flossie and apparently they had cloned it, had sequenced it and they were a little bit unsure about a couple of things at that point."[47]

It was almost Christmas before Pasteur's sequence paper was finished. Despite David Klatzmann's unhappy experience with *Nature*, Wain-Hobson summoned the courage to offer the manuscript to Peter Newmark. "We phoned them up the evening of December twenty-third," Wain-Hobson recalled, saying "'You'll have our paper tomorrow.' And they didn't want it."[48]

Without missing a beat, Wain-Hobson turned to *Cell*, a weighty tome then published by the Massachusetts Institute of Technology. "We received an inquiry from the French group," recalled *Cell*'s editor,

Benjamin Lewin, "saying that they had been intending to send the paper to *Nature*, that *Nature* had told them that they wouldn't consider it, and they were naturally somewhat upset about this.

"They felt they had been working pretty much evenly with Gallo's group, and suddenly they were not going to get their paper published maybe until months afterwards. So we said to the French people, yes, we thought the sequence of the first isolate of the AIDS virus was a significant event, that we thought it was appropriate for *Cell*, and that if they wanted to submit it we'd be glad to consider it in the usual way. The usual way meaning, 'We will look at the paper and we will then decide whether or not it is something we ought to publish.'"[49]

The day after Christmas the Pasteur paper was on Lewin's desk. "It was pretty straightforward," Lewin recalled. "Sequence papers are very easy. Either they've sequenced the right thing, or they haven't. And since you don't actually go and look at sequence gels anymore, sequence papers are among the easiest papers we have to review. It didn't take us very long to decide that we should publish the paper and that we should publish it very quickly, because this was a competitive situation. We thought the fair thing would be if the paper came out more or less contemporaneously with Gallo's paper."

Cell's editorial deadlines didn't permit it to publish again before the third week in January, and the French expected to see Gallo's sequence in *Nature* before then. By mid-January the Gallo paper still hadn't appeared, which Ben Lewin thought a bit strange. "*Nature* can publish stuff in about ten days," said Lewin, who had been an editor there before moving to Boston. "The paper was in press longer than one would have expected, given how significant it was."

In the interim, a story had begun circulating that, shortly after Wain-Hobson's talk, the Gallo group had changed its genetic interpretation of the HTLV-3B sequence to match Pasteur's interpretation of LAV. "The story," Cy Cabradilla said, "goes that because there were significant differences, somebody went back to the lab and resequenced. It took them about three weeks. They were really trying to steal the thunder from the French again. When they subsequently resequenced another variant, it turned out that yes, they got what Wain-Hobson got."

Ben Lewin also recalled hearing "stories about someone from the Gallo mob flying over to London and changing these proofs on the spot." Peter Newmark had "some fairly dim recollection of something happening" to the Gallo sequence paper after it had been submitted. "In retrospect," Newmark said, "it would have been a very important event. But at the time? You know, people change things at the last minute because they've found something different. It wouldn't have stuck in my mind because it's not so unusual."[r]

According to Lee Ratner, the paper that eventually appeared in *Nature* was "almost identical to what we mailed in," the only differences being cosmetic. "The first printout, when we saw the galleys, it just wasn't readable," Ratner said. "We retyped the figures so that they would look much better." But Ratner emphatically denied having flown to London. "I talked to London," Ratner said, "but nobody went to London as far as I know. I would have liked to have gone."

The DNA sequence of HTLV-3B appeared in *Nature*'s issue of January 24, three days after *Cell*'s publication of the sequence of LAV.[50] But *Cell* wasn't fast enough for the National Cancer Institute, which released advance copies of the Gallo article to the press with a five-page commemoration of "an important milestone in AIDS research."[51] "Now we see the face of the enemy," Bill Haseltine told the *Washington Post*.[52] As drawn by Gallo and Haseltine, the face of HTLV-3B was virtually the same as the face of HTLV-1. But it was dramatically different from the face of LAV.[s]

In less than a month the gene wars were over, with victory accorded to the French. The gene map of ARV, decoded by Paul Luciw and his California team, was a dead match for LAV, which meant Gallo's map was dead wrong.[t] "In contrast to earlier reports," Luciw wrote in *Science,* the AIDS virus had no more in common with HTLV-1 and HTLV-2 than with any of the animal retroviruses — so different from the HTLVs, observed Montagnier, that "it cannot even be considered a cousin."[53]

The cake was iced by a sequencing team at San Francisco's Genentech, whose gene map of Gallo's HTLV-3B looked like those of LAV and ARV — and where researchers agreed that HTLV-3 seemed "entirely unrelated" to HTLV-1.[54] "It was anybody's bet, and we proved wrong," said a chastened Roberto Patarca, who had played a key role in formulating the Gallo sequence in Bill Haseltine's lab. "We just took that calculated risk of going for it. Of course, the French didn't go for it."

Once the sequences were in print, it was easy to see why nobody else had been able to find the genetic similarities between the AIDS virus and the HTLVs that Gallo had been claiming for nearly a year.

They didn't exist. Of the 9,213 nucleotides that contained the DNA code for the AIDS virus, there were eighty-three matches with HTLV-1, and only seventeen with HTLV-2.

Moreover, the AIDS virus was bigger than HTLV-1, had a different-shaped core, and ultimately proved to have three times as many genes. The AIDS virus killed the T-cells it infected, grew well in culture, and could exist outside its host. As a delighted Abraham Karpas put it, the AIDS virus and HTLV-1 were "as different as cheese and chalk."

Peter Newmark realized, too late, that by declining the Pasteur paper *Nature* had missed the story. "Had we *seen* your paper," Newmark wrote Montagnier, "and had it, too, differed substantially from Gallo/Haseltine (as I gather it does), I am certain we would have been persuaded."[55] But Wain-Hobson had chosen to telephone London rather than simply sending the manuscript, and *Nature* hadn't asked to see the Pasteur paper before saying no.

"We lived to regret our decision," Newmark said later. "I can't remember what we were thinking. I assume that it was 'a sequence is a sequence,' and that they would be the same. It so happened that we had just taken an editorial decision based on a number of occasions on which we had found that we were publishing the same sequence over and over again. I've forgotten what it was, but it kept happening that we were finding that we would accept a paper and before it was published somebody else would send us another paper with the same damn sequence."

John Maddox, who disclaimed any knowledge that the French had offered their sequence to *Nature,* found Newmark's letter of explanation to Montagnier "a bit laconic. He doesn't say, 'Exceedingly sorry,'" Maddox said. "He simply says, 'Here's the explanation in case you wonder.'"

"In retrospect," Maddox said, "it was an unfortunate decision, and we quickly abandoned the policy, of which Montagnier was the only victim. Or *we* were the only victim. We became aware of it when Gallo, I think, called up and said, 'Look, we want to put out a press release. Because you're not going to publish our sequence until the week after *Cell* publishes Montagnier's.' And so I said, 'Why don't we have Montagnier's?' And then I get the story that Wain-Hobson had called. I was very angry, particularly because there was the earlier instance with Montagnier, the earlier paper. I knew about that too."

Ludwik Gross, an elderly virologist from the Bronx VA Hospital whom Gallo credited as "an inspiration through much of my career," had been chosen to write a review of the NCI symposium for *Cancer Research.* When someone slipped Montagnier an advance copy of Gross's review, he found it extraordinary that Gross failed to mention Wain-Hobson's presentation at all.

"This was the first report on the entire sequence of LAV," Montagnier wrote to Gross. "Of course, you have the right to take or not to take into account these remarks. But I should be very grateful to you if you could still modify your text on the galley proof. Perhaps I will find another opportunity to meet with you again and to tell you more about the LAV story! A very strange affair where extra scientific factors are playing a great or even greater part. . . ."[56]

Gross, whose claim to fame was the discovery three decades before of a mouse leukemia virus, admitted to Montagnier that he hadn't really understood much of the molecular biology presented at the symposium. "I am sort of an old-timer in virology," Gross explained, "not quite aware of the most recent methods." He had tried "very hard to be honest and to give credit where credit belongs," Gross said, "but it is very difficult to please everyone."[57]

When Gross's review appeared in *Cancer Research,* it contained no indication that the first-ever genetic map of the AIDS virus had been unveiled at the meeting by the Institut Pasteur. Nor did the proceedings even contain Simon Wain-Hobson's paper.[u] The proceedings did, however, contain a gene map of HTLV-3B, as part of the symposium presentation by Flossie Wong-Staal. Odd, since Wong-Staal hadn't presented any gene map at the symposium.

Odder still, the map in Wong-Staal's paper wasn't the erroneous map Gallo had published in *Nature* a month after the symposium. In fact, it looked *exactly* like Simon Wain-Hobson's map of LAV in *Cell.*[58] According to a footnote, however, the data contained in Wong-Staal's paper had been "presented at the HTLV Symposium, December 6 and 7, 1984, Bethesda, MD."[v] As far as historians of science would be concerned, Gallo, not the French, had won the race to map the AIDS virus.

The publication of the DNA sequences had rendered irrelevant the more rudimentary comparisons of LAV and HTLV-3B that had occasioned so much angst during the spring and summer of 1984. In early January of 1985, Montagnier sent Gallo the draft of Jean-Claude Chermann's paper, written for *The Lancet,* detailing the structural similarities between LAV and HTLV-3B that Chermann and Sarnga-dharan had found at the Pasteur eight months earlier.[w] Gallo hadn't replied, and now the protein comparisons had been overtaken by the sequences. So had Flossie Wong-Staal's restriction maps showing that HTLV-3B and LAV were indistinguishable, and Montagnier agreed with Gallo that the Wong-Staal paper was also "obsolete."

The third of the erstwhile joint papers, written by Don Francis, recounted the CDC's comparisons of the Gallo and Pasteur ELISAs.[59] "I understand the consensus now is that it should be pub-lished," Francis told Gallo at the end of October 1984. "Also enclosed is the original printout of the results. . . . Please send me comment, authors and corrections as soon as possible."[60] But Gallo didn't want to see the CDC's blood-testing data in print. "As you know," he replied to Francis, "our agreement was made with the ideas that the comparisons of the viruses would be published first by the Pasteur group and my lab. Until this occurs neither you nor anyone else should be making serological comparative papers."[61]

Had the comparative papers been published, they would have belied Gallo's many declarations during 1984 that he hadn't had enough LAV to compare with HTLV-3. They would have shown that the French and American viruses were one and the same —"quasi-identical," in Simon Wain-Hobson's terminology — and that Gallo had known as much in the summer of 1984. The Wong-Staal paper, moreover, proved there hadn't been a contamination in Paris.[62] Per-haps most important, the papers would have shown that the French had been first to make a blood-antibody test and use it to establish the cause of AIDS. But none of the papers was ever published, and all that was lost to history.

"Let Them Bark in the Wind"

When People *profiled the world's twenty-five "busiest bees"* Robert Gallo made the list, along with Queen Elizabeth, Bob Hope, Jesse Jackson, and Dr. Armand Hammer, the millionaire philanthropist who had recently honored Gallo with the Armand Hammer Cancer Research Award. Gallo, just back from a week in the West Indies and preparing to depart for Colorado and Hawaii,[1] was accorded the maximum of three bees, the same degree of busyness as the Queen herself.[2]

"The search for a desperately needed AIDS vaccine keeps the top medical sleuth in his laboratory at Bethesda, Maryland's National Cancer Institute six days, 72 hours a week," People said. "Naturally he sets his clocks five minutes ahead. His assistants are accustomed to grabbing time with Gallo in elevators, parking lots and the doc's Nissan Stanza, which he races across town — often ignoring stoplights — to Capitol Hill appointments. Twice a month or so Gallo travels to medical conferences abroad. Then, without a second for sightseeing or a night on the town, it's back home to the lab in Bethesda. Sighs his wife, Mary Jane: 'Bob's addicted to adrenaline.'"

Gallo hadn't been spending much time searching for an AIDS vaccine. Most of his energy was being devoted to fending off suspicions that his historic discovery was really somebody else's discovery. With the DNA sequences in print, many of the French scientists who had disdained the work of Luc Montagnier and his group at the Institut

Pasteur now understood that Montagnier had been right from the start, and that the virus discovered in Paris in 1983 was the same virus Gallo claimed to have discovered in 1984. At the annual Park City AIDS meeting in February 1985, Gallo was confronted by a senior Pasteur scientist, Gerard Orth, the codiscoverer of the human papilloma viruses, who demanded to know exactly what Gallo had done with the LAV sent by Montagnier.

Orth's question prompted a tirade, which Gallo regretted after returning home. "What did I do with the virus of Montagnier?" Gallo wrote Orth from Bethesda. "My answer was based on the interpretation that you people were pushing the question whether we 'took' 'his virus.' I reacted to this insult in a way that I felt was complete, appropriate, and conclusive. However, now I have reason to believe that this question was also asked in a manner that is more subtle, technical, and quasi-legal: i.e., we used his virus to learn something which helped us for the blood test. I did not address that question. I will address it here and now. . . . I am far from sure we learned anything useful to us, to AIDS research, or for the blood test."[3]

People hadn't mentioned that one of the principal questions surrounding the discovery of the AIDS virus had been resolved, not in Gallo's favor, by the publication of the DNA sequences of LAV and HTLV-3B. With the genetic structure of the AIDS virus uncloaked, it was the uncontested opinion of the scientific community that HTLV-3 and HTLV-1 belonged to different families of viruses. Gallo wasn't saying so in public, but the revelation had come as a huge surprise. "The sequence data was a shock to us," Gallo admitted later, "basically because we were thinking the virus was going to be closer to HTLV-1. We just were amazed at the amount of differences."[4]

As the *New York Times* observed, "In the world of science, as among primitive societies, to be the namer of an object is to own it."[5] If Gallo could no longer lay a clear claim to the discovery of the AIDS virus, he at least could see that it remained a nominal member of his "HTLV family." Despite his private astonishment at the manifold differences between the AIDS virus and the HTLVs, Gallo continued to insist that the right name for the AIDS virus was HTLV-3. "LAV is clearly an inaccurate name," Gallo wrote a colleague at the beginning of 1985, adding that Jay Levy's AIDS-related virus was "the dumbest name I have heard yet." In Gallo's opinion, HTLV-3 was "as accurate, as innocuous, and as consistent with the past as any name possible."[6]

When Montagnier objected, Gallo reminded him that "eighteen scientists from United States, Japan and Europe" had agreed at Cold Spring Harbor that the next human retrovirus would be named HTLV-3. But the Cold Spring Harbor Agreement, which had only nine signatories, not including Montagnier, merely stated that future *leukemia*-causing human retroviruses would be named HTLV-3, HTLV-4, and so on. To Gallo, the fine points didn't matter. "Any impartial scientist," he declared, "will adopt the name HTLV-3. In fact, almost everyone in the United States and most people in Europe have already done so. I hope we would save our energy in trying to contain the virus and the disease rather than to beat a dead horse over nomenclature."[7]

Montagnier retorted that it was Gallo's laboratory, not the Pasteur, which had "spent a lot of energy, time and money" to find similarities between the AIDS virus and the HTLVs. "In renaming this virus HTLV," Montagnier said, "you have induced a lot of confusion amongst unaware people. It will help them and not diminish your prestige if you state clearly that your earlier interpretation has to be corrected. If you believe in sequence data, why don't you leave off your previous dream and admit that the AIDS virus is not an HTLV strain?"[8]

Montagnier suggested keeping LAV and changing what the initials stood for, to lymphadenopathy AIDS virus.[9] Montagnier remained "open to any better proposal"— though not the one from Flossie Wong-Staal, who thought the AIDS virus should be called HALV, for human AIDS/lymphotropic virus. Her name, Wong-Staal wrote *Nature*, was "the perfect solution for the two groups to meet *halv* way."[10] When the French protested that the Americans were making light of a serious matter, Gallo replied that "Flossie's letter had been sent 'with tongue in cheek.' I did not even know she wrote it. She was saying it in the lab as a joke. To emphasize to you how silly it is, such a name would not be acceptable to me."[11]

To settle the dispute, the scientific community turned to Harold Varmus, who chaired the taxonomy committee of the *Retroviridae* Study Group. Varmus responded by forming a fourteen-member sub-committee that included Gallo, Montagnier, Max Essex, Robin Weiss, Jay Levy, and, for some *gravitas*, Howard Temin. When Gallo challenged the Varmus committee's right to involve itself, Varmus reminded Gallo that it had been Dani Bolognesi who urged the committee to step in and settle the matter. No sooner was the panel assembled than Gallo sent each of the other members a list of twenty arguments why the name HTLV-3 was "fair, accurate, and safe."[12]

The fuss over the naming of the virus overshadowed the elephant in the parlor: the no-longer-avoidable reality that HTLV-3B and LAV differed by only eighty-seven nucleotides out of 9,213, less than 1 percent. That singular genetic identity, hinted at by the still-unpublished data from Marty Bryant and Flossie Wong-Staal, inspired Gallo to replace his contamination-in-Paris hypothesis with a new explanation of why HTLV-3B was an independent discovery. According to Gallo, Frédéric Brugière had become infected "at a similar time and place" as one or more of the patients in the Popovic pool.[13]

In Gallo's version of history, Brugière had visited New York City around the time the blood and tissue samples were being obtained from the pool patients. Either he had sex with one of them, or someone who had recently had sex with a pool patient. However it happened, Brugière had gone back to Paris carrying an AIDS virus indistinguishable from the one that infected his American partner. That was the reason LAV looked so much like HTLV-3B.

The French dismissed Gallo's explanation as balderdash, pointing out that Brugière's only visit to New York City had occurred in 1979, more than *four years* before the creation of the Popovic pool.[a] That Brugière hadn't experienced the first symptoms of pre-AIDS until the summer of 1982 suggested he had become infected in the spring of that year — *three years* after his visit to New York.

Instead of further confusing science, Montagnier suggested Gallo settle the question himself, by sequencing, or at least mapping, the individual AIDS viruses that had infected Popovic's pool patients. If even one of the patients had a virus that matched LAV, then HTLV-3B was indeed an independent discovery. But if Gallo ever took Montagnier's suggestion, he never said anything about the results.

The DNA sequences of LAV, HTLV-3B, and ARV were scattered across several journals, and the nuances of their similarities escaped anyone who hadn't studied the literature with a magnifying glass. Thinking it might be instructive to pull the data together in an article for *Cell,* Mal Martin declared it "surprising, in view of their independent isolation," that HTLV-3B was no more different from LAV than Beatrice Hahn's various clones of HTLV-3B were from one another.[14] Martin's inference was clear, but his article stopped short of asking how two virtually identical AIDS viruses had been isolated ten months and three thousand miles apart. "Mal had the data," a frustrated George Todaro said later, "but he didn't have the guts."

With Martin's article bound to raise more questions among those who caught its meaning, Gallo stepped up efforts to demonstrate that his lab did indeed possess AIDS virus isolates that were different from HTLV-3B and LAV — the implication being that, with other AIDS viruses at hand, there hadn't been a motive to steal the virus from France.

Within days of Martin's paper, Robin Weiss and a number of other researchers received an unexpected announcement: samples of the R.F. virus, and another called M.N., from a New Jersey infant born to an intravenous drug user, were now available to anyone who wanted them.[15] "I wrote to him," Weiss recalled, "saying, 'Look here, we've been asking you for ages and you never sent any. Now you're offering them to all and sundry. Can you include us on the list?'"

Only those with access to Gallo's lab records could have seen that neither R.F. nor M.N. conferred priority for the discovery of the AIDS virus. R.F. hadn't begun growing in a continuous cell line until the end of December 1983, just as Popovic was turning his attention from LAV to MOV.[16] M.N. hadn't been put into a continuous culture until three weeks before Margaret Heckler's news conference.[17]

The R.F. culture reported in *Science* had faltered, and it had been reisolated in the more productive H-9 cell line.[b] Throughout the fall and winter of 1984, Popovic had worked feverishly to increase the production of R.F. to the point where it could be "distributed in some selected laboratories."[18] Not until March of 1985, nearly a year after the Heckler news conference, had there been enough R.F. to make available to other labs. The researchers who finally got it were chagrined to discover that the R.F. culture was full of mycoplasma, a type of bacteria whose proclivity to contaminate cell cultures is the bane of virologists.[19]

Ironically, one of the last to receive R.F. was Jim Hoxie, the University of Pennsylvania oncologist who had gone to the trouble of sending Gallo R.F.'s cells, but who hadn't been a co-author on, or even mentioned in, Popovic's *Science* article. "I felt somewhat screwed," Hoxie said later, "because I was scrounging to get grants, and having my name on a paper of that import would have been very helpful to me at that point in my career."

The *Washington Post* was still calling the AIDS virus a "Human T-Cell Leukemia Virus,"[20] and most of the rapidly expanding battalion of science and medical writers assigned to the AIDS story had missed the message of the DNA sequences. Not among them was Omar Sattaur, the London-based reporter in charge of the *New Scientist's* AIDS coverage.

Although a biologist by training, Sattaur was as intrigued by the politics of science as by science itself, and in February of 1985 he declared that "the world has ignored the true discoverers" of the AIDS virus, "and has given Gallo the credit instead." Why, Sattaur wondered, "does the myth that Gallo is the discoverer of the AIDS virus persist? The reason is that it seems to make a nice story." But he suspected there was more to it than that.

"Deciding who has priority on the discovery of the virus is important for reasons other than to glorify the discoverers," Sattaur wrote. "The total US market for diagnostic kits alone, to screen blood for the presence of the AIDS virus, is estimated at $80 million. Who receives the money from patent rights obviously depends on who first patented the procedure for isolating the AIDS virus."[21]

Sattaur, a native of Guyana with a degree from the University of London, had first encountered Gallo at a medical conference in Boston a couple of years before, and remembered having been "really impressed. He was so full of charm. He's bright, really quick-witted. And also, he has this kind of camaraderie. I remember going to dinner with him. Haseltine was there, dressed extremely elegantly — great long trench coat and a hat, an amazing character. Gallo got a bit tipsy. In fact more than tipsy — came out of the pub, threw his arm around me, and invited me to one of his famous pool parties. And I thought, 'Oh, you know, just what Americans would call a regular guy.'"

For some months after that, Sattaur and Gallo "had a very good relationship. I'd ring him up and say, 'What's new?' And he'd just spout. A lot of the things scientifically would be a lot of rubbish. But it's a very interesting read. I just told people, 'This is speculation, this is what he's thinking about at the moment.' At that time, he was the one who had the most to say. Once I'd started to publish things that he didn't like, he started to change radically."

Acting on a tip from Abraham Karpas, the *New Scientist* had begun looking into the dispute between Gallo and the Pasteur. "He contacted us," Sattaur recalled, "and he said, 'Look, I'm convinced that Gallo has cheated.' And the editor put me onto it because I'm a life scientist. So I said, 'Great, now I'll go and interview Karpas.' I was quite intrigued by it, because I'd just done another story about plagiarism."

Following a memorable afternoon in Karpas's lab, Sattaur had flown to Paris. "An extraordinary visit," Sattaur said later. "I would not have been taken with the story had Montagnier turned out to be anything like Karpas. If you see what I mean. Karpas is this man who has a deep vengeance to satisfy, which made me dubious. But the precision of his work, for whatever motive, was so good that I had to listen to him.

"Now if I'd gone to Paris and found that Montagnier was the same kind of person, I would have thought, 'Well, is it really sour grapes?' But no. Montagnier was actually distressed. He was distressed that his very poor institute had just been sort of disregarded. It must have felt awful for Montagnier. He was very forthcoming, and what he said was said in a way that was very diplomatic. He was perturbed, and he didn't try to hide that. But that made me think, 'There's something in this.'"

The trail led Sattaur from Paris to Atlanta and the CDC, where he encountered V. S. Kalyanaraman, a talented Indian virologist who had discovered HTLV-2 while working in Gallo's lab, but had jumped ship when Don Francis offered him a higher salary grade and a less "intense and competitive" working environment.[22] Gallo protested Francis's recruitment of Kalyanaraman as "unfair, if not outrageous,"[23] and threatened to prevent Kalyanaraman from publishing anything further on retroviruses if he abandoned the NCI for the CDC.[c] When Kalyanaraman accepted the CDC's offer, Gallo decreed that Kalyanaraman wouldn't be taking any of Gallo's cells or viruses to Atlanta.[24]

"He's great, actually," Sattaur said of Kalyanaraman. "I really liked him. He had a kind of fascination with Gallo, but also a slight fear of the man. Kalyanaraman said that everybody in Gallo's lab felt paranoid in some way, and that it was quite an awful place to work. Because it was very high-pressure and he ran it like an autocrat. They were all his minions."

According to Sattaur, Kalyanaraman had told a "most extraordinary" story. "He had befriended Popovic," Sattaur said. "Popovic had very few people he could talk to. He said that Popovic is the man whose neck is on the line. Because Popovic was instructed by Gallo to mix up the viruses — the Pasteur isolate and their own isolates. The rationale for doing that was that there would be some synergistic effect in growing this virus that's extremely difficult to grow. The unknown, as it were."

The *New Scientist* article was the first publication on either side of the Atlantic to suggest a darker side to the "nice story," and Sattaur recalled that "We had everyone down on us like a ton of bricks. There were extremely nasty letters. We had a phone call from Walter Bodmer, the head of the Imperial Cancer Research Fund. Nobody bothered to dispute any claims that I made. They just said, 'How dare you write this stuff?'"

Robin Weiss thought Sattaur's article "the nastiest piece of writing I have seen in twenty years of studying retroviruses."[25] Dani Bolognesi warned the *New Scientist* that Sattaur's "inaccurate, misleading, grossly biased, remarkably uninformed, and naive remarks" would "accomplish nothing more than to discredit your journal."[26] The only kind word had come from Abraham Karpas, who complimented Sattaur "on his illuminating article on what may become 'Gallogate' in spite of a *Weisswash*."[27]

Sattaur hadn't printed Kalyanaraman's remarks about Popovic, which Kalyanaraman's lawyer later denied had been made.[d] But Gallo thought Sattaur's story defamed him anyway. "Gallo said he ought to get the government to start a libel action," said Sattaur. "Then he goes through his whole history. I've got a quote: 'You're getting manipulated for goddamn money. We published forty-eight isolates — they published a picture. They had no publications in the field. I had two hundred, three hundred. We had the virus before they ever worked in the field, but they couldn't propagate it.'"

Gallo went on rewriting history. "They did not *isolate* the virus in May 1983," he told Sattaur, "They *identified* it. They did not think [LAV] was AIDS. *I* did. *We* linked it to the disease. They're only linking it now, with people from CDC. In January '84 I called Jim Curran to say that the etiology was sound. And he was overwhelmingly convinced. Not one fucking picture, but forty-eight isolates. You're being taken for a ride because of big, commercial, economic reasons. The French simply followed my reasoning and followed me."

Years later, Sattaur shook his head at recalling the conversation. "Gallo has this ability to just absorb everything," Sattaur said. "He's wonderful at it. He's so good at manipulating things that I'm pretty sure that unconsciously he's doing it most of the time. If you talk to him about other people's work, he'll say, 'Well, he worked in my lab for six weeks. I taught him everything he knew.' He's a real megalomaniac. I think that's why I got quite angry with myself — I felt I'd been duped, when I found out the other side of things."

Margaret Heckler's October 1984 deadline for putting the AIDS blood test into service had come and gone, with Abbott Laboratories and the other licensees still field-testing their ELISAs in cities where significant numbers of potential blood donors were presumed to be infected with the AIDS virus.[28] Lowell Harmison, the senior HHS official charged with getting the blood test to market, had promised the blood banks the ELISA would be at least 98 percent accurate.[29] But the computer printouts Abbott was sending the Food and Drug Administration showed that at least 60 percent of blood samples scoring positive contained no AIDS virus antibodies at all.[e]

So inaccurate was the American ELISA, the FDA conceded, that it would be necessary to use a more complicated and expensive test, the Western Blot, which registers the presence of antibodies to specific viral proteins, to confirm any ELISA-positive result.[f] When health groups threatened lawsuits to keep the AIDS test from being licensed until its accuracy could be assured,[30] the FDA, which had planned to license all five tests simultaneously, shifted its strategy to putting at least one reasonably accurate test in the hands of the blood banks as quickly as possible.[31] The American Red Cross, which collected more than half the blood donated in the United States and which was the world's biggest purchaser of blood antibody tests, announced that it would buy its AIDS tests from whichever company received the first FDA license.

By the end of January 1985 Margaret Heckler was promising that the AIDS test would be licensed by mid-February. Attempting to assuage concerns about the risk from unscreened blood, Heckler assured Americans that infection with the AIDS virus didn't mean most people would get AIDS. Only "a small number of those with positive test results," Heckler said, would go on to develop the disease itself.[32] It wasn't true, but it wasn't Heckler's fault. Three days earlier, the Public Health Service's Executive Task Force on AIDS had estimated that only 5 to 20 percent of those infected with the AIDS virus would ever get AIDS.

When mid-February arrived with no AIDS test in sight, Heckler explained that the FDA needed still more field data from Abbott and the other manufacturers.[33] The Red Cross was already negotiating a draft contract with Abbott Laboratories, whom the FDA had pushed to the front of the line.[34] But the Red Cross technicians working with the prototype Abbott test were finding it "extremely cumbersome and labor intensive," and the Red Cross's Boston blood center had "major concerns" about the test's ability to catch every virus-infected blood sample.[35] The Abbott ELISA, a senior Red Cross official complained, had "the potential for causing undue concern for a number of healthy donors" by registering too many false positives, "while not removing from the blood supply all the units that are potentially infectious for AIDS."[36]

In the Reagan administration's view, any AIDS test was better than no test, and on a Saturday afternoon in early March 1985, timed to make the Sunday papers, Margaret Heckler announced that the FDA at last had approved a blood-antibody test for HTLV-3.[37] Jack Schuler, the Abbott executive, recalled being summoned to meet with Heckler early that morning, then watching from her anteroom sofa as a delegation from Electronucleonics, one of the other licensees, filed out of the secretary's office.

Schuler's first thought was that both Abbott and Electronucleonics were being approved at the same time, which would have cost Abbott a substantial share of Red Cross business. Once the Electronucleonics team departed, Heckler reassured Schuler that the FDA had decided to approve Abbott first. She had merely been explaining to Electronucleonics that the approvals were being issued in alphabetical order.[38]

The following day, Abbott closed a deal to supply the Red Cross with a year's worth of ELISA kits at the cut-rate price of ninety-three cents apiece. When the stock market opened on Monday morning,

Abbott's shares began a long upward climb that would see them more than double in price over the next two years.[g] The first blood bank in the world to get the AIDS test was the Red Cross Blood Center on Ohio Street in downtown Chicago, a thirty-minute drive from Abbott's North Chicago headquarters.[39] Accompanying each of the two thousand test kits delivered that Saturday afternoon was a warning that "false positive test results can be expected with a test kit of this nature."[40]

Because of the delays in field-testing, Abbott only had sixty thousand ELISA kits on hand, not nearly enough to fill the nationwide demand. The AIDS test would be rationed among fourteen cities,[h] with no tests available for the rest of the country. A month after the test was approved, the Red Cross was still testing only half its new blood donations, and none of the blood that had been stored in its freezers when the test became available.[41] Testing the stored blood might raise concerns that the blood was unsafe and discourage hospitals from buying it.[42]

Such concerns would have been justified. At the end of March, an Arkansas patient received a pint of blood donated four days after Abbott received its FDA license. Although routine blood testing in Arkansas had begun five days *before* the patient's surgery, the blood used for the man's transfusion hadn't been screened. He later got AIDS. There were other such cases,[43] and not until mid-April of 1985, after nearly three million AIDS tests had been distributed, was Heckler able to report that the domestic backlog had been filled. "As a result," she told researchers attending an international AIDS conference at the CDC, "our manufacturers will now be able to turn their attention to *your* needs — meeting the foreign demand for the test, which has been significant. That is a contribution to the international community we are very proud to make."[44]

Some eight thousand Americans had been diagnosed with AIDS.[45] But there were less than four hundred cases in France, barely two hundred in Germany, and fewer than that in Great Britain. There was plenty of AIDS in Africa, but those cases weren't the result of hospital transfusions, and in the countries whose health systems could afford it, the demand for an AIDS test was less than overwhelming. Gallo reminded a physicians' convention in London that, because of the long lag-time between infection and disease, the number of reported cases was no guide to the number of people actually infected with the virus.

Two million Americans, Gallo declared, were already carrying the AIDS virus — a number that later proved to be far beyond the actual scope of the epidemic.[i] In another two years, Gallo predicted, a half million British would be infected with HTLV-3. Although the actual numbers in Britain would never surpass a tenth of that figure,[j] the headlines generated by Gallo's warning —"British doctors told of massive new AIDS crisis," cried the *Observer* — prompted questions in Parliament and elsewhere about why there was no AIDS test in Britain.

In fact, there was a British AIDS test. Months before, Robin Weiss had developed a laboratory ELISA and used it to test nearly two thousand Londoners, including a thousand randomly selected blood donors, for Weiss's *Lancet* paper concluding that LAV and HTLV-3B were both the cause of AIDS.[46] That none of the randomly selected blood donors had been positive suggested there wasn't much AIDS virus circulating in England. But the National Health Service, hoping to head off what might be an incipient epidemic, wanted to begin precautionary screening of donated blood at a few of its Regional Transfusion Centres.

Weiss had made his ELISA with HTLV-3B, and like everyone who received Gallo's virus he had been required to promise not to use it for commercial purposes. The National Health Service was an agency of the British government, not a private company, and an NHS blood test hardly fit the description of a commercial product. But when British officials asked the Reagan administration for permission to scale-up Weiss's ELISA, they were told to buy their AIDS tests from Abbott or Electronucleonics.[47]

"We are prevented from using a perfectly good and reliable test because the Americans want to make money," one of Weiss's assistants, Angus Dalgleish, told the *Daily Telegraph*. "The American test is worse than useless. It has produced false negative results and even false positives. It's not surprising that the American health department delayed giving it a license. Commercial considerations are absolutely hampering the containment of the disease in Britain. We've allowed AIDS to get a year's start."[48]

A *Daily Telegraph* reader who happened to be a hemophiliac sent a copy of the article to President Reagan with a demand for an explanation. Replying on the president's behalf, Lowell Harmison explained that unfortunately no British company had applied for a license to sell the Gallo ELISA, and now no more licenses were being issued. The writer and his fellow hemophiliacs would simply have to await the arrival of the AIDS test from one of the American manufacturers.[49]

An angry Robin Weiss responded to the American rebuff by putting "more effort into growing our own isolates." In short order Weiss had isolated an AIDS virus called CBL-1, named for the Chester Beatty Laboratories where Weiss was scientific director, that appeared to grow even better in culture than HTLV-3B. What Weiss did with his own discoveries wasn't governed by his agreement with Gallo or the American government, and CBL-1 was licensed to the British pharmaceutical firm Burroughs Wellcome, which lost no time producing an ELISA — only to receive a stern warning from the United States Department of Commerce that the company had not "been granted any rights under our pending patent rights to market such a kit" in the United Kingdom.[50]

When a rival British company, Amersham Laboratories, announced its intention to make an ELISA with an AIDS virus obtained from Don Francis, the HHS lawyers warned Amersham to cease and desist.[51] Although the CDC virus had been isolated independently of Gallo, the HHS decreed that any competing blood test "would discourage the development of the inventions already made by our licensees."[52] Amersham turned to Abraham Karpas, who provided the company with his own AIDS virus isolate, C-LAV.

The American laboratory and blood-bank technicians called upon to deploy the Gallo AIDS test had little information about how it performed under real-world conditions. When Murray Gardner compared the commercial ELISAs, he found that both Abbott and the new test from Electronucleonics "repeatedly" scored antibody-negative blood samples as positive.[53] The Red Cross was finding the same. Of every four positive blood samples tested with the Abbott ELISA, three were antibody-negative when tested by the Western Blot.[54]

The excessive number of false positives produced wasn't due, as first thought, to technician error or variation in the quality of the test kits, although there was plenty of both. As it happened, the source was Gallo's "revolutionary" method of growing the AIDS virus, the H-9 cell line, which Abbott and the other licensees were using to produce the virus for their ELISAs.

The H-9 phenomenon had first been noticed in Germany, where a surprising number of middle-aged women had begun testing positive for the AIDS virus —"staid matrons who had only ever been married to one man," said Robin Weiss.[55] "They turned out to have the same HLA group, these women, as H-9 cells. Or their husbands had, and they had had children with their husbands, so they had made antibodies against their fetuses. So they had this antibody that gave positive reactions." So, apparently, did thousands of Americans, including a group of black farmers in rural South Carolina, whose risk for AIDS was virtually zero and who had exhibited a false-positive rate of 300 percent.[56]

Despite efforts to purify the virus from which the tests were being made, some debris from the H-9 cells inevitably remained, apparently including the HLA protein in question.[57] "All five of the licensees who were making virus out of that cell line had this contamination," said Bob Nowinski, whose Genetic Systems was gearing up to manufacture the Pasteur ELISA with virus grown in a different cell line. When the Red Cross sent Nowinski fifty coded blood samples, it discovered that the Genetic Systems test didn't share the false-positive problem —"complete concordance," Nowinski said later, "between the Western Blot and our test."

Like the Pasteur in Paris, Genetic Systems was growing virus in the C-30 cell line David Klatzmann had cloned from CEM, which didn't have the errant protein that was causing all the trouble with H-9.[k] The C-30 clone had grown out of another of Klatzmann's precocious discoveries, that a particular molecule on the surface of T-4 cells seemed to disappear a few hours after those cells were infected with LAV. This, Klatzmann reasoned, must mean the molecule, called CD-4, was the receptor, or portal, through which the AIDS virus found its way to the interior of the cell before beginning to reproduce.

To prove his hypothesis, Klatzmann exposed a batch of uninfected T-4 cells to a synthetic antibody designed to adhere only to the CD-4 protein, then tried infecting the cells with LAV. When no infection occurred, Klatzmann concluded the antibody was blocking the pathway used by the virus. "Maybe because I was not such a hot scientist at that time, it came very easily in my mind," Klatzmann said. "I saw the patient — no T-4 cells. I looked for the tropism, I saw decreasing CD-4 on the cells. It's disappearing because it's the receptor. I started reading a little bit about receptors. All my experiments were very simple."

The identification of the AIDS virus receptor represented a major advance, since once the virus's pathway into the T-4 cell was known, various strategies could be considered for blocking its entry. Robin Weiss and Mika Popovic also were struggling with the receptor problem, but Weiss had taken a more circuitous route, methodically testing scores of monoclonal antibodies one at a time.

"We didn't know which was which," Weiss recalled. "We went through 150 and we picked out fourteen that blocked, and they were all CD-4. Klatzmann got the same results, but we thought our work was a little bit nicer." Popovic had tried the single-antibody approach, but unlike Klatzmann he had used the wrong antibody. "Mika was unlucky," Weiss said.[58]

Having identified CD-4 as the point of entry for the AIDS virus, Klatzmann sorted through CEM looking for the cells with the most CD-4 proteins, on the assumption that they would the best for growing LAV. "Some cells had quite a lot of CD-4," Klatzmann said, "and some not at all. We made clones, I and the technician in Montagnier's lab. She picked up cells and gave me back the clones. I came out with the C-30 clone, and that was a good virus producer."

The Pasteur might have the best cell line and the most reliable AIDS test, but it didn't have an FDA license or an American patent. In May of 1985, with the French patent application filed seventeen months before still pending before the United States Patent and Trademark Office, the American patent was awarded to the Gallo AIDS test.[59]

The Gallo application had been approved in near-record time — thirteen months, less than half the average for biotechnology patents. The reason, it would later develop, was that the American application had received expedited handling from a special branch of the patent office which examined patents related to national security and nuclear energy.[60] The AIDS test didn't have anything to do with national security, but the number of pending applications in that group was much shorter than in the biotechnology group, where the Pasteur application still languished near the end of the line.[61]

The day after the Gallo patent was awarded, a patent office supervisor named Charlie Van Horn got a call from Bert Rowland, a biotechnology specialist with the Pasteur's San Francisco law firm of Townsend and Townsend.[62] How, Rowland demanded to know, could a patent have been issued to Gallo and the HHS, who had filed *last*, instead of the Institut Pasteur, which had filed first?

Rowland's call was the first Van Horn had heard about a French AIDS test. When the Pasteur application was tracked down and dusted off, the cardboard "wrapper" around the application and its attached documents told the story. The first examiner to whom the Pasteur patent was assigned had protested her lack of qualifications in that particular area of biotechnology. The application had been reassigned to a second examiner, who soon afterward had quit the patent office. A third examiner had inherited the Pasteur file, but had put it aside for later consideration. Now *he* was about to leave. The French application had fallen between the cracks, and nobody at the patent office seemed to have noticed. Or at least that was the story.

To keep track of potential conflicts, the patent office compiles a short description of each application in a central index. As she was expected to do, the examiner who issued the Gallo patent had searched the index to see whether anyone else was claiming to have invented a blood test for AIDS. But the examiner hadn't found any trace of the Pasteur application, because it had never been indexed.[1] Had she known there was a competing application on file, she said later, rather than issuing the Gallo patent she would have requested an "interference," an administrative proceeding intended to sort out competing claims.[63]

Bert Rowland had no idea what had happened to the Pasteur application when he called the NIH patent coordinator, Tom Ferris.[64] Looking at the government's case in the best possible light, Rowland said, the most Gallo could claim was that he had been first to establish a cell line in which the AIDS virus could be continuously grown. But the H-9 cell line was the subject of a separate patent, and considering the false positives H-9 was causing, the Americans were welcome to it. The ELISA was another question, and the Pasteur thought it deserved the patent on the blood test. In Rowland's opinion, the simplest solution would be for HHS to add Montagnier, Chermann, and Barré as co-inventors on the Gallo patent and to split the royalties fifty-fifty with the French.

Rowland asked for a chance to carry the Pasteur's complaint to NIH higher-ups, and Ferris suggested he call Peter Fischinger. When Rowland replied that he would prefer to speak to someone "less apt to be biased," Ferris suggested Lowell Harmison. When Rowland rang Harmison, he was assured that the HHS was as interested in an amicable settlement as the French. Suppose, Harmison said, HHS agreed to add Montagnier and the other French inventors to the Gallo patent. Would Pasteur be willing to add Gallo, Popovic, and Sarngadharan to its own application? No, Rowland replied. The French had developed the AIDS test first, and without any help from Gallo, whereas Gallo had developed his AIDS test second, and with considerable help from the French.[65]

Another Pasteur lawyer, Gerard Weiser, tried to explain to the patent office that LAV and HTLV-3B were two names for the AIDS virus, and that the blood tests made with those viruses must be the same invention. With the DNA sequences in print and Gallo's own acknowledgment in *Nature* that HTLV-3B and LAV were "variants of the same AIDS virus,"[66] Weiser's task should have been easy. But the patent office hadn't been persuaded.[67] Fischinger, Harmison, and other senior HHS and NCI executives had seen copies of Gallo's correspondence with Montagnier, Barré, and Chermann, and they had known for more than a year how angry the French researchers were. But the calls from Rowland and Weiser were the first indications the government might be in for a serious fight with the Pasteur Institute itself.

Gallo, on a visit to Paris when the French began tossing grenades, had erupted himself upon learning that Rock Hudson, the American actor, was being treated for AIDS at the Institut Pasteur.[68] "Something is very wrong," Gallo wrote Vince DeVita, "when this man and many other Americans are heading to the Pasteur for treatment." According to Gallo, the National Cancer Institute had "much retrovirus talent, much more molecular biology talent, considerably greater facilities, [and] much more experience" than the Pasteur, not to mention "far more ideas."[69]

DeVita, who had just finished responding to inquiries from at least two senators whose constituents were complaining of "scientific impropriety" surrounding the discovery of HTLV-3,[m] lost his patience when he saw Gallo's memo. "I hardly need to be reminded of your accomplishments," he shot back, "since I have watched them with great interest and have played a role in assuring you receive proper credit including the national recognition that has come with the receipt of many prizes in the past three years. I believe that Dr. Montagnier would probably feel that he has been under recognized if one would look at scientific recognition in the form of prizes as an index of the scientific community's feeling about who has played a major role in the HTLV-3 field." [70]

Besides the dispute with the French, Gallo's personal life was also consuming more of DeVita's time. A couple of months before, Flossie Wong-Staal had separated from her husband, Steve, after fourteen years of marriage. The reason for the breakup, no surprise to many of Wong-Staal's coworkers, was stated in the couple's separation agreement: "The Husband believes and therefore avers that the child, Caroline, born March 21, 1983, is not his but is the child of the Wife and Robert Charles Gallo." Under the agreement, Wong-Staal would receive custody of Caroline, and Steve Staal custody of the girl's thirteen-year-old sister, who would be permitted to visit her mother only if Wong-Staal agreed "to keep contact between the parties' minor child and Robert Charles Gallo to an absolute minimum, and to ensure that the parties' minor child will never be alone in his company."[71]

"She was *the* most important person in the lab," complained Zaki Salahuddin. "If she made a decision, that was supreme. The lady was given a merit award and the best salary and the title of section head and all kinds of things. It was a tremendous conflict of interest. Why? Because she was sleeping with the boss." But if the relationship posed a conflict of interest, Vince DeVita didn't see it.

"Flossie's husband and Bob's wife used to call me with great regularity," DeVita said. "I told them that as long as they produced scientifically we would continue to support them, and if they didn't they would go. In Bob's case, he was put in the hands of a psychiatrist for a while, to talk over the issue of the child and sort it out. But Flossie was a functional scientist. There was no sign that Flossie was unraveling. Maybe Flossie worked harder because of the relationship, maybe she worked less. I can't tell. All I know is Flossie's a pretty damn good scientist. She did good work and she probably doesn't get enough credit."

One of the French journalists with whom Gallo had done battle was Claudine Escoffier-Lambiotte, the redoubtable medical editor of *Le Monde*. At the Palais des Congrès meeting two years before, Escoffier had appeared to side with Gallo at the expense of Luc Montagnier and LAV. Since then, enough new facts had emerged to lead Escoffier to the conclusion that Gallo and NCI had at least stolen the credit for an important French discovery. As the most influential medical journalist in France, Escoffier's turnabout had done more than anything else to marshal the French public, and the French government, behind the Institut Pasteur.

A slight, silver-coifed woman in her early sixties, Escoffier had pursued her medical studies while serving with the Resistance in her native Belgium during the Second World War. "A few professors would give us our teaching in very extraordinary conditions," Escoffier recalled in her throaty voice, "completely underground, with false papers and everything. And then every year we would pass our exams before a kind of national jury. A very difficult way, I must say. Only six of us remained in the underground university, because it was extremely dangerous. But it was fantastic, to have your medical training in private lessons for five years."

Escoffier survived the war to become one of the first female doctors in France. After a postwar fellowship at Columbia-Presbyterian Hospital in New York, she returned to Paris to work with her husband, Jean-Bernard, a surgeon and grandson of August Escoffier, the creator of modern French cuisine. After practicing for several years, Escoffier had been persuaded by *Le Monde* to become the first journalist in Europe to regularly cover medicine for a daily newspaper. In America, however, her famous name was something of a liability. "Wherever I go, I have to eat and eat and eat," Escoffier said, rolling her eyes, "and go in the kitchen and see the cooks, and so on."

Gallo responded to Escoffier's reporting with what she described as "a letter written with a gun."[72] To Escoffier's observation that Gallo had Montagnier badly outgunned in terms of resources, Gallo warned that the French should take care not to become "a victim of the Viet Nam syndrome, i.e., 'poor me, poor me, look at the big big Americans.'" But Gallo wanted Escoffier to know he had no interest in a fight with the French. "I am working on this problem," he said, "and once in a while I am distracted by articles pushing disputes that are atrocious, sensationalistic, and harmful to science and the resolution of this problem. The only controversy is in the naming. It can be settled, and it is trivial. Remember, my colleagues and I discovered T-cell growth factor, called it that, but today most people call it interleukin-2. I lost but I don't cry nor care."

Anyone who knew Escoffier would have expected her to answer Gallo in kind. "I told him, 'If you want to explain yourself, come here,'" she recalled. "'But don't send letters like this to people you don't know.' Because at that time, and still now, Bob Gallo would write to every journalist in the world who would publish an article that wouldn't be completely in favor with his point of view. He would explode. He would immediately conclude that the journalist who had written the article that was not in favor of his genius was prejudiced, was poorly informed, was a friend of Pasteur, or something like this. I said, '*Le Monde* is a paper which is open to everybody. I know you come quite often to Paris. We'll meet whenever you wish to, and organize an interview.' He first answered saying, 'I never give any interviews.' I said 'OK, then don't complain. Stay in your nest in Bethesda and leave me alone in mine.'"

But during one of his visits to Paris, Gallo had a change of heart. "I had a call from Daniel Zagury," Escoffier recalled, "saying 'Gallo desperately wishes to see you, he is completely depressed.' With Gallo, everything is such an emergency. Wherever Gallo is, he takes all the air for himself. Daniel Zagury is crazy in love with Bob Gallo. He forgives Gallo everything. Gallo calls and says, 'You must come immediately, drop everything.' Zagury goes, and Gallo is not there."

To the interview at Zagury's home Escoffier brought a short list of questions prepared with the help of Montagnier, and after a few pleasantries she turned on her tape recorder.

"When did your laboratory culture the isolate of LAV virus sent to you by the Pasteur team in September 1983?" Escoffier asked.

"At the end of 1984 [*sic*]," Gallo replied. "We never put LAV in a continuous culture."

"When did you compare it with your own isolate?"

"When we were able to obtain mass production of the pool of viruses in sufficient quantity. The LAV was in the freezer and we then compared all our specimens, including the forty-eight that I had isolated. That was in April 1984."

Escoffier wondered how there could be a 99 percent genetic similarity between LAV and HTLV-3B, "when the differences are very much greater with other isolates from other labs?" Easy, Gallo replied. The real similarity between the two viruses wasn't 99 percent. It was only 98.3 percent.[73]

The interrogation over, Escoffier predicted that if the Americans refused to permit the French AIDS test to be sold in the United

States, the French would go to court. "I told him the French government was ready to sue the American government on the business of the patent," she said. "His eyes got like this. He said, 'I never heard about it.' Unless he was playing a role, but I don't think so. Because he was so petrified. He said, 'What can I do? It's not to be believed, it's an awful situation, something horrid, and I don't want that.'"

"I told him, 'If you are ready to do something, call François Gros, who was at that time the director of the council of trustees of the Institut Pasteur. Which he did immediately, in front of me, from Zagury's house. François Gros was the adviser of the prime minister, and of François Mitterrand. François Gros told him 'Yes, there is a big problem.' And Gallo answered, 'I will do anything to avoid it. As soon as I come back to Washington, I will see the people involved.' He said he didn't want the patent, that the American government pushed him, that his only interest was in science. That he actually fought against the patent."

Claudine Escoffier was more than the medical editor of the most prestigious newspaper in France. She served on any number of boards and committees, including the general assembly of the Pasteur Institute — a relationship that for an American journalist would have been a clear conflict of interest, but which Escoffier saw as an opportunity to head off an impending Franco-American crisis. "I tried to do my best so that an arrangement could be found," Escoffier said. "I had the feeling it was no good for French-American relationships. I love America, so I was very disturbed about it. And secondly, it was no good according to the layman, as far as the image of science was concerned."

Invitations to dine at Escoffier's home in the 8th arrondissement, with its museum-quality furnishings and Monet-style views of the Parc Monceau, were not often refused. To join her at dinner Escoffier invited Gallo, Zagury, and Jean Bernard, a distinguished Paris physician and the head of the French national council on medical ethics. "Gallo didn't know how to get out of the mess," Escoffier recalled. "So he said, 'We could get out of the mess in writing down the history of the discovery. We'll come back to the ethics of science and we'll get away from all these financial considerations — patents, governments, institutions.'"

A history of sorts was written that night over cognac. "Then I translated it in English," Escoffier said, "and Bob Gallo added a few things that would reinforce his role in the whole thing. Nothing for Montagnier and the Pasteur group, but several points for him." Afterward,

Escoffier said, "Bob Gallo sent a long letter to Jean Bernard, of which I still have a copy. In that letter he said, 'I cannot accept this, I cannot accept that. I didn't dare say so at the home of the charming lady' — which is completely ridiculous and has no meaning whatsoever — 'I didn't dare say anything, but I don't accept this and that and that.'"

Escoffier dutifully arranged a second Gallo dinner, this time with François Gros and François Jacob. "Jacob was quite tough that evening," Escoffier said. "From the very beginning, François Jacob had the feeling that Gallo's behavior was not fair and was absolutely unethical. He told that to him. He said, 'You didn't behave in an ethical way as far as science is concerned.' François Gros was a little more indulgent, I would say, in trying to fix things and to avoid a lawsuit. He knew that it would be very tough, financially, for the Pasteur Institute, so he wished to avoid that."

Nothing was accomplished that evening, and Gallo's next attempt at codifying the discovery was with the help of Jean-Claude Chermann. "Daniel Zagury invited Chermann for dinner," recalled Escoffier. "We all knew Chermann since a long time, and I'd seen Chermann with Bob Gallo at Zagury's place several times. Chermann was not as tough and angry, was more friendly with Bob Gallo, than Montagnier was. So all of a sudden they got this scientific history of the discovery countersigned by Chermann, which was something nobody could have accepted. I was extremely mad about it. I sent it back to Chermann, and I said, 'What happened to you? You know very well that nobody could accept such a way to describe the discovery.' It was more favorable to Bob than the first one was. Chermann said, 'We had a lot to drink. They were very kind to me. I didn't realize it was something that they intended eventually to publish. It was a very informal conversation.' I told him, 'But didn't you realize they were taking notes and that everything was written down?'"[n]

Afterward, Escoffier warned Gallo that if he made the Chermann history public, Chermann's career at the Pasteur would be in ruins. Gallo promised the document would never see the light of day. Back in the United States, Gallo sent a copy to Jim Wyngaarden and began deluging Escoffier with "a huge pile of documents, tons of documents" to buttress the American position.

Among the documents was Chermann's response of the year before to Gallo's letter claiming that he had discovered the AIDS virus in November of 1982. Something about that particular letter struck Escoffier as odd, and she showed it to Chermann. "I said, 'This is very strange,'" Escoffier recalled. "'How is it that you sent that letter?'" When Chermann compared the letter sent by Gallo to the original in his files, he saw that someone had cut out his signature and pasted it at the end of the third paragraph, transforming what had been a scathing two-page critique of Gallo's behavior into a one-page testimonial.

"The next time Bob came to Paris," Escoffier said, "I told him, 'This is outrageous.' He read the thing and said, 'I didn't know it was cut. I will call my secretary immediately.' So in front of me he called, and she said 'Yes, we thought that the end of the letter was not relevant to the whole problem.' I don't believe it, I'm sure. He did nothing but take care of the whole thing at that time. He was very emotional about it. Unfortunately, this is very typical of some aspects of Bob Gallo's temper. He's too impulsive, and this is not compatible with science."

• 9 •

"I Don't Want to Go to Jail"

Accompanied by four lawyers, Professor Raymond Dedonder descended on Washington on the afternoon of August 6, 1985, a Tuesday. The contingent of Americans assembled to meet the director of the Institut Pasteur included Lowell Harmison, Peter Fischinger, Berge Hampar, *five* lawyers, several NIH and HHS executives, and the patent licensing coordinator from the Department of Commerce.

"The NIH side was very heavily represented," recalled Bob Nowinski, whom the French had brought along as their scientific expert. "There were eight of us and fifteen or sixteen of them. We went in expecting a modest meeting, and there was big firepower."

For more than a year the French had been chafing over Robert Gallo's claim to have discovered the virus that caused AIDS, followed by the revelation that Gallo's HTLV-3B was indistinguishable from the AIDS virus the French called LAV. Now the American patent on the AIDS test had been awarded to Gallo's HTLV-3B ELISA. Hoping to calm the international waters, Margaret Heckler had visited the Pasteur a few weeks before and met briefly with Dedonder, but her visit hadn't mollified the French.[1]

Beneath his jovial exterior Dedonder was a Gaullist to the core, and he was determined that his institute not get run over by the Reagan administration. Dedonder had asked Heckler for a more formal meeting in which to present Pasteur's position to the appropriate American officials, and his opening statement in Washington made clear where the French stood.

It was "a well established fact," Dedonder declared, "that the virus responsible for AIDS has been discovered by the group working at the Pasteur Institute. This is supported by competent scientists all over the world including in this country. We think that we are entitled to a full recognition of this fact and consequently to a full recognition of our right to a patent, which was filed here, in the United States, in December 1983. We are confident that our position is legally strong. Therefore we are expecting that a common proposal for a satisfactory settlement can be attained before the end of next month."

If that deadline wasn't met, Dedonder continued, "the Pasteur Institute is prepared and determined and even compelled to utilize all the available procedures to obtain complete recognition of its rights."[2] But before Dedonder could finish speaking, he was interrupted by the senior American official present, Lowell Harmison, known among his subordinates as "Harmful Lowellson."

"Harmison cut him off," Bob Nowinski recalled, "and said that HHS was of course going to cooperate, and how it was looking for the best for the world. It was apparent that Dedonder was not being well received. There was a language barrier, and there seemed to be a reasonably set position on the other side. Rather than a discursive meeting, which we expected, the government representatives were fairly well aligned in their view of how they were going to handle it, which was basically to hardball the issue."

Nowinski had come to talk about the science behind the AIDS test. But when he saw the direction HHS was heading he made a statement he hadn't intended. "It wasn't a prepared statement," Nowinski said later. "I referred back to the fact that there had been in Gallo's laboratory, many years ago, a claim that he had discovered a human retrovirus which turned out to be a monkey virus. I said, 'This happened once before, and this may be the origin of what happened here.' I said, 'No one is claiming that Dr. Gallo has purposely taken this virus. This may have been inadvertent. But no virologist I know of would ever mix culture fluids together. You would never mix, because there would be no way of knowing what you'd derived. You do things one at a time and you work things through methodically.'"

To Nowinski's suggestion that Gallo had simply "reisolated" the French virus, the reaction from the American side was caustic.[3] "I believe it was Fischinger," Nowinski said, "who responded by saying that the difference in sequences were sufficient so that the viruses were clearly different from each other. There was steam across the table. The reception was pretty much a shut-down."

Trying to refocus the discussion, the Pasteur's Gerard Weiser warned that the French were prepared to sue the United States government for breach of contract, the contract in question being the non-commercialization agreement signed by Mika Popovic that accompanied the September 1983 shipment of LAV. In case that failed to get the government's attention, the Pasteur was contemplating an action for fraud against the government lawyers who had filed the Gallo patent.[4]

To avoid this, Weiser said, the Americans would have to acknowledge Luc Montagnier's team as the true discoverers of the AIDS virus *and* the inventors of the AIDS test, and allow Pasteur to sell its ELISA in the United States without being sued for patent infringement. Finally, the Reagan administration would have to hand over to the French the patent royalties it already had collected from Abbott and the other American licensees.[5]

As the meeting broke up with halfhearted handshakes, the Pasteur's patent coordinator, Danielle Berneman, remarked to herself how little Lowell Harmison had seemed to know about the facts of the case. "It was impossible for us to believe he looked at the file," Berneman recalled. "Five people are coming from France, including the director of Pasteur. You have to prepare your meeting."

After the French had gone, Harmison suggested they were bluffing, "gambling that HHS's fear of adverse publicity will cause us to meet their demands rather than litigate."[6] Peter Fischinger assured everyone that the AIDS-test patent wasn't in jeopardy. The key to the invention of the ELISA, Fischinger said, had been Mika Popovic's discovery of the H-9 cell line. As for the Pasteur's claim to have discovered the AIDS virus, Gallo had evidence that *he* had discovered the AIDS virus in February 1983 — three months before the Pasteur's first paper in *Science*.

Everyone agreed it would be helpful to have an internal review of exactly what had been done in Gallo's lab and when, and that Peter Fischinger was the man to conduct it. A Yugoslav Catholic who fled the Nazis at the age of twelve, Fischinger had earned an M.D. and Ph.D. at the University of Illinois, and done his postdoctoral work at the Max Planck Institut in Heidelberg with Dani Bolognesi, followed by a job with George Todaro during the early cancer-virus years.

Fischinger had published a couple of papers about oncogenes that were still remembered as insightful. But he hadn't shown tremendous promise as an experimental scientist, and he had been unhappy in Todaro's lab. When the cancer-virus program ended, Fischinger had been rescued by Vince DeVita, and as a scientific bureaucrat he had succeeded admirably, earning a reputation as an ultracool, unflappable administrator whose tinted glasses lent him a slightly Strangelovian air. Behind his back Fischinger's subordinates referred to him as "the Fish," but anyone who discounted his intelligence usually regretted it later.

One of the Americans at the meeting was Berge Hampar, a bluff New Yorker of Lebanese descent, who managed the NCI's Frederick satellite facility and who was the only senior NCI scientist with a law degree. As Hampar and Fischinger drove the fifty miles back to Frederick, they hashed the meeting over. The following morning Hampar telephoned John Roberts, an attorney who had worked with Bill Bundren on the drafting of the Gallo patents. Doubts were being raised about the legitimacy of the Gallo patent, Hampar said. Roberts should know that the veracity of the attorneys who had written the application was also being questioned. As Hampar talked, Roberts switched on his tape recorder.[a]

"I said I was quite surprised that they blatantly were accusing Gallo of stealing the virus," Hampar recalled. "We tried to get them to put something in writing and they didn't want to. I said, 'Pasteur is willing to put its reputation on the line to back Montagnier. Are we going to put our neck out to defend Bob Gallo?'"

"Yeah," Roberts replied.

"And, of course, our position was through the meeting that the actions of the department were in response to a public health problem and we're not involved in the issues of priorities with respect to patents."

"Right," Roberts said.

"Basically what I said is, before we decide to change that stance and become defenders of Gallo, I said somebody better get the hell in his lab and find out what the real scoop is on what went on. See, the whole trouble is no one really knows."

"We have some pretty good leads on it," Roberts said.

"But that's all after the fact. The question is, what did Bob do before the date — the priority date? At least it can be established by the French. And I keep telling Fischinger, before you put your neck out defending Bob Gallo, you better make sure that what you're saying is really the case."

"True," Roberts said.

"We didn't file until April of '84. In their application of September of '83, we were surprised they have ELISA data in there. They had not published anything on that prior to that time. So we were somewhat surprised. In looking at their application, they did have ELISA data. So, I mean it'd be pretty hard to argue that point. The patent at issue was the first patent that issued, not the one on the cell line."

"Yeah," Roberts said.

"Peter keeps bringing that one up. Everybody told him the same thing, 'But that's not the patent. That is a different patent.' I think we finally got that point across." Hampar mentioned Gallo's interview in *Le Monde*, "when he starts sort of putting the blame on the government with this patenting stuff: 'I have nothing to do with patents'— that type of thing. 'I am a scientist' attitude."

Roberts laughed.

"And the SOB even has the gall to make a statement, that's quoted in there, is that he said 'I don't gain anything personally from these patents.' I look at that and I say, 'Well, I didn't see him turn his checks down when they came in to him.'"

Roberts laughed again.

"Monday's *Wall Street Journal*," Hampar said. "Did you see that?"

"No," Roberts replied.

"There was a big article that started on page one. At the end of the article, and this is a typical Gallo, they quote Gallo here: 'Dr. Gallo says he is currently told everyone will probably pay them.' And then in parentheses, the French royalties. I mean, essentially . . ."

"Conceding," Roberts said.

"Conceding. I showed it to Peter and I said, 'Look at this.' He looked at it. He said, 'Gallo, why can't you keep your mouth shut?'"

"Jesus," Roberts said.

"My feeling still is that he's been less than candid with the [cancer] institute as to what occurred."

"Less than a good soldier," Roberts said.

"On the other hand, I think things could've occurred in his lab that he doesn't know about. Now, it's funny, you know, because the way Bob Nowinski sort of presented the scientific evidence. Basically what he's saying is that LAV and HTLV-3 are identical viruses. And there's no way they would be identical viruses if they were separate isolates, because all the other isolates aren't the same.

"Now that's a scientific question. We could question the scientific validity of that statement. But he then says that must have probably happened, he said that someone in Bob's lab inadvertently contaminated his cultures with the LAV. But then Nowinski and Todaro know NCI very well. Todaro, see, is out at Seattle too. And he got kicked out of the institute essentially. And he knows Gallo very well and he knows what's been going on there. So then he follows that statement about this contamination, the fact that the same thing occurred in Gallo's lab several years ago.

"Of course Peter and I knew about it, because we were familiar with his referring back to when they contaminated cultures with a primate virus. Anyway, he says some scientists will be publishing papers soon that indicate that the two viruses are the same."

Hampar brought up something Weiser had mentioned about Montagnier's May 1983 *Science* paper.

"Bob Gallo received a preprint from Montagnier around April 17th," Hamper said. "Bob doesn't deny. In fact, they said Bob made some corrections on the paper. And then you know, for Montagnier, and actually helped get it published, what Peter told me. But what Weiser says is that this occurred April 17th, which is equivalent to a public disclosure and therefore is a one-year bar in terms of our filing"— in other words, that the Americans had had only a year from April 17, 1983, to file their own patent application, a deadline they had missed by a week.

"Yeah," Roberts said.

"Well, you know, that's kind of where we stand," Hampar said. "We are keeping it very quiet. But I wanted you to know since you're the attorney of record on this thing. And I don't know what the department's position is going to be. As of yesterday we don't know. I think now we're waiting to try and get something in writing from the French. I think that decision is going right up to the secretary. I mean, this thing has sort of gotten up to the secretary's level."

"Jesus," Roberts said.

Gallo remained adamant. He had been "the first inventor" of the AIDS blood test.[7] But Peter Fischinger hadn't any better idea than Lowell Harmison or Berge Hampar of how the blood test had emerged from Gallo's lab, let alone the virus from which it was made. Fischinger's first move was to send Gallo a long memo summarizing the French allegations and requesting the data to refute them. Fischinger also wanted copies of Gallo's correspondence with Montagnier, every piece of paper reflecting Popovic's work with LAV, and "adequate documentation from your laboratory data that you have isolated an HTLV-3 agent(s) prior to the receipt of LAV."[8]

Before many days had passed, the media got wind that the Pasteur dispute had taken a serious turn.[9] "Peter, for your records," Gallo wrote in mid-August of 1985, "I received a call from a Mr. Corky Johnson. He told me he works for columnist Jack Anderson. He told me he was given information from someone who attended an Institut Pasteur/NCI-NIH meeting regarding a possible law suit on HTLV-3 concerning patent rights, and he told me of the slimy statements of possible accusations."

Gallo told Johnson he hadn't been at the meeting, and that "'I know nothing about patents and what could I possibly say.' I talked perhaps two minutes about science. He *seemed* to understand the truth and *appeared* sympathetic."[10] A few hours after Johnson's call, a reporter for *Time* told Gallo "that one or more key people at CDC were prompting her to bring up the French-NCI 'problem.' If true, it is one more example of this kind of self-serving political behavior we have seen which is not in the government interest."

Pasteur scientists kept the records of their experiments in the European style, in sequential hardbound volumes that made it impossible to insert or remove pages after the fact and constituted a verifiable chronological record of what had transpired in their labs. Montagnier had a closet full of such volumes. So did Françoise Barré, whose notebooks were minor works of art, her experiments carefully laid out and accompanied by hand-drawn graphs and charts in multicolored inks. But when Gallo asked Mika Popovic to see notebooks reflecting the discovery of HTLV-3B, Popovic said he didn't have any notebooks.

"We were finding stuff in drawers, pieces of paper," Gallo recalled. "I mean, we pulled out stuff that Mika didn't even know he had, and there it was. You know, old stuff, old archaic papers with scribbles on them."[11] The scraps proved to be the only records Popovic could produce of what the government now counted as a landmark achievement. "They told me I have to give all notes," Popovic said later,

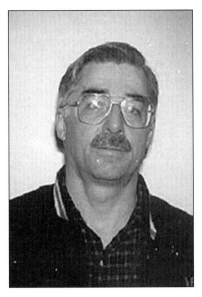

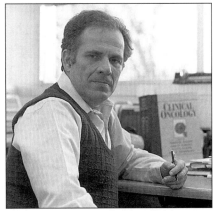

ABOVE: Frank Ruscetti
(National Cancer Institute/Bill Branson)

Bernard Poiesz *(Courtesy B. Poiesz)*

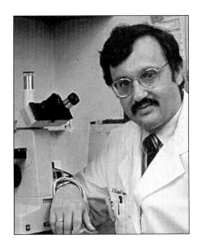

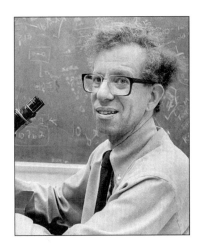

LEFT: Sam Broder *(National Cancer Institute)*, RIGHT: Howard Temin *(Michael Kienitz/University of Wisconsin–Madison University Communications)*

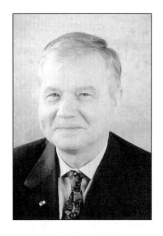

Luc Montagnier *(Institut Pasteur)*

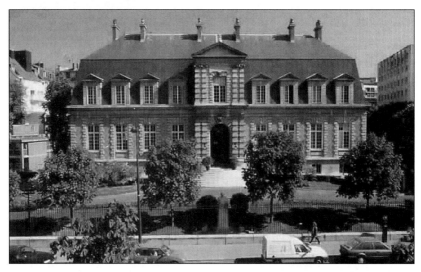

The historic administration building of the Pasteur Institute in Paris. The apartment of Louis Pasteur on the top floor has been preserved. *(Institut Pasteur)*

Luc Montagnier, Françoise Barré-Sinoussi, and Jean-Claude Chermann, 1983 *(Institut Pasteur)*

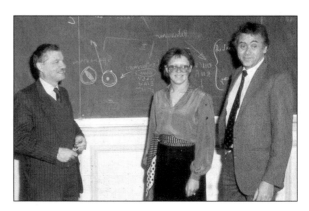

David Klatzmann
(Courtesy D. Klatzmann)

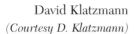

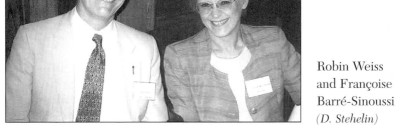

Robin Weiss
and Françoise
Barré-Sinoussi
(D. Stehelin)

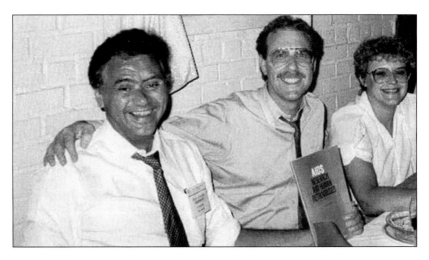

Jean-Claude Chermann, Michael Gottlieb, and Françoise Barré-Sinoussi,
Third International Conference on AIDS, Washington, D.C., 1987
(Courtesy M. Gottlieb)

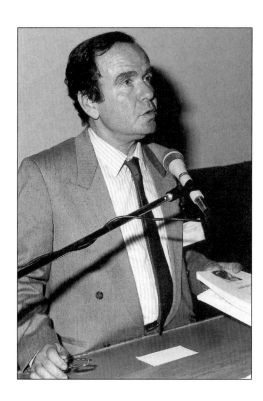

Abraham Karpas
(Courtesy A. Karpas)

Cirilo Cabradilla, Don Francis, and James Curran, CDC AIDS Task Force
Meeting, 1982 *(Centers for Disease Control)*

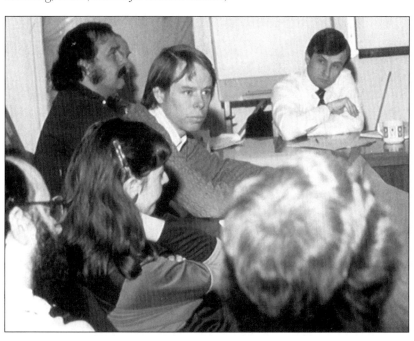

Don Francis, smallpox eradication in India, 1975 *(Courtesy D. Francis)*

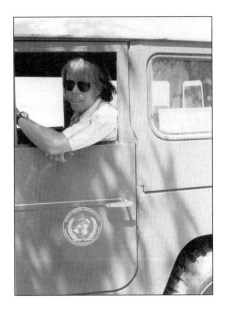

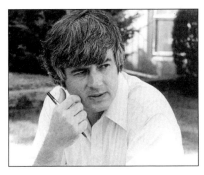

ABOVE: Myron "Max" Essex at the Cold Spring Harbor HTLV meeting, May 1983 *(Joan James/Cold Spring Harbor Laboratory Archives)*

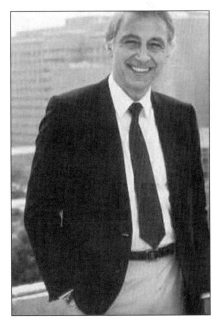

Robert Gallo
(National Cancer Institute)

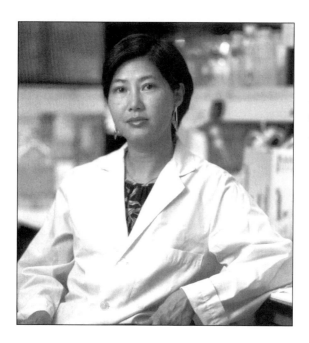

Flossie Wong-Staal
*(National Cancer
Institute/Bill Branson)*

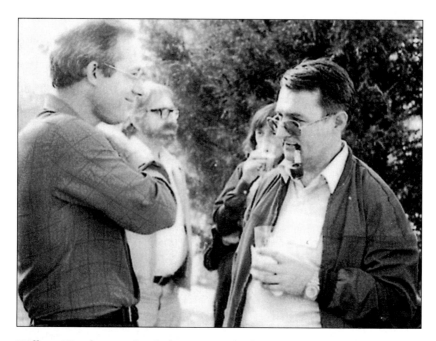

William Haseltine and Mikulas Popovic at the Cold Spring Harbor HTLV
meeting, May 1983 *(Joan James/Cold Spring Harbor Laboratory Archives)*

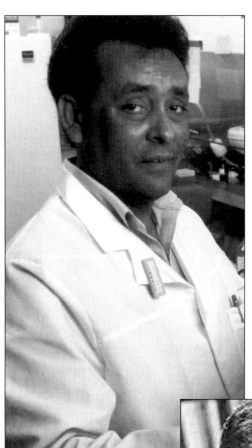

Zaki Salahuddin
(National Cancer Institute)

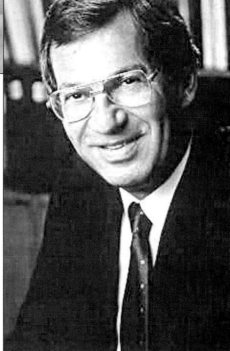

Vincent DeVita
(National Cancer Institute)

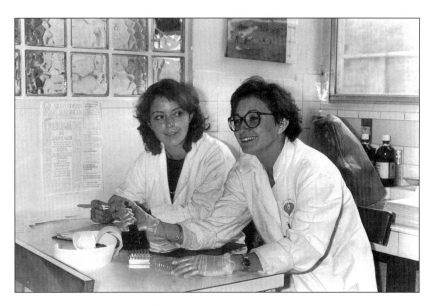

Françoise Brun-Vézinet and Christine Rouzioux *(Institut Pasteur)*

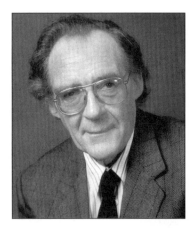

John Maddox *(Nature)*

Jay Levy
(David Powers)

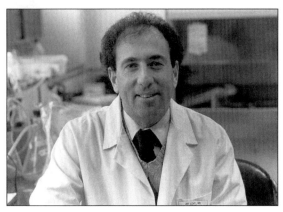

"otherwise I would go to jail. So I told, 'Take whatever I have. I don't want to go to jail.'"[12]

His lab never had intended to keep "records of legal standing," Gallo explained to Peter Fischinger, and the records that did exist were "often incomplete."[13] In contrast to this "rather normal behavior" was "the meticulous and apparently premeditated documentation of others interested, it seems, more in patents and notoriety." Even if it couldn't be documented, Gallo assured Fischinger that HTLV-3B had been discovered by Popovic in material "pooled from several patients who showed high R.T. activity in primary culture."

Popovic's own chronicle of his work left out a good deal of the story, beginning with the delivery of LAV by Montagnier to Gallo's house in July 1983. Popovic described only his use of the second LAV shipment in September 1983, and admitted using the French virus only to infect cord blood cells.[14] But it was the July LAV that had first been grown in cord blood cells, first been photographed by Matt Gonda and used for the Eureka! experiment that had led Popovic out of the virological wilderness.[b]

Popovic's memo, which read as though it had been written by Gallo, also omitted to mention that the September LAV had grown in more than cord blood cells, namely in two continuous cell lines, and had been photographed yet again by Gonda.[15] Such omissions wouldn't have been evident to anyone not familiar with Popovic's work firsthand. But according to Vince DeVita, Fischinger hadn't made a concerted effort to verify the information provided by Gallo and Popovic.

Whatever he thought privately,[c] Fischinger assured Lowell Harmison that there was "no substantive support for the French claims" to have discovered the AIDS virus and invented the AIDS blood test.[16] The French didn't even *have* an effective test, Fischinger said.[d] Nor could there have been a motive for Gallo or Popovic to steal LAV, since they had had "ample isolates" of their own AIDS viruses, including two dating from December 1982 — a month before LAV was discovered in Paris.[e]

As for Pasteur's assertion that HTLV-3B and LAV were so close genetically they could only have come from the same patient, according to Fischinger the point was moot. Gallo had just isolated two viruses from a couple of AIDS patients in New Jersey that were genetically as close "or closer" than LAV and 3B.[f] With the advent of the "New Jersey Pair," it seemed entirely possible that LAV and HTLV-3B had come from different patients.

DeVita remembered that Fischinger hadn't been quite as confident in person as he sounded in his report, which DeVita thought had been "more prepared for the patent attorneys than anything else. Peter did go and look through the notes, and I think he came to pretty much the conclusion that he couldn't basically tell. He found no evidence that there was a clear misrepresentation. But the notes were not in the greatest of order, and Peter knew that they had thrown in several viruses, not one. He was not pleased with it."

DeVita also recalled wondering why, if Gallo had identified the AIDS virus in December of 1982, he, DeVita, hadn't heard anything about it until March of 1984. Nor, until he read the Fischinger report, did DeVita have any idea Popovic had been working with LAV. "That's obviously a question we asked many times," DeVita said later. "My understanding was they could not grow the French virus, that they had isolates that were separate from the French virus before they had the French virus, and so on. The issue at hand was, 'Did Bob take that virus and use it purposely?' And we were assured that that was not the case. I was assured that HTLV-3B was not LAV."

The dispute over who deserved the patent didn't depend on which virus Gallo had used to make his AIDS test, only on whether he had done it first.[17] But as the HHS lawyers sifted through the Fischinger report, they realized it was full of holes. Among the missing items was the *date* on which Gallo's lab had first performed an ELISA for AIDS virus antibodies. The lawyers also wanted "the exact sequences and timing of the events which led to the virus-producing line HTLV-3B that is now in current use."[g] In passing on the latest requests, Fischinger thought it would be helpful to have a written statement from Popovic that LAV had never been "used in any connection in that complex infection sequence which led to the isolation of the HTLV-3B line." He also thought the time had come to identify the patient who had been the source of the H-9 cell line.[18]

Following Raymond Dedonder's return to Paris, Margaret Heckler's chief of staff, Mac Haddow, moved to put the French on the offensive, demanding that Dedonder document the Pasteur's "extremely serious allegations" against Gallo and HHS.[19] Jim Mason, who had been released from the doghouse to replace the departing Ed Brandt as the assistant HHS secretary for health, was dividing his time between Washington and Atlanta, where he retained the directorship of the CDC. Before the government gave the French its final response, Mason thought Lowell Harmison should visit Atlanta and find out what the CDC had done with LAV.

With a Public Health Service lawyer in tow, Harmison began his visit by warning Jim Curran and the CDC's AIDS staff that everything relating to the Pasteur dispute should be considered "administratively confidential," the closest HHS could come to Top Secret. For Harmison, Curran recounted the CDC's enthusiasm over Chermann's presentation at Park City, the equivalent scores of the French and American blood tests, and the dawning recognition that the viruses from the CDC's transfusion pair were indistinguishable from LAV.

Fred Murphy remembered the Harmison visit as "a full trip through the record with no holds barred, with all the data points described. A lot was said about the CDC data. All Curran's log books were made part of the record." But Curran thought Harmison seemed mostly uninterested. "We were trying to show this guy our data," Curran said, "and he wasn't even paying attention. He kept running in and out of the room and talking on the telephone."

The only person missing was Don Francis, who had requested a transfer to the San Francisco Bay Area after his proposal for expanding the CDC's research on retroviruses was shelved. Installed as the CDC's liaison with the California Department of Health Services in Berkeley, Francis attended the meeting via speakerphone. In anticipation of Harmison's visit, Francis had shipped Curran a box containing his lab notes, letters, memos, and other relevant documents from late 1983 and early 1984. On top of the pile was a strongly worded letter.

"I am not familiar with the legal issues being addressed by the French litigation," it began, "but there are really important ethical and scientific issues that the Public Health Service should consider before putting up a strong defense. I am sure that I am not alone in believing that Bob Gallo exceeded ethical bounds in his dealings with the French. If this litigation gets into open court, all of the less-than-admirable aspects will become public and, I think, hurt science and the Public Health Service. The French clearly found the cause of AIDS virus and Dr. Gallo clearly tried to upstage them one year later."[20]

Francis's letter, said Fred Murphy, illustrated "how we all felt. But only Don would take that extra step of bluntness."

For more than a year, John Maddox had watched as Gallo and the AIDS research community published article after article in *Science,* some of which Maddox wished had been published in *Nature.* At least one of Gallo's *Science* articles on the discovery of HTLV-3 had been cited as a reference in nearly every subsequent paper published on AIDS, and those articles had done more than any others to help *Science* enhance its visibility at *Nature's* expense.

In hopes of drawing Gallo back into *Nature's* fold, Maddox offered his juiciest plum: a review of human retrovirology, in which Gallo would be able to set down for future scientists and historians an extensive account of his own discoveries. But the nine-page article, long even for *Nature,* was little more than a scholarly sounding version of the ersatz history Gallo had been propounding to Peter Fischinger, heavily larded with arguments for why the AIDS virus should be a member of the HTLV family.[h]

Annoyed that *Nature's* editorial board had agreed to publish such a distorted account, Montagnier objected to Peter Newmark that Gallo's article was the farthest thing imaginable from an objective survey of the discovery of the AIDS virus.[21] Montagnier reminded Newmark that *Nature* had just published a paper from Stu Aaronson confirming Montagnier's longstanding contention that the AIDS virus was indeed related to the equine infectious anemia virus, and therefore a lentiretrovirus.[22] "Yet readers of the Gallo review article," Montagnier said, "will ignore this and instead see an imaginary tree, where HTLV-1 and HTLV-3 are put arbitrarily in the same box. This is only an example among many inexactitudes. . . ."

As the dispute with Pasteur gained momentum, *Science* assigned its best reporter, a British writer named Colin Norman, to sort the matter out. In a lengthy interview with Norman, Gallo gave the French some credit for having been first to recognize that the AIDS virus killed the T-cells in which it was cultured.[23] "We just didn't believe that that is what this kind of virus could do," Gallo said. "It is certainly true that in that period of time, in summer and certainly by early fall, Chermann had recognized the [cell-killing] effect of that virus and I had not. As I look back now, I could bang my head against a wall that we were so stubborn in trying to grow those cells long term in IL-2. We went through loss of months with that problem."

That was as far as Gallo was willing to go. When Norman wondered whether HTLV-3B was LAV by another name, Gallo became incensed. "Gallo indignantly disputes this allegation on several counts," Norman wrote, "including the fact that the viruses are not identical and that the amount of virus Montagnier sent would not have been sufficient to infect a cell line."

While Norman took notes, Gallo and Popovic repeated the story they had told Peter Fischinger about Popovic's failure to grow the July LAV, or to achieve continuous growth with the September LAV. "Gallo says no reverse transcriptase activity could be detected in the [July] sample," Norman wrote, while "Popovic, a cell biologist in Gallo's lab, says he tried twice to infect fresh lymphocytes but failed." The September LAV had produced some reverse transcriptase in fresh T-cells, but "they could not get continuous virus production, so they put the material in the freezer."

Norman suspected he hadn't been given all the facts. But he could only write what he had been told, and articles like the resulting two-part series in *Science* were costing the French the battle for the minds of the scientific community. For decades the Pasteur Institute had fought to retain its independence from the French government, insisting that the government's contribution to its treasury never exceed half the institute's total budget. Now Dedonder recognized that if Pasteur was going to prevail against the Americans it needed official help.

The previous August, Montagnier had led a delegation to plead the Pasteur's case before the cabinet.[24] The French had a number of pressing disputes with the United States, from agricultural trade matters to whether American military aircraft could overfly France on missions to North Africa and the Middle East. But an affront to French scientific pride was also serious, and in September 1995 the Quai d'Orsay informed Washington of its surprise that the patent application filed by Pasteur was "still under consideration while NIH, who applied for a patent four months later, received a positive answer from the Patent Office."

Despite the French government's "strong desire" that the patent issue be "promptly resolved,"[25] Washington couldn't understand the problem. "We have carefully reviewed the written material you furnished and the oral representations made during your visit to the Department," Haddow wrote Dedonder following the French diplomatic note. "Based on that information and our own review of the laboratory records and other documents relating to this matter, we can find no basis to support your position that United States Patent No. 4,520,113 is invalid or that the actions you requested be taken by the Department are warranted."[26]

In private, the HHS lawyers were less confident. Signing off on the Fischinger report, one HHS attorney cautioned Lowell Harmison that "my initialing of this report should not be interpreted as an indication to you, Dr. Mason, or other officials in the Department that I am fully comfortable that the Department would prevail if the French were to proceed to press their claims through litigation." The attorney's reservations stemmed primarily "from our lack of information regarding the details that the French may have to support their claims and from our lack of expertise to fully understand the complex scientific issues that have been raised."[27]

The lawyers were still getting their information indirectly, from Gallo and Mika Popovic through Peter Fischinger, and on his way to Sweden Gallo stopped by the lab to help Popovic craft some answers to Fischinger's latest set of interrogatories.[i] Although ignoring the lawyers' questions about when the first blood test had occurred, Popovic revealed that the pool had sprung to life on November 15, 1983, the day he infected the HUT-78 cell line with fluids from the cultured T-cells of three AIDS patients.

A week later, Popovic had re-inoculated the pool with more material from the same patients. At the beginning of January, material from seven new patients had been added. At some point thereafter — Popovic didn't say when — the virus called HTLV-3B had emerged. But HTLV-3B couldn't be LAV, Popovic said, because his work with the pool had been "almost entirely confined to the *tissue culture* room 6B03A *where no LAV was ever used.*"

When Lowell Harmison's fact-finding expedition showed up at NIH, Mal Martin laid his suspicions on the table. LAV and 3B, Martin declared flatly, had come from the same patient. "And Harmison said would I please put in writing what I'd just told him. He said it would be treated as administratively confidential."

Reluctantly, Martin agreed. "When you're asked to do something by somebody in the department downtown you jump," he said later, "and

Lowell Harmison was probably the single most powerful person in the government on issues pertaining to health. I had seen him in action, and I saw people jump very high, including the director of NIH. So I prepared this report and gave it to them."

Martin was the well-regarded chief of a good-sized lab at the NIH's Institute of Allergy and Infectious Disease. Like Robin Weiss, Martin had been on the periphery of some significant discoveries. But Martin had made important contributions of his own, and neither the veracity of his research nor his scientific expertise had ever been questioned. Even Gallo conceded that Martin was "better analytically, whereas I'm more impulsive than analytical."

Martin's report to Harmison began by recalling the session at Cold Spring Harbor, in May 1983, where Martin had permitted Françoise Barré to speak about the discovery of LAV.[28] That meeting, Martin pointed out, had occurred almost six months after the December 1982 date in Fischinger's report for Gallo's first isolations of the AIDS virus. To Martin, it wasn't conceivable that Gallo's lab had found the AIDS virus in December but was still talking about HTLV-1 in May.

Next Martin described how the LAV sample he was given by Montagnier in April 1984 contained "two discrete species of the AIDS virus," one with the maverick *Hind*III restriction site and one without. Martin recounted his surprise upon learning, at the Pasteur's Thanksgiving meeting, that one of Beatrice Hahn's HTLV-3B clones contained the same exact site, while Hahn's other clone did not.

To his report Martin attached a paper he had submitted recently to *Science,* comparing HTLV-3B and LAV with ten other AIDS viruses, seven isolated from patients in North America and three from Zaire. Of the ten, only LAV and HTLV-3B had contained the *Hind*III site. "Informed virologists," Martin wrote, "will certainly draw certain obvious conclusions."

The paper was a collaboration between Martin's lab and Paul Feorino, the veteran CDC virologist who had isolated the LAV-like viruses from the transfusion pair. In subsequent experiments, Feorino had been surprised to discover that the virus from the male blood donor wasn't exactly the same as the one from the female transfusion recipient. Although he hadn't recognized it at the time, Feorino was simply seeing the natural genetic changes the AIDS virus undergoes as it reproduces itself ten million–fold, the result of the frequent mistakes in transcribing its RNA into DNA.

When the woman received her transfusion, in late 1982, the virus she got was virtually identical to the virus that her donor was carrying on the day he gave blood. Since then, it had undergone genetic changes while replicating in the woman's T-cells; the virus that infected the donor had continued to change for the same reason. Following their isolation in December 1983, both viruses had reproduced in culture in the CDC's lab, changing their relative genetic makeups even more. By September 1984, when Feorino made his first restriction maps, the transfusion pair already diverged by 5 percent.

Feorino had expected them to be the same. "We were wondering," he recalled, "'What the hell is going on?'" When he decided to compare genetic similarities across a range of AIDS viruses from Zaire and the United States, Feorino had chosen both HTLV-3B and LAV as his controls —"trying not to take sides," Feorino said later. "That was the dumbest thing I've ever done." Whether Feorino looked at an AIDS virus from North America or one from Africa, "every strain was different from every other strain." The only exceptions were the control viruses, HTLV-3B and LAV.

"Once I saw the results, there was no way I could not publish it," Feorino said. "I knew it was trouble when I saw it, but the data is the data." The implication, unstated in the paper, was bad news for Gallo's scenario that had Frédéric Brugière becoming infected in 1982 by one of the pool patients in New York. Had that been the case, by the time LAV and HTLV-3B were isolated in Paris and Bethesda there would have been at least a 5 percent difference between them, perhaps 10 percent. But when the sequences of the known AIDS viruses were placed side by side, 3B and LAV stood out like a pair of identical twins at a family reunion.

The paper reporting the comparisons, on which Mal Martin was senior author, had been submitted to *Science* in June of 1985.[29] By the time Martin finished his report to Harmison, it still hadn't been scheduled for publication. "It took us six months to get that thing published," Feorino said. "Someone got sick. Someone's mother died. It got to be Halloween, it got to be St. Swithin's Day. I had to threaten the editor that we would take it away and put it in another journal."

Not long after filing his report to Harmison, Martin was in Cold Spring Harbor for a meeting on AIDS vaccines. On the shuttle returning to Washington, Martin took a seat next to his new boss,

Anthony Fauci, the recently appointed chief of NIAID. "Tony said to me, 'Malcolm, what did you write in that report?'" Martin recalled. "I said, 'Well, I just told the facts. I thought it was sort of a smoking gun.' At this meeting, Max Essex, Bill Haseltine, and Dani Bolognesi had all come up to Fauci and said that I had written a devastating report to 'get Gallo.'"

"I was a fool," Martin said later, "to have even put anything on paper. I thought it was going to be treated in a discreet way. I said to myself, 'Look, you didn't do anything wrong, these guys are a bunch of worms.' I said, 'I'm tough, I can take this heat.' But that's when I realized there was no way to deal with it from the inside."

Harmison thought Martin's report held "very, very little, if any" significance for the American position in the dispute with the French.[30] But once it was part of the record, the HHS had no choice but to address the issues Martin raised.[31]

"The Department requests a prompt reply to these questions," Fischinger wrote Gallo in mid-September 1985. Why, if Gallo had discovered in 1982 the existence of a retrovirus in AIDS patients which wasn't HTLV-1 or HTLV-2, hadn't he mentioned his discovery "in your many ensuing publications" over the next year? "Ostensibly," Fischinger said, "all of the papers mention HTLV-1 association with AIDS, but none address the fact that you were aware of the existence of other agents which were of the HTLV-3 type."

Gallo found Fischinger's memo waiting upon his return from Sweden. Before departing for Italy to accept the Premio Internazionale Tevere Roma,[32] Gallo replied that detecting the presence of a virus wasn't the same as isolating that virus — a distinction Gallo hadn't paid much attention to before now. To do anything with a virus, one first needed to isolate it, to extract it from the cells in which it was originally cultured and transmit it to uninfected cells where it could be examined and characterized.

To accomplish that, one needed first to grow the original cells. But Gallo hadn't been able to grow any of his virus "detections." Because he couldn't isolate whatever viruses were there, he hadn't been able to characterize them. Without any characterization, Gallo admitted to Fischinger, he hadn't been able to say what they were, much less whether they were the cause of AIDS.[33]

It was a different story altogether from the one Gallo had been telling in public and in print. "What good would it do me or the field,"

Gallo asked Fischinger, "to slip in a few sentences that another retrovirus is occasionally detected (at that time it was only occasional) and that it is not HTLV-1 or 2; but we have no evidence that each time this new virus is detected it is one and the same virus, i.e., this could have been an HTLV-3 in patient one, no virus detected in patient two, three, four, five, six . . . and when detected again in, say, patient seven it could have been an HTLV-4, i.e., not the same as HTLV-3 and only an opportunistic infection."

Fischinger had noted that "some researchers" were suggesting that the first clear linkage of the virus to AIDS had been reported by Jean-Claude Chermann at Park City in February 1984, three months before Gallo's papers in *Science*. "Some researchers," Gallo sniffed, "especially those who publish in non-reviewed places, e.g., *MMWR*" (the CDC's *Morbidity and Mortality Weekly Report*), "are of the impression that stating something is the same as publishing in a *reviewed scientific journal*. It is not. It is as if they have no experience in established scientific documentation. Even if stating something is acceptable as a claim of priority, how is fairness established when we go through the time and effort of writing the papers, submitting, getting the reviews, revising, resubmitting, and then waiting for the publication to come out?"

Gallo questioned whether Chermann's Park City data really had linked LAV to AIDS. "First of all, it is true his data improved a lot," Gallo said, although "probably with the help of Kalyanaraman who, as you know, was hired from our group by CDC and sent to Paris at that time." The only reason Gallo hadn't said anything about his own discoveries at Park City, he told Fischinger, was "because our papers were being prepared for publication, and our data was not yet in the hands of Dr. DeVita or Dr. Wyngaarden."

Had Fischinger troubled to check, he would have discovered that Kalyanaraman hadn't arrived in Paris until late April 1984, nearly three months after Park City.[j] Even then he hadn't played any part in the development of the Pasteur ELISA, which had been finished in early March.[34] A glance at Betsy Read's notebook would have revealed that nearly all the data Gallo published in *Science,* including his ELISA results, hadn't existed until weeks after Park City.

Fischinger had saved Mal Martin's smoking gun for last. "Because of the scientific nature and the nonscientific implications and seriousness of the next concern," Fischinger wrote, "the allegation below is presented in almost verbatim form. The scientist's name is not mentioned."

After summarizing Martin's memo to Harmison, Fischinger asked whether Gallo had seen more than one "species" of AIDS virus in any isolate from a single individual — for example, the LAV/HTLV-3B clones with *Hind*III, and those without. Gallo replied that hairline genetic mutations did exist, but they took so long to develop in culture that even if Popovic *had* grown the LAV sample from Paris there wouldn't have been time for mutations to have arisen.

"We received an extraordinarily small amount of Montagnier's virus September 24, 1983," Gallo told Fischinger, although how much virus came in the door was less important than what happened to it afterward. "Mika developed the H-9 clone in early November 1983. Can anyone possibly imagine mass production of this amount of virus in five weeks? Further, can anyone possibly imagine 150 nucleotide changes, deletions, and additions coming into a genome in six weeks of culture."

Gallo's math was off,[k] and anyway the Paul Feorino–Mal Martin paper said otherwise. But if Fischinger had seen the preprint of that paper, he hadn't passed it on to Gallo. In any case, Gallo didn't care about hairline mutations or distinctive genetic signatures. It wasn't necessary to deal with such complex questions, Gallo said. The mere existence of R.F. precluded any motive to steal LAV. "We isolated, mass produced in H-9 cells, patented and published on a major variant, HTLV-3$_{RF}$, (Haitian isolate)," Gallo said, which wasn't true. "Very different from LAV, at exactly the same time, making all this crap irrelevant."

Besides responding to Fischinger's memo, Gallo had been spending a good deal of time in Europe, where his favorite stopping place was Italy. When Oliver Varner of the University of Genoa invited Gallo to speak at a symposium, what he described sounded more like a millionaire's vacation. "We will wait for you and your friends at the airport," Varner wrote Gallo, "and drive you to Pordenone in Friuli. Being aware of your long traveling, we will organize a simple characteristic evening welcome party and dinner.

"On the next day, there is the symposium with 30 minute talk, interrupted by a rural local lunch. The dinner will be our challenging opportunity to offer you the products of our region. The next day, we will visit wineries, castles, and after a short press conference, we will go to Forgaria. At 2.00 pm we will embark in the ship 'Ausonia,' directed to Barcelona and Tulone in a scientific cruise . . . the ship will change the course to meet a shuttle boat, which will take you to Imperia, where a car will be waiting for you to go to Nice." In case Gallo ran a little short, he would "receive cash in Genova Li 1,500,000, about $1,100, for your traveling expenses without asking you the flight coupon, and cash in Pordenone Li 500,000, about $350, as pocket money."[35]

Gallo had been invited to return to Italy before the end of the year, to address the hematological institute in Naples, but the welcome there wasn't likely to be as warm as what was offered in Genoa. Among the other scheduled speakers was Abraham Karpas, who had just sent Jim Wyngaarden yet another multipage, single-spaced letter accusing Gallo of stealing the French virus.[36] When the president of the Naples institute, Mario D'Angelo, who happened to be visiting the NIH, stopped by Gallo's office to say hello, he was met with what D'Angelo later described as "a rambling tirade."

Gallo "was very angry with Karpas and Montagnier," D'Angelo said later. "He told me he would never come, because we had arranged things in such a way as to tear him to pieces, despite the presence of many American scientists." D'Angelo remembered being nonplussed by Gallo's appraisal of his colleagues. "About one of the speakers, he said, 'He is a shameless fraud. He is a researcher worth but four cents.' And then, 'Who is he? Who is he? I don't know him! I only know that he is a megalomaniac.' About another, he said: 'He is an old imbecile.' He acted as if he was going to attack me. I tried very hard to remain calm, and since I could not make myself understood I asked the lady doctor present to translate what I was saying: 'In order to have you come to Naples, I am willing not to have Karpas or someone else, provided Montagnier will be present.'

"He calmed down immediately and appeared to accept this possibility and he asked me the following question: Change the date of the conference to January, cancel all the names from your list. I will bring to Naples all the scholars you want, even a hundred scientists, and I will do it without charge. I answered that his proposal was unacceptable, because we already had committed ourselves. He answered me, 'There are no problems, I can personally telephone your president.'

At this point I told him he was behaving not as a scientist and that his presence in Naples was no longer of interest to me. He invited me to leave. A few days before the seminar, a letter was received by the Naples newspaper where he said that we had fabricated everything and that he did not even know us. We had exploited his name without his knowledge for publicity purposes."[37]

The blood test for AIDS was proving even more profitable than its manufacturers had predicted. During the first four months of testing, Abbott Laboratories had sold $8 million worth of ELISA kits. Despite Margaret Heckler's assurance of a few months before that American manufacturers were prepared to meet the foreign demand for the AIDS test, Abbott still couldn't make enough tests to satisfy the domestic demand.[38] Unable to increase its inventory beyond a one- or two-day supply, Abbott had asked the FDA for permission to change its method of producing the AIDS virus.[39]

The change increased the amount of available virus, but it did nothing to resolve the false positives the test was producing. During the last six months of 1985, the Red Cross blood center in Springfield, Illinois, reported that two hundred blood donors had tested positive after the first Abbott ELISA. Only eighty-six remained positive after a second ELISA. When the eighty-six double-positives were run through the Western Blot, only two donors proved actually to be infected with the AIDS virus — an astounding false-positive rate of ninety-nine in every hundred.

The FDA required that donated blood be discarded if the first ELISA was positive,[40] and the Abbott test had cost the Springfield Red Cross 198 pints of perfectly good blood.[41] Nationwide, nearly four out of five Red Cross blood samples testing positive by the Abbott ELISA were falsely positive, and in addition to losing blood the Red Cross and the other blood banks were losing donors.[42] Anyone who was ELISA-positive was no longer permitted to donate blood, even those who were subsequently negative by Western Blot.[43]

Despite its increasing alarm, the Red Cross was finding it difficult to get Abbott's attention. "It has taken us over two weeks to convince persons at Abbott Laboratories that indeed a crisis situation does exist," the head of the Los Angeles blood center wrote Abbott in early November.[44] Not until the Gallo ELISA had been on the market for eight months did Abbott form an "HTLV-3 Task Force" to address the false positive problem.[45]

The Red Cross contract with Abbott didn't prevent it from evaluating other AIDS tests, and in mid-November of 1985 a competition was arranged: blood samples from thousands of donors would be tested in sequence by the Abbott ELISA and the Pasteur test from Genetic Systems.[46] Genetic Systems won the competition hands down. Not only was the Pasteur test far more precise, the Red Cross technicians found it much easier to use. "WE LOVE IT!!!!! Easy to learn. Easy to run," exclaimed the Red Cross blood center in San Jose.[47]

The superiority of the Pasteur ELISA was well-confirmed by independent studies.[48] But the Red Cross wouldn't be switching to the French AIDS test any time soon. A year before, Genetic Systems had applied to the FDA for permission to sell the Pasteur ELISA in the United States, and the company still didn't have an FDA license.[49] Considering Mac Haddow's rebuff of Raymond Dedonder, it seemed unlikely that a license would be forthcoming soon, and without a license the Pasteur ELISA couldn't be employed for the testing of human blood.

The more intransigent Washington became, the more Dedonder's resolve stiffened. "I am left with no choice," he wrote Haddow in September 1985, "but to turn the matter over to our attorneys. They are instructed to proceed quickly and efficiently. We are now compelled to present all the facts to the community, so it may judge the actions of those involved."[50]

It wasn't the solution Dedonder would have chosen. "At the beginning," he said later, "we did not want to start a big fight. We wanted to share. We were really aware of the importance of the AIDS problem, of the fact that such kits to test the people who were contaminated by the virus were very deeply needed. I didn't want to stop the production of any of the firms that were putting kits on the market, because of the important public health problem of AIDS."

Not really expecting a reversal, Dedonder appealed Haddow's rejection to Jim Mason, who privately put the government's chances of winning a lawsuit against the French at no better than sixty-forty.[51] "I think Mason was rather sympathetic," Dedonder said, "but he was not in a position to do something." Most of what Mason knew about the dispute came filtered through Lowell Harmison, and Mason's knowledge was fragmentary. "I was peripheral," Mason said later. "I think I know pretty well what [Harmison] found out from Fred Murphy and his people in Atlanta. But I do not know what he discovered in Bob Gallo's lab."

Realizing he would have to make good on his threat to take the United States to court, Dedonder retained a brace of New York City law firms and set them on parallel paths. The out-of-court negotiations would be handled by Weil, Gotshal & Manges, whose managing partner, Ira Millstein, sat on the board of the American affiliate of the Pasteur Foundation, and who had a longstanding relationship with the French government that previously had brought him the Legion of Honor. "For something else I did for them," was all Millstein would say about the rosette in his buttonhole, except that "it gets me better tables" in Paris restaurants.

If the negotiations failed, Dedonder wanted a lawsuit ready to file, and his New York connections introduced him to James B. Swire, a senior litigation partner in the Manhattan firm of Townley & Updike. The offices of Weil, Gotshal, on the upper floors of the General Motors Building in Midtown Manhattan, were modern, light, and airy, and housed many, many attorneys. Townley, on the twenty-sixth floor of the Chrysler Building a mile away, was smaller and more conservative, all dark wood and polished brass. The Weil, Gotshal letterhead listed trendy branch offices in Miami, London, Singapore, and Budapest. The letterhead of Townley & Updike, which had no branch offices, bore only the names of its partners.

A product of Princeton and Harvard Law and a Reagan Republican to the core, Jim Swire once had been interviewed for a job by Richard Nixon's White House counsel, John W. Dean 3d. The interview took place a few months before the Watergate break-in, and Swire recalled with amusement Dean's interest in an article Swire had written on wiretapping for the *Harvard Journal on Legislation*. To his everlasting relief, Swire turned Dean down, only to find himself later helping to defend Nixon's onetime FBI director, L. Patrick Gray 3d, against lawsuits by members of the Weather Underground.

Jim Swire was to be the Pasteur's stick, Ira Millstein its carrot. If HHS didn't give Millstein what Pasteur wanted, Swire would get it in court. "We fought in both directions," Dedonder said.

Before becoming Ronald Reagan's HHS Secretary, Heckler had represented Massachusetts in the House of Representatives, where her principal distinction had been her seniority among the female members of Congress. Heckler thought her political career had ended when she was beaten by a Democrat, Barney Frank. But Reagan, under pressure from progressive Republican circles to appoint a few women to high office, had invited her to join his cabinet.

Heckler's stewardship of HHS, the largest and most complex of all cabinet departments including the Pentagon, had been marred by what her subordinates described as a mercurial temperament and a difficulty in grasping the functions of the manifold agencies that comprised HHS. To get her out of the picture, Heckler was offered the post of American ambassador to Dublin.

Jim Mason, who had never found his balance as assistant secretary, announced that he, too, was leaving Washington, to return to Atlanta as full-time director of the CDC. "As soon as I heard Margaret was going to Ireland," Mason recalled, "I saw that as my window of opportunity." No sooner had Mason walked out the door than Lowell Harmison stepped in to fill the power vacuum. Harmison was now the man to see about the Gallo case, and in mid-November of 1985 one of Ira Millstein's lawyers, Nancy Buc, informed him that the Pasteur had asked the patent office to declare an interference.[52]

Buc, who had served as the FDA's general counsel during the Carter administration and wasn't intimidated by high-ranking government officials, expressed considerable doubt that Gallo had discovered the AIDS virus before the French. Given Gallo's personality, Buc thought it "quite unlikely that Gallo would really have remained silent" about such a discovery, because "too much glory would have attended even a preliminary announcement." If, on the other hand, Gallo's claim were true, Gallo had "done a serious disservice to scientific progress" by keeping quiet about such an important breakthrough. Either knowingly or unknowingly, Gallo had used a French discovery to make the blood test on which the United States government was now collecting patent royalties.

One of the HHS lawyers at the Buc-Harmison meeting was Darrel Grinstead, with whom Buc had worked closely during her years at the FDA. Buc considered Grinstead "honest, hardworking and quite intelligent." But Grinstead wasn't a scientist, and he had been assigned to defend the Gallo patent, not conduct a scientific inquiry. According to Buc's account of Grinstead's remarks, "Dr. Gallo asserts that he never used the virus which was delivered to Dr. Popovic in September of 1983, that it had simply 'remained in the refrigerator,' metaphorically speaking, and that since Gallo had never used the virus there could be no question of a breach of contract even assuming that the document signed by Popovic constitutes a contract."

If that were true, Buc replied, the government shouldn't mind giving her copies of Popovic's notebooks and a narrative showing that he had done his published experiments with viruses other than LAV. When word came down from HHS that yet another declaration would be required from Mika Popovic, Gallo complained that he didn't understand why he had to answer so many questions about his research when the French didn't have to answer any questions about theirs.

"Time spent on pulling this information together takes away from critical work on the AIDS projects," Gallo complained to Lowell Harmison.[53] "I would like to see documentation of what the Pasteur group did with materials that they received from us. . . . I believe this exchange of information should be a two-way street, and that we should not be constantly subject to responding to their accusations, and it is certainly peculiar that this is the way it is being managed."

Gallo didn't seem to understand that the Reagan administration wasn't accusing the French of having misappropriated HTLV-3B. But despite Gallo's railings, Popovic's latest memo provided some of the details missing from his earlier accounts. Now Popovic acknowledged growing LAV in Ti7.4 and one other cell line, though without mentioning HUT-78 by name. Moreover, the successful infection of Ti7.4 had been confirmed by immunofluorescence on December 14, 1983, nearly two months after it had begun growing. The same LAV-infected cell line, Popovic said, had been used later by Beatrice Hahn for the "comparative studies with H-9/HTLV-3B" reported in the unpublished Wong-Staal paper.[1]

Had it become public, Popovic's memo would have closed the case. No longer could Gallo insist that Popovic hadn't been able to grow or work with the French virus, or that there hadn't been enough LAV to compare to his own isolates — or to contaminate Popovic's own cultures. More to the point, the virus Gallo received from Paris in 1983 had proven indistinguishable from the virus he called HTLV-3B in September 1984.

The memo stayed under lock and key. But when HHS moved to settle the dispute, it offered Montagnier and his team equal credit with Gallo for the discovery of the AIDS virus and the AIDS test, and an FDA license that would allow Genetic Systems to sell the Pasteur test in the United States. The French wouldn't receive royalties from Abbott and the other licensees, but they wouldn't have to pay any royalties to the American government.

A few days before tendering their offer, the HHS lawyers had responded to Buc's request to see the government's cards with a sheaf of Popovic's note pages.[54] That none of the pages mentioned LAV anywhere appeared to buttress the government's claim that Popovic hadn't done anything with the French virus. Stuck in among the pages, however, was a copy of the letter Matt Gonda had sent Popovic in December of 1983, reporting his success in photographing what looked like a lentivirus in two of Popovic's cultures.[55] Either the HHS lawyers hadn't read the Gonda letter carefully, or they hadn't recognized its significance, because the two lentivirus-producing cultures were named *HUT-78/LAV* and *Ti7.4/LAV*. Nancy Buc told the government her client would see them in court.[56]

A young attorney from Jim Swire's firm spent most of December 12, 1985, a Thursday, waiting at the United States Court of Claims, a few blocks from the White House, and checking in with Swire on the hour. In his Manhattan office Swire was waiting as well, for instructions from Paris. Just before the court closed for the day, Swire told the young man to file the lawsuit he carried in his briefcase.[57]

The complaint stopped short of accusing anyone in Gallo's lab of stealing LAV. Rather, it described the French virus as the "master key" that had allowed Gallo's lab to "unlock the safe" containing "the secret of the cause of AIDS." Left unstated was the possibility that the unlocking might not have been serendipitous, but for the purposes of Pasteur's case it didn't matter whether a theft had been committed. What mattered was that Gallo and the government were enjoying the scientific credit, and commercial profits, that rightfully belonged to France.

The Department of Health and Human Services dismissed the Pasteur's allegations as "absolutely without basis." There wasn't any question, the HHS said, that the United States was the rightful owner of the patent for the AIDS test — or that, "without the work and the discoveries of the National Cancer Institute, we would not today have an effective, reliable and commercially available blood test serving to protect Americans and others against the spread of AIDS."[58]

Tracked down by the *Wall Street Journal* in Jerusalem, where he was about to receive the Rabbi Shai Shacknai Cancer Prize, Gallo explained that his lab couldn't have stolen LAV, because there hadn't been enough LAV to steal. The virus sample sent from Paris, Gallo said, had been "too small to be of practical use."[59]

Suggestions that Mika Popovic's cultures might have become contaminated with LAV were "the height of outrage," Gallo said. There hadn't been anything to contaminate Popovic's cultures *with*, because it had been "physically impossible" to grow the virus sent by Montagnier.[60] "We helped them a lot more than they helped us," Gallo told the *New York Times*. "They didn't receive a patent because they didn't have a working blood test."[61]

"French Virus in the Picture"

The dispute with Pasteur raised Robert Gallo's profile to the point where Gallo could complain that "I get press calls every day. Every day. I'm invited on 'Good Morning America,' 'Hello America,' 'Wipe-the-Dust-Out-of-Your-Eyes America.'"[1] According to the *Washington Post,* Gallo was "tired of all the fury, but is caught up in it as one story adds to another, and as rumors become 'facts' because they are published repeatedly. He is also caught up because he is a competitive, emotional man who has difficulty not fighting back. 'Gossip occurs about people who are visible,'" Gallo said. "It can give you a bad weekend sometimes."[2]

Gallo's disposition improved in early February of 1986, with a visit to Bombay and Delhi as an honored guest of the Indian Oncological Society,[3] a trip he later described as one of the best he had ever taken. "They treated me like a maharajah," Gallo said. "They put garlands of flowers around my neck and sprinkled me with oil. What a place."[4]

While Gallo was out of the country, the Food and Drug Administration notified Genetic Systems that the company had been approved to make and sell the Pasteur AIDS blood test in the United States. Abbott Laboratories had gotten its license in just nine weeks; it had taken Genetic Systems nearly nine months.[a]

In the interim, a Red Cross task force had christened Genetic Systems its "test of choice" and recommended that the company be awarded at least 80 percent of the Red Cross business currently going to Abbott.[5] "Our test brings a new accuracy standard to AIDS testing," declared Bob Nowinski. "With this accuracy, it should be possible to virtually eliminate the transmission of AIDS virus through the blood supply system."[b]

The lack of an American patent didn't preclude Genetic Systems from selling the Pasteur test in the United States, since the most the Reagan administration could do was to sue the French for patent infringement. Indeed, several of the companies selling the Gallo AIDS test had begun pushing for such a suit.[6] But patent infringement cases can take years, and the French, who had been first to apply for an American patent, stood an excellent chance of winning.

In the meantime, the FDA license made the sales legal, or so Bob Nowinski imagined. But when the company tried to bid on the enormous military contract for AIDS antibody tests, Genetic Systems representatives couldn't even get a meeting with the Pentagon brass. It would be un-American, they were told, for the United States military to buy a French AIDS test. The Pentagon contract went to Electronucleonics, whose false-positive rate was many times higher than the Pasteur's.

The French found it a further insult that their FDA license described the Pasteur ELISA as a test for antibodies to HTLV-3.[7] "The FDA knows perfectly well," Dedonder protested to the FDA commissioner, Frank Young, "that the Genetic Systems kit works with LAV, the virus isolated by the Pasteur group in January, 1983, more than one year before the description of HTLV-3 by Gallo and his co-workers. Thus, requiring Genetic Systems to call its product HTLV-3 is simply wrong, both historically and scientifically . . . it also does a disservice to the discoverers of the AIDS virus, *Montagnier et al.*, who, though having made an important scientific breakthrough, are apparently not to be allowed the ordinary right to see in everyday use, on their own product, the name they chose for the AIDS virus."[8]

Young replied that if Pasteur wanted to sell its AIDS test in the United States, HTLV-3 was the name it would have to use. "Please be assured," he told Dedonder, "that it is not in any way meant to slight the very important work of scientists like Dr. Montagnier and others on whom research advancement is depending."[9] It sounded like a conciliatory letter. But within a few days the FDA was warning Pasteur that its advertising shouldn't mention any of the independent studies showing the Pasteur test to be more accurate than the Gallo version.[10]

That information might have been welcome at the Blood Center of Southeast Louisiana, where two-thirds of the donors testing positive with the Gallo/Abbott ELISA weren't infected with the AIDS virus at all.[11] Or at the North Colorado Medical Center in Greeley, where false positives were running over 70 percent.[12] Or in tiny Hays, Kansas, where there was no AIDS, but whose town doctor complained to the FDA that unless something were done about the false positives there soon wouldn't be anyone left who was eligible to donate blood.[13]

With the advent of blood screening for the AIDS virus, the ramifications of false positives reached far beyond the relatively small number of prospective blood donors. The military had begun testing all new recruits and active duty personnel, the State Department foreign service officers and their dependents, the Peace Corps and Job Corps anyone who applied to join. The state of Illinois, where Abbott had its headquarters, was gearing up to require mandatory AIDS tests for anyone who wanted to be married.[14]

The consequences of a false positive AIDS test could prove horrendous. A Michigan college student, advised by his county health department to begin making final arrangements on the basis of a false-positive test, dropped out of school and spent what he thought were his last months on earth working for an AIDS support group.[15] A Philadelphia man, having taken a required premarital blood test for syphilis — and been tested, without his knowledge, for the AIDS virus — lost his fiancée when the test proved falsely positive.[16]

A Los Angeles teacher with a false-positive test lost his job.[17] A pregnant soldier who volunteered for an Army blood drive discovered her positive test was false only after having the abortion urged by her doctor.[18] An Alabama housewife became celibate, stopped kissing her children, and started seeing a psychiatrist until she, too, was discovered to be the victim of a false-positive ELISA.[19]

The FDA official in charge of monitoring the performance of the AIDS test was Tom Zuck, a hematologist and army colonel from Letterman Army Hospital in San Francisco who had been temporarily assigned to FDA headquarters in Rockville, Maryland. "They wanted a blood banker," said Zuck, "and they couldn't find anybody on short notice, and I was available. So I got the job."

Zuck had been in San Francisco when the Abbott test was approved, and he believed that the decision had been made in haste.

"There's no doubt that Abbott was rushed to market," Zuck said. "Absolutely no doubt about it. Part of the problem with those tests was *because* they were rushed to market. They were bound to be lousy tests. They were hastily concocted. The issue was, is it better to have a bad test than no test at all? And I think everybody involved said, 'We'll worry about the nonspecificity later.'"

Later was now, and Zuck saw the false positives as a huge problem, not only because they were costing the blood industry money but also because of the human consequences. Even when the follow-up Western Blot was negative, the news that their initial "AIDS test" had been positive unhinged donors who didn't comprehend the complexities of blood-antibody diagnostics. "A lot of blood centers told people, 'You're repeatedly reactive but you don't confirm, so you can't give blood,'" Zuck said. "A lot of these people were hysterical and believed they really had some kind of unusual AIDS."

When the complaints about the Abbott test began piling up on Zuck's desk, he ordered the company to send him its "action plan" for eliminating the false positives.[20] The Abbott test was an old-style configuration, in which tiny polystyrene beads coated with inactivated AIDS virus are placed in small indentations, or wells, on a plastic plate, each filled with a tiny drop of the blood being tested. If the blood contains AIDS virus antibodies, in theory the antibodies adhere to the virus on the bead, triggering an enzyme to change color.

To eliminate the aberrant H-9 cell proteins on the bead that were adhering to nonviral antibodies and triggering false-positive reactions, Abbott had enhanced its virus-purification techniques. That hadn't worked, and now the company was proposing to reduce the length of time the bead was exposed to the blood.[21]

When Zuck saw the company's newest proposal, he realized that Abbott was trying to reinvent the AIDS test from the ground up. "You don't know what's wrong, do you?" Zuck told Marijane Sidote, Abbott's liaison with the FDA.[22] Sidote admitted Zuck was right, and that Abbott was worried. The company had been hearing rumors that the FDA had put Abbott "on probation," Sidote said — or, worse, that it was about to pull the Abbott test off the market. Zuck replied that there was no such thing as "FDA probation," and that in order to withdraw the license the FDA would have to take Abbott to court.[23] The FDA just wanted Abbott to fix its test.

Zuck's decision to award a license to Genetic Systems hadn't been well received by the executive hierarchy at HHS. In mid-March of 1986,

Zuck was summoned for interrogation by no less than Lowell Harmison, whom Vince DeVita had come to view as "hostile toward the French" because he thought they were "stealing American technology."[24]

"It got really kind of ugly," Zuck recalled. "I had to show cause, actually defend myself, for licensing a French test. Remember, we're in the middle of this lawsuit at the time. It was a very difficult meeting. You've got one active-duty army colonel in uniform, surrounded by a whole bunch of one- and two-star Public Health Service officers. The meeting was a political meeting, but the science won the day."

According to notes taken by one of the HHS lawyers present, Zuck explained that the greater a blood test's specificity, the fewer false positives it will record. The Pasteur ELISA was "widely regarded as superior," Zuck said, because "it was considerably more specific" than the Gallo test. In fact, the accuracy of the Genetic Systems test approached "the benchmark criteria," the Western Blot.

The main reason the French test was so much better, Zuck told Harmison, was the Pasteur's CEM cell line, which meant the test resulted in less wasted blood. But the blood banks also liked the test because there were no little beads to deal with, and because the Genetic Systems kits were "more complete than any of the other licensees."[25]

Moving quickly to head off the notion that the French had made a better AIDS test, Gallo declared that *his* lab had been first to grow the AIDS virus in CEM, a claim with which Robin Weiss would have taken issue.[c] The problem with CEM, Gallo told Harmison, was that it had to be reinfected periodically with virus — which happened to be precisely how Genetic Systems was growing huge quantities of pristine LAV in Seattle. Gallo nonetheless insisted that CEM "offers no intrinsic advantage in virus production and may have yet to be discovered disadvantages. Therefore, I would strongly urge our FDA officials to get input from very experienced people (like us) before making public quality pronouncements."[26]

Momentarily, Zuck had a call from Gallo. "Every time you dealt with Lowell," Zuck said, "it always seemed there was a Gallo connection somewhere. Gallo called and shouted at me that the French virus was 'incompletely integrated' in their cell line, which is bullshit. The Public Health Service, particularly in the person of Lowell Harmison, tended to always side with Gallo. There were a whole lot of financial interests floating around there too, which I don't even want to touch. But we all know there were royalties on this and royalties on that."

Developing a blood test that could accurately detect antibodies to a single AIDS virus had proved difficult enough. But there was no reason there should be only *one* kind of AIDS virus. If the virus had come into man from African monkeys, as most researchers believed, many monkeys must have been infected before the first human acquired the virus.

Waiting to leap the "species barrier," an event which probably occurred sometime in the 1940s, the virus would have mutated in each of those monkeys. Nobody could say how it had finally crossed over — a monkey bite, a wounded hunter, incompletely roasted monkey meat — but Gallo had his own ideas. "Maybe there's some ritual with monkey blood," he suggested. "Who knows? They do a lot of funny things in Africa, like when they make the lower lip stick out or when they put things through their noses."[27]

However it had happened, there was no reason to think the AIDS epidemic should have been confined to a single monkey virus that had passed into a single human. Why not two or three such viruses, or even more?

The second AIDS virus, like the first one, was discovered at the Institut Pasteur in Paris, this time by a genial, thirty-one-year-old doctor named François Clavel. Like David Klatzmann before him, Clavel had given up clinical medicine to pursue a fascination with research. Clavel counted himself lucky to have landed in Montagnier's lab, where one of his first assignments was to search for a virus in T-cells from an AIDS patient languishing in a Lisbon hospital.[d]

Nobody was sure what it meant, but the man's cells had tested positive for reverse transcriptase and negative for antibodies to LAV. Clavel began by hybridizing the cells to a LAV DNA probe. When the probe failed to detect any LAV, he repeated the experiment under increasingly less stringent conditions, searching for the point at which some annealing was bound to occur. Eventually he could see some genetic similarities between LAV and whatever was growing in the Lisbon cells, but they were faint.

According to his doctors, the Lisbon patient, code-named *Mir*, had come to Portugal from one of that country's former African colonies,

Guinea-Bissau. He unquestionably had AIDS, and the positive reverse transcriptase assays by Montagnier's technician, Denise Gué-tard, suggested the man was infected with a retrovirus. But François Clavel's radiographs were saying the retrovirus had hardly any genetics in common with LAV.

When Clavel mentioned to Montagnier the possibility that he had discovered a new human retrovirus, "he politely suggested that I repeat the experiment. So I made a number of different DNA probes to different regions of LAV. When we saw that the patient's serum was negative for most of the viral proteins, we got really excited, Montagnier and everybody else in the lab. It turned out that it was really a very different virus. It was completely different than LAV."

A few months before, François Clavel had been listening to patients coughing through a stethoscope. Now he had discovered LAV-2. "I started to be extremely thrilled by this whole thing," Clavel recalled. "This is great science: 'Let's discover a virus, then let's clone the virus.' For me it was completely new. I was coming up from the clinical field. Clone the virus — it was magical."

A few miles from Clavel's lab, at the Hôpital Claude Bernard, Françoise Brun was discovering the same virus. Among Brun's vast collection of blood samples was one from an African man who had made his way to Paris after coming down with AIDS, and who now lay close to death. Brun's patient, code-named *Rod*, had suffered from AIDS for a couple of years. But like the Lisbon patient *Mir*, *Rod*'s blood was negative for antibodies to LAV. When Brun learned *Rod* had come from the Cape Verde Islands, she had to look at a map. "I did not know where the Cape Verde Islands were," she said, "but I learned that — in West Africa, just near the coast of Guinea-Bissau."

The Guinea-Bissau virus had been isolated in September 1985, the Cape Verde virus at the beginning of December.[28] At the end of December, a paper appeared in *The Lancet* from none other than Max Essex. Following the demise of HTLV-MA, Essex had begun testing blood from Senegalese prostitutes. Although none of the prostitutes had AIDS, they all appeared to have antibodies to the core protein of the AIDS virus.

But antibodies to the virus's envelope protein, which should have been strongest, were significantly weaker than those of American AIDS patients. Even more curious, when the prostitutes' blood was tested for antibodies to an AIDS-like virus Essex's lab had discovered in African green monkeys,[29] the reaction was off the scope — indirect evidence, as Essex was now reporting in *The Lancet,* that "certain healthy Senegalese people have been exposed to a virus" more closely related to a monkey AIDS virus than the human AIDS virus.[30]

What that virus might be, Essex couldn't yet say. But the mystery virus might represent the "missing link" in the natural history of AIDS, the transitional step between monkey and man, a truly seminal discovery. In case the possibility needed further underscoring, Essex pointed out that African green monkeys were thought to be "reservoirs" of viruses that cause disease in humans, like Ebola fever, Marburg disease, and African yellow fever.[31]

By the time Essex's paper appeared, *Mir* had been growing in Montagnier's lab for more than four months. François Clavel didn't need to look at a map to know that Senegal was next to Guinea-Bissau. "It was obvious to us from Max Essex's paper," Clavel said, "that our virus was the same as that infecting the Senegalese prostitutes. We knew we had to rush to publish our results."

The Senegal connection was a fortuitous consequence of the arrival in Essex's lab of a visiting French scientist, Francis Barin, who knew a Senegalese physician who was collecting blood from prostitutes in Dakar. When Clavel saw the *Lancet* article, he decided to find out "exactly what they were doing at Harvard. So I called Francis Barin on the phone. I told him we had a virus. But the difference was that our patients had AIDS, whereas they claimed these prostitutes didn't have AIDS. He said there was work going on with the virus, and that there was another paper about to come out. I said, 'Well, why not exchange reagents?' He said, 'I have to talk with Max.' I said, 'Well, I have to talk with Montagnier.'"

When no reagents were forthcoming from Essex, Clavel asked another Harvard researcher, Ron Desrosiers, for a sample of a related monkey virus Desrosiers's lab had isolated from rhesus macaques. "As anticipated," Clavel said later, "we found that LAV-2 was very close" to the macaque virus, STLV-3$_{MAC}$.

While François Clavel and Françoise Brun wrote up their discovery for *Science,* Essex's lab was isolating a virus from three of the Senegalese prostitutes. Essex's report of the new virus, HTLV-4, went to *Science* at the end of January, three weeks ahead of the French manuscript announcing the isolation of LAV-2.[32] Waiting to learn whether *Science* would publish both papers — or, if not, which one it would choose — Clavel got a call from Barin. "He asked me, 'Are you guys preparing something like a press conference?' I said, 'No, we're not going to have any press release. I want the thing embargoed.' The paper had been submitted to *Science,* and the last thing I wanted was to ruin its chances of being published because of some media hype."

Two days later, at a scientific meeting in Lisbon, Montagnier announced the discovery of LAV-2.[33] Reporters rushed to the Institut Pasteur, and Clavel had to "spend the whole day answering the press," sure by that time "that my *Science* paper would be rejected." Montagnier didn't want to jeopardize the publication of the Pasteur's discovery in *Science,* but neither was he prepared to let the Americans take credit, once again, for something discovered at the Pasteur. The city where *Mir* had died seemed an appropriate place to report the discovery of the virus that had killed him.

"I called the *Science* editor from my hotel," Montagnier said later, "and I asked her, 'Have you made the decision? Because I would like to know before talking about this virus.' She said, 'Well, your referees are negative. We won't publish that paper.' I was very upset." Having suspected that *Science* might confer priority for the discovery on Essex's group, Montagnier had sent an abbreviated account of the LAV-2 story, in French, to *Comptes Rendus,* the journal of the French Academy of Sciences.[34] By the time of Montagnier's talk in Lisbon, the *Comptes Rendus* article was already in press.

Max Essex had planned to announce the discovery of HTLV-4 the day after Montagnier's Lisbon talk, at a meeting of the American Society of Microbiology in Washington, D.C. But Essex sent advance copies of his announcement to a number of journalists, with instructions that the story be released in the event of "a similar story about which we've heard rumors from Paris." As a result, the next day's news reported competing discoveries from both sides of the Atlantic.

According to the *Washington Post,* Essex's announcement had been "hastened" by news reports from Pasteur of "a distinct new form of the AIDS virus that may be responsible for rare forms of the disease."[35] Essex complained that he had been "outjockeyed" by Montagnier, whose behavior he found "slightly sordid." Gallo thought it "unorthodox at best" for Montagnier to have preempted Essex's presentation in Washington.[36] After the story broke, Montagnier got a call from *Science.* "They were saying, 'We are ready to accept your paper,'" Montagnier said with a laugh.

The competing announcements fostered predictable confusion. Had both laboratories discovered the same virus, or something different? The confusion was compounded by Essex's isolation of HTLV-4 only from healthy individuals, whereas the French had found LAV-2 only in people with AIDS. The explanation favored by Essex's principal assistant, Phyllis Kanki, was that the two labs had discovered different viruses. "We believe there is a variety of viruses in Africa and some are pathologic and others are not," Kanki said.[37]

When Clavel ran into Kanki at Cold Spring Harbor, he got the same explanation. "She told me, 'Well, we might be both right,'" Clavel recalled. "'We might have different viruses — yours is pathogenic, ours is not.' I said, 'No, I don't think so. They're so much alike that it's very unlikely. I think there's one kind of virus circulating in humans in Western Africa.'"

The illustrations in Essex's paper included Western Blots comparing the proteins of HTLV-4 with those of Essex's African green monkey virus. As Clavel studied the blots, he remembered his own comparisons of LAV-2 with the rhesus macaque virus. There had been similarities, but also some notable differences. But no matter how long Clavel stared at Essex's blots, he couldn't see *any* differences between HTLV-4 and the green monkey virus. "I was struck," Clavel said later. "The sizes of the proteins of this HTLV-4 thing were *exactly* the same."

Of all the disputes in AIDS research — and there were many that didn't make the newspapers — none was more contentious, or less necessary, than the consuming row over what the AIDS virus should be called. While the Varmus committee pondered the question, Gallo had continued to call the AIDS virus HTLV-3/LAV, and he thought the least Pasteur could do was to call it LAV/HTLV-3. When Gallo discovered the French were using the term LAV alone, he sent Montagnier a peevish letter.

"I thought an oral agreement with you meant something," Gallo said. "I have written to all my colleagues and asked my co-workers to generically use the double name for the virus as we agreed. Nonetheless, you yourself as well as some of your co-workers have gone straight ahead with LAV alone, now coyly calling it lymphadenopathy-AIDS virus. This will re-initiate some tensions. I hope your oral words with me have meaning. In any case I would like to see a written response from you within the week that you do or do not accept our original plan."[38]

The way Montagnier saw it, LAV had existed many months before there was an HTLV-3, and he couldn't imagine why the French should call their virus LAV/HTLV-3. Neither could Harold Varmus, who found it "a frequent source of irritation" that Gallo continued to invoke the Cold Spring Harbor agreement, which Varmus considered irrelevant, as having mandated the use of the name HTLV-3.

In the spring of 1986, the Varmus committee acted. Henceforth, the AIDS virus would be known as the human immunodeficiency virus, or *HIV*. The original strain would be HIV-1; Max Essex's HTLV-4 and Pasteur's LAV-2 would become HIV-2. The only exceptions were existing individual isolates that would retain their original names, including LAV-Bru, HTLV-3B, HTLV-3$_{RF}$, and ARV-2.[e]

Montagnier thought HIV a fine solution, since it amounted to a clear signal from the scientific community that the AIDS virus wasn't an HTLV. Gallo refused to abide by the committee's decision, which he dismissed as "purely advisory." In future Gallo articles, the AIDS virus would continue to be HTLV-3. But the only member of the Varmus committee to side with Gallo had been Max Essex, and the motion for HIV carried eleven to two.[f] When Gallo discovered that Robin Weiss had voted with the majority, Weiss said, "he stopped speaking to me for two years."

In case anyone thought it odd that a celebrated AIDS researcher should care what the AIDS virus was called, the *Washington Post* explained that the naming dispute was "part of a wider controversy, involving backbiting rumors, publicity campaigns and court suits, between two competing groups of American and French researchers over who discovered the virus, who proved its relationship to AIDS, who borrowed whose results and who should be allowed to make and sell blood tests to screen for signs of AIDS infection."[39]

As summarized by the *Post*, the dispute seemed one-sided: the French had reported finding a new virus "in one pre-AIDS patient," whereas Gallo's group had "published numerous papers [reporting] that it had found the causative virus, worked out a way to grow it and study it and was readying a blood test to detect signs of AIDS virus infections." The current trouble had started only after "members of the French group began to claim that they had not only found the virus first but that Gallo's team had either secretly taken the French virus and called it their own or used the virus to help make, patent and market the profitable blood test." In the end Gallo had prevailed, thwarting Pasteur with "'solid evidence' of his group's independent work with the virus in late 1982 and 1983." The explanation for the current legal contretemps, Gallo told the *Post,* was that "'public relations firms and lawyers are trying to cause us embarrassment.'"

The *Post* didn't mention a three-paragraph correction from Gallo that had just appeared in *Science.*[40] "We recently reexamined the electron micrographs used in our publications," it began, "and discovered that in the composite micrograph of *Schupbach et al.* (figure 4) the panel labeled HTLV-3 was inadvertently composed from photographs of a HUT-78 culture transiently infected with a sample of LAV-1 provided by Luc Montagnier's laboratory."[g]

Not many readers of *Science* were likely to recall that Mika Popovic's article of two years before claimed LAV had "not yet been transmitted to a permanently growing cell line." Readers of the *Los Angeles Times* might not have noticed Peter Fischinger's recent assurance Gallo had "tried to work with" the French virus "and it didn't grow. So he didn't do much with it."[41] Only two months before, Gallo had assured Jean Bernard, the dean of Paris physicians, that Popovic had *never* grown LAV in a continuous T-cell line.[h]

Now all such assurances were, to resurrect a phrase from the Watergate era, inoperative. LAV had not only grown in HUT-78, but grown long enough and well enough for Matt Gonda to micrograph it. Gallo insisted he hadn't known the pictures were LAV, or even that his lab *had* any pictures of LAV.[i] But the pictures published by Gallo had been described as having come from an otherwise unidentified "patient with pre-AIDS," which happened to be Frédéric Brugière's diagnosis. If nobody in Gallo's lab had known the source of the micrographs, how would they have known the patient's diagnosis?

Science acknowledged that Gallo's correction was "likely to raise a few eyebrows," and that it "could also have some legal ramifications" in the patent dispute.[42] Gallo grumbled that it was much ado about nothing.[43] "If it were any other field," he said, "without the dirtiness this involves, I wouldn't be spending ten seconds on this."[44]

But Gallo's correction put the government in an awkward spot. Only a few days before it was published, the HHS lawyers had assured the Court of Claims that "the full story" of Gallo's scientific accomplishments had been "told in the scientific literature." The Pasteur's suggestion that HTLV-3B was LAV by another name, protested the lawyers, was an "indefensible" slur on Gallo's reputation.[45] Now Gallo was admitting that his *pictures* of HTLV-3 were pictures of LAV by another name.

Using the phone in his daughter's dorm room at Wellesley, Jim Swire told the *New York Times* that "the story the United States government has put out is falling apart."[46] Swire didn't mention that he had played a role in precipitating the events leading to the correction, which had begun a few months before with an unexpected telephone call from George Todaro in Seattle.

From an unnamed scientist at NCI-Frederick, Todaro had learned that Gallo's pictures of "HTLV-3" were really Gonda's pictures of LAV. "Gonda works at the Frederick Cancer Center," Swire informed Montagnier, "and apparently knows that the label 'HTLV-3' on the photograph was applied over the original label, 'LAV.' Dr. Todaro gave me the names of additional people who are supposedly aware of the cover-up.

"Obviously," Swire continued, "this information, if true, is extremely significant. However, we are not sure how reliable Dr. Todaro is since we have heard that he left NCI under strained circumstances. In any event, until we decide how to attempt to confirm Dr. Todaro's information, it is of the utmost importance that it be kept confidential and limited to a small number of people. We should discuss this with you and Dr. Dedonder at your earliest convenience."[47]

Following Todaro's call, Swire obtained from Nancy Buc a copy of the Gonda-to-Popovic letter from December of 1983. Attached were copies of Gonda's micrographs of LAV, which to Swire's eye looked identical to the pictures of HTLV-3 in *Science*. After debating various scenarios with Montagnier and Todaro over dinner at the Metropolitan Club, Swire concluded that his next move was a conversation with Gonda. It would have been improper for Swire, having sued the United States government, to approach a government employee involved in the case without the approval of the court. But Gonda worked for a private company that operated parts of the Frederick facility under an NCI contract, and that made him fair game.

On the afternoon of February 6, 1986, in response to a telephone inquiry about a possible consulting job, Gonda walked into the Washington, D.C., offices of the Weinberg Group, a firm of consultants that assists attorneys in litigating complicated scientific issues. When Gonda learned Swire was representing the Pasteur, according to Swire's recollection of events, "he expressed no outrage and made no attempt to leave or to terminate the conversation. He said that the thought occurred to him while he was driving down from Frederick that we might be Pasteur's lawyers."[48]

Swire began by saying he had heard that Gonda was "uncomfortable with what had happened," and that some of Gonda's friends were afraid that the government "would protect Dr. Gallo at all costs" and make Gonda the "fall guy" in the Pasteur dispute. According to Swire, Gonda replied that he had nothing to worry about. He had kept excellent records, he said, in a big "AIDS book" locked up in his office.

Gonda recalled receiving cells from Popovic bearing the designation "LAV," but said he assumed the letters were a patient's initials. Despite having heard Montagnier talk about LAV at the NCI task force meeting, and been sufficiently impressed by the French micrographs to have identified LAV as a lentivirus, Gonda told Swire he hadn't known LAV was the Pasteur's term for the AIDS virus. Nor, Gonda said, had he cared what it stood for. Gonda received samples of cells and viruses from many labs at NCI, and his job was to micrograph whatever he was given and send back the results. "He operated in a vacuum," Swire wrote later. "He has no idea what information or motivation Dr. Gallo had when he reached any conclusions."

As for the misidentification of the LAV micrographs as HTLV-3, Gonda remembered a telephone request from Zaki Salahuddin for pictures, not specifically pictures of LAV but of any AIDS virus that had been grown in the H-9 cell line. Of one thing, however, Gonda was certain. He had never received any specimen from Gallo's lab on which the name "LAV" had been overwritten with something else.

"We got the impression," Swire's memo concluded, "that Dr. Gonda has no great love for Dr. Gallo but fully recognizes the power Dr. Gallo wields. He made some rather bitter references to the fact that he has encountered difficulty in getting work published and that he doubted that he had many friends at NCI. He stated openly that he hoped he wouldn't be damaged by this affair. . . ."

Gonda claimed later not to have understood what Swire was driving at when he asked whether the pictures of HTLV-3 in *Science* were really pictures of LAV.[49] "At first," Gonda recalled, "I thought that they were playing on the fact that they represented the Pasteur and that they were going to call this photograph of the AIDS virus LAV instead of HTLV-3. Later, I thought that they were asking if I could discriminate between HTLV-3 and LAV morphologically."

When Gonda got back to Frederick, he called his immediate boss, a former Todaro postdoc named Ray Gilden, who called Berge Hampar, who met the two men in Gilden's office. "They told me they had found that the pictures that were published were LAV and not HTLV," Hampar recalled. "I said, 'How did you find this out? How all of a sudden did this thing come to light?'"[j]

The NCI evidently wasn't aware the HHS general counsel had given Nancy Buc the Gonda-to-Popovic letter and the attached micrographs of LAV; according to Hampar "the question that was being asked by everybody was, 'How did the French get the pictures?' Some of them weren't the ones that were published. They had copies of the actual micrographs. That led to everybody blaming everybody else. They wanted to blame us at Frederick. I said, 'It's more likely it came from Gallo's lab.'"

More important than when the mislabeling of the pictures was discovered was the question of how it had happened. Gallo told the *Boston Globe* that Gonda's technician had "picked the wrong picture,"[50] but that wasn't what Gonda and Hampar were saying. "What Gonda told me," Hampar recalled, "was that he sent down pictures initially. Apparently these pictures came from samples that were supplied by Salahuddin. Salahuddin, he wasn't one of the authors on that particular paper. He called Gonda and said, 'You can't use my pictures, you have to get other pictures. Get Popovic's pictures.'"

The pictures that had emerged from Gonda's files were Popovic's pictures all right, but they were Popovic's pictures of LAV. "We sent them what they asked for," Gonda declared. "They just called out the numbers, some log number that we gave them, and I pulled the stuff out and gave it to them. I wouldn't have known what it was at the time. Because, you know, it's a secret. It's their business. I get coded samples, I give them an answer. I don't have to know what it is. I give a viral diagnosis, and that's all. I remember the plate being made, and I actually selected the photographs. But I didn't know what the samples were."[k]

However the mislabeling had happened, and however it had been discovered, the revelation dealt a major blow to the NCI's credibility. One of the "HTLV-3" pictures had been reproduced so often in newspapers and magazines that it had become an icon of the AIDS epidemic, even appearing on the cover of Vince DeVita's own textbook on AIDS.[51] According to Zaki Salahuddin, Gallo had a copy of the collage, framed in gold, on his office wall amidst dozens of photographs of Gallo with every notable person he had ever met, a gallery described by a visiting Swedish journalist as "like looking in a thousand mirrors." When Gallo found out the virus in the collage was LAV, Salahuddin recalled, "he took it down from the wall and threw it on the floor, smashing all the glass everywhere."

The most troubling question raised by the mislabeling was Where were *Gallo's* pictures of HTLV-3B? In the four *Science* papers, the only picture of an AIDS virus isolated in Gallo's lab was the dim image of Zaki Salahuddin's virus, J.S., which had followed the arrival of LAV by several months.[1] According to Popovic's article, electron micrographs had also been made of three of his five patient isolates, S.N., B.K., and L.S. But if those pictures existed they hadn't been published in *Science* — odd, given the consternation that had attended the last-minute search for a picture of the AIDS virus — and they weren't being brought forward now.

Neither, for some reason, were the pictures Gallo claimed to have of MOV.[52] Asked whether any photographs of HTLV-3B had ever been taken, Gallo replied: "I am of that opinion, but I have some answers that were given to me as to why not. I don't want to go into them. I think it raises a can of worms again. It's a no-win situation."[53]

Vince DeVita remembered thinking it "a little odd that we didn't have the pictures of Gallo's virus, but we had them of Montagnier's virus." Gallo had assured DeVita that LAV hadn't played any role in his research, and now DeVita was determined that Gallo would correct the record. "I remember saying to him, in front of these people, 'Either you do it or I will, on your behalf'— that this was something that wasn't going to be allowed to go untended. His initial reaction was 'OK, we'll do it, but I want to write a long historical account of why in fact it didn't make any difference, and when we had the virus, and why we didn't have to do this.' And of course he felt that other people had done this to him on purpose, as a way of making him look bad, and that sort of thing.

"So there was a lot of 'I'll explain why it wasn't my fault and doesn't make any difference.' And what I wanted was a letter retracting it, pure and simple. We were interested in the minimum amount of information in the letter. Just retract it and get it over with. This was a recurring theme with Gallo. 'Don't go into this defensive posture, don't explain things that are not relevant. Don't try to shift the blame. It's an error, you're the author, you made a mistake, and you retract it. Be honest and open about it.'"

Despite DeVita's directive, the drafting of the correction hadn't gone smoothly. "Gallo wanted to blame it on PRI," Hampar said.[m] "There was lots of hassle, but after a couple of weeks the letter was finally drafted. Gilden hadn't seen the final version, so they fax it up to him. Gonda says it's a bad copy, so NCI sends one up by messenger. And it has these micrographs with it."

The pictures were tiny images of what purported to be an AIDS virus particle emerging from the T-cells of Claude Chardon — Gallo's way of trying to show the world that he really did have his own picture of the AIDS virus after all. But Gallo had reported Chardon in *Science* as a French AIDS patient infected with *HTLV-1*. "Gilden and Gonda looked at the micrograph," Hampar recalled, "and they both said, 'That's not HTLV-3.' My impression was that Fischinger had had more to do with picking the EM than Gallo had, and that Gallo said, 'OK, we'll get rid of it.' So Gallo calls *Science* that same night and pulls back the letter and the picture."[n]

Under the headline "French Virus in the Picture," *Nature* termed Gallo's correction "acutely embarrassing," an admission that would "do nothing to help the Americans in their battle with the *Institut Pasteur.*"[54] But *Nature* hastened to reassure its readers that despite the slip-up, Gallo had his own AIDS virus pictures "dating from as early as February 1983, before Montagnier's first publication of a photograph of LAV." Those pictures would soon be published in a "recognized journal" and should "lay to rest the suggestion made by Montagnier's lawyers that Gallo used LAV simply because that was his best source."

The "recognized journal" turned out to be *Nature* itself,[55] which at the beginning May 1986 published a lengthy letter from Gallo entitled "First isolation of HTLV-III." The letter, which included most of the material Vince DeVita had ordered left out of the *Science* correction, began with the observation that it "should not be surprising" that Gallo had pictures of the French AIDS virus. To verify that LAV was a retrovirus, Gallo said, his lab had "wanted to check the material received from Dr. Montagnier by electron microscopy."

The real reason for the letter was the accompanying table listing ten patients from whom Gallo claimed to have "isolated" the AIDS virus in late 1982 and 1983.° There hadn't yet been a ruling from the patent office on the French request for a patent interference. But if the Pasteur's request were granted, it would be up to Gallo to prove he had recognized the existence of the AIDS virus before May 20, 1983, the day the Pasteur's Brugière paper appeared in *Science*.

Tom Byrnes, a senior attorney in the Justice Department's civil division who was coordinating Gallo's defense, had warned Gallo that "the dates set forth in this letter will be perceived as our earliest dates. For this reason, the dates must be as early as possible."[56] According to the *Nature* table, blood and tissue samples from the first four patients on Gallo's top-ten list had been received by his lab prior to May 20.

The first was G.W., the Houston man whose blood Gallo had received from M. D. Anderson in December 1982. According to the *Nature* table, G.W. had tested negative for HTLV-1 and positive for reverse transcriptase,[p] retrospective evidence, in Gallo's opinion, that he must have been infected with the AIDS virus — which, being an AIDS patient, he no doubt was. Now Gallo was claiming to have *isolated* the AIDS virus from G.W. But no AIDS virus had ever been found in G.W.'s cells, because Gallo had been looking for HTLV-1.[57] When G.W.'s cells yielded no HTLV-1, they had been discarded.

Forgotten as well was the second patient on the list, the French journalist B.U., whose cells were among those delivered by Jacques Leibowitch. Like G.W., B.U. had yielded some reverse transcriptase, but no HTLV-1 or any other virus. As with G.W., the *Nature* letter marked the first time Gallo had ever mentioned B.U. in print.

The third patient in the table was another Leibowitch contribution: M.A., the Haitian woman, who appeared to have undergone a postmortem transformation. In Gallo's May 1983 *Science* article, M.A. and Claude Chardon had been the two AIDS patients from Paris in whom Gallo claimed to have detected HTLV-1.[q] Now M.A. was listed as HTLV-1 *negative*. But Gallo's lab records showed that her cells had never yielded either the AIDS virus *or* HTLV.

Claude Chardon followed M.A., and the *Nature* letter revealed, for the first time, that Chardon had been infected with both HTLV-1 *and* HTLV-3. What Gallo's letter didn't mention was that the only virus to have grown out of Chardon's cells in 1983 — or for that matter in 1984 or 1985 — was HTLV-1. The AIDS virus hadn't been isolated from Chardon until two weeks before Gallo's letter was mailed to *Nature*.[r]

Accompanying Gallo's letter were six tiny photographs of AIDS viruses, including Matt Gonda's first picture of LAV, a picture of R.F., and a picture of the Chardon virus dated February 15, 1983. If Gallo had a picture of the AIDS virus taken before May 20, it would go a long way toward persuading the patent office that he had recognized the existence of a new human retrovirus before the French made their own discovery known in *Science*.[s] But February 15 wasn't the date the Chardon virus was photographed. It was the date Leibowitch brought Chardon's cells to Gallo's lab. The Chardon micrograph hadn't been made until May 26, 1983 — six days *after* the French had published the first picture of LAV_{Bru} in *Science*.[t]

Some *Nature* readers might have wondered why, if Gallo had had a picture of the AIDS virus in the spring of 1983, he hadn't published it then, or with the *Science* articles the following year — or said anything about it until now. Gallo's European colleagues might have asked why, with such a picture in hand, he had assured them in the fall and winter of 1983 that he had "never seen the virus that Luc Montagnier has described."[58] Even Peter Fischinger could have been excused for wondering why Gallo had told him the year before that there weren't any pictures of his early AIDS virus "isolates."[u]

The answer, not hinted at by anything in the *Nature* letter, was that the technicians who made the Chardon micrograph in May of 1983 had identified it as a picture of *HTLV-1*.[v] The day before the Pasteur lawsuit was filed the technicians had gone back, at Gallo's urgent request, for another look at the musty, two-year-old micrograph. Even then they hadn't been sure what it showed. Only after consultations with Gallo had the picture which now appeared in *Nature* been re-labeled as "HTLV-3."[w]

Upon closer inspection, Hampar recognized the Chardon micrograph in *Nature* as the same one Gallo had tried to publish with the *Science* correction.[59] "This thing was all retrospective," he said later. "No one prior to the critical date said, 'There's another virus there.' Subsequently they found HTLV-3. They went back and looked at these things, and they all said 'Oh, look, there it is.' They didn't come out and say at that time to anybody, 'Hey, there's another virus here.'

They didn't recognize any particles as different from HTLV-1 until long after they knew about HTLV-3.

"When we saw *Nature*, we laughed," Hampar said. "We said, 'Is this the only photograph they got? They're staking all their claims on one photograph with two particles in it?' That's when I said to myself, 'These people are really crazy.'"[60]

• 11 •

"Bingo. We Win"

In the spring of 1986, two thousand scientists descended on Paris for the largest-ever international conference on AIDS. Covering the congress for *Le Monde,* Claudine Escoffier marveled at the reporters who clustered around Gallo. "The groupies," Escoffier called them. "There is no other word. Groups of young journalists, from Sweden, from Norway, from America many of them, begging him for a little hello. And they were so proud when they could call him Bob. I realized then that it had not been easy for American journalists to examine the problem."

The week Gallo's *Nature* letter appeared, the patent office, concluding that nine of Gallo's ten claims for inventorship had been made first by the French, had granted the Pasteur's request for an interference with the Gallo patent.[1] In the corridors of the Palais des Congrès, *Pasteur v. Gallo* was Topic A. According to Larry Altman's dispatch in the *New York Times,* the dispute was bigger than Gallo and Montagnier, going to "the very fabric of what makes scientists tick, their altruism as well as their egos, their fierce desire for independence, their yearning to gain respect from peers, and the competition for Nobel Prizes and other public recognition for themselves and their institutes."[2]

In Paris Gallo tossed another log on the pyre, deriding the Pasteur's contribution to the search for the cause of AIDS as inconsequential. "They had not mass-produced the virus," Gallo told CBS

News. "They had not linked it to disease. They had not characterized it." Appearing on the same broadcast, Jim Swire upped the ante by accusing someone in Gallo's lab of having stolen LAV. "They simply studied it," Swire said, "concluded we were correct, renamed it, and claimed it as their own."[3]

Temporarily distracted from his feud with Robin Weiss, which was approaching the dueling stage,[a] Abraham Karpas had composed a long and complicated reply to Gallo's letter claiming the "first isolation" of HIV.[4] John Maddox replied that Karpas's charges of "general dishonesty" on Gallo's part "would, if published, be potentially libelous." In any case, "enquiries" *Nature* had been making for several months "suggest that the matter is more complicated than your letter says. Nevertheless, the subject with which you deal is of course a matter of great importance as well as public interest. I am hoping that in the next few weeks we shall be able to do something to throw light on the matter."[5]

Slipping into an auditorium where Sarngadharan was about to begin speaking, Karpas managed to grab a seat just behind Gallo. As Sarngadharan finished and called for questions, Karpas rose, waving a copy of the *Science* article, on which Sarngadharan was a co-author, concluding that Max Essex's HTLV-MA was a viral protein.[6] With Gallo "jumping up and down in his chair," Karpas demanded to know why, if Essex had been detecting HTLV-1 in all those AIDS patients, Sarngadharan and Gallo had abandoned HTLV-1 in favor of HTLV-3 as the cause of AIDS.

A more ominous confrontation occurred following Mika Popovic's talk, where the first question came from Marc Alizon. "I don't think I would have said anything," Alizon recalled, "but Popovic started with some really bad jokes about how American research was killing the French. So I asked Popovic if he could give any information about these different patients he put in the pool. He didn't provide any clear answer to that. He said he tried later to check out which were the patients that contributed to HTLV-3. I don't know if he did that, but they never published it."

Alizon didn't buy Popovic's explanation for having created the pool in the first place. "The major point was," Alizon said later, "was it or wasn't it necessary to mix isolates, which seems a heresy to a virologist. If you mix, you do not increase the titer. If you take one milliliter from the blood of different individuals, some infected and some not infected, you will get less. You should take *ten* milliliters from the guy who was infected. This is what Popovic said he had tried directly on each of these individuals, but he didn't get anything. So he mixed them and got something. My point was, you cannot get a higher titer by mixing a small fraction of blood from ten individuals. You will not get more virus."

In Alizon's opinion, what mattered most wasn't what had gone into the pool, but what had come out. An acknowledgment by Popovic that, purposely or not, LAV had gotten into the pool would be "the only honorable explanation," Alizon said. "If it's not an accidental contamination, what can it be? There is no way that two viruses so similar can be isolated."

There hadn't been time for Alizon to press the point before Gallo showed up to rescue Popovic. "Gallo was trying to cool things down," Alizon recalled, "saying, 'Poor Popovic, he's in a very bad time, you shouldn't be nasty with Popovic.'" But wherever Popovic ventured in Paris, the question hung in the air. Paul Luciw remembered sitting in a café with Popovic and Kalyanaraman when the subject came up over a beer. According to Luciw, after some hemming and hawing Popovic confided that he had kept his LAV culture in the same incubator with the flask that contained the pool, and that he "might have mixed them up."

Montagnier wasn't buying mixed-up cultures as an explanation. "We must remember," he told *Paris Match,* "that, on two occasions, in July 1983, and September 1983, we have sent to Dr. Gallo samples of LAV viruses. Afterwards, he has been continuously informed of our work and its evolution. What is singular and gives me trouble is the fact that Professor Gallo did never communicate any precise information concerning the patient, or the patients from whom he isolated this virus."

Montagnier regretted the Pasteur's lawsuit against the American government, which was burning money that could have been used for AIDS research. "But it is a question of principles," he said, "a question of ethics. If France does not do anything, it means that there is a group, across the Atlantic, which is above the laws."

"Including scientific fraud?" the interviewer asked.

"It is you who are saying this," Montagnier replied.

When Gallo and Montagnier finally met, it was on the terrace of a country-style restaurant near Port Maillot where Danielle Berneman had arranged an off-the-record lunch with Lowell Harmison. According to Montagnier, Gallo's first words after shaking hands were "'Believe me, I didn't steal your virus.' He was very upset." The conversation that followed was strained until Harmison suggested, halfway through the meal, that a public pronouncement by Montagnier that HTLV-3B and LAV had come from different patients might be worth a million dollars.

Where such a sum of money might come from, Montagnier recalled, "was not really said in proper words." But he remembered thinking that if the Americans were willing to pay him a million dollars, "something was being hidden by the NIH." Berneman quickly interjected that any payment from the Americans would have to go to the Pasteur, not to Montagnier directly. But, Berneman said, money alone was not enough to resolve the dispute. At a minimum, the Pasteur wanted the lion's share of the patent royalties and co-inventorship for the blood test.

Jim Wyngaarden received the same message over lunch from Michèle Barzach, the French minister of health. When Wyngaarden got home, he warned the HHS lawyers they were in for a tough fight. The French were "going all out for a share of [the] patent," Wyngaarden said. "It is open and shut." Not only did the French see the dispute as "a bell-weather [sic] patent case," they were saying they could "prove that HTLV-3 was cultivated from LAV."[7]

According to Wyngaarden, the view from within NIH and HHS had been that the French "were trying to take credit for Bob's work. Everyone felt that — of course, relying on Bob's account of what he had done."[8] But the HHS lawyers were coming to the conclusion that the French had a case. "A significant part of this dispute is whether LAV and HTLV-3 are the same virus," one HHS attorney wrote. "NCI is very firm in its view that HTLV-3 is different. However, they are very similar viruses and this is a weak thread to rely on . . . we might better settle now."[9]

Among the speakers in Paris was the head of the Red Cross's bloodtesting laboratory, who presented his evaluation of the five AIDS blood tests on the market. Of the five, only the test made with LAV recorded a perfect score, both for false positives *and* false negatives. But the false-positive rate for the Abbott ELISA was still through the roof.[10] While Abbott experimented with reducing the bead-coating time from three hours to fifteen minutes, Mike Ascher was boarding a plane for Florida and the Second Annual Clinical Virology Symposium. Ascher was deputy chief of the Viral and Rickettsial Disease Laboratory at the California Department of Health Services. For more than a year, Ascher's urgent preoccupation had been developing an accurate HIV-antibody test for the state's diagnostic blood laboratories. Now he had some bad news.

Ascher had used Jay Levy's ARV to search for viral antibodies in a unique set of blood samples, drawn from hundreds of San Francisco men for a hepatitis-B study in the mid-1970s. Although the existence of AIDS wouldn't be recognized for another six years, some of the men were already infected with HIV at the time their blood was taken. Fortunately, the blood samples from the "City Clinic cohort" had been preserved in the freezers of the San Francisco Health Department, an invaluable serological archive of the natural progression of the AIDS virus. Using a home-made blood test, Ascher had been able to identify with great precision which of the samples were infected with decade-old HIV and which were not. But when Ascher tested the same HIV-positive samples with the commercial Abbott ELISA, several had been *negative.*

There had been indications from the start that the Gallo ELISA produced *false negatives* as well as false positives, but they had been overlooked or ignored.[b] Before the Abbott test was licensed, the Boston Red Cross had expressed "major concerns" about its sensitivity.[11] Murray Gardner had done the same shortly afterward.[12] Gardner had been joined by the Canadian CDC, which discovered that the Abbott ELISA couldn't detect HIV antibodies in blood samples from seven AIDS patients.[13] Even Max Essex, whose Cambridge BioScience was attempting to market its own version of an HIV ELISA, warned that the Abbott test was failing to detect one HIV-positive sample in every twenty — a false-negative rate of 5 percent.[14]

It was Murray Gardner who first recognized that all the false-negative blood samples contained antibodies to a single HIV protein, p24. The Canadians had found the same thing. When Mike Ascher ran *his* false negatives through the Western Blot, the only antibody that showed up was anti-p24. In every case, the false-negative samples had come from men infected with HIV a relatively short time before their blood was drawn. The reason some HIV-infected people were showing up as negative on the Abbott ELISA was that the Gallo test simply couldn't see antibodies to p24.

After warning California's public health laboratories about a "gray zone" in the commercial AIDS tests, Ascher had presented his data in Clearwater.[15] A number of people at the meeting expressed interest, but Ascher recalled that two seemed more interested than the rest: the representative from Abbott Laboratories, and Gallo's deputy lab chief, Prem Sarin.

When Ascher performed his initial tests, the Pasteur ELISA hadn't been approved by the FDA. Now that it was approved, Ascher was curious to see how the French test handled blood samples containing only p24 antibodies. The Pasteur test scored all twelve samples positive. The new prototype Abbott ELISA with the reconfigured bead missed every one. In fine-tuning the test to reduce the number of false positives, Abbott had somehow increased its propensity for false negatives, which meant the Pasteur test was now more precise than Abbott at both ends of the scale. Bob Nowinski thought it was the batch virus production process about which Gallo complained to Lowell Harmison that accounted for the advantage in false negatives.

"You grow up a batch of CEM," Nowinski said, "put in the virus, and it releases a large amount of virus. You grow huge liters of it, you let it go through a cycle of ten days and you harvest the fluid. You purify the virus from it, and then do a second infection, a third infection, and so on. You can do this forever." The only reason Gallo used a continuous cell line like H-9, Nowinski said, "was that in all retroviruses up to then, everyone had used continuous cell lines. But you grow as much virus by our method as you grow in any other method. Genetic Systems could produce enough virus for the entire nation without any problem."

Five weeks after the Clearwater meeting, the FDA approved the reconfigured Abbott test for clinical use. In granting certification, the agency agreed that Abbott could advertise its new ELISA as providing fewer false positives, and no more false negatives, than the original ELISA.[16] When Ascher heard what the FDA had done, he asked Tom Zuck "'What the hell's going on?' I said, 'Why did you relicense Abbott?' "He said, 'Ascher, what's your problem?' "I said, 'My problem is that we're still getting false negatives with Abbott, and the improvements you just licensed have made the problem worse.'"

Zuck retorted that the FDA had been checking for false negatives too, and *it* hadn't found any difference between Abbott and Genetic Systems. When Ascher asked *how* the FDA was measuring sensitivity, Zuck explained that it was using the standard laboratory method, by successively diluting blood samples and testing for antibodies at ever-lower levels of virus concentration.

No, Ascher said. Dilution might work for ordinary viral antibodies, but it was the worst possible way to measure sensitivity to HIV antibodies. With the AIDS virus, Ascher explained, it wasn't a question of how *many* antibodies there were in a given sample of blood, but rather *which* of the viral proteins had given rise to them. The only way to measure HIV sensitivity was with blood samples from recently infected individuals, "early seroconverters" who had just begun producing antibodies. Still skeptical, Zuck asked Ascher to test more sera and send him the results. When Abbott scored eight out of eight early seroconverters as HIV-negative and the Genetic Systems ELISA scored the same samples positive, "the FDA was fairly responsive," Ascher said.

Before the summer of 1986, the unnecessary expense and wasted blood caused by false positives had seemed a more pressing concern than the likelihood of false negatives, which remained largely theoretical. False positives were immediately visible, by comparing ELISA results with Western Blots. Because AIDS often took years to develop, there hadn't been any way to know for sure whether HIV-contaminated blood was passing through the ELISA screen and into transfusion patients or hemophiliacs who might remain healthy for years.

That changed in mid-June of 1986, when the CDC reported the case of a thirty-one-year-old Colorado man who had made a donation at his local blood-transfusion center the previous August.[17] Tested with the Abbott ELISA, his blood had registered HIV-negative. When the man donated another unit three months later, he was HIV-positive. According to what the donor told local health officials, he had had only one male sex partner in his entire life, and their first contact had occurred three months before the first donation.

The records of the hospital to which the first donation had gone showed it had been divided between two middle-aged patients, both of whom had undergone cardiac surgery. The first recipient was now HIV positive, but because he was also a homosexual there was no way to say whether he had acquired the virus from the donated blood. The second recipient, a sixty-year-old man, had been married for thirty years and denied any extramarital sexual contacts with either sex, as well as intravenous drug use. But when the second man's blood was tested by Western Blot, it too was HIV-positive. The only way he could have become infected with HIV was from the blood the Abbott ELISA had scored as HIV-negative.

The same thing happened on a more devastating scale two months later, following the fatal shooting during an armed robbery of a Virginia gas station attendant, William "Pete" Norwood. Before he died, Norwood's mother agreed to donate her son's vital organs for transplantation, and Norwood's blood was tested twice for HIV. Both tests were negative, but both negatives were false. At least seven recipients of Norwood's organs and tissues, including his heart and kidneys, contracted the AIDS virus.[18] "It's like Petey died all over again," his aunt Emma said.[19]

Three months later, in nearby Richmond, a thirty-three-year-old woman underwent surgery to remove a uterine cyst, not a life-threatening condition but a procedure her doctor said was necessary if she wanted to have children. The blood the woman was given had tested HIV-negative; it, too, was infected with the AIDS virus.[20] Such cases, the Red Cross declared, didn't represent "a test failure," because no ELISA was capable of detecting antibodies in early seroconverters. "We know the test can't do the impossible," a Red Cross official said.[21]

Mike Ascher had data showing that what was impossible for the Gallo AIDS test was possible for the Pasteur/Genetic Systems ELISA, and Ascher was no longer alone. At the NIAID in Bethesda where Mal Martin worked, a researcher named Al Saah was coming independently to the same conclusion. Saah was working with a collection of blood samples as unique in their way as the City Clinic cohort, taken from gay men in several cities over a period of years beginning with the dawn of the AIDS epidemic. At the outset of the study, the subjects had been healthy. As it progressed, many had become infected with HIV and developed symptoms of AIDS. By studying the samples in chronological order, it was possible to construct a time-lapse picture of how the human immune system responded to the AIDS virus.

Saah and his collaborators noticed that the earliest postinfection samples didn't always test positive by ELISA. Or, rather, that *some* of those samples tested positive only with *some* of the commercial ELISAs. When Saah tried to figure out what was different about the positive samples, he discovered what Murray Gardner and Mike Ascher already knew. The earliest samples contained only p24 anti-bodies, whereas those taken from the same subjects later had antibod-ies to a host of HIV proteins.

When Saah used the ELISA from Litton Bionetics to test thirty early seroconverters, it scored only two HIV-positive, next to useless for blood-testing purposes. The test from Electronucleonics did scarcely better, only four positives out of thirty. Abbott recorded thir-teen of the thirty samples positive — better than the others, but still a false-negative rate of 57 percent. The Pasteur/Genetic Systems ELISA caught twenty-five of the thirty samples.[22]

A major blood-testing conference was about to convene at NIH, the first time in a year that the test manufacturers and blood bankers, including a large contingent from the Red Cross, would be in the same room at the same time. When Al Saah got a postcard from *Science* rejecting the paper reporting his blood-test comparisons, he packed up his charts and graphs and joined Mike Ascher at the NIH conference. Neither was on the conference program, and they lis-tened from the audience while one speaker after the next described a world in which the blood supply had been made as safe as possible from HIV. When the time came for questions, Ascher and Saah asked permission to present their data from the floor.[23]

The reporters covering the conference hadn't heard much about false negatives, and the impromptu presentation made headlines. "Despite a concerted effort to screen blood donations," the *Washing-ton Post* reported, "a small percentage of blood throughout the coun-try remains contaminated with the AIDS virus." The *Post* quoted Saah's boss, Anthony Fauci, as saying the bad news was "something that we have suspected for a long time. It tells us that we have got to get a better test."[24]

Not until the eighteenth paragraph did the *Post* reveal that there already *was* a better test, made by "the French [*sic*] company Genet-ics [*sic*] Systems." The story didn't say that, a month before, the Com-merce Department had begun preparing a patent infringement suit against Genetic Systems.[25] An Abbott spokesman said the company needed "to look at the methodology" used by Ascher and Saah before commenting on their data. But the Abbott representative at the conference informed his superiors in Chicago that "Litton and ENI [Electronucleonics] clearly take a dive on this, and the implications for our test are not exactly favorable."[26]

The United States market for the HIV ELISA, once estimated at $20 million a year, had passed $34 million and was headed upward,[27] and the news had implications for Abbott's bottom line. As it happened, Abbott had known about the false negatives for months. The company had seen Mike Ascher's data in the middle of June.[28] The previous April, the Red Cross chapter in Burlington, Vermont, had encountered a false negative on a blood sample with the newly configured Abbott test.[29] When the Burlington sample, from a man recently infected with HIV, was tested by Western Blot, it had antibodies only to p24. In May, Abbott had learned that the Red Cross blood center in Syracuse, one of the sites testing the new ELISA, had found another false-positive blood sample from another early seroconverter.[c]

Abbott hadn't told the FDA.[d] Now, however, the story was out, and Abbott headquarters was on maximum alert. "Action plans" were drafted to "immediately address the critical need for increased sensitivity" in the Abbott ELISA. Project teams were formed, under orders to meet daily until the crisis was resolved.[30] Having no idea what was causing the false negatives, Abbott decided to make *two* new ELISAs, one spiked with extra p24 and the other with extra gp41, the transmembrane protein that connected to the HIV envelope.[31] But new tests meant new field trials, and new field trials would take months, and the Ascher-Saah revelations put the American Red Cross in a bind.

Months before, the Red Cross task force had selected the Genetic Systems ELISA as its "test of choice." Sensitive to the political implications of buying the French test over the American version, senior Red Cross officials had reversed the recommendation. When the second-year contracts were signed, Abbott had 80 percent of the Red Cross business, with 20 percent split between Genetic Systems and DuPont — the opposite of what the task force had recommended.[32]

The new Abbott–Red Cross contracts had been signed only a few days before the NIH conference. Now the *Washington Post* was telling its readers that the Abbott test, whose principal user was the Red Cross, missed more than half of all HIV-infected blood samples. When the Red Cross blood centers demanded to know what headquarters was doing about the situation, Gerry Sandler invited Al Saah to present his data to the monthly meeting of the Center Directors'

Council. "What we learned from Al Saah's presentation was that there was a better way to determine sensitivity than the way we had been doing it," Sandler said later. In the end, the Red Cross had "agreed with Saah's analysis." The Abbott test "did not pick up samples that could be picked up."

Among the Red Cross officials alarmed by Saah's presentation was the director of its Miami blood center, Peter Tomasulo. "It is not impossible," Tomasulo wrote to a Red Cross executive after returning home from the meeting, "that, within the next month, we will run across another seronegative viremic donor. We know we have a better chance of detecting such an individual by using the Genetic Systems assay. Delaying the switch even one month may be wrong. Should we move ahead as quickly as possible to use the best p24 test that is now available? If one person in South Florida develops AIDS from a seronegative blood donor after July 30, 1986 which was processed by Abbott, I will wonder if I did everything I could have done."[33]

The American Red Cross wasn't a government agency. But it was a public trust, chartered by Congress. Although the Red Cross's original purpose had been wartime disaster relief, its real business had become the selling of blood.[e] While paying no taxes and collecting tens of millions of dollars each year from United Way and other charities, the Red Cross used free television advertising to persuade Americans to roll up their sleeves, for free, at blood centers, Bloodmobiles, and office blood drives. The millions of pints of donated blood were sold to hospitals for a "processing fee" approaching $400 a pint, affording the Red Cross an annual operating profit of nearly $40 million. Now the Abbott test had placed that business in jeopardy.

The Red Cross contract had an escape clause that could be invoked if another test became available that was more sensitive by at least 5 percent, and the Pasteur ELISA was much more sensitive than that.[34] Seizing the opportunity, Genetic Systems told the Red Cross it was "willing and able to expand to additional Red Cross centers," whenever the Red Cross wished.[35]

"When the Saah study came out," Bob Nowinski recalled, "Genetic Systems received an inquiry from the Red Cross asking to submit a bid for one hundred percent of all their business. Just before the bid was ready, they called back and said, 'Don't submit the bid.' They then held a closed session of which no minutes were taken, which is unusual at the Red Cross. At that point Abbott made a representation to them that they could correct the test in a certain period of time. So the Red Cross took Abbott at its word. I think Abbott promised them three months."[36]

A few days after Saah's presentation to the Red Cross, a thirty-year-old North Carolina man was admitted to Moses Cone Memorial Hospital in Greensboro following an auto accident. The man was in a coma, and his condition was critical. As part of the hospital's admitting procedure, a blood sample was drawn for typing. Over the next eleven hours, the man's doctors transfused him with fifty-six units of blood. Despite the transfusions, the man's condition worsened, and his name was added to a list of prospective organ donors. A second sample of blood was taken for HIV antibody testing. The Abbott ELISA scored it negative for HIV.

Forty-eight hours later the man was declared brain dead and his heart, kidneys, and liver were distributed to other medical centers for transplantation, each accompanied by another blood sample to be double-checked by the receiving center for HIV. At three of the four centers the blood tested negative, and the donor's liver and kidneys were transplanted into waiting patients. At the fourth center — the only one to use the Genetic Systems ELISA — the blood tested positive.[37] Within weeks, the patients who had received the donor's other organs were also HIV-positive.

While Gallo and Montagnier parried in Paris and Genetic Systems did battle with Abbott and the Red Cross, the Institut Pasteur and the Reagan administration were crossing swords in the Court of Claims. None of the government lawyers was a scientist, and in characterizing Gallo's research for the court they depended on Gallo and his people to interpret his data and explain its significance.[38]

Not only had Gallo *not* stolen LAV, the government declared, the French virus hadn't contaminated Popovic's cultures, even by accident. The scientific evidence was "clear" that HTLV-3 and LAV had come from different patients,[39] and it showed "conclusively" that "HTLV-3 is *not* LAV by another name."[f] Finally, neither the Gallo blood test nor the H-9 cell line had "depended on," much less been "derived from," LAV.[40]

The claims court judge, James F. Merow, perceived the existence of "a major factual dispute" as to whether LAV, in the Pasteur's view, had provided the "master key" for Gallo's research, or whether the discovery of HTLV-3 and the Gallo AIDS test were "the result of independent NCI research." Before that dispute could be addressed, Merow had to decide whether his court had jurisdiction over the question. That depended on whether the United States had breached a contract with the Institut Pasteur, which depended in turn on whether a contract had existed in the first place.

Tom Byrnes, the lead Justice Department lawyer, argued that there couldn't have been a contract, since neither Gallo nor Mika Popovic — particularly Popovic, who had been a visiting scientist at NIH, not a career government employee, and not even an American citizen — had the authority to enter into binding agreements on behalf of the United States.[41]

Jim Swire countered that Popovic had been paid by the NIH to work in Gallo's lab, and that in signing the agreement accompanying the September LAV he had bound his employer to use LAV only for noncommercial purposes, not including the making and selling of a blood-antibody test. "It would be a shocking result indeed," Swire intoned, "if Drs. Popovic and Gallo could induce Pasteur to send them LAV, sign the standard scientific agreement limiting its use to research purposes, then rename the virus claiming it as their own and renounce the agreement on lack of authority."[42]

Judge Merow seemed to agree. The Pasteur hadn't given Gallo the LAV samples for no reason, Merow said. It had expected research results in return, including Gallo's opinion about whether LAV was the cause of AIDS. That opinion, Merow went on, "would appear to have substantial monetary value." By accepting LAV from Paris, Gallo's lab had entered into a contractual relationship with Pasteur. The fact that Pasteur hadn't received any research results from Gallo was beside the point.

In Merow's view, the Pasteur's problem was a federal statute, the Contract Disputes Act, intended to resolve civil claims against the government. Under the statute, the first step for an aggrieved party is to submit a bill for damages to a government contract officer. Pasteur hadn't submitted such a bill, and Merow concluded that "because plaintiff has not complied with the mandatory requirements of the CDA, this court lacks jurisdiction over this litigation and the complaint must be dismissed."[43]

Merow wasn't telling the French they didn't have a case — he seemed to be suggesting they might well have a case. He was telling them that they had to go through bureaucratic channels before they could argue their case in his courtroom — in essence, to get in line with the people who sold paper and pencils to the government. "That ruling was like a body blow," said Jim Swire, who announced that Pasteur was filing an immediate appeal.[44] It was "a sad day for international scientific research," Swire said, "when the National Cancer Institute openly disavows the written agreements of its principal investigators."[45]

The principal downside to Merow's decision was the wrench it had thrown in the Pasteur's efforts to obtain evidence via the channels of civil discovery. Swire had been able to interview Matt Gonda because Gonda wasn't a government employee. But he couldn't just invite Gallo or Popovic to drop by for a chat. They would have to be formally deposed under oath, and without an active case Swire had nowhere to obtain court orders for depositions or the production of documents, like the laboratory notebooks kept by Popovic, Ersell Richardson, and Betsy Read. Thanks to Judge Merow, the only avenue left open to Swire was the same one available to any citizen: the Freedom of Information Act.

Swire's six-page, single-spaced FOIA request demanded a copy of virtually every document in the possession of the NCI related to Gallo's work in "recognizing, conducting research on, detecting, isolating, discovering, identifying, growing, cloning, developing, commercializing, or otherwise working with" the AIDS virus.[46] It took the government five months to produce 1,600 pages of documents that were even remotely relevant. But those were only a fraction of the 16,000 pages the government claimed to possess, and several of the documents that were produced were missing key pages or attachments.[g] Popovic's memo describing the development of the H-9 cell line, and identifying the ten patients Popovic claimed had made up the HTLV-3B pool, referred to an "attached statement" by Betsy Read and to lab notes prepared by Popovic and Ersell Richardson. But none of the attachments was included with the memo.

The government provided Swire with a handful of the memos written by Gallo and Popovic during Peter Fischinger's investigation in the fall of 1985. But the memos that would have been most helpful to the Pasteur's case — and most detrimental to the government's — were withheld, in some cases without any indication they even existed.[h] Among the missing documents were Mika Popovic's notes from the Eureka! experiment, and the August 1983 memo in which

Gallo informed Vince DeVita that a minor variant of HTLV-1 was the cause of AIDS — a crystal-clear declaration, in Gallo's own words, that he hadn't identified a LAV-type virus prior to May 20, 1983.

Several of the other withheld documents would have done equal damage to the revised history Gallo was inscribing in the scientific literature, and which was being parroted by the Justice Department and the HHS lawyers to the patent office and the court of claims. In one withheld memo, Gallo admitted to Fischinger that he hadn't had any AIDS virus isolates in late 1982.[47] Another contradicted Gallo's published claims that HTLV-3$_{RF}$ had been discovered "between November, 1982 and early 1983"[48] — a year before the actual date — or that HTLV-3B had been isolated from the Popovic pool "in December 1982 or January 1983"— ten months before the "Popovic pool" existed.[49]

But the document that would have closed the circle for the French remained buried deepest in the government's vault: Gallo's November 26, 1985, memo to Lowell Harmison containing Mika Popovic's account of having "successfully transmitted LAV into permanent cell lines in December of 1983."

The task of responding to Swire's FOIA request had fallen to the NIH's Freedom of Information officer, a tall, no-nonsense New Englander named Joanne Belk, who recalled her first conversation with Gallo as "a stunning experience." Belk, whose strongest epithet was "Jiminy Christmas," had never spoken to Gallo, and she was utterly taken aback. "I didn't know how rude he was," Belk said later. "This man called me and started blasting me on the phone. 'Who the hell do you think you are?' That kind of thing. I was absolutely shaken. He was terribly profane. Nobody had ever talked to me like that. That was my introduction to this so-called eminent scientist."

Belk took the Freedom of Information Act seriously, and she tried her best to obtain the notebooks and other records that were covered by Swire's request. But like all FOIA officers throughout the government's Executive Branch, Belk had no power to make Gallo or anybody else actually hand over documents. "I'm in the disclosure business," Belk grumbled. "Everybody else around here is in the withholding business. We have a lot of information here, but not much freedom. We have to depend on the offices that contain the records to produce them for us. I can't march in there like a storm trooper and say, 'I want to look at your files.' One, I wouldn't be admitted. Two, I've never seen these files and I wouldn't have a clue where to look for them."

Terminally frustrated, Belk had paid a visit to Gallo's office, but had gotten nowhere. "It was impressively messy," she said. "Gallo wasn't there. I talked to Howard Streicher," one of Gallo's administrative assistants. "He gave me all this double-talk, and all he was giving me were published articles. Nothing else. I had a whole list of things I wanted. 'Oh, we'll take care of that.' It was just a blatant stall. Nothing ever came. For a long time I was told, 'Those are in file boxes and we can't get to them.' Or, 'Dr. Gallo says he doesn't have the personnel to look through his records.' Then he'll also say, 'I don't keep anything.' He would tell me, 'I'm here to develop an AIDS vaccine.' Well, that's not really the way the Freedom of Information Act works."

A month after Judge Merow's dismissal, Jim Swire filed a second lawsuit against the Department of Health and Human Services, charging that relevant documents relating to Gallo's AIDS research were being improperly withheld under the law.[50] The lawsuit evidently got HHS's attention. According to Joanne Belk, Peter Fischinger "put his hand on Gallo's shoulder. He told Gallo, 'Look, you've gotta give this stuff up.'"

On a late-summer afternoon in 1986, Belk got a call telling her the records were waiting for her — not in Gallo's lab, where they had originally been, but at Biotech Research Laboratories in Rockville, which Belk thought surpassingly odd. "Usually the records come into this office," Belk said. "One doesn't usually have to go out to some contractor to pick up NIH records." Fearing the window would soon close again, Belk drove to Rockville, put the records in the trunk of her car, and deposited them at HHS headquarters downtown, where they became somebody else's problem. "And let me tell you," Belk said later, "I have never been so glad to be rid of anything in my life as Dr. Gallo's records."

The records Swire got went beyond those the HHS lawyers had provided Nancy Buc in the days before the initial lawsuit was filed. Considering the stakes for HHS, Swire had expected Popovic's notebooks to be models of completeness and lucidity, a carefully documented scientific record of Gallo's published and patented claims about the independent origin of HTLV-3B and Popovic's inability to grow LAV. The notebooks were anything but lucid — so cryptic and disorganized, Swire complained, "as to make them difficult, if not impossible, to comprehend."[51] Some pages were completely black; some were completely white. Some had been photocopied so often (on purpose, Swire suspected) they had been reduced to hieroglyphics.

Swire's scientific consultant, Myron Weinberg, a Ph.D. chemist who had kept his own laboratory notebooks for years and scrutinized many others in previous court cases, couldn't recall ever having seen a notebook that didn't identify its owner. But none of Popovic's pages was signed. Neither were any of the pages evidently kept by others in Gallo's lab, something Weinberg found "simply incredible."[52]

Swire assumed that two sets of accompanying pages, in feminine handwriting, belonged to Ersell Richardson and Betsy Read. Whoever their authors were, those notes appeared more or less standard. Popovic's notes, written in an unmistakable Middle-European hand, resembled a diary or a journal, filled with retrospective observations and abbreviated descriptions of each day's work, but scarcely any experimental protocols or raw data.

HHS assured Swire that the laboratory notebooks had been copied "in the order in which they were maintained."[53] To Swire, it looked as though they had been "shuffled like a deck of cards." When he tried to assemble the notes in chronological order, he found that the follow-up results for one experiment were dated three weeks *before* the experiment itself. Another page, dated Jan. 19, 1984, was continued on a page dated Nov. 7, 1983. Several of Popovic's pages weren't dated at all. A few contained the handwriting of more than one person, and parts of several others had been whited out. The top half of one page bore an entry dated 11/21/83, and the bottom half an entry dated 11/22/84. In a sequential log of laboratory specimens, the year "84" had been crossed out and replaced by "83." Many people mistakenly wrote the previous year at the beginning of a new year. But Swire hadn't heard of anyone using the upcoming year's date before the end of the current year.

More significant than what the Popovic notes contained was what they didn't. There were entries for only five days in December 1983, and only seven days of notes the following month — the period later described by Gallo as the most intense in the history of his lab. In the notes that did exist, Swire and Weinberg could find no support for many of the experiments described in Popovic's *Science* article.

The article purported to show data from an AIDS virus culture that had been producing reverse transcriptase for a little over five months. But nothing in the notes reflected anything approaching five months of virus production. Nor could Swire find any evidence that the AIDS virus had been isolated from G.W., B.U., M.A., or Claude Chardon, as Gallo claimed in his letter to *Nature.* Either Gallo hadn't had any AIDS viruses in 1982 and 1983, or the relevant notepages were being withheld from Pasteur — odd, since they alone would have been enough to send the French packing.

Gallo didn't have any authority under the Freedom of Information Act to withhold documents from the French. That decision was Joanne Belk's alone. But one of Jim Swire's assistants, Julie Finch, quoted the HHS Freedom of Information officer as warning that Gallo had been "playing games and running risks," by insisting that he, Gallo, personally approve the release of documents from his laboratory.[54] Gallo denied it. "I didn't touch or get involved with anything that was given out," he said. "Private letters, anything, they got it all."[55]

After weeks of work by Myron Weinberg and the scientific detectives of the Weinberg Group, the notebooks, memos, and correspondence of Gallo and his staff began to yield some clues to what had transpired in Gallo's lab. But for every question the documents answered, two more were raised. For most of 1983, the records showed a single-minded focus on the search for HTLV-1 as the cause of AIDS,[56] followed by what appeared to be a sudden change of direction in October 1983.

Although the direction change had been prompted by Popovic's Eureka! experiment, the page reflecting that experiment was among the documents withheld by HHS. So, unbeknownst to Swire, were all of the pages reflecting Popovic's subsequent success with LAV.[i] "We were told not to put the LAV stuff" in the package of FOIA documents," recalled Betsy Read. "They wanted the other stuff."[57]

Now that Gallo had been forced by the *Science* correction to admit growing and photographing LAV, HHS turned over the page, headed "Lav transmission" and dated October 24, 1983, on which Betsy Read had listed the five continuous T-cell lines to be inoculated with the French virus during Popovic's visit to Switzerland. What happened to those cultures wasn't clear, because the term "LAV" didn't appear anywhere else in the Read or Popovic notes. What *did* continue to appear, however, were the names of HUT-78 and Ti7.4, the two cell lines in which LAV had grown best.[j] On one of the Popovic pages, Swire found a mystifying entry:

$$HUT78/v; Ti7.4/v = MOV.^{58}$$

There hadn't been anything called "MOV" in Gallo's *Science* papers. Swire wasn't sure what it was, or even sure how to pronounce it. But MOV must have been a virus, because on November 29 Popovic had harvested MOV supernatant — virus-containing culture fluids — to infect one of his HUT-78 clones:

$$Infection sup HUT78/MOV \rightarrow Htu4 \text{ usual procedure}$$

On December 5 the MOV culture was again harvested by Popovic, who concentrated it in a centrifuge and sent the concentrated liquid to Sarngadharan. Just before Christmas, Popovic informed Montagnier by telephone that he had "learned how to handle" the French virus.[59] Within days of that call, Sarngadharan had received a larger shipment of MOV,[60] followed by another batch at the beginning of 1984.[61] Sarngadharan was employed by Litton, not the government, and his notebooks hadn't been produced along with the others from Gallo's lab, which meant Swire couldn't see what Sarngadharan had done with MOV. But judging from Sarngadharan's *Science* paper, he had spent the early months of 1984 developing the Gallo ELISA.

Anyone looking at Popovic's notes would have concluded that Popovic himself had never touched LAV, but had spent his time working with cultures called "HUT-78/v," "Ti7.4/v," "HUT-78/inf," "Ti7.4/inf"— and, of course, "MOV."[k] The designations would have been incomprehensible to Jim Swire, except that he had gotten the Rosetta stone from Nancy Buc: the December 14, 1983, letter in which Matt Gonda informed Popovic that he had photographed lentiviruses in Popovic's LAV-producing cell lines.

When Popovic sent those samples to Gonda, on November 15, he had identified them by their right names, HUT-78/LAV and Ti7.4/LAV.[62] When Gonda reported his positive results on December 14, he naturally used Popovic's designations: HUT-78/LAV and Ti7.4/LAV. The problem was, Popovic's lab notes for November 15 didn't contain any references to "HUT-78/LAV" or "Ti7.4/LAV."

Instead, the cultures were identified as "HUT-78/inf" and "Ti7.4/inf"—"inf" being Popovic's shorthand for "virus infected."[63]

Why, Swire wondered, would someone working with the same two virus cultures day after day refer to them by different names on different days? Or, for that matter, by different names on the same day, as seemed to have happened on November 15?[l] To be consistent with Popovic's transmittal letter to Gonda, the November 15 entries in Popovic's notes should have read "HUT-78/LAV" and "Ti7.4/LAV." To Swire, it looked as if somebody had systematically tried to replace the evidence of Popovic's work with LAV with something that would appear innocuous to the Pasteur lawyers.

Swire decided he was right when the HHS FOIA office handed over yet another copy of the December 14 Gonda-to-Popovic letter. The first copy, given to Nancy Buc by the HHS lawyers months before, recorded "HUT-78/LAV" and "Ti7.4/LAV" as virus-positive. A second copy, obtained later by Swire from the HHS general counsel's office, was identical to the first.

But in the copy of the letter included with the FOIA materials, somebody had whited out "HUT-78/LAV" and "Ti7.4/LAV", leaving a suspicious-looking blank space. Who had done it Swire couldn't say, but he knew which batch of FOIA documents had included the redacted copy. "The batch which came from Gallo's lab," Swire said.[m]

Next, Swire tried to reconstruct the isolation of HTLV-3B. On November 15, 1983 — the day Popovic sent his LAV-producing cultures to Gonda — Swire found an entry in Popovic's notes that appeared to reflect the creation of the Popovic pool.

The first patient into the pool was 6233, a married carpet salesman from Long Island named Seymour Engler who had become infected with HIV during heart-bypass surgery in a New York hospital. Engler was followed by patient 6367, a Jamaican immigrant named Max Anglia, and then by patient 6592, a hemophiliac.[n] None of the three, Swire remarked to himself, was likely to have had sex with Frédéric Brugière.

A week later — the day "MOV" made its first appearance in Popovic's notes — the pool was boosted with a second infusion of material from the same three patients.[64] On January 2, 1984 — the same day Popovic sent Sarngadharan a large batch of MOV — Popovic had spiked the culture he now called "HT/v pool" with material from seven more patients. That made ten pool patients in all.

Gallo had assured Peter Fischinger that HTLV-3B was isolated from material "pooled from several patients who showed high R.T. activity in primary culture."[65] But Myron Weinberg couldn't find any evidence in the FOIA materials that any of the ten patients except Seymour Engler had been RT positive prior to pooling.[66] In view of that, it wasn't surprising that the pool had sputtered and required two rechargings.

But why, Swire wondered, had Popovic bothered to struggle with the pool at all, when his MOV cultures were producing large quantities of virus? Beyond that, why had Popovic chosen to pool so many patient samples that, according to his own records, were negative for RT and EM?[67] Wouldn't it have made more sense to pool material from cultures that were already producing virus? Unless Popovic hadn't *had* any virus-producing cultures besides MOV and LAV.

Popovic's notes for most of January and February didn't mention the pool, his attention evidently having been refocused on trying to isolate a single-patient AIDS virus, and on finding a continuous cell line in which the virus could grow. Swire could see that a number of single-patient cultures had been started, but without immediate success.[o] Not until February 25, two weeks after Gallo's return from Park City, did the pool virus reappear in Popovic's notes, when Popovic used it to infect eight of the newest T-cell lines he had cloned from HUT-78. By the beginning of March, all eight T-cell clones were producing the virus Gallo would later name HTLV-3B. The most productive clone was the ninth one created, H-9.

In November the pool had gotten off to a shaky start. By the beginning of January, it was still flagging. To save it, Popovic had spiked it with seven patient cultures, none of which had displayed any evidence of a replicating virus. Nevertheless, in barely a month, the pool had become a potent source of AIDS virus — an AIDS virus indistinguishable from LAV.

Gallo's lab didn't have the capacity for mass virus production, but his contract laboratories did, and Gallo had been using Biotech Research Labs, Electronucleonics, and Litton to grow the AIDS virus Popovic called MOV. At the end of March 1984, a Biotech researcher had sent a shipment of MOV to Gallo's lab. One of Gallo's molecular biologists, Sasha Arya, logged the shipment in his notebook as "LAV." A week later, on April 5, Biotech delivered a second MOV shipment. Again, Arya recorded the shipment as LAV.[p]

In a note dated April 12 — eleven days before Margaret Heckler's news conference — Swire found what he was looking for, the first reference to HTLV-3B. Two days before, on April 10, three liters of MOV culture fluids had been collected at Biotech and sent to Electronucleonics, where they were centrifuged into a single milliliter of super-concentrated virus. The concentrate was sent back to Biotech on April 11, which sent it to Gallo on April 12. This time, however, Arya recorded the shipment of MOV as HTLV-3B.[q]

George Todaro, brought in by Genetic Systems to examine the Gallo lab's notebooks, thought the serial name changes were "the most incriminating thing" in any of the notes. The way Swire and Todaro saw it, LAV had been renamed MOV, and MOV had been renamed HTLV-3B. Perhaps there really had been a Popovic pool. Perhaps the notes purporting to show the creation of a pool had been dummied up. Either way, the pool now seemed irrelevant. "When I saw LAV equals MOV equals HTLV-3B," Swire recalled, "I said 'Bingo. We win.'"

"A Small Guy Who Stumbled"

Had John Maddox been inclined to print the venomous exchanges between Robert Gallo and Abraham Karpas, they would have consumed an entire issue of *Nature,* and offended Maddox's sensibilities as well. "In Britain," Maddox said, "excessive zeal in the pursuit of other people's reputations is regarded as a very bad thing. People cringe from it." Rather than publishing Karpas's latest attack, Maddox sent it directly to Gallo, who responded with what Maddox termed "an over-generous but effective reply" of four-and-a-half single-spaced pages.

"I appreciate that Karpas is capable of reading our 'multiple papers,'" Gallo wrote Maddox, "and we are pleased that we are fortunate enough to have our work regularly accepted for publication. We wish, however, that Karpas would read them carefully and with less malice. Mostly, we are astonished to see how regularly he suspects the integrity of his scientific colleagues. . . . Enough is enough! We wish to work in peace solving problems and not to be preoccupied with malicious, petty, ignorant, jealous sentiments."[1]

Karpas replied that Maddox, "as an outsider of retrovirology," might believe that Gallo's reply was effective, but that "none of his claims are valid when one actually checks the published record. Dr. Gallo still believes that in this age of communication and science he can get away with not only saying, but even writing, that black is white and vice versa."[2]

"Thank you for your letter, which is really quite helpful," Maddox replied to Karpas, "but I am afraid that I have decided not to publish your letter or indeed anything about the Gallo/Montagnier issue until we have completed, written and published our account of the investigation I told you about."[3]

Nature's investigation consisted mainly of a long conversation between Maddox and Luc Montagnier in Paris, followed by a visit by Maddox and his deputy, Peter Newmark, to Gallo's lab, where they were joined by *Nature*'s Washington correspondent, Joe Palca. Gallo, who had just returned from giving a talk in Toronto, greeted the delegation in his office on a Friday afternoon. After shaking hands all around, Maddox placed a tape recorder in the middle of Gallo's conference table and began asking questions.[a]

Of particular interest to Maddox were the lab notes, obtained by Palca, which appeared to record numerous experiments from early 1984 comparing HTLV-1 and HTLV-2 with LAV — the virus Gallo had insisted couldn't be compared with anything, because it hadn't grown.

"You said that the second sample, the second LAV sample, grew," Maddox said.

"It grew," Gallo admitted.

"What investigations did you make with it?"

"Mika passed it in cord blood cells," Gallo said. "Let me — you could ask specific questions: Did we ever use it to clone genes? Did we ever use it to make antibodies? Did we ever use it to raise reagents? No. We used it for nothing like that. Although to be honest there would be nothing wrong with doing that. We used it for nothing, other than showing it was a retrovirus, getting RT, getting EM, passaging it for a while in cord blood, getting it into HUT-78 for a short period, then seeing that we couldn't maintain it in HUT-78. And then, quite frankly, at my request to Mika, 'Get rid of it.' Not throw it away, but, you know, 'I don't want to do more with this now.'"

"Nothing but HUT-78?" Palca asked.

"Nothing but," Gallo replied.

"Not Ti7.4?"

"Um, yeah," Gallo replied. "That's an M. D. Anderson cell line. Yeah, that one too. Transient. That one doesn't produce at all, very much. Just a little."

"How many of your own viruses were you then growing?" wondered Peter Newmark.

"R.F.," Gallo said, "and one of what came out of the ten samples."

"So, the one called 'B'?" Newmark asked.

"Yes."

"So those two were growing."

"Those two were growing," said Gallo.

Maddox wondered when Popovic had stopped working with LAV.

"You know what?" Gallo replied. "I got caught sometimes by not saying something accurately. It looks like you're then bullshitting. The answer is, I don't know. But what I'm sure of, it's not the spring. And what I'm sure of, it's not January. So it ends in '83. If we carried it over to January, I'd be very, very surprised. But I would like Mika to answer that question, or Betsy Read. They could tell you precisely."

Maddox remarked that the LAV comparisons in the unsigned lab notes were dated in February and March of 1984. "Somebody thrust these documents on us," Maddox explained. "I don't know whose lab notes they are. But they're from this lab, obviously. And this looks like something being done with LAV in February."

"Yeah, sure," Gallo replied, contradicting what he had said a minute earlier. "There was a lot done. That was to compare the viruses. That was when we were going to have the meeting with Chermann. That was the material that never got published. People are throwing things on people's desks. Wonderful. We have a lot with LAV done. Because that's when we agreed with Chermann to make the comparisons. Immunologically and the nucleic acids."[b]

"Which LAV was that?" Palca asked.

"That's really interesting," Gallo replied. "See, what I wonder . . . I just wonder — excuse me for my interpretation — but how many people have been twisted? You're presented a series of documents like that. 'Look, they didn't grow LAV.' 'Look, here's LAV in their notebooks.' Our guy goes into their office. They have by Freedom of Information Act everything I have here. You know what my role — you know that we're being sued again for not giving it out in time? Every document in here some contract people gave. I didn't touch or get involved with anything that was given out. You can look. Private letters, anything, they got it all. There are boxes, like over here. Some contract people came in and took all our files. So they have everything. They don't have to break in anymore."[c]

"We've had these papers for a couple of months, is it?" Maddox said. "We haven't done . . ."

"But," Gallo interrupted, "you *could* do something with them. The interesting thing is *why* you have them, and what does somebody want you to believe?"

"That's why our colleague Joe Palca smelled a rat," Maddox said.

"I had a call from Marilyn Chase at the *Wall Street Journal*," Gallo said. "Their litigation lawyer, Swire — some of the things that you may not know, that we have to put up with. This guy had not only tried entrapment of a witness. Berge Hampar, a lawyer-scientist at Frederick, had two pages for the record he gave to the attorney general of the United States which formally say that Swire tried to bribe him. . . .[d] Sam Broder told me that some young man directly told him that Swire was hiring people to come to restaurants to sit where I go to eat, to try to hear what I say. This is a fantastic situation."[e]

Joe Palca wondered whether the Pasteur lawsuit had affected Gallo's ability to discuss his research. "I don't particularly care, you know?" Gallo replied. "I've never been told what to do or not do by the lawyers and I don't talk to the lawyers.[f] He [Montagnier] talks to the lawyers regularly and so he gets a lot of advice, including how to have the Lasker written. The blood test, if he had a blood test right away, and so on. So he got that in there. No, the lawyers don't tell me. They just say they wish I would tell them. They know that I operate independently. I'm not going to be told by a lawyer that I can't say something."

Maddox wondered whether the DNA sequence differences between LAV and HTLV-3B were large enough to justify Gallo's claim that they had come from different patients. "The impression that Montagnier gave me about the sequences," Maddox said, "is that — he used the phrase 'sequencing noise' to imply that there is a kind of built-in error."

"That's the noise in France," Gallo said. "It's quieter in Bethesda. We sequenced it three times. We didn't have any differences . . . the very line that he's arguing, what I want you to understand is that he's denying this to me in the presence of witnesses. He's lying, see? If I make a mistake I'm not going to directly lie to you. I don't tell a deliberate lie. This guy's lying, because in my presence, with Harmison, and with his patent lawyer, he swore he never made that innuendo. That is, you know, that we could have taken his virus or that we had his virus."

"When we were talking," said Maddox, "he said he believed you had done that with the first, or the second sample."

"The final point," Gallo said. "Why would I — just a little bit of common logic. Why would I then rush into print with this goddamn sequence, be the one who discovers heterogeneity, and call that son of a bitch on the phone and tell him? I called him on the phone and said, 'Look, these viruses show heterogeneity.' We were observing heterogeneity. And I must say I was struck by the similarity of ours with theirs, with the B strain. And I called them about it.

"I said, 'You know, our B strain looks a lot like LAV by the restriction map. And we have some other ones that don't look so similar.' But I told him they both came from New York about the same time. So I was telling him not to be worried, because I thought he had a contaminant, since we had brought the cell line into his lab, and that he probably cross-contaminated with his cell line. And I assumed that could never happen to me, it would happen to him.

"He tells you one story," Gallo said, "he tells me another story. People don't know these things, or understand them. I mean, I was yesterday at McMaster [University], in the guest house. There was a physicist there from Germany and a geophysicist from England. They say to me, 'It's such an exciting field, are you the guy with Pasteur?' The orchestration now is fantastic. They've had public relations lessons, they've been told how to behave at meetings, to be more aggressive with the Americans, to shave off your mustache.[g] They only talk about HTLV-3 and never with B after it, as if all viruses are that from our lab. Always, every goddamn talk, no matter where they go."

"Well," Peter Newmark observed, "it was the first one."

"Yes," Gallo said, then caught himself. "No. R.F. was the same time, the same week. It was — OK, I'll tell you what it was. It [3B] was the virus that was handed out to the companies. That's the lasso on my neck. You want to get Mika to go off the wall? Why did he select that versus R.F.?[h] R.F.'s a Haitian. He knew from day one that B was the worst thing to send out because it came from ten people and he'd always be asked which patient. He wanted to go with R.F., but first it was a Haitian. So we were concerned, not an American.[i] The second point was although all criteria were that it was positive and high producing, the EM report from Frederick was strangely negative."

Montagnier "cannot be that stupid," Gallo said. "He knows we signed the document. He has in his hands that we labeled the virus LAV from Pasteur. They have that. Proof. Mika sent it up labeled black as can be. "I mean," Gallo said, "why wouldn't we give out the

R.F. if we had any suspicions? He must realize that. He knows that R.F. is available. These are the things I find hard that a rational person could really believe down deep. Who in their right mind with an IQ of 3 would play their cards that way? What could we have been thinking of? I told him a long time ago, go call American Tissue Type Culture, when did they get R.F.?"

"That would have been in December?" Maddox asked.

"Whenever we sent the viruses," Gallo replied.ʲ " So I don't understand how far you could go in that attack. Does he think he needs more visibility? More credit? Did a man ever get so much credit for one paper? I mean, I want to be as calm as possible."

"I think it's very difficult," Maddox agreed. "I think it's to some degree the French sense of constantly being put upon by superpowers, the United States."

"The David and Goliath syndrome," offered Flossie Wong-Staal, who had just entered the room.

"You know how I look at it?" Gallo asked. "They ran rampant on everyone. They did as much as they could. I don't really feel that terribly American. You gotta understand the difference between me and a Frenchman. I feel very European in a very American, sort of, like, here we are all Europeans here, Chinese and Indians. I mean, what is my lab but foreign people? Who am I but a descendant of somebody who came from Northwestern Italy? I don't feel like I identify with flags here or anything else. I like this country. It's treated me well, and my father too.

"I look at the French capitalizing on their food industry from some places where my ancestors came from," Gallo went on. "They package it better and they sell it. I look upon them hyping in their wine to a degree. What's great is super-great, what's mediocre is very good and what's awful is fine. I look at the way they sell perfume to all the Japanese in the airports like for $50 a smell. As if it's the only perfume in the world. I think they do great in getting credit for nothing half the time, more than any people I've ever seen. That's the bias I would have against France. I like a lot of Frenchmen, and I like some of my days there. But I think they get plenty of credit. Boy, oh boy. They told us what to do about flying into Libya. They helped get us into Vietnam."

"Honestly," Maddox said, "I think he's a reasonable guy."

"I just can't agree with you," Gallo said. "I just don't agree with that. I talked to Simon Wain-Hobson at lunch the other day. He says

[Montagnier] hasn't a single collaborator left, because no one trusts him. Because he screws every collaborator he has. Chermann's not even talking to him anymore. Wain-Hobson won't work with him anymore. I see what he did to me when I told him what my problems were. I find him extremely political, always not sure what he believes. People who are full of distrust and see the world as everybody scheming to screw them. That's the way I look at that guy. . . . Montagnier's an example of a small guy who stumbled into shit, and he got famous. More than he deserves. He can't handle it, sees everybody as plotting against him."

"Who's the Englishman who does the sequencing?" Newmark asked.

"Simon Wain-Hobson," Gallo said. "He's straight as an arrow. If he criticizes me, I believe it. If Simon Wain-Hobson said, 'Bob did this,' as far as I'm concerned, I can't criticize Wain-Hobson. He's always been direct and straight with me in any conversation. I have never seen him do bad politics."

"I think the only thing we can be accused of," said Wong-Staal, "is that we didn't do the comparisons right away."

"I told them that," Gallo said. "That was deliberate. I mean, I admit it. It can be criticized. I said that to a professor at the Karolinska about three months ago. I admitted it. I said, 'We had the ability. We didn't have the data but we could have gone forward. It was our prerogative but it wasn't generous. . . . I made a decision. And so I have to take full responsibility."

Having sat quietly since returning from a seminar, Popovic now wanted to speak. "I have a few things," he began hesitantly. "I thought that before we had the EMs it was the same thing. This can be checked because it was . . . May 26. In July. Before we submitted the paper we . . . February '84. Also negative. Also by EM."

"Mika," Gallo interrupted. "Don't drive John Maddox crazy. Just summarize."

"We used also their serum. . . ," Popovic went on. "BRU serum . . . for comparison. . . ."

But nobody was listening, and Popovic stopped talking.

Despite a number of misstatements, Gallo had been remarkably candid. The comparisons of HTLV-3B with LAV, Gallo said, *could* have been done — a stunning contravention of Gallo's declaration at Margaret Heckler's news conference, that he couldn't say whether LAV and HTLV-3B were the same because there hadn't been enough LAV to compare with HTLV-3B.

Nature had previously assured its readers that Gallo had grown LAV "for one week only and in small quantity."[k] Now Gallo admitted that LAV had grown for at least three months,[l] and there had been plenty of virus. Also on the disabled list was Gallo's claim of forty-eight AIDS virus isolates. Besides HTLV-3B, Gallo said, the only AIDS virus growing in his lab had been HTLV-3$_{RF}$.

Had the Gallo interview been reported, it would have dramatically changed the face of the dispute with Pasteur. But *Nature* never published a word of what Gallo had said — or anything else about its investigation. "We gave it up," John Maddox said later. "I think that it literally is impossible to tell who's right and who's wrong. You know, each side has reasons for being frenetic about the other. Transgressions of good manners, to say the least, on both sides, are very, very hard to understand. At the stage we were looking at this, it was very hard indeed to discover what the truth was."

Maddox wasn't sure how Gallo's extended absences from the laboratory, and Flossie Wong-Staal's role as Gallo's alter ego, might have contributed to whatever had gone on. "Here you have a man of great ambition and great enthusiasm," Maddox said. "And people say to him from time to time, 'Come and give us a talk. Come and accept the gold medal from our society, come and do this, that and the other, and tell us how famous you are.' And Bob would say 'Yes, I'll go, I'm off to Houston in the morning.'"

"On one extraordinary occasion," Maddox said, "he came and talked on short notice at a conference we were holding in Tokyo. And the conditions were that he had to be able to catch the plane to be able to talk in Houston the following day. With somebody like that, it's plain that he couldn't succeed unless he had somebody in the lab who could keep the ball rolling, keep the research work going on, tell the people what to do. And, indeed, to keep in touch with him, tell him what was happening. So I think that Flossie probably slipped into that managerial role naturally. There had to be somebody to do it and she was the one who did it."

Gallo had mentioned to *Nature* that Montagnier was being advised by the Pasteur lawyers about "how to have the Lasker written." The meaning of his remark became clear the following Monday, when the Lasker Foundation announced that Gallo, Montagnier, and Max Essex would share the Albert Lasker Clinical Medical Research Award for their "immense contribution to the central discovery that a retrovirus is the cause of AIDS"— in Essex's case, the discovery of the second AIDS virus, HTLV-4.[4]

A few days before the announcement, one of Gallo's administrative assistants, Ann Sliski, had sent Jim Wyngaarden a draft of what Sliski described as the "slanted" Lasker press release. Montagnier was listed as "discovering the retrovirus responsible" for AIDS, Sliski complained, "and Bob is listed as 'unique contributions to understanding AIDS.' We feel that either all three should read for 'contributions toward the identification of family of viruses that are the etiological agent of AIDS' or more clearly reflect in Bob's case that he proved the cause of AIDS and developed a blood test that has made the blood supply safe."[5]

More offensive, in Sliski's view, was the declaration that while "other investigators hypothesized that the known human T-cell leukemia retroviruses (HTLV-I and HTLV-II) might cause AIDS, Dr. Montagnier based his research on the premise that a different retrovirus is involved." That sentence, Sliski said, "implies that Bob and Max were on the wrong track and that Montagnier was the only one on the right track. We feel this sentence should be removed."

When the release was issued, Montagnier's discovery of "the retrovirus responsible" for AIDS had been changed to read "the retrovirus *later shown* to be responsible for this major new threat to world health." Now it was Gallo who had performed the "seroepidemiologic studies proving it to be the agent that causes AIDS," and done the work which "led to the development of a test for antibodies to the retrovirus in the blood, for screening transfusions and preventing bloodborne spread of the disease."

"It is a fair award," Gallo told the *Washington Post*.[6] According to Vince DeVita, who sat on the Lasker jury, the inclusion of Essex's name had been a "complicated" affair. "There were other people who had something to do with Max," said DeVita. "I don't think Max really has done a lot. He was always around the edges. I think when you're around discoveries, you have a different view of what your role is. When AIDS hit, Essex's claim to fame was that he was one of those viral oncologists who was doing work that was relevant to the new problem of AIDS. And he played it very well."

. . .

While Gallo's lab celebrated the Lasker Prize, Sasha Arya was frantically reconstructing the genesis of his laboratory notes. Arya, who worked for Flossie Wong-Staal, had been the principal author of the paper in *Science* reporting nonexistent similarities between HTLV-1 and the AIDS virus — the same paper that had first identified the source of HTLV-3B as a patient pool.[7] According to the paper, HTLV-3B had been the AIDS virus used in Arya's comparisons with HTLV-1. But the notebook pages John Maddox had brought to the Gallo interview identified the AIDS viruses with which Arya had been working as "LAV" and "MOV."[m]

Following the interview, Gallo demanded an explanation. Arya replied that he hadn't known anything about the provenance of the AIDS virus Mika Popovic had been sending him. Sometime in January 1984, Popovic had told him the virus was called LAV, and Arya had simply adopted the term. Arya had continued working with Popovic's virus preparations through most of March, and Popovic hadn't ever told him to *stop* calling them LAV. The first Arya ever heard of HTLV-3 was from Flossie Wong-Staal, a few days before the Heckler news conference.[n]

Arya's claim that he used "LAV" as a "generic designation" for the AIDS virus didn't explain the single, unsigned notebook page bearing the designation "LAV from Paris." Nor did it explain how experiments recorded as done with "generic LAV" and "MOV" could have been performed with HTLV-3B, as the paper claimed, since HTLV-3B hadn't existed when those experiments were done.[o]

It certainly didn't explain why the notebooks of Beatrice Hahn and George Shaw were also peppered with references to "LAV" during the first months of 1984. According to Shaw, the source of the term had been Mika Popovic, "because he was the only person we were working with at the time on these kinds of things."[8] Had *Nature* persisted in its inquiries, it might have solved the mystery of LAV and HTLV-3B. Shaw's notes contained a critical clue, a single reference to "LAV/Htu-4"— Htu-4 being the fourth HUT-78 clone, H-4, that according to Popovic's notes had been infected with AIDS virus the previous November — not with HTLV-3B, but with MOV.[p]

Time magazine thought the dispute between Gallo and the French "one of the more unseemly rivalries to sully the scientific community in decades."[9] Money aside, said *Time*, "no one doubts that Gallo is as eager as the French to get the glory for one of the more important discoveries in late-20th century medicine. 'It's what we call the race for the Nobel Prize,' says one cynical scientist."

Gallo didn't deny wanting a Nobel Prize, but he didn't care about the money from the AIDS test patent. "My father's a successful metallurgist," Gallo said. "I'm the only child; my sister had leukemia and died, so my father's money will go to me. He's very happy that I went into research, very proud of it, and my needs are small. I have a little Datsun. I have my house, paid for by my father, so I have no bills to pay. What do I need? I have my office, I have my work. People pay for me to travel to go to meetings to give lectures. I like to read and play tennis — all almost free. That's it. I don't need any more money."[10]

It was the French, Gallo said, who were interested in the American dollars the blood-test patent would bring them. "The fight is theirs to get the money," Gallo protested. "I don't get any money. My name is used in vain. If I wanted to make money, I wouldn't work at NIH. If I get any money from this at all, I will give it to charity. This patent is the worst thing that ever happened to me. What am I getting out of it? I'm getting nothing out of it but a lot of pain."[11]

That was about to change. A few months before, the House of Representatives had passed a bill intended to make technology developed in government laboratories more accessible to the private sector.[12] One aim of the Federal Technology Transfer Act, inspired by President Reagan's challenge to privatize portions of the federal government, was to retain government scientists who were being lured by higher salaries to universities and private companies. Government salaries would never reach competitive levels in the private sector, since the best-paid university researchers already earned more — with stock options many times more — than the president of the United States.

One thing the government could do, however, was let its scientists share whatever patent royalties were generated by their inventions. Because most NIH patents weren't terribly valuable, the average earnings of most NIH scientists were token at best. Beatrice Hahn collected an annual royalty of $813.38 on one patent; Berge Hampar got $8 a year on another. But with the AIDS blood test earning millions, both Gallo and Popovic qualified for the maximum payment — $100,000 a year during the lifetime of the patent, a total of $1.5 million apiece over fifteen years. The AIDS test had made them millionaires.[q]

"Just Show Us the Proof"

By the autumn of 1986 the Red Cross had been aware for months that the Abbott ELISA produced false-negative results. But Red Cross blood banks had continued using the Abbott test while the company searched for a solution. When Abbott's Marijane Sidote called the FDA to report that the false-negative problem at last had been solved, the FDA's Tom Zuck wasn't persuaded. "I told him we have process change to improve sensitivity," Sidote wrote in her telephone notes.[1] "He asked what? I said enriched with p41. He said no, it's p24 we miss. I explained our position. He said he doesn't believe it, that we have a circular argument. He said it will be hard to convince."

Zuck was "upset," Sidote told Abbott executives a few days later, "that he has been asking for confirmation of 'What's on the bead' for seven months and we still haven't told him. He said he can't work the science of the assays for dealing with lawyers and executives. He said he's so angry with Abbott, 'There are several stacks to work on, and we won't pick Abbott first.'"[2]

At the end of July 1986 a flock of specialists from Abbott headquarters descended on the FDA. Zuck's concerns about p24 aside, the data presented by the Abbott group seemed to show that the more gp41 on the bead, the fewer false negatives. Mike Ascher, now employed as a consultant to Abbott, surmised that antibodies to *both* gp41 *and* p24 must be produced early in the infection, but that for some reason only p24 antibodies showed up on a Western Blot.

In the FDA's view, it wasn't necessary to understand what was going on serologically as long as the Abbott test improved its reliability and sensitivity. Then Abbott confided that while gp41 enrichment had worked with its laboratory model test kits, the company didn't have the capacity to purify enough gp41 to make the same change in its product line.[a]

Abbott asked the FDA to approve a lesser bead modification without additional field testing, but Zuck refused. Abbott would have to present the gp41-enriched bead as an entirely new product, rather than an improvement on a product that already had an FDA license. That meant more field tests.[3] But no sooner had those evaluations begun than Abbott told the Red Cross to put everything on hold. A new problem had cropped up — an unexpected reappearance of the false positives Abbott thought had been resolved.[4]

When the Red Cross Blood Center Directors' Council met in Washington in October, the topic was the performance of the new Abbott ELISA. The new test was clearly better than the one the Red Cross and the blood banks were still using. The bad news was that it still missed nearly half the samples the Western Blot called HIV-indeterminate. Considering the manufacturing challenges involved, Abbott couldn't say when it could put the new test on the market. In the meantime, sentiment was growing among the Red Cross blood bank directors for dumping Abbott altogether in favor of Genetic Systems, whose AIDS test was already being used on a trial basis by seven of the fifty-five Red Cross blood centers.[5]

The Red Cross lawyers warned that dropping Abbott completely would probably violate the Abbott contract, and someone suggested using the Genetic Systems ELISA to back up the Abbott test. But if the Red Cross were going to buy the Genetic Systems test anyway, it didn't need the Abbott test. In the end, the blood center directors agreed that Abbott would be given an ultimatum: If the company's new test hadn't been approved by the FDA in ninety days, the contract with Abbott would be terminated. Less than a week after that decision, the Red Cross blood-testing chief, Gerald Sandler, assured the American public that "the blood supply is as safe as it can possibly be made."[6]

Bob Nowinski, the head of Genetic Systems, knew it wasn't true. "Statistically, bad blood got into the system," Nowinski said. "You can make a calculation, which in fact we did. If one test is twelve weeks later in picking up a newly infected individual and you make various suppositions of what's the rate of new infection, then you can calculate given the number of transfusions, given the number of new infections, and given whatever the latency is. You can come up with a number that can be anywhere from eight hundred to several thousand a year."

As the Red Cross directors reconvened in San Francisco in November, Sandler was saying something quite different from what he had been telling the news media. The Red Cross lawyers, Sandler said, had decreed that if the agency wanted to protect itself from lawsuits down the road, it "could wait no longer" before putting a better HIV-antibody test into service. The formal ninety-day notice had never been given to Abbott, but the company had been made "aware" that the Red Cross was ready to replace it if the new test didn't become available "in the immediate future."

In the meantime, one council member suggested that the Red Cross stop making reassuring public statements and admit that the AIDS test was flawed. That might at least discourage people who thought they were HIV-positive from giving blood. His suggestion was rejected out-of-hand. But France Peetoom from the Portland Red Cross, one of the seven centers using the Genetic Systems ELISA, implored his colleagues to take "rapid action" in switching the entire system to Genetic Systems. If they didn't, Peetoom warned, it would soon be a full year since the Red Cross had learned about the false-negative problem.[7]

In mid-November Abbott sent the FDA its latest field data on the new ELISA, which now had a gp41 enriched bead, a new diluent *and* an improved conjugate.[8] The new test, Abbott assured the FDA, no longer would misread any blood samples containing HIV antibodies as antibody-free. When Tom Zuck saw the data, he fired a broadside at Abbott.[9] "You threw us a curve," he told Marijane Sidote. "You've made more changes — bead, diluent, buffer. It may be a new product. We can't keep putting Abbott before other reviews. We've been asked to take Abbott off the market because of poor sensitivity. We've had complaints that we handle Abbott changes as amendments instead of as a new product. You've made too many changes. You wasted our time with enriched bead and it didn't work. Now you have more changes coming. You've got to stick to an assay configuration for at least 60 days and quit changing it!"

The FDA had tried to tell Abbott "you had a sensitivity problem," Zuck went on, "and we told you the enriched bead would cause a specificity problem. Heller heard us, but the rest of you wouldn't listen. We wasted half a day talking to the Red Cross about your improved bead. Now we're concerned with the cell lysate. We don't know what it will do to the product. I've now been hauled in front of the Commissioner three times. We tell him you don't know what's in your product. You gave us 4 manufacturing options and asked us to help and we're not going to design your product for you . . . if you can't produce [the new test] then why should we approve the change? We don't think you've got a product you can make."

While Abbott sweated and Zuck fumed, the Red Cross continued to stall. At the beginning of October, the blood center directors had voted to give Abbott ninety days. Now it was nearly Christmas, and Red Cross headquarters executives hadn't even obtained a price quote from Genetic Systems for supplying the entire Red Cross system, as the directors' council had also requested. In a late-December conference call, the center directors demanded that Abbott be given an ultimatum. Headquarters promised the company would be told the following day that its contract would be canceled if the new test didn't receive a license within sixty days.[10]

On the second day of January, seventeen-year-old Kandra Kae Crosby of Fort Walton Beach, Florida, gave birth to her first child, a son she named Michael. During childbirth, Kandra Kae received four units of blood. One was from an early seroconverter who had tested HIV-negative prior to transfusion.[11] "She's never going to see her son graduate from high school," said her attorney, Dennis Webb.

While Jim Swire awaited the appeals court's ruling, the Institut Pasteur and the Department of Health and Human Services prepared to square off before the United States Patent and Trademark Office. According to *Time,* the PTO's decision to grant Pasteur's request for an interference represented a "minor triumph" for the French.[12]

On its face, the question of who deserved credit for inventing the HIV blood test seemed open-and-shut. The first-ever ELISA for AIDS virus antibodies had been performed in Paris in July 1983, using LAV from Frédéric Brugière. In September of that year the French had applied for a European patent on their blood test. In December they had applied for an American patent. The following month, Sarngadharan had performed the first AIDS blood test in the United States, using the virus Mika Popovic called MOV. When the Centers for Disease Control compared the performance of the French and American tests, the French results had come in first and they had been more precise. Two weeks later, the Reagan administration had applied for a patent on the American test.

The Americans had won the patent, but now the patent office wanted to have a second look. Because both the French and American applications appeared to describe the same invention and had been filed less than six months apart, they had been declared in "interference" with one another.[13] The fact that the Pasteur had filed first gave the French senior status and a "priority date" of September 15, 1983, the day Montagnier had spoken about the LAV ELISA at Cold Spring Harbor. As the junior party in the interference, the burden would be on the United States to show that Gallo, Popovic, and Sarngadharan were the first, true, and only inventors of the HIV-antibody test, as they had claimed to be.

In patent law, an invention is "reduced to practice" when it is first used successfully for its intended purpose. With the AIDS test, reduction to practice would have occurred when the first blood sample was tested for AIDS virus antibodies. If Gallo were going to prove priority, he would have to demonstrate that somebody in his lab had conducted at least one ELISA with the AIDS virus before September 15. But on September 15 Gallo had been at Cold Spring Harbor, speaking about HTLV-1 as the likely cause of AIDS and deriding Montagnier's blood-test data with LAV.[14]

Pressed by the government's lawyers to come up with the earliest possible reduction date, the best Gallo could do was October 6, 1983,[15] the date of Mika Popovic's Eureka! experiment. Although the immunofluorescence tests Betsy Read conducted that day weren't ELISAs, and although they employed LAV as a reference virus and Frédéric Brugière's serum as the antiviral reagent, they nevertheless represented the first AIDS-virus-antibody testing in Gallo's lab.

But October 6 was still several weeks too late, and if the government wanted to save the patent it would have to come up with another approach. One strategy considered by the Justice Department was the argument that the Pasteur and Gallo ELISAs were really different inventions. By definition, only Gallo could be the inventor of the Gallo ELISA, and only HHS would therefore be entitled to the patent on that invention.[b]

The strategy was not without risks. If the patent office declared the inventions substantially different, the Gallo patent would stand. On the other hand, Genetic Systems would be free to sell the Pasteur blood test in the United States, since it wouldn't be infringing on the Gallo patent. Considering the trouble the Red Cross and the other blood banks were having with the Gallo test, once the infringement roadblock was lifted the American manufacturers were certain to lose business to Genetic Systems.

To represent it before the patent office, the Pasteur had chosen Charles E. Lipsey, a veteran patent attorney with the Washington law firm of Finnegan & Henderson. In Lipsey's opinion, the only difference between the Pasteur and Gallo AIDS tests was that Pasteur called its virus LAV and Gallo called his HTLV-3B.[16] Both tests were made with the AIDS virus, both were designed to detect human antibodies to that virus, and the French test had existed months before the American version.

The Material Information Disclosure filed with the patent office by the government hadn't mentioned LAV — an omission that, in Lipsey's opinion, amounted to gross negligence at best by HHS.[17] It was "hard to imagine," Lipsey said, "that the failure to cite [Pasteur's initial *Science*] article and explain its significance on the record was anything less than intentional." Most egregious, in Lipsey's eyes, was the failure of anyone in the Reagan administration to inform the patent office about the CDC's comparative study of the Gallo and Pasteur tests.[18] When Lipsey asked Montagnier and Chermann to give him affidavits recalling the tripartite meeting at the Pasteur, Montagnier swore "that as of April 6, 1984, Dr. Gallo was aware of substantial evidence of the similarity of LAV and HTLV-3," including the fact that "a large number of specimens from patients with AIDS or related conditions show similar results when either of the prototype viruses is used as antigen."[c]

Who had invented the HIV blood-antibody test was a separate issue from whose test was best. Under the patent laws, an invention didn't have to be *perfected* to merit a patent. It only had to be *novel*, meaning new, as well as "not obvious," not anticipated by the "prior art," and of course workable. One couldn't invent what was merely a different size or color of wheel. Nor could an invention be anticipated, or *taught,* by someone else's previous discoveries, or *prior art.* That made it an adaptation, not an invention.

It wasn't necessary for the interference proceedings to address the question of whether LAV had been renamed HTLV-3B. LAV had made it possible for Gallo to confirm that the AIDS virus was a new human retrovirus, that AIDS patients had antibodies to that virus, and that those antibodies could be detected with an ELISA. For Gallo, Lipsey argued, the mere existence of LAV in Gallo's laboratory represented *de facto* prior art. Far from being a novel invention, Gallo's AIDS test was nothing more than an adaptation of the Pasteur AIDS test.[19]

The HHS lawyers were aware that the government's arguments about significant differences between the French and American tests were weak, since both tests currently were being used by the Red Cross to screen the blood supply for antibodies to the AIDS virus. But there was another way HHS might yet prevail over Pasteur. Because the Pasteur's first *Science* paper had been published less than a year before the Gallo patent application was filed, the patent laws allowed Gallo to try to prove that even if he hadn't had a working AIDS test before the French, he had conceived the *idea* first.[d] For that strategy to prevail, Gallo would have to prove he had become aware of the existence of the AIDS virus prior to January 1983, when LAV was first isolated in Paris.

Gallo had claimed to Jean-Claude Chermann that his lab had found the AIDS virus at the end of 1982 — ahead of the French.[e] To Peter Fischinger he had admitted his late 1982 and early 1983 virus isolations were wishful thinking.[20] Now, before the Patent Office, Gallo's claims were resurrected under oath.[f] According to Gallo's sworn declaration, in December 1982 "our group at NCI detected a new retrovirus in AIDS sera which appeared to be different from HTLV-1 and HTLV-2." In February 1983 "a further detection of the virus which would later be called HTLV-3 was made which this time included electron microscopy as well as RT."[21]

Gallo was treading dangerous ground, because there hadn't been any electron micrographs of the AIDS virus in Bethesda in February of 1983. Then, and for months to come, the only AIDS virus EMs had been in Paris. But Gallo's declaration went farther, claiming "approximately 25–30 instances of the detection" of the AIDS virus between May and September of 1983 — a claim that didn't square with Gallo's statements about HTLV-1 during the summer of 1983,[22] Popovic's concern about Gallo's HTLV-1 "mindset," or his Eureka! experiment.[23]

As for LAV, Gallo swore that the July 1983 shipment used in the Eureka! experiment had been useless because it hadn't contained any "detectable virus." Despite the CDC blood-test comparisons, on the day of the Heckler news conference Gallo hadn't considered LAV and HTLV-3 "to be the same, or even substantially the same, virus." *That* didn't square with Gallo's remarks in Zurich two weeks before, that the Pasteur's serology "has gotten very good, almost as good as I know we have with these."

But the declaration's biggest gaffe was Gallo's assertion that he had seen "no evidence" LAV was the cause of AIDS "up through the allowance of the Gallo patent" in May 1985. As Gallo must have remembered, three months before the patent was issued he had affirmed in a letter to *Nature* that LAV and HTLV-3B were "variants of the same AIDS virus."[24]

When Jim Swire saw the declaration, he didn't understand how the government's lawyers had allowed Gallo to sign it. If Gallo had had "twenty-five or thirty" AIDS virus detections prior to Cold Spring Harbor, HHS certainly hadn't provided the evidence to the French.[g] Nor had HHS given Swire a picture of an AIDS virus taken in February 1983 — or, for that matter, any picture of any AIDS virus except LAV.[h] "We told them from the beginning," Swire said, "'just show us the proof and we'll go home.'"

Swire thought it only a question of time until the French went home with the patent in their pocket. But the interference alone could last two years or more, not including appeals, and even if the French were victorious all they would gain was a patent without any back royalties. Reparations and damages would have to be worked out in claims court, and it was there that the question of whether HTLV-3B was LAV really mattered.

In asking the appeals court to reverse Judge Merow, Swire laid it on the line. "Dr. Gallo and certain of his colleagues," Swire said, "essentially took LAV, renamed it HTLV-3 and then claimed and exploited it as their own. . . ."[25] Tom Byrnes, appearing for the government, recoiled at such suggestions. "Egregious," Byrnes said, an "outrageous attempt to impugn the reputations of one of the world's foremost virologist and his coworkers."[26] A theft of the sort suggested by Swire simply hadn't occurred, because "continuing research" had revealed that LAV and HTLV-3B were "two different isolates of the

AIDS virus." For the French to say otherwise was "like saying that because John Wilkes Booth and Abraham Lincoln were both people, they were identical. People they certainly were, identical they equally certainly were not."[27]

The government's lawyers claimed later they had been prisoners of the information provided to them by Gallo. "Here's this guy," one lawyer said, "almost a Nobel prize winner, you walk in his office and see all these awards all over his walls. If he tells us he did something, are we going to question it?"[28]

Although they evidently didn't understand what they were seeing, the HHS lawyers had unmistakable evidence in their files that much of what they, and Gallo, were telling the patent office and the courts simply wasn't true. The HHS General Counsel had the letter from Electronucleonics stating that the Chardon micrograph hadn't been made in February 1983, but on May 26 of that year.[i] It had the box of documents Don Francis had sent Jim Curran in anticipation of Lowell Harmison's visit to CDC.[j] The HHS lawyers even had a copy of the CDC printout showing virtually identical results for Gallo and the Pasteur in the AIDS test comparison.[29]

In addition to the Department of Justice and the HHS Office of General Counsel, Gallo was represented by the NIH legal adviser and, at government expense, the law firm of Cushman, Darby & Cushman.[30] Also at Gallo's disposal were the NCI's Office of Cancer Communications and the Public Affairs Offices of NIH and HHS. But Gallo was nevertheless offended by the Pasteur's employment of "base litigation lawyers and a propaganda ('public relations') firm from New York, designed to promote Montagnier and to hurt me in a way that is unprecedented in science and a bit disgusting."[31] The Pasteur's "malicious treatment" of him, Gallo complained to André Lwoff, and its "deception of the public" must be "unprecedented in contemporary scientific history."

Scarcely had his admonition to Lwoff gone into the mail before Gallo sent off an article to *Scientific American*, declaring that the first blood testing for HIV antibodies had been done not in Paris but by "my colleague M. G. Sarngadharan."[32]

As the patent case ground forward and the principals skirmished in public, Jonas Salk checked into the Ritz Carlton Hotel in Washington and began making phone calls. Salk's wife, Françoise Gilot, a former mistress of Picasso, still kept an apartment in Paris, and at one of Gilot's *soirées* Salk had listened to Don Francis's version of the intractable dispute between Gallo and Pasteur. In the twilight of his career, denied the Nobel Prize and even membership in the National Academy, relegated to the role of figurehead and fund-raiser at his own Institute for Biological Studies near San Diego, Salk was in need of a last triumph.

Salk was a veteran of his own bitter dispute with Albert Sabin over who deserved the credit for eradicating polio from the developed world. Sabin, a veteran laboratory researcher, had publicly derided Salk's less elegant inactivated-virus vaccine, which killed a number of children, as dangerous "kitchen chemistry."

Other colleagues accused Salk of grabbing the spotlight and taking credit for the work of others — allegations reminiscent of those lodged against Gallo.[k] Perhaps for that reason, Salk thought engineering a settlement between Gallo and the French sounded like something he could manage. Jonas Salk's name still opened the most tightly sealed doors. For legal assistance Salk could command the *pro bono* services of a major Washington law firm, and he had only to call the Republican senator from Maryland, Charles McC. Mathias, Jr., to arrange an audience with Otis T. Bowen, a former Indiana governor who had replaced Margaret Heckler as secretary of Health and Human Services.

With his bow ties and white hair, Bowen resembled the country doctor in a Norman Rockwell painting. In fact Bowen was a doctor, the first physician ever to head the cabinet department charged with safeguarding the nation's health. Bowen had cared for his wife of forty-one years during her long, terminal illness with bone cancer, in the end giving her THC, the hallucinogenic ingredient in marijuana, to ease her pain — a fairly radical act for a Republican governor from Indiana.

While Bowen and the HHS lawyers listened, Salk observed that the only impediment to a settlement seemed to be the Pasteur's insistence that it must receive a United States patent for its AIDS test.[33] What did the government really have to lose, Salk wondered, by granting a patent to the French? The American companies licensed to make the Gallo test could continue to sell that test, just as they were doing. The only difference was that Abbott and the other licensees would have some competition, and wasn't the Reagan administration in favor of competition?

Under Salk's proposal, there would be two patents: the existing patent, which would remain in force, and a second patent that would be issued to the Pasteur. Although both would be for the same invention — a situation that would ordinarily necessitate an interference proceeding — Salk's lawyers had assured him that the two patents could co-exist as long as they were owned by a single entity. The entity suggested by Salk was a joint foundation, governed by directors from HHS and the Pasteur. Acting independently of either government, the foundation would receive, pool, and then distribute the royalties generated by both AIDS tests.

A third of the money would flow back to HHS, and another third to the Pasteur. As a public relations gesture, the final third would be used to fund AIDS research projects in the Third World. To resolve the dispute over scientific credit for discovering the AIDS virus, Salk proposed that Gallo and Montagnier co-author an official history of the discovery of HIV.

In order for the dual-patent part of the Salk proposal to fly, Gallo would have to show that he had invented the AIDS blood test independently between September 15, 1983, the date the Pasteur filed its patent application in London, and December 5, when the French filed in the United States. If that were the case, neither the French AIDS test nor the Gallo test would represent "prior art" against the other. But it wasn't the case, because Sarngadharan hadn't performed the first ELISA until January of 1984.

In early September 1986 the HHS lawyers got the news from their outside patent counsel that "The factual predicate underlying the Salk proposal is not met."[34] At the end of September, the HHS sent the French a settlement proposal:[35] Gallo would write a *unilateral* scientific history of his discoveries, to be published by HHS with no input from Montagnier or the Pasteur, which would nevertheless agree to add Gallo's name to its pending patent application — thereby granting HHS co-ownership of the Pasteur AIDS test.

The names of the Pasteur inventors wouldn't be added to the Gallo patent, but Pasteur could continue, through Genetic Systems, to make and sell its test in the United States and to keep the resulting royalties. In return for not very much, the Pasteur would agree to withdraw the interference and drop the claims court case and all other proceedings against the government.[36]

The French reaction was evident in the next communiqué from Michèle Barzach, the minister of health.[37] The French weren't willing to settle for next to nothing, Barzach said. It was still her government's hope that Bowen would reconsider HHS's position, and do it as soon as possible. "Rather than risk a failure that would be incomprehensible in the eyes of public opinion," Barzach told Bowen, "we must pool our efforts to arrive at an additional and particularly outstanding example of Franco-American cooperation in the service of humanity."

Bowen's noncommittal reply reflected his limited understanding of the case, which depended mainly on briefings and memos from the HHS lawyers.[38] The Pasteur AIDS test, the lawyers assured Bowen, "was so unreliable as not to be patentable"— which would have come as news to the FDA and the Red Cross. Allegations that Gallo had used LAV to develop his AIDS test were "totally without merit." LAV was different genetically from HTLV-3B.[39]

Whatever they were telling the secretary, privately the lawyers acknowledged that their primary goal was to keep the French tied up in court. Not settling the case, one lawyer wrote, "keeps Pasteur's position uncertain and could inhibit [the French] from expanding operations out of concern for the HHS patent friction." A settlement would simply enable the French to make more money, whereas keeping the dispute alive placed a "financial burden on Pasteur to maintain the interference and other actions."[40]

Not many scientists thought courtrooms were the right forums for allocating scientific credit, and the scientific community agreed that the Gallo-Pasteur dispute was doing serious harm to the image of science. Two days after the November 1986 elections, a group of Nobel laureates that included David Baltimore, Renato Dulbecco, Salvador Luria, and Howard Temin urged President Reagan to "bring the power of your office, your wisdom, and your humanity to bear in helping to achieve a solution" to the dispute. "Given the grave crisis which AIDS presents," the laureates wrote, "it does not befit the scientific community to be engaged in what appears to be a self-serving dispute."[41]

In appealing to Reagan to do the right thing, the Nobelists were implying that it was up to the American side to find an equitable solution. When Otis Bowen met Michèle Barzach in Paris just before Thanksgiving, the temperature seemed to have warmed. It was absolutely imperative, Bowen said, that the dispute be resolved as quickly as possible.[42] With so many lawyers and scientists filing briefs and giving interviews, it had been impossible for either side to negotiate with a single voice. What was needed, Bowen told Barzach, was a principal who could speak for the Americans and one who could speak for the French. As his point man, Bowen nominated the HHS general counsel, Ron Robertson. The Pasteur chose Ira Millstein. "They would call me up and say, 'Gallo said this, and this one said that,'" Millstein recalled. "I'd say, 'I don't care. Until Robertson tells it to me, I don't hear it.'"[43]

The day before Christmas 1986, the Red Cross's vice president for medical operations, Victor Schmitt, sent the blood center directors a telegram.[44] "We share your concern," it said, "over the continued delay with licensure of Abbott Test Kits. Be assured that if Abbott has not received licensure . . . by 9:00 AM January 19, 1987, we will be prepared to inform you of contingency plans made to ship HTLV-III test kits from an alternate supplier effective January 20, 1987." On January 16, 1987, with only three days left to go, the FDA granted Abbott a product license for its "second-generation" AIDS blood test.[45]

The blood center directors tried to ensure their agency would never again place itself at the mercy of a single supplier.[46] The current contracts for purchasing test kits — 80 percent from Abbott, 15 percent from Genetic Systems and 5 percent from DuPont — would expire on July 1, less than six months away. Henceforth, said the Red Cross ELISA task force, Genetic Systems must "have a significant part of the Red Cross reagent business." No company should be awarded a contract of longer than one year's duration.[47]

The Red Cross invited Genetic Systems to submit a bid for what Terry Bieker, the company's sales manager, described as "mega-volumes" of ELISAs, between three and five million tests a year.[48] Bieker caught the next plane to Washington, where he met Red Cross executives face-to-face and received what Bieker said were personal assurances that the Red Cross would "not return to its exclusive supplier relationship with Abbott."

Less than a month after Bieker's visit, the Red Cross signed a deal with Abbott Laboratories to supply all its AIDS test kits for the next two years.[49] Schmitt explained that Abbott had simply offered the

Red Cross a deal too good to pass up. Genetic Systems would have charged the Red Cross eighty cents per test, while the Abbott test cost the Red Cross only seventy-six cents.[50] "In negotiations," Schmitt reminded Gerry Sandler, "we must avoid letting the benefits available to the majority be compromised by the preferences of the few."[1]

Eight days after the exclusive contract with Abbott took effect, a unit of blood was donated at a community blood bank in Lafayette, Louisiana. According to the new, improved, fine-tuned Abbott ELISA, the blood was negative for HIV. It was shipped to the local hospital, where it became one of fifteen units transfused into Otto Boutte during heart bypass surgery.

The blood had been donated by an early seroconverter, and Otto Boutte later died of AIDS.[51] A few months after Boutte's surgery, Abbott notified the FDA that it was sending the Red Cross yet *another* redesigned AIDS test for evaluation. Enriching the bead with gp41 evidently hadn't done the trick, because the bead in the newest version was enriched with p24, the principal antigen in the Pasteur AIDS test.[52]

"We Were Going to Get Killed"

Determined to lay the groundwork for some kind of settlement, Jonas Salk spent the end of 1986 and the beginning of 1987 shuttling between Robert Gallo and Luc Montagnier, in search of a shared version of history. "It was a very long process," Montagnier said. "Jonas Salk went to see Gallo, he went to see me. We had one or two meetings with all three together, but mostly he went back and forth. Of course we did not agree on all things, and that's why this took so long. The point was the contribution of each party, you see. We didn't see these things from the same point of view."

Gallo was willing to afford the French credit for isolating LAV from Frédéric Brugière, and for Montagnier's presentation of the first blood-test data at Cold Spring Harbor. But in Gallo's version of history the Pasteur's contribution stopped there, while Gallo had crossed the goal line carrying forty-eight isolates of HTLV-3, the H-9 cell line, and the first workable blood test.

In November of 1986 Salk flew to San Francisco, where Montagnier was attending the annual meeting of the American Association of Blood Banks, which like the Red Cross was struggling with the question of whether to continue using the Gallo AIDS test. Between jousts with Max Essex over credit for HIV-2, Montagnier provided Salk with more additions and revisions to the chronology, including more credit to third parties.[a] The last entry in Gallo's latest version concerned the sequencing of HTLV-3 and LAV. "The nucleotide sequence of the AIDS virus genome," it read, "was determined independently at the Pasteur Institute, at the NIH and at Genentech, Inc." To which Montagnier added, ". . . to reveal similarities of isolates examined."

While Salk stitched the history together, a federal appeals court in Washington concluded that Judge James Merow had erred in dismissing the Pasteur's lawsuit and remanded the case to Merow for trial. "Scientists engaged in collaborative research relating to deadly diseases such as AIDS should not be required to await compliance with procurement regulations," the court said, in what sounded like a rebuke.[b]

Now that the French were back in court, Jim Swire could take sworn testimony from Matt Gonda, Sarngadharan, Prem Sarin, Zaki Salahuddin, Ersell Richardson, and Betsy Read. Don Francis, Murray Gardner, and Montagnier could be deposed about the April 1984 meeting in Montagnier's office, and Swire had a long list of questions for Gallo. But Swire most wanted to give Mika Popovic an opportunity, under oath, to resolve such mysteries as how he had chosen the ten samples for the Popovic pool, and what he had meant by $HUT78/v; Ti7.4/v = MOV$. Civil discovery was considerably broader than the Freedom of Information Act, and Swire might even convince the court to order production of the Gallo-Popovic memos and other documents that were being withheld under FOIA.

The prospect of court-ordered discovery gave the Americans a new incentive to settle, and the framework for such a settlement was being assembled by Ira Millstein and Ron Robertson along the lines suggested by Salk, but with a few key modifications.

The names of Luc Montagnier, Françoise Barré, Jean-Claude Chermann, Françoise Brun, and the rest of the Pasteur group would be added as inventors on Gallo's patent, and the names of Gallo, Popovic, and Sarngadharan to the Pasteur's still-pending application, which the patent office, hopefully, would agree to issue. Rather than the two competing but co-existing patents envisioned by Salk, there would be two shared patents. The deal depended on the PTO's willingness to overlook the existence of two patents for the same invention, which might be made easier by the fact that both would be owned jointly by HHS and the Pasteur.[1]

Because the Red Cross had been using the Gallo test almost exclusively, the $4 million in annual royalties being collected by HHS was several times the $500,000 earned by the French. After the redistribution imposed by the settlement, HHS would end up with some $2 million a year, and the Pasteur with about $1.5 million. The French still would hold the short end of the money stick. But it wouldn't be quite so short, and they would have an American patent. All the settlement lacked was an official history.

Jonas Salk had nearly given up hope of working out a history acceptable to both Gallo and Montagnier. "Insanity afloat," was the way Salk described the process to Don Francis. The latest sticking point, Salk said, was the fact that the history mentioned Gallo's name nine times and Montagnier's only eight. Somehow another reference to Montagnier would have to be added, and Gallo had other issues he wanted resolved.[2] Under pressure from their respective governments, Gallo and Montagnier agreed to meet one last time, with no intermediaries present, to make a final stab at resolving their differences.

What proved to be the synergistic moment occurred on Sunday, March 22, 1987, the day before Gallo's fiftieth birthday, in Gallo's room at the Intercontinental Hotel in Frankfurt. Montagnier had been met at the Frankfurt airport by Prakash Chandra, an Indian scientist from the University of Frankfurt who was collaborating with Gallo on the testing of anti-AIDS drugs, and who had driven Montagnier to the hotel.[3]

"We had a meeting in the bar," Montagnier recalled, "and then Gallo came, and we went up to his room. The Intercontinental is like the Hilton. The rooms are not very big. He had a small desk and two chairs. I bought at the airport, at the free-tax shop, a bottle of cognac for him, because I knew it was his birthday. He said that he would not open the bottle of cognac before we finished."

It would be hours before Gallo and Montagnier were finished. Montagnier went straight to the airport and caught the last plane back to Paris. Before leaving, he suggested that Gallo delete two references to his own articles in order to make the number of citations more equal. Gallo agreed, but back in Bethesda he changed his mind.

"Regarding a balance," Gallo wrote Montagnier, "yes, I agree with you, we have 19 and you have 13 on AIDS only. However, you have the earliest and included in my 19 AIDS references are four which have to do with a putative HTLV-1 variant and not with the causative agent. Moreover, in fact there is not a more or less balance in number of lines on the key AIDS papers. Your group has 52. Mine has 33, which is only a little better than half.

"If you include my HTLV-1 (presumed variant) AIDS papers (which does not help me), then we have 39 lines, which is only 3/4 of yours. Finally, not that our group is better, but we did publish many more papers during that key period than any other group. So Luc, it appears it all depends on the angle one looks from. Therefore, I suggest we keep it as we agreed. I think it is fair to both in balance. I have signed it, and please do the same, and let's send it to John Maddox immediately. I have spoken to everyone here and everyone agrees to send it in now."[4]

Gallo ended his letter with "kind regards and looking forward to many future discussions and happy meetings with you." Weary of the fighting, and under mounting pressure from Pasteur to let the settlement go forward, Montagnier let Gallo have his way. "The next thing," John Maddox recalled, "was Bob called up, saying 'We've got our chronology now.' And as I remember, that's how it went. Nothing in writing, entirely by telephone. The stuff came in by fax. They left out a lot of people like Jay Levy. I asked Bob about that afterwards — 'Why did you leave Levy out?' He said, 'He did nothing of any importance at all. Just trivial work.'"

According to Maddox, the chronology that appeared in *Nature* at the end of March 1987[5] was published without peer review, which may explain why it contained a number of factual mistakes, why several names were misspelled, and why portions of the text read as if they had been translated from Chinese.[c] The history also began with a lie. "Both sides wish it to be known," the preamble read, "that from the beginning there has been a spirit of scientific cooperation and a free exchange of ideas, biological materials and personnel between Dr. Gallo's and Dr. Montagnier's laboratories. This spirit has never ceased despite the legal problems and will be the basis of a renewed mutual cooperation in the future."

Thanks to Maddox, Jay Levy was back in. But there was no mention of Gallo's discovery of any AIDS viruses in 1982 or electron micrographs from February 1983, or any of the other representations Gallo and the HHS had made about his research, in court and under oath. Missing as well was Gallo's claim to have first proposed a retrovirus as the cause of AIDS at Cold Spring Harbor in February 1982. The lapses on the French side included Montagnier's omission of Françoise Brun's conclusive results with Peter Piot's Zairian samples in February 1984, and Jean-Claude Chermann's seminal presentation at Park City. "We had so many versions at the end," Montagnier said later. "When you write something many times, you don't see things."

With the history at last in print, the stage was set for the resolution of a dispute that had consumed nearly three years, the attention of two governments, hundreds of thousands of tax dollars,[d] and a healthy portion of scientific credibility. But the same day the history appeared in *Nature*, Gallo informed Otis Bowen that his concern "for the integrity of science" prevented him from agreeing to a settlement, "unless Institut Pasteur officially and Dr. Montagnier specifically dis-associates [*sic*] themselves from the charges made against me and the laboratory in writing."[6]

The cause of Gallo's distress was a ten-page article in the *New Scientist*,[7] the same magazine where Omar Sattaur had raised the first questions about HTLV-3 two years before. The latest issue contained an article by Steve Connor, a thirty-two-year-old Oxford graduate who had inherited the AIDS beat following Sattaur's departure for India in search of personal enlightenment.

Connor had worked on his story for weeks, traveling to Paris for interviews at the Pasteur and to New York to examine the documents obtained by Jim Swire under the Freedom of Information Act. Connor even had wangled an interview with Gallo, during a telephone conversation Connor described as "an uninterrupted half-hour stream of abuse and invective — language like I've never heard in my life, before or since."

While Connor was en route to New York, Gallo's office telephoned his editor, Michael Kenwood, in London to say the interview was off — something Connor discovered only after checking into his Manhattan hotel. When Connor called HHS to protest, he was told he could meet instead with the deputy HHS general counsel, Robert Charrow, the NCI's Peter Fischinger, and Jim Wyngaarden's deputy, William Raub — an experience Connor later described in a letter to *Nature*.[8]

> During this meeting I presented the details of my investigation into allegations that Gallo's virus isolate was one and the same as that of Montagnier, which Gallo insisted had failed to grow in his laboratory. I made it quite clear that, in the opinion of virologists I had interviewed, Gallo had not discovered any new virus and that the only matter to be cleared up was

whether it was deliberate or accidental contamination. The attitude of Dr. Fischinger was of mild amusement. He dismissed the possibility of contamination, despite the strong evidence to the contrary, arguing that the genetic similarities of the two virus isolates was due to chance. He said the suggestions about contamination and the evidence I supplied were nothing new. . . . None of the three officials gave any indication in the course of the discussion that they were interested in pursuing the truth about what went on in Gallo's laboratory at the time of his "discovery." They were more interested in finding excuses and arguments they could use in a court case against the Pasteur. Truth, it seemed to me at the time, was just an inconvenience.

John Maddox declined to publish the letter, but Connor's article in the *New Scientist* reflected the same sentiments.

"In the war against AIDS," it began, "scientific truth was among the first casualties. No one listened when Luc Montagnier at the Pasteur Institute in Paris said that he had found the virus that causes AIDS. Scientific journals and scientists preferred to hear what Gallo was saying from the National Cancer Institute in the US. Gallo said that the AIDS virus belonged to the group of viruses, the HTLVs, on which he established his reputation. He was wrong, but it took a year for people to realise it. In the interim, blood went unscreened, spreading the virus further, a climate of distrust among the key scientists developed, spilling over into the courts. Scientific collaboration itself joined the list of victims."

Connor's article included the pictures of LAV that had been published by Gallo as HTLV-3, and a photocopy of the Gonda-to-Popovic letter from which Gonda's references to LAV had mysteriously been excised. It also quoted Abraham Karpas declaring that "a full year was wasted" because of Gallo's misguided focus on HTLV — a year, according to Karpas, in which "many lives could have been saved, many infections could have been prevented."

The article's centerpiece was the one aspect of the dispute that had been most assiduously avoided by the American press: a sophisticated explication of the genetic identities of LAV and HTLV-3B, and what that implied. But Gallo assured Connor he would "soon publish data on two separate AIDS viruses from two New Jersey men that are even closer to each other than HTLV is to LAV." The "New Jersey pair," Gallo said, would show that it was "possible for such similarity to occur by chance."

Dani Bolognesi, who had tangled with the *New Scientist* over the Sattaur article two years before, expressed "anger, revulsion and disgust" at Connor's account,[9] circulating a "Dear Colleagues" letter imploring Gallo's friends "to respond to the *New Scientist* attack on Bob."[10] It was impossible, Bolognesi wrote the *New Scientist,* "to ignore the damage that Connor's article does, not only to Gallo but to the entire scientific community which is doing its best to unite as it must, in the face of this deadly epidemic of AIDS and its stark prognosis."

Under "pressure" from the Reagan administration,[11] Raymond Dedonder joined HHS in condemning the *New Scientist* article as typical of the "sensationalist journalism and the gross inaccuracies which have appeared recently describing the dispute between the two parties."[12] But just as no one had been able to find anything wrong with what Omar Sattaur had written, no one could say what inaccuracies Connor's article contained.

Gallo demanded that the Pasteur's disavowal be made part of the settlement agreement, and a confidential "side-letter" was drafted. Montagnier refused to sign, but Dedonder did, binding everyone at the Pasteur to a formal, but secret, renunciation of "any statements, press releases, charges, allegations or other published or unpublished utterances that overtly or by inference indicated any improper, illegal, unethical or other such conduct or practice" by any scientists employed by HHS, NIH, or NCI."[13]

With the stroke of a pen, the accusations and contentions of the past two years had been erased. "We signed that we will not go back to court," Dedonder said later, "no matter what evidence comes. That was one of the conditions of the settlement." Jim Swire, who hadn't played a role in the negotiations, thought the Pasteur had been railroaded by HHS. "The disavowals and the secrecy clauses and all that weren't for the benefit of Pasteur," Swire said later. "They were for the benefit of NIH."

Despite his own ultraconservative politics, Swire found himself horrified by the Reagan administration's behavior. "I expected a hard fight from the government," Swire said, "but not the degree of hardball I wound up with. I'm a conservative Republican, and this was a Republican administration we were dealing with. I voted for Ronald

Reagan, twice. But the things his people did were absolutely outrageous — in court, and out of court. Absolutely beyond the pale."

The war was over, and Swire's team of litigators was ordered to stand down and stack arms. Scientific comity was the order of the day, and the impending settlement was blessed by the high priests. In a letter to *Nature,* David Baltimore and the other Nobel laureates decreed that Montagnier and Gallo together had "contributed most to the discovery of HIV and its relation to AIDS. Their work needs to be celebrated and separated from the legal dispute which is being settled through the clarification of the rights and responsibilities of their respective institutions."[14]

Befitting its significance, the official peace proclamation was to be consecrated at a joint White House ceremony by President Reagan and the French prime minister, Jacques Chirac. When Gallo learned of the president's planned announcement, he warned that Reagan shouldn't try to take credit for the settlement. "Gallo said that if the White House tried to imply that they had any hand in forcing the agreement he will go public to denounce such an idea," a worried NCI official informed her boss. "He claims that HE did the lion's share of work to get things settled."[15]

The complexities of retrovirology, not to mention patent law, were beyond most of the reporters who crowded into the White House on Tuesday morning, March 31, 1987, to hear Ronald Reagan herald the beginning of "a new era in Franco-American cooperation." Although the agreement concerned only the patent rights to the AIDS test and nothing else,[e] the media insisted on presenting it, incorrectly, as the resolution of a long and contentious dispute over who had discovered the AIDS virus.

According to the *Washington Post,* the settlement "assigns credit equally to the two labs for discovering the virus and developing the test to detect it."[16] The *Los Angeles Times* read the history as concluding that the French had failed to prove that LAV was the cause of AIDS, "while Gallo's later work enabled researchers to pinpoint the virus as the agent responsible for the deadly disease."[17] Even the usually astute *Wall Street Journal* described the pact as having ended "a 16-month dispute in which the French claimed credit for the discovery of the virus."[18]

Only *Newsweek* got the story right. "Most 'who got there first' disputes in science concern nobody but the scientists," *Newsweek* said.

"But the three-year tussle between United States and French medical researchers over who discovered the AIDS virus and developed the AIDS blood test involves big money for both countries — at least $100 million annually, and probably more as the disease spreads. That may explain why the argument ended last week, not in the pages of a medical journal, but in the Rose Garden of the White House. President Reagan and visiting French Prime Minister Jacques Chirac announced an agreement in which both countries could share profits from the blood test — and historians could decide who found the AIDS virus first."[19]

The settlement resolved the question of who invented the HIV blood antibody test. The names of the French inventors were added to the Gallo patent, and Gallo, Popovic, and Sarngadharan were added to the Pasteur's still-pending application, which the patent office then issued. Each side now owned a United States patent. But the Pasteur's patent bore a filing date of September 15, 1983, seven months before Gallo's patent. It had taken four years, but the French had won the patent race.

To anyone who would listen, Ira Millstein explained that the settlement had *deliberately* failed to address the question of who had discovered HIV and identified it as the cause of AIDS. "We leave that to history," Millstein said. "The scientists felt there had to be winners and losers. People wanted to be vindicated — that they had discovered it, or that they hadn't done anything wrong. There were all sorts of people involved who felt it was extremely important to vindicate their respective national honor, their respective medical honor, the contributions they had made to the state of the art. It was clear we had to settle without saying X won and Y lost."[20]

Gallo celebrated with French champagne.[21] "This has not been good for me or my lab or our state of mind," he said. "We won't have to worry about lawsuits or debates or rivalries. Now, instead of being distracted by all the legal business, I'll be able to return full time to trying to do something about this disease." Before leaving on a post-settlement tour of Europe,[22] Gallo expressed his gratitude to Otis Bowen, "for your support throughout the difficult period and for keeping faith in me and my co-workers. . . . I can tell you that you have a group of scientists with high morale and much enthusiasm for facing the challenges ahead."[23]

Berge Hampar thought the settlement had come just in time. "The government was going to lose," Hampar said later. "We were going to get killed. How can you say Gallo did it before Montagnier did it? You don't have to look at laboratory notebooks. If someone would take the time to read the published literature, it's obvious that he didn't do what he claimed he did at the time he did it. If you look at the published literature, he did not have anything before September of 1983, when he got the French isolate."

Gallo's claim of forty-eight virus isolations had been resurrected in the official history, but Hampar scoffed. "There were forty-eight frozen samples," Hampar said. "I wouldn't argue that. He could have had a hundred and forty-eight, but they were in his freezer because he couldn't do anything with them. They would get this stuff out and they would get it in culture, but what was happening was the cells were dying. He got some AIDS cells and he saw some reverse transcriptase activity, which by itself doesn't mean anything."

Officially, Gallo and the French were codiscoverers of the blood test for HIV. The concept of codiscovery was not unknown to science, but it never had been stretched nearly so far. Watson and Crick, who had worked side-by-side in the same lab, were universally acknowledged as codiscoverers of the double helix. Temin and Baltimore, who had worked independently half a continent apart, would be remembered as the codiscoverers of reverse transcriptase. But Watson and Crick had published together, and Temin and Baltimore within days of one another. Whatever the settlement decreed, it didn't alter the fact that the first AIDS virus had been isolated in Paris a year before its counterpart in Bethesda, or that the first HIV blood-antibody test had been performed at Pasteur six months ahead of Gallo's lab.

Jean-Claude Chermann couldn't comprehend why someone who had chased the wrong virus for so many months was now being anointed in the press as a codiscoverer of the right virus. "Gallo is the winner," Chermann said. "He can be happy. I cannot help thinking, deep inside me, that it was a surrender. With time, everyone would have seen that we were right. Chirac pushed Pasteur to make a compromise."

Raymond Dedonder was well aware that many of his Pasteur colleagues thought he had brought home half a loaf. "Some people in France said that it was not a good agreement," Dedonder recalled, "that we have abandoned everything. It was not perfect, it's true. But if you consider the difficulty to fight in the States — it's a country which is very well protected. It's not a liberal country at all, from that point of view." Dedonder thought the American patent system was weighted too heavily in favor of American inventors — something with which many patent lawyers agreed — and he reminded his critics that he had started out in search of a compromise, not an all-out victory.

"At the beginning," Dedonder said, "I went there to arrive to an agreement. We wanted at the beginning to fight for the principles, and for the public recognition of the work which has been done by the French team. And that I think is now something which really is obtained. At the patent office we probably could have won. It was a good case. Because we had the proof that one year in advance, really, the facts were known on American territory."

Abraham Karpas thought Dedonder's rationalizations were poppycock. "If de Gaulle had been alive," Karpas said, "the French would have gone to court."[24]

High in the mountains of northern New Mexico, a soft-spoken, bearded scientist named Gerald Myers listened as the AIDS virus spoke of where it had been and where it was headed. The Los Alamos National Laboratory, where Myers worked, was the place where the nation's nuclear weapons had been designed — and, at the very beginning of the nuclear age, tested as well. But as the Cold War wound down, Los Alamos had been forced to find other uses for its vast intellectual resources and its formidable supercomputers. In shifting its focus toward the biological sciences, Los Alamos had begun compiling a number of genetic databases.

Since taking charge of the HIV Sequence Database, Gerry Myers had learned to decipher a DNA sequence the way he had once translated Latin and Greek as a classical scholar at St. John's College in nearby Santa Fe. The slightest change in the genetic makeup of the virus — the insertion or deletion of a single nucleotide, the exchange of one nucleotide for another — left a genetic trail that Myers could follow like footprints in the snow.

Myers's rapidly expanding database represented a tapestry of the historical evolution of the AIDS virus, from its presumed beginnings in African monkeys to its current infestation in humans on four continents. The HIV sequence database was an invaluable tool for Myers's principal research interest, tracing the genesis of HIV and its spread across the globe. But it had the more immediate mission of providing AIDS vaccine researchers with information about the virus they hoped to vanquish.

Because the polio virus doesn't mutate very quickly, a polio vaccine made with a virus isolated in Minnesota in 1955 can still protect African children against polio three decades later. The virus influenza A, which changes very fast, requires a new vaccine every year. How long a vaccine made with a particular strain of HIV would remain effective, even against that same strain, depended on the "velocity" of HIV's genetic variability. One of Gerry Myers's goals was to find out how quickly the AIDS virus changed its stripes.

The answer appeared to be very quickly indeed — so quickly that an individual with HIV harbored not just one variant of the AIDS virus, but many distinctive mutants of the original virus with which he or she had become infected. The only known cases where near-identical viruses purportedly had been isolated from different patients were HTLV-3B and LAV, and the New Jersey Pair.

Identical AIDS viruses from separate patients would have represented vitally important knowledge about how HIV behaved. Although Gallo had been talking and writing about the New Jersey Pair for nearly two years, he had refused to publish their DNA sequences.[f] When Gerry Myers finally wrangled the sequence data from Gallo's lab, he understood why. The second member of the pair wasn't an independent isolate after all, just another laboratory contamination.[25]

With the evaporation of the New Jersey Pair, Gallo turned to new data from Lee Ratner, now running his own lab at Washington University in St. Louis, which showed a less than 1 percent genetic variation among thirteen HIV clones from a male blood donor and the two newborn infants who had received his blood.[26] But Myers didn't believe Ratner's data either. "There's something wrong with that paper," he said. "All thirteen of the sequences have the same premature 'stop' codon in exactly the same place."

Myers had fashioned the DNA sequences of each of the genuine HIV isolates into a kind of tree, called a dendogram, illustrating the genetic distances, and therefore the relative degrees of mutation, between viruses isolated at different times and places. Each isolate was represented as a branch attached to the trunk, with HTLV-3$_{MN}$ about in the middle of the tree and HTLV-3$_{RF}$ near the bottom, close to Jay Levy's ARV-2.

It was the general assumption among AIDS researchers that since HTLV-3B had come from a patient in the eastern United States and LAV from a patient in Paris, they must represent a common world-wide strain of HIV. If so, a vaccine made from either 3B or LAV would be most likely to offer wide protection against infection with HIV.

On Myers's tree, however, HTLV-3B and LAV were together at the very top, three or four mutational years away from ARV-2 and R.F., and seven or eight away from the African HIV isolates. Quite apart from being representative strains, 3B and LAV were practically in outer space, which made them the *worst* viruses to use in vaccine development.

But there was something else. When Myers told his computers to treat LAV and 3B as though they had been isolated from different patients, the computers balked. Only when he allowed the two viruses to be viewed as isolates from the same patient did the other branches of the tree fall into place. Like the New Jersey Pair, LAV and HTLV-3B were too much alike to be real.

"Not only were the French being cheated," Myers said later, "the research community was being led to think that the virus was more stable than it was. I was angry, because I felt that, if one made the argument that 3B arose from a pool of blood, it gave the misimpression that the variation of the virus was not so great." As for the origin of HTLV-3B, Myers said, "if you're going to try to reconstruct what happened back in 1983, you better think about contamination."

A week after the announcement by Reagan and Chirac, Gerry Myers sat down at his keyboard. A "double fraud" had taken place, Myers wrote Mal Martin and several of Martin's colleagues at NIAID.[27] The initial fraud had occurred when HTLV-3B and its various clones were declared by Gallo and Popovic to have origins independent of LAV. The second was Gallo's insistence that 3B had been derived from the pooled blood of several patients.

"The probability of either account being true is very very small," Myers said, "and I predict that it will become smaller with each United States isolate sequenced in the future. I suggest that we have paid for this deception in more than the usual ways . . . which we can ill afford during the dog days of an epidemic let alone during halcyon times."

When Myers informed Mal Martin that he intended to present his virus-tree data at the upcoming Third International Conference on

AIDS, he predicted that there would be "realizations." The conclusion that HTLV-3B and LAV had come from the same patient, Myers said, was "hard to avoid, impossible to disguise even if we chose to do so."

At the first international AIDS conference in Atlanta two years before, the focus had been the CDC. The second international conference, in Paris, had been intended to honor the Pasteur. The third international, set to open in Washington, D.C., in June of 1987, was Gallo's moment.

More than six thousand AIDS researchers, three times the number that had gathered in Paris, assembled in the grand ballroom of the Washington Hilton to hear Vice President Bush predict, incorrectly, that the number of heterosexuals infected with HIV would increase dramatically over the next five years.[28] Bush was followed by Lowell Harmison and then by Gallo, who used his keynote address to tell the world of an important new discovery: a third type of AIDS virus, HIV-3, that had been isolated in Nigeria.[29] "New virus tied to AIDS is found in Africa," warned the *New York Times*, which reported that the new virus had been isolated from ten patients in Nigeria, seven of whom had "a disease indistinguishable from AIDS."[30]

Although he hadn't finished characterizing the new virus, Gallo told his audience that it "looks like it can cause AIDS . . . but with less efficiency than the real AIDS virus."[31] The main significance of the discovery, said the *Times*, lay in Gallo's having added "yet another member of the family of viruses that can cause AIDS-like diseases in humans." Montagnier was quoted as "reserving judgment" until more details were forthcoming. But no details would ever be forthcoming, because the "Nigerian AIDS virus" didn't exist.[g]

Partly to Myers's relief, partly to his chagrin, the viral trees he had put on display at the conference attracted virtually no attention. Dendograms were so difficult conceptually that most of the scientists who bothered to examine them didn't comprehend that HTLV-3B and LAV had come from the same patient. Even Lee Ratner, who had presided over the DNA sequencing of HTLV-3B, complained that "I don't understand these trees."

But Myers remained convinced that "time is against Gallo. Every year, as new sequences come out, it becomes clearer and clearer that the LAV and the original NCI isolates had a very recent common ancestor, are closer and closer together," Myers said. "Nobody believes any more that 3B represents pooled distinct viruses. Everybody at NIH has given up on that."

Major medical conferences resemble small, hastily erected cities where thousands of physicians and researchers spend four or five days eating, drinking, sleeping, and attending lectures together before checking out of their hotels and rushing back to their laboratories, clinics and hospitals. Because there are many more attendees than opportunities to speak, most of the research presentations are displayed as printed abstracts mounted on posters that can be inspected at leisure by passersby.

Among the hundreds of abstracts submitted for the Washington conference was one from Jim Mullins at Harvard. Although Mullins was a member of Max Essex's department, the program committee, which included Essex and several of his friends, had consigned his abstract to the conference graveyard, the last "poster session" on the last day, when many researchers would have already departed.

What Mullins's data showed was that HTLV-4, the "second AIDS virus" Essex claimed to have discovered the year before, and for which he had shared the Lasker Prize with Gallo and Montagnier, wasn't a human virus after all.

A few months before the Washington conference, Mullins and his colleagues had published a paper in *Nature*[32] that raised a red flag about the provenance of $STLV-3_{AGM}$, the African green monkey virus Essex also claimed to have discovered,[33] observing that it was virtually identical to a virus called $STLV-3_{MAC}$ previously discovered in rhesus macaques.[h] But when Mullins's graduate students compared HTLV-4 with the green monkey virus, they too were identical.[i]

The recognition that his own departmental chairman had experienced, at best, an accidental three-way contamination put Mullins in the most awkward position of his young career. "I was worried," Mullins admitted. "I remember sitting here in my office with about five of my students and saying, 'If we decide to do this, it's going to be a nightmare.' But we couldn't let it go. It was too exciting. So we decided to do it and boy, do I regret it. I regret the anguish very much. If I had to do it over again, I wonder. I would do it again, only I would do it a lot quicker and cleaner."

Similar comparisons were under way in Gallo's lab that included Essex's green monkey virus, HTLV-4, and $LAV-2_{FG}$, a virus isolated in Paris from a Guinea-Bissau native named Fernando Gomez. Because there weren't any West African AIDS patients in the United States, for Gallo coming up with a LAV-2 isolate had proved a challenge. According to Françoise Brun, who had isolated LAV-2$_{FG}$, Gallo had prevailed on Daniel Zagury to acquire a sample of Gomez's blood, without her knowledge or the permission of the hospital where Gomez lay dying.[j]

In honor of Zagury, Gallo renamed the Gomez virus "NIH-Z."[k] When Beatrice Hahn compared the green monkey virus with HTLV-4 and NIH-Z, she got the same results as Jim Mullins: the monkey virus and HTLV-4 differed "only by a few restriction enzyme sites," while NIH-Z — really LAV-2 — was quite different from both.[34] It looked like the French had found the second AIDS virus and Max Essex had another big problem.

Gallo, who had ordered Murray Gardner to leave the comparison of HTLV-3B and LAV alone, showed Max Essex no quarter. Beatrice Hahn's paper professed "surprise"— the scientific equivalent of raised eyebrows — at "the remarkable similarity" between STLV-3$_{AGM}$ and HTLV-4. The two viruses, the paper concluded, were "not independent isolates"[35] — precisely what François Clavel had suspected on seeing the blots in Essex's HTLV-4 paper the year before.

As events unfolded, a few months before his "discovery" of the green monkey virus, Essex had asked the discoverer of the rhesus macaque virus, Muthiah Daniel at Harvard's New England Regional Primate Center, for a sample of STLV-3$_{MAC}$. In Essex's lab, Daniel's macaque virus had somehow been transformed into Essex's new green monkey virus, which had somehow become HTLV-4, the second human AIDS virus isolated from Senegalese prostitutes. But both of Essex's discoveries were just Muthiah Daniel's STLV-3$_{MAC}$.

Essex and his principal assistant, Phyllis Kanki, continued to write and speak about HTLV-4, later renamed HIV-2, as though it were a new human retrovirus.[36] That ended when *Nature* published the last word on the Essex affair from Muthiah Daniel and his colleagues at the Harvard primate center.[37] "Isolates previously referred to as STLV-3$_{AGM}$ and HTLV-4 by others," the group declared, were "not authentic." Both had been "derived" from a sample of STLV-3$_{MAC}$. Cross-contamination of viral cultures, observed Daniel's boss, Ron Desrosiers, who had given Essex the STLV-3$_{MAC}$ over Daniel's objections, "could happen in any lab. But it's unfortunate that it has been so extensive."[38]

To *Nature*, Essex and Kanki gingerly acknowledged "the results of others," agreeing "that certain isolates initially reported by us as

HTLV-4 should be considered [STLV-3] unless proven otherwise."[l] An embarrassed Harvard dropped its claim for the American patent on HIV-2, which was promptly awarded to Pasteur and François Clavel.[m] When a Japanese group isolated the real African Green Monkey virus a couple of years later, it proved to be vastly different from the human AIDS virus.[39] The "missing link" between monkey and man turned out to be a chimpanzee lentivirus, analyzed by Simon Wain-Hobson, closely related to HIV-1.[40]

Within a year, Jim Mullins was running a lab at Stanford. When Harvard chose a director for a new university-wide institute designed to expand and accelerate its AIDS-related research, it picked the man Harvard president Derek Bok referred to as "that nice Dr. Essex."[41]

Marc Alizon didn't see why the genetic relationship between HTLV-3B and LAV had been exempted from scientific scrutiny, while the same questions about Max Essex's research received a full airing in the scientific journals. "HTLV-4 and STLV-3$_{MAC}$ had more than 99 percent sequence identity," Alizon said, "so everyone concluded they were identical and HTLV-4 was a contaminant.

"If you compare LAV and HTLV-3B you have the same sequence similarity. Many, many isolates have been sequenced now, and no one has found two viruses so close. But you cannot conclude anything, because there is a settlement between the Pasteur Institute and NIH."

It had taken several months to put the pieces of the Franco-American settlement in place, but before the ratification ceremony could get under way in Paris a few items still required resolution. In September 1987, HHS filed a petition with the patent office to "correct" the inventorship of the Gallo patent; to the administration's relief, the PTO concluded that HHS, "through error and without deceptive intent," had incorrectly limited the inventors of the AIDS test to Gallo, Popovic, and Sarngadharan. The "error" was corrected by adding Montagnier, Chermann, Françoise Barré, Françoise Brun, and Christine Rouzioux as co-inventors on the American patent, and Gallo, Popovic, and Sarngadharan to the French application — the same application which, the government had assured the patent office during the interference, failed to disclose a method of detecting AIDS antibodies.

Two weeks before the ratification ceremony, the Institut Pasteur was awarded United States Patent No. 4,708,818 for its blood-antibody test for HIV. The filing date on the French patent remained December 5, 1983, four months before the date on the Gallo patent. Although the AIDS test was now a joint discovery, the French had discovered it first.

The settlement notwithstanding, the newspapers and magazines continued to laud Gallo as the discoverer of the AIDS virus, while rarely mentioning Montagnier. As one of the few scientists whose name was immediately recognized by most newspaper editors and television producers, whatever Gallo said was likely to make news. Not counting his $100,000 annual patent royalty, Gallo's salary reportedly topped $208,000, a handsome sum for a civil servant.[42] His laboratory's budget had swelled to $10 million a year, enough to support a dozen university research labs.[43] Still, Gallo complained to David Remnick of the *Washington Post* that the settlement hadn't dispelled "the bizarre accusations" and "the flashes of hatred" from some of his colleagues.[44]

"I can't tell you how much the criticism hurts," Gallo said. "Even the outlandish, absurd stuff from people who don't know the least thing about science. My colleagues say I should let it pass and concentrate on science. But it hurts. Why should I tell you any different? It wounds. The people that know — they understand I'm doing everything I can. And we've had amazing success.

"But then the other stuff," Gallo went on. "I'm telling you, there are days when I wake up in the morning and feel like the archangel Gabriel. By the time I go to bed at night, I feel like Lucifer. What's going on? Please, tell me why they do this to me. Why do they say these terrible things about me? Do you know? Do you?"

• 15 •

"The Whole Thing Was Sordid"

Exiled from the Centers for Disease Control in Atlanta, Don Francis had been given a hastily created job as the CDC's liaison to the California Department of Health Services, across San Francisco Bay from Marin County where he had grown up. In helping to coordinate California's response to the AIDS epidemic, Francis had gotten to know Randy Shilts, a reporter for the *San Francisco Chronicle* and the first American journalist to cover AIDS as a full-time assignment.

As Francis gradually unburdened himself of the previous four years, Shilts realized there was an important story to be told. Guided by Francis's correspondence and memos, Shilts, who was HIV-positive himself, wove a chronological account of the early years of the epidemic, the response of the government and the blood banks, and the decimation of the gay community.[a] The *New York Times* called *And the Band Played On* a "heroic work of journalism." The *Boston Globe* compared it to Truman Capote's *In Cold Blood*.

More than any other event, Shilts's book moved the AIDS epidemic to the center of the public policy stage. The search for the AIDS virus was only one of several interlocking themes, and Shilts's characterization of Robert Gallo was relatively mild, a portrait of an intensely focused researcher whose "temper and arrogance" made him "a formidable enemy to disease." Gallo had been the target of less kind words, but when he saw Shilts's book he went on the attack. "It never ceases to me to be a source of great wonder," Gallo said, "how people such as a gay young man on the West Coast can think they know more when they're stimulated by the same two people over and over and over and over again. Namely Don Francis and what I would regard as a psychotic who lives in Cambridge."

After years of sparring with Francis in the press, Gallo thought the time had come to confront him directly. "Thank you for your letter of October 6 and your good intentions," Gallo wrote Francis after Shilts's book had been in print for less than a month.[1] "I must ask you to do more, however. The 'old wounds,' as you described them, are reopened weekly with further republication in new books and articles of the false and defamatory statements that plague me and my staff, deeply hurt us and distract us from the collaborative conquest of AIDS to which we are so committed. We must now spend all of our time gaining a complete understanding of and control over AIDS, and we must develop a vaccine. But the libels are interfering, and each time I examine an author . . . about his preconceptions, your name comes up as the principal source in every single case. I want to truly put this behind us in a way that helps secure the future."

Gallo attached a letter for Francis to sign. "I have reviewed in considerable detail," it began, "the public record setting forth the history of the discovery and characterization of the virus causing AIDS. This record unequivocally sets out the fine cooperative efforts between you and the National Cancer Institute on the one hand, and Luc Montagnier and the Pasteur Institute on the other. Unfortunately, I realize that a number of my comments concerning the work leading to the discovery of HTLV-3/LAV . . . are incorrect and were made without full knowledge on my part. Accordingly, I wish to set the record straight as to my understanding of your work. . . . I do not believe that your original isolates of HTLV-3 were contaminated, either accidentally or on purpose, by LAV. There is no evidence whatsoever to support the notion that HTLV-3 was pilfered in this fashion."

The letter ended with a profuse apology from Francis "for the tone of many of my remarks in the past. They have done you, our colleagues and the international scientific collaboration against AIDS an unwarranted disservice. NIH and the Pasteur Institute have worked to clear the air and I wish to join with others, like the scientists whose Correspondence appeared in the March 1987 *Nature,* to congratulate you in your work, and to urge you to continue to devote your fullest efforts in [*sic*] the fight against AIDS."

When Francis didn't reply, his secretary got a telephone call from Gallo.[2] Unless Francis signed the letter, Gallo had a "plan to take action against Don Francis." Gallo had "tapes and letters," and he was prepared to "expose" Francis's financial dealings "and his profit with Randy Shilts's book." If Francis wanted "notoriety," he "should work harder in his field." People inside and outside the government "have things written about Don Francis" that Gallo intended to "expose." Above all, Francis should understand that this was "the most important thing in my life."

Potentially most damaging was Gallo's accusation that Francis stood to gain financially from the considerable success of Shilts's book. From Shilts and his publisher, Francis obtained written denials that he had ever been paid any money, or ever would be paid.[3] But there was nothing Francis could do about Gallo's insinuations that there were "a couple of things in Don Francis's personal life that shouldn't see the light of day."[4]

When it became clear Francis had no intention of signing Gallo's letter, word reached Berkeley that he was being transferred back to CDC headquarters in Atlanta — to work not on AIDS, but on tuberculosis. Francis had just bought a house in the San Francisco suburb of Hillsborough, and his wife, Karen, had an important job at Genentech and detested Atlanta. Only appeals for clemency from Jonas Salk and several California politicians saved Francis's career at the CDC. As one of Francis's supporters recalled, "California told HHS, 'We spend more than any other state on AIDS and you haven't done a damn thing for us except send us Don Francis.'"

The day after his call to Francis's secretary Gallo was en route to the University of Toronto, to collect the prestigious Gairdner Prize, Canada's top award for medicine, with Luc Montagnier. From Toronto Gallo flew to Paris, Vienna, Florence, Rome, and Jerusalem,[5] and when he returned to Bethesda he dropped a bombshell. To the *Washington Post*, Gallo confided that he was on the verge of leaving NIH and the National Cancer Institute, to run an AIDS research institute of his own at Johns Hopkins University in Baltimore.[6] "I have never crossed the emotional boundary lines before," Gallo said. "But now I have. It will be an emotional thing for me to leave here. It has been my home."

There had been rumors for years about Gallo's impending departure from NIH, and the cumulative effect on Gallo's staff was unsettling. "Every year that I worked there, there was a rumor that he was going somewhere," recalled one Gallo assistant. "To Duke. To Hopkins. To Europe. To California. And when I was supporting my husband in medical school and needed this job, this used to send me into a tailspin. Because the tuition was very expensive. So I used to go into his office and say, 'What the hell is going on here? I just heard you were leaving and I'd appreciate some notice. Because if I'm losing my job I'd like to know about it.' And he would always say, 'Oh, yes, I'm considering going there and I have this offer and that offer. But I certainly haven't made up my mind. And if I do make up my mind I'll sure tell you about it.' So after year six, when he was still there, I stopped listening to these rumors."

If Gallo's leak to the *Post* was a trial balloon, it was quickly punctured. A Johns Hopkins spokesman denied that the university had made Gallo such an offer, and members of the Hopkins faculty seemed less than eager to welcome Gallo into their ranks. "There are a lot of egos in Baltimore," one faculty member observed. "His would take up a lot of room."[7]

Vince DeVita had grown weary of seeing Gallo's name in the newspapers. "He was always creating problems," DeVita said. "There was always some crisis with Bob Gallo. There was always a problem with the press. I used to tell him not to talk to the press. He has an arrogance about him, that he felt he could talk to you and persuade you to his way of thinking. And he almost always failed. There was always some crisis in the newspaper with Bob Gallo having said something about Africa. I was dealing with one crisis after another."

The latest was a complaint from Howard Temin, who had noted a "general impression in the community" that Gallo was reluctant to share his viruses and other research materials with potential competitors.[8] Gallo had been chary of releasing HTLV-1 to other labs, and overly careful about who received HTLV-3 and H-9. But Gallo's refusal to contribute his HIV isolates to an NIH AIDS repository prompted David Baltimore to join Temin in worrying that "Bob's way of handling himself does significant harm to both himself and to the national AIDS effort."[9]

Gallo "controls so many resources," Baltimore reminded DeVita, "that he has a special responsibility to be cooperative." DeVita assured Baltimore that he was "very much aware of [Gallo's] tendencies," and that he had "worked hard to box off any abuse of resources" relating to "the personality conflicts you mentioned earlier."[10] But by the end of 1987, DeVita had concluded that if his star scientist were to leave the NCI, "it wouldn't be the end of the world."

"If they wanted Bob," DeVita said later, "they, being Duke and Johns Hopkins and so on, they could have him. We couldn't do any more for Bob Gallo than we'd already done. There were plenty of people behind him that were really quite good, a lot of young talent. No matter what happened, should he win a Nobel Prize or anything like that, he had done his work at the cancer institute. You go to NCI, you spend a period of time there, you do a piece of work in that special environment, and you move on. I would not have been unhappy to see him leave."

Parrying DeVita's thrust, Gallo let the *Wall Street Journal* know he was also "in discussions" with Robert Maxwell, the British publishing magnate whose holdings ranged from the lowbrow *Daily Mirror* to the highbrow Pergamon Press.[11] Despite his reputed billion-pound fortune, a Military Cross for gallantry in the Second World War and service as a member of parliament, Maxwell, a Czech émigré whose birth name was Jan Ludwig Hoch, had never won from his British peers the respect he felt he deserved. Dubbed the "Bouncing Czech," both for his avoirdupois and his frenetic business style, Maxwell was approaching the end of his career and wished to leave as his legacy a cure for AIDS.

Maxwell had pledged $75 million to fund a Maxwell Institute for AIDS Research, and Lowell Harmison had convinced Maxwell that Gallo was the man to run it — with Harmison's help. "Maxwell first met Harmison at an AIDS conference Maxwell hosted," recalled Peter Jay, the former British ambassador to Washington, who had signed on as Maxwell's chief of staff. "Harmison was there as the HHS representative, a very high-profile guy. He made a very strong impression on the people at this conference."

Yale and Johns Hopkins weren't interested in Gallo, but Robert Maxwell evidently was quite serious. In mid-September 1987, a corporation named MC-270 ("MC" for Maxwell Communications, "270" for I-270, the biotechnology corridor between Bethesda and Frederick) paid the Gillette safety razor company $16 million for a warehouse in North Bethesda. A few days after the sale Gallo was in Oxfordshire, where Maxwell maintained his country manse and where Gallo found the billionaire "a charming, brilliant man."[12] According to Peter Jay, shortly after their meeting papers were drawn up, paving the way for Gallo to become scientific director of the Maxwell Institute for AIDS Research.

Faced with competition for Gallo's services, the NIH director, Jim Wyngaarden, began searching for some way to hold on to "the single most active and productive and creative person in AIDS research,"[13] the scientist the *New York Times* described as "a strong candidate" to become the NIH's first Nobel laureate in more than a decade.[14]

When Wyngaarden asked Gallo what it would take to keep him at NIH, Gallo replied that he wanted his own NIH institute. Besides his profound annoyance at Wyngaarden's intercession in what DeVita considered an NCI personnel matter, DeVita felt his own authority being undercut. "It irked me," DeVita said later, "that NIH, which at the time of HL-23 would have been happy to see Gallo go, now was asking me to make commitments to him that I couldn't make, including the creation of a private institute on the NIH campus. There were lots and lots of people — congressmen, Senator Kennedy, anybody who thought they, for whatever motive, should get involved, who were trying to think of ways to save Bob Gallo at the NIH."

In the end, Robert Maxwell was dissuaded by what Peter Jay termed "Gallo's ability to attract controversy." Not long after the deal evaporated, workers arriving on a Monday morning at HHS headquarters discovered that Lowell Harmison had resigned abruptly the previous Friday and spent the weekend cleaning out his office. Harmison's office was sealed and the locks changed, but it was too late.[15] Gone were all of Harmison's files relating to Gallo's research and the Pasteur dispute. The missing files were never recovered.[b]

Without Gallo at his side, Harmison made a seamless transition to his new job as a senior aide to Robert Maxwell. "Lowell was building his empire," recalled Steve Mendel, who then headed the Western America division of Maxwell Communications. "He was going to be the grand master of the medical sciences wing of the Maxwell organization." But Maxwell's fascination with science and medicine seemed to wane as quickly as it had come, and soon Harmison was gone as well. "I felt a little sorry for Lowell," Peter Jay said. "As the relationship seemed to cool he found it difficult to get answers to his communications."

What seemed a lack of interest on Maxwell's part may have been simply a cash-flow crisis. Following his November 1991 death from a heart attack after plunging from his yacht into the Mediterranean, it was discovered that Maxwell had looted the pension funds of his newspaper and other holdings to prop up the stock price of Maxwell Communications and provide collateral for an increasingly tenuous portfolio of bank loans. At the time of Maxwell's death, his assets were significantly less than his liabilities.[16]

While rumors of Gallo's imminent departure swirled in the American and European press,[17] a regiment of senior American officials converged on Paris for the ratification of the Franco-American accord. Despite the egalitarian tone of the settlement, Gallo was once again claiming full credit for the discovery of the cause of AIDS. Montagnier might have been first "to describe what would *later* be demonstrated to be the AIDS virus," Gallo said.[18] "But in this business, it is not enough to believe that you know something. You have to demonstrate it to your peers by publishing in the scientific literature." Gallo's favorite quote had become one from Sir William Osler: "Credit belongs to the man who proves a discovery to the scientific world."[c]

The ranking American official in Paris was Don Newman, the undersecretary of Health and Human Services, and the ceremony was tightly scripted. "The United States Delegation," the scenario read, "will depart from the Embassy at 10:30 A.M. The Ambassador and Mr. Newman will depart from the Embassy at 10:40 A.M. in the Ambassador's car. Upon arrival at the Historic Building of the Pasteur Institute, #25 rue du Docteur Roux, the cars will drive into the compound, past the guardhouse and up to the main entrance stairs.

"The Ambassador and Mr. Newman will then proceed up two short flights of stairs to enter the building. At this point there should be greeters to direct Ambassador. After entering the building, the Ambassador and Mr. Newman will enter the door to their immediate left. This is the 'Grand Bibliothèque.' There will be a table along the back wall, facing the door, with place cards indicating where each participating dignitary should sit."[19]

A general welcome would be offered by Raymond Dedonder. The HHS general counsel, Ron Robertson, and his Pasteur counterpart, Alain Gallochat, would explain the settlement agreement. Montagnier and Gallo would make "statements of collaboration." Robert Windom, a portly Florida physician known as "Doc," who had replaced Jim Mason as assistant HHS secretary, would announce the creation of a French and American AIDS foundation to receive the patent royalties.

Ira Millstein would explain the World AIDS Foundation, the entity created to disburse the royalties.[d] Newman and Michèle Barzach would deliver closing remarks, after which Dedonder would host a festive champagne luncheon.

It was as if the preceding five years had been wiped from the calendar. With Newman's opening statement, the Reagan administration seemed to renounce the solemn representations it had made to the news media, the patent office, and the courts about the failure of the French to have discovered anything.

"Seven years ago," Newman began, "we were unaware of the disease's existence. Within three years scientists at Pasteur and NIH not only hypothesized the cause of the disease, but also isolated the viral agent and then unequivocally proved the causal link. Following that, scientists at both Pasteur and NIH, men such as Luc Montagnier and Robert Gallo, were able to develop the antibody test kit which would be used not only to screen blood to ensure its safety, but also to assist physicians in diagnosing the ailment."[20]

Even the National Cancer Institute seemed to have forgotten the Fischinger report and the assurances it had permitted the government to make on Gallo's behalf. "The antibody test," the NCI's briefing memo read, "was the joint discovery of the Robert Gallo (American) team and the Luc Montagnier (French) team."

Had HHS and NCI taken the same stance on the day Raymond Dedonder arrived in Washington twenty-eight months before, there would have been no dispute. Now the French were semivictorious, but the Pasteur's immediate gain from the fifty-fifty royalty split was wiped out by the legal bills from Jim Swire, Ira Millstein, and Charlie Lipsey. "The whole thing was sordid," said Claudine Escoffier. "Millions of dollars were spent on both sides to pay lawyers. It would have been much better to invest them in science."[e]

Once the ratification was in the can, Gallo began denying — again — that Popovic had ever succeeded in growing the LAV samples from Paris. HTLV-3B *couldn't* be LAV, Gallo told *JAMA*, because Popovic had never received "enough LAV to infect a cell line and so grow out the virus in amounts needed for an antibody test to be developed."[21]

Not long after the American delegation returned to Bethesda, an urgent-sounding fax appeared on Peter Fischinger's machine.[22] One of Gallo's friends in Europe, Fritz Deinhardt of the Max von Pettenkofer Institute in Munich, had sent Fischinger several pages from a book that had just been published in Germany. "There is concern," Fischinger warned Bob Windom, that the book "is damaging to the perception of the U.S. contribution to the discovery of the AIDS virus."[23] According to Fischinger, the book not only resurrected "many old allegations which have been dealt with in our Franco-American agreement," it offered "a particularly negative picture of the NIH's role, to the degree where many of the innuendoes of the earliest French legal assertions are taken as fact."

The author of *AIDS — Vom Molekul zur Pandemie — "*AIDS — From Molecule to Pandemic"— was a soft-spoken physician named Michael Koch, who had emigrated from Germany to Sweden in the late 1960s and spent twenty years as chief medical officer of a Swedish health district. Koch, whose four previous books included the first medical textbook in Swedish on AIDS, had met Gallo at a conference a few years before, and he remembered how Gallo's demeanor had changed when he discovered that Koch lived in the land of the Nobel Prize. "Suddenly he began to be very, very friendly," Koch said, "and without any distance anymore. I was his 'good friend,' and 'please come,' and 'keep in touch,' and so forth. I felt a little bit uncomfortable, because many Swedes have had similar experiences. There is a certain suspicion which is created by this behavior."

Koch's next encounter occurred shortly before the Naples meeting from which Gallo had withdrawn after learning Abraham Karpas was on the program. "Gallo saw my name on the list of speakers," Koch said, "and he told me not to go there. 'They are criminals,' he said. I laughed. He said, 'I warn you, there will be terrible consequences for your scientific work.'" Koch was not easily deterred, and in Naples he was surprised to find "a lot of distinguished scientists" from around the world, including Montagnier and Simon Wain-Hobson.

"You were the first one who ever tried to manipulate me," Koch wrote Gallo upon returning home. "When it didn't work, I was removed from your list of 'cooperative' Swedes and placed on some other list. Did you really think this would change my mind? In so [*sic*] case you don't know much about this part of the world. . . . You got me to consider that the opinion of others about you might be right."[24]

Koch was already at work on *Vom Molekul zur Pandemie,* an account of the AIDS epidemic and the current state of knowledge about the virus. After his run-in with Gallo and conversations with other scientists about Gallo's research, Koch expanded his chapter on the discovery of HIV to take account of Gallo's early AIDS research. "Gallo had the wrong idea and the Paris group had the virus," Koch said later. "He was so fond of his own ideas that he saw evidence when there was no evidence. He fought one year, and then he gave up. He suddenly understood: Gonda was right, the Paris group was right, this damned Karpas was right."

In dissecting Gallo's publications, Koch uncovered some anomalies and discrepancies that others had missed.[f] But the focus of the chapter was the genetic identity of HTLV-3B and LAV. Koch stopped short of accusing Gallo of having stolen the French virus. "I would never claim that Gallo did a scientific fraud," he said. "They could be real mistakes, laboratory contaminations. This field of research is very difficult. Of course you can have laboratory contamination. Of course you can publish wrong data. But the question is, how do you react? Do you recall it and say it was a mistake? Or do you try to talk about it as if you never said it?"

A few months before Koch's book was published, he encountered Gallo for the last time, at a symposium in Geneva. "He tried to put real pressure on me," Koch recalled. "He told me that we should be friends and he would like to be my friend. But then suddenly he changed his tone and took out an envelope from his pocket. He said, 'But on the other hand here is a five-step program to destroy you. You, your job, your position, your damned Carnegie Institute in Stockholm.' Then, after three or four minutes in this style, he suddenly put it back again and became very warm and friendly. He said, 'But you see, I don't want to do all this. Please tell me if I have made a mistake.' It was cold, hot, cold, hot — a changing bath of threats and flattery. Really extraordinary."

According to Peter Fischinger, Koch's book threatened the settlement with the French, as well as "scientific reputations." Gallo liked what he read even less. "At first glance," Gallo said, "the work appears only to be a popularized picture-book about the AIDS crisis; initial translations, however, reveal that *Herr Koch* has adopted and is spreading some of the more pernicious lies about the work undertaken at our laboratories and the integrity of both the scientists here and the Department itself."[g]

In hopes of neutralizing Koch's book, Gallo began firing off letters to a number of prominent Swedes. "In view of the author's background and complete lack of primary knowledge on the history," Gallo wrote, "I do not feel he was qualified to write such a book. Moreover, Koch has no experience in retrovirology and when I recently met him, it was clear that he lacked an understanding of the field. . . . [I]t is particularly disturbing to realize that this report comes from Sweden, since I feel the Swedish scientific community is highly regarded for their neutrality. . . ."[25]

Despite Gallo's failure to identify any "pernicious lies," HHS dispatched a menacing, six-page letter to his German publisher.[26] Signed by Robert Windom and Ron Robertson, the letter expressed "serious concerns" that Koch's book contained "significant scientific, historical and legal errors which may not only undermine its overall utility as a legitimate scientific publication, but also reflect adversely on your firm's reputation."

Such a letter to any publisher from two senior executives of HHS was by itself extraordinary. More extraordinary were the assertions Windom and Robertson made in Gallo's behalf. Gallo had never "suggested, let alone advocated, that HTLV-1 was the cause of AIDS," the letter declared. Nor had he been "less than fully candid when he stated that the LAV specimen sent to him by Montagnier did not survive." The only actual error to which Windom and Robertson were able to point was Koch's statement that the Gallo AIDS-test patent had been granted in January 1985 rather than May of that year. They nevertheless urged Koch's publisher to "seriously consider deleting any polemic statements that impugn the integrity of the United States, its agencies and by implication its employees."

If that weren't enough, the letter concluded with a threat: "It should be noted that the errors in question may be viewed by some as defamatory, thereby possibly subjecting the author, your firm and its distributors to such civil actions as the aggrieved private individual may deem appropriate." In case that didn't give Koch's publisher pause, Koch's book, "if introduced into commerce" in the United States, "would violate certain provisions of the United States Copyright Act of 1976 and the Lanham Act of 1947."[h]

It was too late to stop the German edition of Koch's book, of which 30,000 copies already were in print, but there was still time to prevent the publication of a far more damaging English-language translation. The ink on the Windom-Robertson letter had scarcely dried when the Oxford University Press, which had commissioned a translation, advised Koch's editor that it no longer wished to be his English-language publisher.[27] When Koch approached the Cambridge University Press, Gallo's administrative assistant, Howard Streicher, sent editors there a copy of the Windom-Robertson letter, with the added caveat that the German edition "has created rather widespread concern among our scientific colleagues and public health officials as well as the legal counsel of the Department of Health and Human Services." In Streicher's opinion, Koch's book was "both maliciously damaging to several members of the scientific community and likely to be scientifically, historically and medically unsound."[28] In less than a week, Cambridge had backed off as well; Michael Koch's book was never published in English.[29]

Lost amidst the threats and bluster was a remarkable admission. Responding to Koch's suggestion that the cancer institute had "downplayed the achievements of the Pasteur scientists," Windom and Robertson invoked the CDC's blood-test comparisons as evidence that the United States government had indeed done the right thing by the French.

"Under the auspices of the Centers for Disease Control in Atlanta, Georgia," they wrote, "a series of blind tests was undertaken to ascertain whether the sera from patients with AIDS contained antibodies to HIV. Of significance is the fact that both NCI and Pasteur participated in these tests. Each laboratory was provided with sera and asked to judge whether each specimen contained antibodies to the virus. The results of those tests unequivocally established that HTLV-III/LAV was the presumptive causative agent of AIDS."

Two years before, such an admission from the government would have thrown the patent interference to the French. But the settlement was inscribed in history, and there was no looking back.

By the mid-1980s the proliferation of scientific and medical journals, which by some estimates numbered 25,000, had spawned yet another journal, this one dedicated to reproducing for busy scientists the tables of contents of the most prominent publications. *Current Contents* was the brainchild of the Institute for Scientific Information in Philadelphia, which also kept track of how often published articles were subsequently cited in other articles. On the assumption that the articles cited most often represented the most significant achievements in science, the ISI's *Citation Index* had become the scientific community's index of how its members' careers were faring.

It was a flawed assumption, since the most-cited papers of all are "methods" papers, in which someone reports having worked out a new and better way of performing a standard laboratory task, and which are included as automatic footnotes whenever that experiment is described. The most-cited paper since 1945, referenced 187,652 times in subsequent articles, describes a test for measuring proteins with the Folin phenol reagent.[30] But when the ISI calculated which scientist had been most cited by others during the 1980s, the hands-down winner was Gallo, who had been an author on each of the four *Science* articles published in May 1984, at least one of which was cited in virtually every subsequent article about AIDS — a whopping total of 36,789 citations in just six years.[31]

The trophy of Citation King earned a place on Gallo's mantel next to the General Motors prize, the Japan Prize, the Gairdner Prize, and a brace of Lasker Awards. But the two honors Gallo coveted most were still missing, the Nobel Prize and election to the National Academy of Sciences.

The Academy is divided into sections according to scientific specialty: physiology, microbiology, anthropology, astronomy, and so on. Once a year, the members of each section propose candidates for membership to their respective selection committees, which then choose from those submissions the names to be put forward on that year's general ballot. Gallo had been proposed for membership at the section level several times, but each time the committee had declined to pass his name along. With the Pasteur dispute behind him the moment seemed auspicious, and in May 1988 Gallo joined George Todaro, Harold Varmus, Ed Scolnick, and a few dozen other distinguished cancer researchers as a member of the Academy's section on medical genetics, hematology, and oncology.[32]

Gallo's election came through a rarely used process called voluntary nomination, which circumvented the selection committee and placed his name directly on the general ballot via a petition signed by twenty Academy members. "We had a hell of a time getting him in," recalled one of the signatories, the University of Chicago's Leon Jacobsen, who had circulated the nominating petition along with Ludwik Gross and Hilary Koprowski, an elderly Polish-born virologist at the Wistar Institute in Philadelphia with whom Gallo had been collaborating for years in a futile effort to link HTLV with multiple sclerosis.[i]

"People are jealous of him," said Jacobsen, who had fond memories of Gallo as a young intern. "I think that's the principal problem. He's published six or seven hundred papers, and he runs a big show. He doesn't know that I talked to a lot of people and tried to overcome some of these people who are against him, not because of his work, but just on principle. Whether he was doing too much or publishing too many papers. You know, these things get on some people's nerves, I guess, because maybe they'll put out one a year, and he puts out fifty."[33]

According to Todaro, once Gallo's name was on the general ballot "he was a shoo-in. The people who vote include all the physicists and the astronomers and people like that, who don't know anything about his work. They only know that he's a well-known name."

It was said later that several Academicians, including Todaro and Harold Varmus, considered lodging a challenge to Gallo's election, but decided to let the moment pass. The day after the election, Jay Levy got a call from Peter Duesberg, an Academy member across the Bay in Berkeley. "Peter said, 'Jay, Gallo's in the Academy,'" Levy recalled. "I was so depressed. I couldn't believe it. He told me, 'Don't worry. He's in there with all the other crooks.'"

According to the petition that secured Gallo's election, he had forged the link between HTLV-1 and adult T-cell leukemia, discovered HIV, and invented the blood test that provided the first "definitive proof" of the cause of AIDS. Gallo's most recent accomplishment was described as the discovery of "a new human B cell lymphotropic virus, HBLV, that infects B cells and that is associated with lymphoproliferative disease" in humans. But by the time of Gallo's election HBLV had ceased to exist.

Eighteen months before, Zaki Salahuddin and Dharam Ablashi, who worked downstairs from Gallo in Stu Aaronson's lab, had indeed discovered a new virus in a half-dozen patients, including two with AIDS.[34] Like HIV, the new virus infected human blood cells. But its genetic information was written in DNA, not RNA, and its preferred targets appeared to be B-cells, not T-cells. Gallo christened the new virus HBLV, for human B-cell lymphotropic virus. Any virus discovery was a scientific event, but for Gallo HBLV was a true milestone, the first virus discovered in his lab since Kalyanaraman's isolation of HTLV-2 five years before. The fact that Gallo had managed to link HBLV with AIDS was worth a six-page news release from the NCI press office.[35]

The discovery of HBLV was an accident, stemming from Ablashi's long-standing interest in the Epstein-Barr virus. "Zaki told me, 'I have another EBV isolate in the freezer, if you are interested in characterizing it,'" Ablashi recalled. "I said, 'Sure.' So I started working on it and, after about six months I told him, 'Zaki, this is not an EBV virus.'" When blood testing showed that HBLV appeared to infect at least half of all AIDS patients,[36] Gallo began suggesting it might play an important role as a "co-factor" that made AIDS "more progressive."[37]

It was one of Robin Weiss's London collaborators, Richard Tedder, who gave Gallo the bad news: HBLV wasn't a B-cell virus after all, just another herpesvirus whose preferred target was T-cells.[38] Months before Gallo's Academy election, HBLV had been reclassified and renamed HHV-6, for human herpesvirus number six.[39] Nor was there any evidence HHV-6 caused "lymphoproliferative disease" in humans, as Gallo's petition claimed, or for that matter had anything to do with AIDS. "I was devastated," recalled Steve Josephs, the molecular biologist in Flossie Wong-Staal's section who had done the initial characterization of what once had been HBLV.[40] "It was highly embarrassing to me. We had to change our entire perspective on the virus."

The CDC, the Institut Pasteur, and the NIH had been the focus of attention when Atlanta, Paris, and Washington hosted the first three international conferences on AIDS. But there was relatively little AIDS in Sweden, and no particular reason beyond the obvious that Stockholm should be the site of the fourth international conference. Considering the devastation AIDS was inflicting on Central Africa, that continent would have been a more appropriate venue. But the Swedish capital in the summer is more pleasant than Bamako or Kinshasa, and it is also the site of the anonymous gray-green townhouse at Sturegatan 14 that houses the Nobel Foundation.

As the 7,500 conference delegates descended on Stockholm in June of 1988, to many the time seemed right for a Nobel Prize for AIDS. "I think most people in Sweden feel happy that the conflicts between France and the United States have been settled a little bit, at least on the surface," observed Ingemar Ernberg, a prominent Swedish scientist. Those who looked to the conference program for clues about the current thinking at the Karolinska Institute, which awards the Nobel Prize in physiology and medicine, noted that the first to speak after the Swedish prime minister was Montagnier, followed by Jonathan Mann, the AIDS coordinator for the World Health Organization, and then Gallo. During the boat tours and other sightseeing events that occupied the conference delegates during their off-hours, many engaged in the time-honored game of "who would *you* choose?"

Nobel Prizes have never been shared by more than three, and several possible triplets could be constructed. One was Gallo, Popovic, and Sarngadharan. A second was Montagnier, Chermann, and Barré. But nobody was betting that all the honorees for AIDS were likely to come from the same country. Robin Weiss thought Françoise Barré was "the person who really discovered the virus," and that "she of all people should share the prize with Gallo and Montagnier." Paul Luciw wasn't sure Gallo and Montagnier should be included at all. "Gallo ripped off Montagnier," Luciw said, "but Montagnier ripped off Françoise and Jean-Claude."

Michael Koch was convinced that Barré, being a woman, didn't have a chance — Koch recalled that Lise Meitner hadn't shared the Nobel with the German physicist Otto Hahn, although Meitner had not only done Hahn's prize-winning experiments in nuclear fission but explained them to him afterward. Koch saw the settlement as an attempt by the French and American sides to make the Nobel Prize safe for Gallo and Montagnier alone.

"I think they were frightened that nobody would get it, that people would say, 'This issue is so inflamed,'" Koch said. "Gallo knows his reputation will inevitably be ruined if he does not get the Nobel Prize now and put a lock on everything. He must fight against time. I suppose Montagnier also knew this, and said, 'If I now settle it, I get at least the Nobel Prize to share.'"

Mike Gottlieb, the discoverer of AIDS, thought that whoever got the Nobel, it shouldn't be Gallo. "Really," Gottlieb said, "what Gallo did is actually a very sleazy story. By not giving credence to the French observation — in fact by trying to disparage it — Gallo slowed down the blood industry's recognition that this was an infection. There could have been a test."

Jacques Leibowitch thought *nobody* should get a Nobel Prize for AIDS. "That they should get the Nobel Prize now for this would be an outrageous offense to human beings," Leibowitch said. "I will stand up and raise a lobby against this if it's done, OK? Because at the time when people are dying by thousands, you do not announce the Nobel Prize of medicine for the discovery of a virus that kills. You only do it when there's an alleviation of human pain. I tell you, there will be a rupture between the public and the scientific community if they do this. It will be suicide."

According to Claudine Escoffier, when the Nobel rumors reached Paris, the Pasteur's two living laureates, François Jacob and André Lwoff, wrote to friends in Stockholm "saying that if ever Montagnier were to get the prize, they would send their own Nobel Prizes back. André Lwoff said, 'Never in the history of the Nobel Prize did a man who did nothing important in his lab but see one virus, never before did such a scientist get the Nobel Prize for such a little thing.' That was his argument. I agree completely." But the Nobel is a political prize as well as a scientific honor — ask any scientist who doesn't have one — and AIDS had become the quintessential political disease. Despite Lwoff's objections, as the prospects for an AIDS Nobel loomed the rift over the division of credit within the Pasteur was growing wider.

Shortly after the ratification in Paris, Jean-Claude Chermann had departed for Marseille, 400 miles and several cultural light-years from Paris, whose local university had been glad to add to its modest faculty roster a scientist who was recognized by taxi drivers. "I was the equivalent of professor in Pasteur," Chermann said a few months after taking over an enormous new laboratory in the sere hills above Marseille. "When we start, it was the virus of Barré, Chermann, Montagnier. The following year it was Montagnier, Chermann, Barré. Then it was 'the team of Pasteur.' Now it's Montagnier."

Chermann was quick to explain that he had left the Pasteur not because of the attention being paid to Montagnier, but for other reasons. "First, Pasteur was not giving us space for research or recognition to fight against the Americans," he said. "And second, Pasteur was taking the profit without doing something. I did not get any money from the patent. The virus had been isolated in my lab. Not only isolated, isolated and characterized. It's in my lab that the first blood test has been made. That is very important."

The wall of Chermann's new office bore a small plaque identifying him as a charter member of the "AIDS Discoverers' Club." Mike Gottlieb, Françoise Barré, Jay Levy, and a handful of others had similar plaques, which they had conferred on one another as a half-joke. Was Gallo also a member of the club? a visitor asked. "Certainly not," Chermann replied. On a filing cabinet next to the plaque stood a bottle of California wine Chermann had received from a woman in the United States. On the label she had written *"C'est un example d'un oeuvre de Gallo."*

"It is the worst wine," Chermann said.

Despite their close personal and professional relationship, Françoise Barré had decided not to join Chermann in Marseille but to remain at the Pasteur, tucked away in a dank and ancient laboratory where she rarely saw or spoke to Montagnier. Like Chermann, Barré blamed Montagnier for having inflated the importance of his own contribution to the Pasteur's discovery.

"I think he wanted to be in front," Barré said. "At the beginning of the AIDS story, I think it was very collaborative work. I don't know exactly how things began to change."[41] Montagnier had asked Barré to remain in his viral oncology unit, but she refused. "I told him, 'No way,'" Barré said. "We got into a discussion, but he said everything I was telling him was not true, it was all in my imagination."

Montagnier felt badly that he was now being portrayed by Chermann and Barré as little more than the chief of the laboratory where the famous discovery had taken place. "I started the work *first*," Montagnier said. "The sample came to my lab. I did the mincing of the tissue myself. Françoise Barré learned some biological and chemical techniques on the mouse retroviruses, and she was able to apply that to LAV. She was the one that found the reverse transcriptase activity in the supernatant I gave to her. But the lymph node from *Bru* was put into culture by me, in my lab. The use of anti-interferon serum was also my idea. I don't know exactly when I gave the culture to them, but I gave them all the techniques to grow the virus in T-cells. They learned that from me."

Montagnier had been rewarded by Pasteur with an entire floor in Pasteur's new state-of-the-art retrovirology building, constructed with a $20 million bequest from the Duchess of Windsor, and a huge ground-floor office expensively decorated in *neo-japonaise*. Although Montagnier's lab employed fifty researchers, nothing of importance had emerged since LAV-2.

"I think he blew his fuses this year," said Marc Alizon. "He says he's one of the greatest biologists of the time. He certainly is not. He could have built a really good lab doing research on HIV. He was not able to do it. Most of this floor is people working on their own projects. Some are doing good work, like François Clavel. Montagnier has no time and no interest for research. He's looking for scoops."

Simon Wain-Hobson, whose much smaller lab was two floors below Montagnier's, agreed with Alizon. "Around here," Wain-Hobson said, "we say, 'He stumbled onto the virus, and he's stumbling still.'"

When Montagnier arrived at the Pasteur each morning in his supercharged black Saab, he often found someone with AIDS waiting outside, hoping that the discoverer of the virus could also provide a cure.

"These poor AIDS patients," Montagnier said, shaking his head. "They regard me as a god, you see." Feeling unappreciated by just about everyone else in Paris, Montagnier was talking about starting his own private institute in America. "My motivation comes back to the patient," Montagnier said. "I want to apply a little basic research to new therapeutics. As I view it now, I won't be leaving the Pasteur. But if I'm forced to leave, I will leave, of course. I want to continue basic research at the Pasteur Institute. The problem is to get sufficient money. I have never received anything from the patent for my research. We should receive some personal money too, but the answer I got from the *direction* of the Pasteur was this money was being used for covering expenses."

Like Jonas Salk, Montagnier hoped to set up shop in Southern California, where he had acquired semi–star status within the Hollywood community, and where plenty of entertainment-industry executives were eager to help bankroll a cure for AIDS. "Luc is somebody who's a hero elsewhere," observed Mike Gottlieb, "but not appreciated in his own land, and California's got a certain allure. La Jolla certainly has a lot of glitter, and Paloma Picasso, and money, and it's a nice place to live and to have a research institution of his own."

But Gottlieb worried "that it's going to turn out to be a bogus thing. He's been doing fund-raising around Los Angeles. I was supposed to go to a dinner at Norman Cousins's house, where Luc was the guest of honor. I declined the invitation because I had something else to do, and I understand it was a total bust. He showed up two hours late, and brought some rowdy people with him. I heard it was just a disaster."

"Einstein, Freud — I'd Put Him on a List Like That"

For many of the players in the HIV story, the fall of 1988 was a time of change. Frédéric Brugière, in whom the virus had been discovered five years before, was dead at the age of thirty-eight. "He had a lot of psychological problems," said Willy Rozenbaum, who had taken care of *"Bru"* until the end. "He was very lonely. Nobody came. No friends, no family."[1] Before Brugière died, Rozenbaum gave him a copy of the *Science* article reporting the isolation of a new human retrovirus from his T-cells. "In the story of AIDS," Rozenbaum said, "he was on a special page. But he said that it was like another person. It was not him, you know?"

For many of the young French scientists who had done important early work, the reward was an American fellowship. Marc Alizon was off to the Whitehead Institute at M.I.T., and David Klatzmann to spend a couple of years at Columbia University. François Clavel had met Mal Martin, who offered him a visiting associate's position in Bethesda. "I liked the guy," Clavel said, "and I said, 'Let's go.' It was great fun to be in the U.S. I became a big fan of the Orioles."

Without much resistance from Vince DeVita, Peter Fischinger left the National Cancer Institute for a make-work job as AIDS coordinator for the Public Health Service. After several months with little to do, Fischinger retired from the government and joined the Medical University of South Carolina.[2] Mika Popovic was leaving as well, for New Mexico State University, where he had been offered a nontenured job at the school's primate research institute.[3] Even Flossie Wong-Staal had one foot out the door. "Gallo thinks it's very likely she will leave," said George Todaro following a dinner conversation with Gallo. "He's resigned to it, but he feels that she's abandoning him. She's a relatively good scientist. For the sake of her own career, she really ought to get away."

Vince DeVita, sure to be replaced as chief of the NCI by Ronald Reagan's successor in the upcoming presidential election, preempted a presidential request for his resignation by accepting the prestigious post of physician-in-chief at the Memorial Sloan-Kettering Cancer Center in New York.[4] Jim Wyngaarden, the NIH director, wasn't unhappy to see DeVita go.

"In the Cancer Act," Wyngaarden said, "there's the statement that the NCI director must inform the Cancer Board of any factors which hinder the progress of cancer research. That's a open-ended invitation for insubordination. Any decision I made that didn't fall DeVita's way was reported to the Cancer Board, and now it was public and it was in the cancer rag [the *Cancer Letter*, a privately published weekly newsletter devoted to inside doings at the National Cancer Institute]. I wanted someone in that job who was going to direct an institute that was a component of NIH in all respects, not just when it was convenient."

The consensus choice as DeVita's replacement was Sam Broder, the NCI lab chief who had organized the symposium where Simon Wain-Hobson presented the gene map of LAV, and who had been among the first NCI researchers to join the search for an effective treatment for AIDS. A forty-three-year-old Detroit native with a reputedly encyclopedic knowledge of rock 'n' roll, Broder shared with Gallo the patent application for Suramin, an old drug for African sleeping sickness that had turned out to kill HIV in the test tube.[5] After Suramin proved not only useless in AIDS patients but also dangerous,[6] Broder had come up with another potential AIDS drug, dextran sulfate, an anticoagulant manufactured in Japan that had been around for twenty years.

Dextran sulfate also proved a bust,[7] and when the NCI, in temporary budget trouble, began scaling back its intramural operations, Broder had nearly lost his lab. Gallo saved Broder's job, and Broder had gone on to make headlines by showing that the AIDS virus could be incapacitated by an anticancer compound called AZT. Clinical trials were initiated, with such apparently dramatic results that they had been stopped in midstream, so that the AIDS patients receiving placebos could be given AZT instead.[8]

The FDA's decision to approve AZT as the only treatment for AIDS had boosted Broder's stock at NCI, and on the day his appointment was announced by the White House Gallo sent his new boss flowers. "We are all very proud to be with you," Gallo said, "and we will help you in every way we can."[9] Broder thought even more highly of Gallo. "One of the paradigmatic figures of the 20th Century," he told the *Washington Post*. "He's influenced things in our daily lives to an incalculable degree. Einstein, Freud — I'd put him on a list like that, I really would."[10]

Despite the problems it was causing for the HIV blood test, the H-9 cell line had survived the dispute with the Pasteur as the single AIDS-related discovery to which Gallo's laboratory could unequivocally lay claim. But Mika Popovic still hadn't identified the patient whose T-cells had been used to establish H-9 — or, more precisely, "HT," the parent line from which H-9 had been cloned.

The NCI's Adi Gazdar thought it strange that when Popovic was asked at scientific meetings where H-9 had come from, he was "unable or unwilling to explain."[11] The origin of HT and H-9 was more than an academic question. "Those four papers in *Science* are an irreproducible piece of work, if you don't know what the cell line is," Paul Luciw said. "If I had gotten those papers to review, I would have said, 'They have to provide either a description of that cell line or an indication that it's available.' Seriously, I would have turned them down."

In the absence of any clue from Popovic, rumors had begun circulating that HT wasn't an original discovery at all, merely Adi Gazdar's HUT-78 cell line by a different name. Frank Ruscetti, to whom Gazdar had given HUT-78 along with HUT-102 in the days before HTLV-1, remembered calling Zaki Salahuddin shortly after Popovic's paper appeared.

"I said 'What is this H-9 cell line?'" Ruscetti recalled. "He said, 'They got it out of your freezer.' I said, 'I didn't have any H-9 cell line in that freezer. The only cell line I had in that freezer was HUT-78.'" When the rumors about H-9 reached Cambridge, Abraham Karpas promptly informed John Maddox that "[b]y changing the name of the cell line as well as that of the virus, Dr. Gallo claims credit for the work done by *two* independent groups of investigators."[12]

For whatever they were worth, Popovic's lab notes showed that he had used the terms HUT-78 and HT interchangeably.[a] On January 19, 1984, the day Popovic created fifty-one new cell line clones, including H-9, his notes read "Cloning of HT cells ~ HUT 78." When Popovic claimed later not to have been certain of the origin of HT, Adi Gazdar wondered why the article had described HT as "derived from an adult with lymphoid leukemia."

"How did they know it was an adult?" Gazdar asked. "It could have been a child. For that matter, how did they know the patient had leukemia? The cells could have been transformed in the laboratory."

A Bombay native who had trained as a doctor in London, Gazdar had been a co-author on Poiesz and Ruscetti's papers reporting the discovery of HTLV-1 in the HUT-102 cell line. But Gazdar's name hadn't appeared on any of Gallo's articles about HTLV-3B and H-9. He hadn't been included as an inventor on the government's patent for the HT cell line, and he certainly hadn't shared any of the millions of dollars in royalties generated by the sale of the Gallo AIDS test made with virus grown in H-9.

When Gazdar told a Public Health Service lawyer he thought Gallo and Popovic had appropriated his discovery, he was advised not to pursue the matter. "I was told, 'There's enough of a fight going on between Montagnier and Gallo,'" Gazdar said. "'Why do you want a fight between NIH and kill any claims we have?'"

Gallo still hadn't deposited a sample of H-9 with the American Type Culture Collection — standard procedure for NIH scientists — where it would have been available to any researcher, including anyone interested in comparing it genetically with HUT-78. "The ATCC had written several times to Gallo," Gazdar said, "and Gallo had never responded. So I wrote Gallo a brief note, saying 'I urge you to deposit in the ATCC, they're really anxious to have it.'[b] Two or three days later I get a call from him, between eleven and twelve o'clock at night, demanding to know why I'm 'ordering him around like a general orders a private.' I said, 'I urge you strongly to consider this course of action' is not an order. He said, 'Oh, yeah, I can read between the lines. You're ordering me.'"

Determining whether H-9 was HUT-78 in disguise was a matter of a few laboratory tests. As one of his departing acts, Vince DeVita decided to resolve the question.[13] Disguised by the code names "Cox" and "Nies," samples of HUT-78 and H-9 were provided to an NCI researcher, Steve O'Brien, with instructions to determine whether the cells had come from the same or different patients. O'Brien, who had no idea what cells he was working with, arranged three separate experiments: a comparison of the HLA proteins on the surface of each set of cells; a comparison of their "alloenzyme signatures" using a technique O'Brien had developed; and a restriction analysis of the cellular genome from each line.

Six weeks later, O'Brien reported that "if Cox were the defendant in a rape case and Nies was a semen sample of the victim, Cox would be convicted."[14]

Speaking in Zurich before the April 1984 tripartite meeting at Pasteur, Gallo had recalled "the breakthrough" in growing the AIDS virus made possible by "a particular cell line developed in our lab. That happens to be HT, a new line." At Margaret Heckler's news conference a few days later, Gallo had described H-9 as "developed . . . in our laboratory." During the patent dispute, the government had argued that Gallo's invention of H-9 was the main thing that distinguished the American AIDS test from the French version.[15]

But Steve O'Brien had proven that HT wasn't a new cell line after all, just the HUT-78 cells Adi Gazdar had given Frank Ruscetti nearly a decade before. "If Gallo had simply said, 'I've taken Montagnier's virus and put it in Adi Gazdar's cell line and grown it up,' he wouldn't be in this fix," said Simon Wain-Hobson. "But he had to make it *his* virus and *his* cell line."

Gallo couldn't see why it mattered. "No one cares if H-9 is HUT-78 or not," he said. "Who gives a pickle?"[16] But Adi Gazdar pointed out that, had the identity of H-9 been known in the summer of 1984, researchers seeking to study the AIDS virus could have obtained HUT-78 from the ATCC for $85 plus shipping, rather than waiting months after signing a collaborative agreement that gave Gallo control over who got H-9 and how it was used. As Gazdar also observed, it was Gallo and Popovic who were getting the credit for his work. "Does it matter who discovered the virus?" Gazdar asked. "That does matter, doesn't it?"

O'Brien wrote up the data on Cox and Nies with the intention of submitting it to *Science*, where Popovic's article on H-9 had appeared, and where, it seemed, the scientific record should be corrected.[c] When the paper finally appeared, it was in Dani Bolognesi's *AIDS*

Research and Human Retroviruses.[17] "Gallo picked the most obscure journal he could find," Gazdar said, "which no one except a few aficionados read, and informed Steve O'Brien in no uncertain terms that it wasn't going to *Science* under any circumstances. Steve O'Brien told me Gallo was fuming — fuming — when he thought that thing might get into *Science.* He wanted to get the least publicity he could get. The world still doesn't know. I meet people every day who don't know a thing about this."[d]

Nor would Adi Gazdar's name be added to the government's H-9 patent. In the opinion of the NIH lawyers, when Gazdar had given HUT-78 to Frank Ruscetti he hadn't predicted that it would someday "be useful for growing the AIDS-causing organism."[18] How Gazdar might have made such a prediction before the discovery of AIDS itself, the lawyers didn't say. In lieu of the $100,000 a year Gallo and Popovic were receiving for an AIDS test made with Gazdar's cell line, Gazdar would have to be content with a one-time payment of $10,000.

"I got a call telling me to be in Sam Broder's office in twenty minutes," Gazdar recalled. "When I walked in there was nobody there except Broder. Broder said, 'I have good news and bad news. The good news is, here's a check for $10,000. The bad news is you have to pay tax on it.' Then he walked out of the room. There was no citation or anything, just the check."

Concluding that his future at NCI was "limited," Gazdar joined John Minna at the University of Texas Medical Center in Dallas, where he proceeded to do groundbreaking work on the genetics of lung cancer. Five years after its publication in *Science,* the H-9 cell line, accurately described as "a clonal derivative of HUT-78," was deposited by Gallo with the ATCC.

A press of the button labeled *Nobelstiftelsen Expedition* opens the heavy steel doors that allow visitors to Stockholm to walk through a deserted lobby and up a flight of stairs, where another bell gains admittance to the sanctum. There, in a glass case, nestled in a blue velvet box, rests the two-and-a-half-inch solid-gold medal that for most of this century has driven science forward.[e]

Precisely how Nobel prizewinners are chosen is known only to those involved in their selection.[f] A few details, however, have escaped the sanctum. Each year, a distinguished group of nominators around the world is asked to name those they believe most deserving of the world's highest scientific honor. The nominators include living Nobel laureates, full professors at Scandinavian universities (including Iceland), non-Swedish academics, and certain other celebrated individuals. The nominations are collated, and those deemed potential winners are put before the Nobel committees of the selecting institutions. When the Karolinska Institute receives the short list for physiology and medicine, it prepares summaries of the nominees' work that are bound between green covers.[g] The summaries can highlight a single discovery, a series of related discoveries, or a string of achievements over a lifetime.

At a secret session in the Karolinska library, eight possible prize-winning "topics" are selected, with up to three potential winners per topic. To maintain absolute security against leaks, eight announcements are prepared, each proclaiming one of the eight finalists to be winners of that year's Nobel Prize. During a last-minute meeting in the first-floor conference room, the senior Karolinska faculty votes to eliminate the finalists one by one. When only one finalist remains, the group emerges to hand the surviving announcement to waiting reporters. Or so the story goes.

Among scientists, mentioning oneself in the same breath with the Nobel Prize is taken as extremely bad form. But Gallo made no secret of his ambition. A former NCI researcher, Sam Waksal, remembered a late-night drinking session during a leukemia conference in Corfu following the HL-23 debacle.

"One night we were up very late," Waksal recalled, "Reinhard Kurth, myself, Bob, Max Essex and Dani Bolognesi, Harvey Eisen, all in Gallo's room, sitting and talking about science and the world. And Gallo was drunk, and he had a tear in his eye. And he said, 'You know, I would do anything — anything — to win the Nobel Prize.' I always thought it was the most telling thing about him. Because in the world of science the goal is the pleasantry of the discovery. And he could never find as much satisfaction in the discovery as he could in the limelight."

Gallo had been nominated for the 1988 Nobel Prize by Leon Jacobsen, the elderly University of Chicago researcher who had helped get him into the National Academy. "My dilemma was to nominate him without doing anything about the Frenchman," Jacobsen said. "So I wrote to one of his colleagues over at the Pasteur and asked them to give me a little information. They gave me some stuff they had written up. It went into too much detail, and had a bunch of junk that I wasn't interested in anyway. So I just had to give up on it. I couldn't really pick it apart."

Over dinner with George Todaro, Gallo had mentioned receiving "a funny smile" from Hans Wigzell, a Karolinska immunologist who sat on the Nobel committee and, not coincidentally, headed the Swedish delegation to the annual AIDS symposium hosted by Gallo in Bethesda. During that year's "Gallo meeting" a few weeks before, a picture of Gallo with Wigzell had appeared in the *Washington Post*.[19] Jonas Blomberg from the University of Lund recalled a particularly liquid dinner during the Gallo meeting at which a Swedish colleague had blurted out, "I know very well why you invite us here. It's because of the Nobel Prize."

According to Blomberg, Gallo laughed the remark off. But in the days before the 1988 Nobels were announced, Gallo was candid in assessing his chances. "I don't know if I'll ever get it," he said. "You can't tell. I think there are theoretical possibilities, but there's a hell of a lot of people that are very good candidates. I received the Lasker in 1982 before ever working on AIDS. That ought to mean something, in view of 70 percent of Lasker winners winning the Nobel Prize. If they do it for AIDS, probably not. If they do it for cancer I suppose I have a modest chance."[20]

Montagnier was more effacing. "It's not for me to say," he said. "The Nobel committee might want to give the prize to the discoverer of the vaccine, although it was the discovery of the virus itself that allowed for its detection in blood and the development of public-health measures that can limit the epidemic, even without a vaccine. The contribution of the American team is also important; so I doubt the prize will go to only one of the virus's 'codiscoverers.'"

Since the 1928 award to a Danish scientist for the misbegotten discovery that stomach cancer was caused by a parasite,[h] the Nobel electors have striven to keep any hint of scandal from tarnishing the prize. To allay whatever concerns might exist in Stockholm that Gallo and Montagnier hadn't reconciled their differences, the two had published a step-by-step account of their research in the *Scientific American*.[21] Credit for discovering the virus was now awarded unequivocally to Montagnier, and Gallo was no longer claiming to have conducted the first AIDS blood test, as he had done only a year before in the same publication.[22] "Contributions from our laboratories," the article said, "in roughly equal proportions . . . demonstrated that the cause of AIDS is a new human retrovirus."[i]

The Nobel announcement handed out on the morning of October 17, 1988, bore the names of three researchers who had had nothing to do with AIDS: the American team of Gertrude Elion and George Hitchings, whose work had laid the molecular basis for drugs to treat cancer, malaria, herpes, and other viral infections, and Sir James Black, the inventor of Beta blockers, the first effective treatment for hypertension. The three would split an award of $428,000, up 15 percent from the previous year thanks to the *Nobelstiftelsen's* shrewd investments.[23]

"All was gloom and doom in Gallo's lab," said Joanne Belk, the NIH Freedom of Information officer, who had kept up her contacts with Gallo's secretaries. "While Gallo was in Stockholm for the AIDS convention he had dinner with the king of Sweden, and he apparently came away convinced he'd win the Nobel Prize." According to some who claim to know what happened behind the Karolinska's closed doors, AIDS had indeed been one of the eight potential prize-winning topics, and Gallo one of the finalist nominees — although which other names had been included with his, if any, wasn't said.

The *Scientific American* article ignored questions about the identity of LAV and HTLV-3B, describing them as merely the same *kind* of virus. Neither the NIH nor the Institut Pasteur seemed interested in reopening that particular chapter of history. But Gerry Myers was still troubled by the "double fraud," and a few weeks before the Nobels were announced Myers had written Gallo a letter.[24]

"From our earliest tree analyses," Myers reminded Gallo, "it was patently evident that the LAV and 3B viruses had to have had a recent common ancestor. We have not suppressed this fact in our publications (or talks); neither have we commented upon it, much as we have been pressed to do so. . . ." Now, Myers explained, he had developed something called a "fine-structure analysis," based on recent findings from Gallo's former postdocs, Beatrice Hahn and George Shaw, a comparison of individual AIDS viruses within the same patient that had recently diverged from one another.

For years Gallo had insisted that the slight genetic differences among Hahn's various clones of HTLV-3B were explained by the fact that the cloned viruses had come from different patients in the Popovic pool, rather than from a single mutating virus. The AIDS virus, Gallo said, didn't change quickly enough to account for the differences that had been observed.[25] But Gallo had never published any data to support his claim, and from their new lab at the University of Alabama Hahn and Shaw had just demolished it.[26] In one patient alone, Hahn had found *seventeen* distinct forms of HIV, the closest of which differed by 3 percent, the most distant by 28 percent.

All were imperfect copies, some more imperfect than others, of the virus with which the patient had been infected, and whose reverse transcriptase made an occasional tiny error in transcription each time it reproduced. After many millions of viral replications, the patient was infected with what Simon Wain-Hobson described as a "swarm" of highly related but distinctive viruses.[27] The results from Hahn and Shaw provided empirical support for what Gerry Myers already knew: All Hahn's clones of HTLV-3B were the progeny of a single virus. The genetic distance between LAV and the 3B clones was the same as among the clones themselves, which could only mean they had all come from the same patient.

Like Marc Alizon, Wain-Hobson hadn't missed the parallels with the HTLV-4 story. "You saw the retraction of Max Essex in *Nature,*" Wain-Hobson said. "One of the arguments was that the viruses were 99 percent identical. You tell me another two viruses that are 99 percent identical except 3B and LAV. As more and more viruses get sequenced, it's becoming increasingly outrageous that those two are so close." To a freezer door in Wain-Hobson's lab, someone had taped a front-page headline from a gay newspaper, the *New York Native:* "Should Gallo and Essex be in jail?"

With Gerry Myers's fine-structure analysis, it was now possible to say which virus, 3B or LAV, was the ancestor of the other. The fact that LAV was "older" could only mean it had existed before there *was* an HTLV-3B. Which could only mean that the virus that entered Gallo's lab as LAV had somehow emerged as HTLV-3B.

If Montagnier understood the ramifications of Hahn and Shaw's work, he remained silent. "We have a settlement," Montagnier said, "and we don't say one is a contaminant from the other." Wain-Hobson was under the same strictures as Montagnier. But Gerry Myers wasn't a signatory to the Franco-American agreement, and Myers's only dilemma was when to go public. "There are many people out there,"

Myers said, "that believe that this should be addressed by the history of science, and are going to make sure that it is addressed at some time. The question is whether this should be brought out now."

"I don't expect you to act now on this in any particular way," Myers wrote Gallo. But he cautioned that "eventually the result will have to be put forward to the community as part of the inquiry into fine-structure variation." Before dropping the letter in the mail, Myers asked officials at NIAID, which funded his HIV Sequence Database, whether they thought he should send it. They didn't. "I was apprised of the policy of getting on with things," Myers recalled, "the post-settlement way, so to speak. As Mal Martin liked to say, the HHS had sprinkled holy water on the whole matter, meaning researchers really didn't have the leisure to brood or look back."

One researcher did have the leisure. Abraham Karpas now had tenure, which meant he was officially a Cambridge don. Karpas also had a fat new grant from the Medical Research Council, Britain's equivalent of the NIH, and a fellowship at Trinity College, around which Cambridge academic life revolves. The Karpas HIV blood test was selling briskly in several Third World countries.[28]

In his spare time, Karpas had continued his take-no-prisoners campaign against Gallo, his latest fusillade consisting of a letter to Jim Wyngaarden accusing Gallo of "grossly misleading the scientific community worldwide."[29] Karpas had also pursued his correspondence with John Maddox — "writing for *Nature*'s wastebasket," said Peter Newmark — as well as the *New Scientist*[30] and *Scientific American*.[31] But on a dark December afternoon in 1988, Karpas discovered that the fingerprint on the smoking gun had been in his own lab all along.

One of Karpas's graduate students, a dour Scottish woman, had set out to sequence LAV as part of her doctoral dissertation. When her preliminary results didn't match the LAV sequence published by Wain-Hobson, the woman concluded that she had somehow selected the wrong virus and put the partially completed sequence in a drawer. As it happened, she hadn't chosen the wrong virus, merely a different clone of LAV.

Wain-Hobson and Alizon had sequenced the LAV clone called J-19 — the same clone of HTLV-3B that Beatrice Hahn called BH-10. But the French had cloned a second and slightly different genome from the LAV culture, J-81, which closely resembled the clone Hahn called HXB2 — and which had the *Hind*III site seen in no other full-length HIV clone — except HXB2.[j]

Because Wain-Hobson hadn't taken the trouble to sequence J-81, it wasn't possible to say for certain whether the *Hind*III site on the restriction map was really in the viral genome. But J-81 was the clone Karpas's student had begun to sequence by mistake, stopping a few hundred nucleotides short of where the restriction map predicted the *Hind*III restriction site would be found. Now immersed in another thesis project, the woman had no interest in picking up the LAV sequence where she had left off, and Karpas had asked two of his other students, Mike Tristem and Fergal Hill, to finish it. After several nights of work, Tristem and Hill reached nucleotide number 6,065 — and found the *Hind*III site waiting on the other side.

With a request that it be included in the upcoming edition of the HIV Sequence Database, Karpas sent his sequence of LAV-J81 to Gerry Myers, who had been meeting with Gallo to discuss the prospects for a joint letter to *Science*.[32] "A very good, a time honored way to say to the world, 'These are the circumstances, these are the data, it looks like this,'" Myers said, but the initial meeting hadn't gone well. At one point, when Myers asked whether it was true that all the samples in the Popovic pool had tested positive for reverse transcriptase prior to pooling, Gallo had "exploded." Myers recalled telling Gallo, "If you don't stop behaving like a child, I'm leaving."

Gallo calmed down, but nothing was accomplished. Three weeks later the two met again in Bethesda, this time with Montagnier, who happened to be passing through.[33] To Gallo, Myers patiently explained that his fine-structure analysis showed that HTLV-3B was LAV, not the other way around, and that whatever had happened had happened in Gallo's lab. Myers recalled "mutterings" from Gallo about "overinterpretation," or "'too much focus on those damn trees.' I've almost given up trying to make sense out of him. One day I said to him, 'Well, I owe it to the French.' And he couldn't stand that. 'But I'm your colleague,' he said. 'We're Americans.' He rather expects people to be loyal to him. He's rather baffled when they aren't."

Gallo saw Mal Martin's hand behind what he considered an attempt to torpedo the settlement. "He believed that Mal was pressuring me," Myers recalled, "which wasn't the case at all. Mal was constantly warning me not to become involved. It was Flossie who was really urging Gallo to do this — I thought very well of her. In a funny way, Flossie can be more acerbic and frank about Bob, although she has a deep loyalty. I think other people around him were saying, 'No, don't do it.'"

Myers made one final plea for a joint letter, "a resolution within the tradition rather than within the press . . ."[k] Gallo refused, but promised to publish such a letter of his own.[34] As the summer of 1989 wore on, no letter appeared in *Science*. Also not forthcoming was the brief statement, promised by Gallo for publication in Myers's database, acknowledging "the distinct possibility" that HTLV-3B and LAV_{Bru} were the same isolate.[35] "He backed off," Myers reported later. "I don't know how close we came."

At one point, Myers heard Gallo had told *Science* he was withdrawing his letter on the advice of Howard Temin. But when Myers asked Temin why he had counseled Gallo to pull back, "Howard didn't know what I was talking about." Mal Martin had bet Myers $25 that the Gallo letter would never see print, and Myers contributed the money to the Christmas party for Martin's lab. When Myers's trees appeared in the 1989 edition of the HIV-AIDS database, they were buried in the middle of a huge compendium of DNA sequences, with no comment or elaboration.[36] Anyone who studied the trees could see that LAV and HTLV-3B were virtually identical. But the trees offered no clue that LAV had existed first, and had somehow been renamed HTLV-3B.[37]

Also buried was Abraham Karpas's short sequence of *LAV-J81*, identified only as "*Brul*20C."[38] With a magnifying glass and enough time, it was possible to discern that "l20C" and HXB2 shared a *Hind*III site that was present in none of the other LAV or HTLV-3B clones. But nobody seemed to have taken the time, and the government's version of scientific history remained intact: HTLV-3B had been independently isolated by Mika Popovic from a pool of American AIDS patients. When Gallo published a short memoir in *Discover*, the magazine described him as "The man who discovered the cause of AIDS."[39]

There matters might have remained, but on Sunday, November 19, 1989, the *Chicago Tribune* published a sixteen-page, 55,000-word account of the discovery of HIV.[40] The *Tribune* reproduced the sequence of Brul20C that had appeared a few weeks before in Gerry Myers's database — probably the first time that a DNA nucleotide sequence had appeared in a newspaper. The article concluded that HTLV-3B was LAV, although without an explanation from Mika Popovic, who declined to be interviewed, of precisely how that had occurred. "What happened in Robert Gallo's lab during the winter of 1983–84," the *Tribune* said, "is a mystery that may never be entirely solved. But the evidence is compelling that it was either an accident or a theft."

What followed was six years of history: the mixed-up micrographs; the CDC's bakeoff of the Gallo and Pasteur blood tests; the still-unsolved mystery of the redacted letter from Gonda to Popovic; Gallo's authorship of the Pasteur *Science* abstract; his repeated assertions that Popovic hadn't grown LAV and the mounting evidence to the contrary; the bogus claim of forty-eight AIDS virus isolates; the renaming of HUT-78 as "HT"; questions about whether Popovic's "lab notes" had been composed after the fact; Gallo's rewriting of history after Cold Spring Harbor and Park City; and, finally, the fact that no AIDS virus in Gallo's lab except HTLV-3B had been capable of growing in the quantities necessary to perform the key experiments that led to the AIDS blood test.

When François Sergent, the Washington correspondent for the Paris newspaper *Liberation,* called Gallo for comment, Gallo said he hadn't read the article. "I know the history," Gallo said. "I know who I am and I know what I did." Gallo admitted that he had had "a temporary bad period. But I think the scientists understand the scientific history and understand the scientific process. I believe that the man who wrote the article has no knowledge of the scientific process and had a motive in his article. Because he never wanted to interview me.[1] He looked for a lot of bad things. He looked under the rocks, trying to create notions of scandal. He didn't find anything."

When Sergent informed Gallo that Montagnier had declined comment as well, Gallo urged him to try again. "Because we talked on the phone a long time," Gallo said, "and I told him 'no comment' leaves an unpalatable taste. Look, let's put it another way. This statement I want to be one statement off record, OK? One statement. If Montagnier and Chermann knowingly sign an agreement for history, if they had any doubts and signed it, they were doing it for some self-gain, correct? That's a worse sin than anything anybody's accused me of. . . . [T]he point is simple. The agreement speaks for itself. If Pasteur knows different than the agreement, then they have been dishonest, not me."

As for whether Popovic had grown LAV in Bethesda, Gallo thought the question moot. "It doesn't matter," he told Sergent. "We had freedom to do anything we wanted with the so-called French virus. There is no 'French virus.' There's HIV. It causes AIDS. Our minds should be on doing something about it, not wallowing in the past. The day I retire from science, and I hope it's when I'm very old, I will give a course for reporters to understand the scientific process."

When Sergent inquired about the forty-eight isolates, Gallo pointed out that his *Science* article didn't say virus had actually been *isolated* from forty-eight patients. "If you look at the title," Gallo told Sergent, "it says '*Detection* and Isolation.'" But Gallo emphatically denied having written the abstract for Pasteur's first *Science* article. "That's nonsense," he said. "You think if I write their abstract, you think any journal is going to accept that? If I wrote their abstract then somebody's stupid on their side, aren't they? I wrote their abstract — what does that mean? That they come to me to write their papers? Or that I own *Science*? . . . the person who allows somebody else to write their abstract — don't you think they look a little odd? They are not being scientists and independent. That's as bizarre as I've ever heard."

Though he claimed not to have read the *Tribune,* Gallo nonetheless took umbrage at a number of the quotes it contained. Lee Ratner's questioning of Popovic's wisdom in pooling patient materials had been "not very helpful,"[41] but Gallo took the greatest exception to the quotes from Françoise Barré and Jean-Claude Chermann. "The article is filled with breeches [*sic*] of our agreement," Gallo complained in a letter to Barré.[42] "That is, once again there are quotes from you and Jean-Claude over old debates. Of course, the article was designed to harm me, and is a one-sided libelous attack."

To Barré, Gallo did admit having written the Pasteur abstract. "The truth," he told Barré, "is that Montagnier asked for my *help,* because he (or you) forgot to send in an abstract. The truth is that we wrote it together, i.e., we discussed *every* sentence by telephone and he agreed with all of them. . . . Of course, as a reviewer, I am supposed to suggest. Furthermore, *your* own data clearly argued that it was not a new virus but a member of the HTLV family. My suggestion to Montagnier was simply, why not call a spade a spade? Six years later I am given hostile treatment in a U.S. newspaper by you for this."

Gallo was most anguished to learn that Robin Weiss had taken a copy of the *Tribune* article to a meeting at Cold Spring Harbor, where it had been passed around and photocopied by a number of scientists. "You must realize," Gallo wrote Weiss, "that when I hear you are saying to scientists that all we had was LAV . . . and when you tell me it was you who brought the article to CSH — I am just a bit concerned about our relationship and your real understanding and/or appreciation of events. Would you be kind enough to clarify things for me? If not, your words will continue to be used — I think grossly unfairly, against me."[43]

"So far as I am quoted," replied Weiss, "none of the citations are inaccurate. Some are taken somewhat out of context. For example, where I said in reference to you 'He misled us all'. . . I was referring to your statements that you had not propagated LAV_{Bru} in your lab, and it was my impression that you had stated that publicly more than once after your four papers appeared in *Science* in May 1984."[m]

"Knowing you as well as I do," Weiss concluded, "it is very difficult to believe you deliberately 'stole' LAV-1 to present it as 3B. It is not, however, beyond imagination that someone in your laboratory tried too hard to please you."

Spying a new opportunity to stir the pot, John Maddox offered to publish responses to the *Tribune* from Gallo and Montagnier, and to write an accompanying editorial. Montagnier agreed, although expressing his regret that Gallo "ought to spend time again in details aimed at increasing (incorrectly and unnecessarily) your contribution to our 1983 work." Still, Montagnier thought it would be in Gallo's interest "to acknowledge the likely possibility that 3B was contaminated by LAV_{Bru} in your lab. . . ." Trying to dream up "more sophisticated and less likely explanations," Montagnier said, "will not help. Best wishes for the New Year."[44]

• 17 •

"I Have Probably Talked
Too Much"

As chairman of the House Energy and Commerce Committee, John D. Dingell was arguably the most powerful member of Congress — "an investigative powerhouse," according to the *New York Times,* capable of bringing "the biggest corporations, academic institutions and federal agencies to their knees." Thanks to Dingell, said the *Times,* everything from "nuts and bolts to blood banks, bottled water and cardiac pacemakers" was "unquestionably safer now."[1] To *U.S. News & World Report,* John Dingell was simply "the most feared Democrat in the land."[2]

Dingell, who had first been elected to Congress when Eisenhower was president, had amassed too many trophies to count, among them the Pentagon's $640 toilet seats and dozens of more serious cost overruns; tainted blood at the American Red Cross; illegal kickbacks at the FDA; and the misuse of federal research funds by universities. But Dingell hadn't gotten to be an eighteen-term congressman from Detroit by annoying the auto industry, and his investigators had spent years trying to prove that airbags were less effective than auto safety advocates maintained.

Dingell's preferred target was the Executive Branch, and he was frankly despised by the Reagan and Bush administrations for the unabashed enthusiasm he brought to his role as congressional watchdog, poking and prodding this agency or that one for evidence of something fetid, then publicly eviscerating the bureaucrats who had squandered, and sometimes stolen, the taxpayers' money.

No one on Dingell's staff could explain exactly how the Committee on Energy and Commerce had gained authority over the National Institutes of Health, except that the chairman wanted it that way. However it happened, in April of 1988 Dingell made history when the full committee's subcommittee on oversight and investigations, which Dingell also chaired, held the first-ever congressional hearing on allegations of scientific fraud.[3]

Dingell's probe focused on a manuscript, published two years before in *Cell,* by researchers at the Massachusetts Institute of Technology. Although David Baltimore was one of a half-dozen co-authors on the manuscript, he had contributed nothing to the research it contained. According to scientific custom, Baltimore's name was included merely because one of the authors was a postdoc in his lab. But a Nobel laureate touched by even a faint scent of scandal was irresistible for the media, and the case inevitably became known as "the Baltimore affair."[4]

That fraud occurred in science was well known among scientists themselves, and most of them preferred to keep it within the scientific family. Research funding was easier to come by if the taxpayers and their elected representatives were able to imagine scientists as high-minded seekers of truth. The reality, that scientists often engaged in the same kind of back-stabbing and throat-cutting as politicians and businessmen, had remained behind laboratory doors. The traditional penalty for scientists caught cheating had been the scientific equivalent of the locked room with a loaded revolver on the table: a loss of research grants, perhaps a quiet faculty resignation, even ostracism by one's peers, but almost never a public denunciation.

Only a handful of cases of alleged fraud had ever come to public attention. One involved Sir Cyril Burt, a British psychologist, who had been accused, posthumously, of fabricating his celebrated data showing that identical twins raised in different families had equivalent IQs, presupposing a genetic basis for intelligence. In a 1974 case, an American researcher had admitted painting spots on mice to falsify the results of skin graft experiments. A few years later, some cancer researchers at Boston University were caught falsifying patient data. In the early 1980s a Harvard cardiologist, John Darsee, had acknowledged faking a series of experiments. Stephen Breuning, a University of Pittsburgh psychologist, actually had been incarcerated for falsifying research on hyperactive children.

The problem of fraud, always present at some level, seemed to have worsened with the advent of biotechnology, which dramatically enhanced the opportunity for financial gain from published research. Not until the early 1980s, however, had the scientific community acknowledged that research fraud was even an occasional problem. That year, the Association of American Medical Colleges issued the first set of guidelines for handling allegations of scientific fraud. The first HHS regulations, published in 1985, authorized specially constituted panels of nongovernment scientists to consider evidence of impropriety in research funded with federal grants.

The NIH was part of HHS, but it had no mechanism for investigating misconduct by the universities it funded, much less its own intramural scientists, which was where John Dingell came in. The data under scrutiny in the Baltimore case had been produced under an NIH grant by another M.I.T. scientist, Thereza Imanishi-Kari, who had spent years working on the genetic regulation of body functions. Dingell's star witness was Margot O'Toole, a former postdoc in Imanishi-Kari's lab, who had ignited the "Baltimore affair" after noticing what seemed to be discrepancies between the results of her own experiments and those published by her boss in Cell.[a]

O'Toole first voiced her suspicions to administrators at M.I.T. and at neighboring Tufts University,[5] where Imanishi-Kari since had taken a new job. The M.I.T. faculty member assigned to look into the matter, a friend of Baltimore's, had concluded that while the Cell article contained mistakes, they were too trivial to warrant a formal correction. Tufts also found nothing amiss. When O'Toole suggested that Baltimore send a correction to Cell, she recalled his reminder that the scientific process was "self-correcting," meaning that Imanishi-Kari's errors, whatever they might be, would be recognized by other scientists. O'Toole should let the matter rest.[6]

The NIH had opened an inquiry of its own, recruiting three nongovernment scientists to assess the evidence in what, fairly or not, had become known as "the Baltimore case." Although the panel found "significant errors of misstatement and omission" and "serious concerns about . . . the reliability of these data and their interpretation," the inquiry absolved Imanishi-Kari and the other authors of intentional fraud.[7] Baltimore sent Cell a letter acknowledging three "misstatements" in the paper, but Jim Wyngaarden thought it hadn't dealt with all of the issues requiring attention.[8] In Wyngaarden's opinion, the number of serious inaccuracies in the paper warranted a formal correction in *Cell,* and Wyngaarden also criticized the manner in which Baltimore had responded to Margot O'Toole's concerns.

"One function of congressional oversight," Dingell declared, "is to shed light on problems of public importance. The apparent unwillingness on the part of the scientific community to deal promptly and effectively with allegations of misconduct is unfair to both accuser and accused. Even more important, it impairs the conduct of research, its present and future value to other scientists, and its benefits to the public."[9] Observing that all three of the scientists chosen by the NIH to assess the Baltimore case had some sort of tie to Baltimore or Imanishi-Kari, Dingell questioned the NIH's commitment to get to the bottom of alleged scientific misconduct.[b] "We don't want cooked figures," Dingell told the senior NIH executives who sat squirming at his witness table, "and we don't want cooked panels judging the people who cook figures."

David Baltimore, who was intimidated by no one, labeled the affair "a tempest in a teapot," and many of Baltimore's colleagues were horrified at the Dingell subcommittee's apparently ferocious determination to illuminate the darker side of science. To allegations of "McCarthyism" Dingell replied that it was Congress which authorized the NIH's $8 billion annual research budget, and Congress which had the responsibility "to make sure that this money is spent properly."

Dingell admitted his staff had "better things to do than police science," and it was the chairman's "fondest hope" that the NIH would one day take on that responsibility itself. Until then, the subcommittee's investigation of the Baltimore affair would continue. "I don't want you to get the impression," Dingell told the NIH officials, "that this committee is going to stage a one-day hearing, bring you up, make you miserable, and then let you go on about your business. When we do these things, we try to see to it that the pain and suffering goes on for a greater period of time, until the abuse that is obvious is taken care of."

To stop the pain and suffering, the NIH had created a new agency, the Office of Scientific Integrity, and charged it with investigating and deciding cases of suspected plagiarism, falsification, fabrication, or other serious scientific misconduct. As its first official act, the OSI assembled a second, and more carefully chosen, panel of inquiry in the Baltimore case.

. . .

Within weeks of Dingell's hearing Jim Wyngaarden announced his resignation, after seven years, as director of the National Institutes of Health. Before long his acting replacement, a tall, genial Ph.D. named William Raub, who had been Wyngaarden's deputy, had a letter from John Dingell on his desk.[10] His subcommittee, Dingell advised Raub, had "recently begun looking into allegations of scientific and financial misconduct on the part of certain staff members in the laboratory of Dr. Robert Gallo at the National Institutes of Health."

Dingell reminded Raub that the NIH had previously "turned a blind eye to misconduct by senior scientists supported by Federal funds. We trust that this will not be the case in the present situation, and that the allegations will be thoroughly investigated and appropriate actions taken if warranted by the investigation developed."

For HHS and NIH, the potential consequences of the unanswered questions about Gallo's research transcended the importance of those in the Baltimore case, and nobody mistook Robert Gallo for David Baltimore. Where Baltimore had done Nobel-winning work and rarely sought the spotlight, *The Lancet* observed that Gallo was "neither modest nor universally revered among fellow scientists," many of whom attributed to him "an unabashed passion for scientific glory and public attention."[11]

Raub directed Gallo's immediate boss, a hulking, baldish NCI bureaucrat named Richard Adamson, to draft a response to Dingell for Raub's signature. As chief of the division of cancer etiology, Adamson's responsibilities included going on television to warn Americans not to overcook their meat and to eat more green and yellow vegetables. Adamson hadn't worked in the lab for years, and he knew less about the details of Gallo's AIDS research than Peter Fischinger had at the outset of the Pasteur dispute.

Adamson nevertheless declared that, despite its "length and detail," the *Tribune* article hadn't contained any new information.[12] "Almost in its entirety," Adamson's letter said, "the evidence presented is circumstantial, misinterpreted, often trivial or moot, and in many places flagrantly misrepresentative." In particular, LAV had never been "intentionally grown" in a continuous cell line in Gallo's laboratory, and HTLV-3B and LAV_{Bru} were "not identical" isolates of HIV. Thinking the letter not very helpful, Raub told Adamson to compile a list of every question raised by the *Tribune* that required resolution.[13] In the meantime, Raub sent Dingell a less combative letter assuring the chairman that the *Tribune* article was undergoing a careful examination.[14]

The news that a congressional panel had reopened "the question of who was first to discover the AIDS virus" was applauded by the *Boston Globe*, which observed that "even for nonscientists, much is at stake."[15] At issue, the *Globe* said, was "not just the timing of the discovery or the huge royalties that are tied to AIDS tests and patents on basic AIDS biologicals. Nor is it who really discovered the remarkable AIDS virus. It is: Under what circumstances did the discovery take place? Was the process or the reporting of the research violated? The central point is that only the AIDS virus isolated by Gallo, among hundreds since isolated, is a genetic twin to the virus found by the French team, which sent samples of it to Gallo's lab. How this could happen is difficult to explain. . . ."

A couple of weeks after the *Tribune* article, the acting director of the NIH's new Office of Scientific Integrity, Suzanne Hadley, was returning from an acrimonious meeting with Imanishi-Kari's lawyers in Boston. Once the plane was in the air, Hadley's traveling companion, the NIH's legal adviser Robert Lanman, pulled the article from his briefcase and began paging through it. Hadley, a diminutive blonde psychologist on loan to OSI from the National Institutes of Mental Health, remembered being "horrified" that no one had informed her that questions were again being raised about Gallo's research. When she got back to the NIH, Hadley went straight to see Bill Raub.

"I told him, 'This should be an OSI matter,'" Hadley recalled. "I said, 'If it were anybody else besides Gallo, it would have been an OSI matter a long time ago.' Bill said, 'Well, if I gave this to you, what would you do?' I said, 'I would immediately inform Dr. Gallo that it was a formal inquiry, tell him what the issues were, get all his notebooks, and begin the interviews.'" Hadley didn't have to argue very hard. "He said to me, 'You're absolutely right, it's an OSI matter.'"

OSI's procedures called for a two-stage investigation: an informal inquiry, in which the evidence was assessed to see whether there was a realistic possibility that misconduct might have occurred, followed by a formal investigation of the possible misconduct. Under the two-tier system, spurious allegations by disgruntled colleagues could be disposed of before the accused was required to undergo a full-fledged investigation that might taint a career regardless of the outcome.

In early January of 1990, almost seven years to the day after LAV$_{Bru}$ was first isolated at the Pasteur, Suzanne Hadley advised Dick Adamson that the OSI had opened an informal inquiry into several aspects of Gallo's AIDS research. The inquiry, Hadley promised Adamson, would be "thorough and fair and also will be able to stand up to scrutiny as having been objective and entirely credible."[16]

Hadley's letter set off alarm bells in the corridors of the cancer institute, the loudest of them in Gallo's lab, where the dispute with the French had been relegated to history. Suddenly an NIH official Gallo had never heard of was preparing to go *back* over Mika Popovic's records of LAV and HTLV-3B, and to interview Gallo, Popovic, Betsy Read, and everybody else involved in the early work on AIDS. After making some inquiries, Gallo seemed more relieved. Suzanne Hadley, Gallo told his staff, was a psychologist, not a research scientist, and word had it that she was "not experienced and not intelligent."[17]

It was true that Hadley's research experience had been limited to rats, and that she didn't know a retrovirus from a restriction enzyme. But Suzanne Hadley had a photographic memory, she was a lightning-fast study, and she was dogged as all get-out. Hadley's first step was to request that the original notebooks kept by Popovic, Read, and Ersell Richardson be removed from Gallo's lab and secured as soon as possible. In addition, Hadley told Adamson, Gallo should be warned about any conversations he might have regarding the investigation. "There needs to be caution exercised," Hadley warned Adamson, "to ensure there is no appearance of an attempt to 'refresh the memory' of any persons that Dr. Gallo might contact."

After studying the *Tribune* article, Bill Raub had identified a number of issues that "may not have been examined fully" during the dispute with the Pasteur. Advising John Dingell of the scope of the Gallo inquiry, Raub included the four questions to which the NCI least wanted answers: the "growth and usage" of LAV in the Gallo laboratory; the possible "contamination" of Gallo's cultures; the invention of the HIV blood test; and whether the Gallo ELISA had been developed with "material obtained from another laboratory."[c]

The OSI inquiry team would be joined by two non-NIH scientists, Paul Parkman of the FDA and an army colonel, Edmund Tramont, from the Walter Reed Army Institute of Research. But to ensure that the outcome couldn't be dismissed as a government whitewash, Bill Raub wanted an additional layer of independent review. In early February of 1990, Raub advised Dingell that the NIH planned to ask the National Academy of Sciences to form a special panel to oversee and advise the Gallo inquiry.[18]

It was an unusual request, but hardly an extraordinary one. Since its establishment by an Act of Congress signed by Abraham Lincoln, the Academy has served as the federal government's adviser on matters of science and technology, obliged by its congressional charter "whenever called upon by any department of the Government" to "investigate, examine, experiment, and report upon any subject of science or art."[19]

If Suzanne Hadley viewed Raub's request as an unwarranted intrusion on the OSI's independence, Gallo thought an Academy oversight panel was a fine idea. Jim Wyngaarden, no longer at NIH but still in touch with Gallo, remembered telling Gallo that matters had reached a stage where "he couldn't be exonerated within the system," and that if he wanted a Nobel Prize his research needed the imprimatur of an impartial body like the Academy. "He said, 'Good idea,'" Wyngaarden recalled.[20]

"I welcome this," Gallo told *Science*. "These allegations have been going on too long. I have done nothing wrong and I have no apprehension or anxiety about the review. And, I'm confident that the only chance I have is the help of independent colleagues."[21]

Behind the scenes, Gallo was already at work to ensure that the Academy panel was as friendly as possible. "Here is a list of academy members," Gallo wrote Sam Broder at the beginning of March 1990.[22] "I list about 60 who I believe would be fair. I list another 10 or so I believe present possible or probable problems." The "fair" list included several of Gallo's friends and collaborators, among them Ludwik Gross and Hilary Koprowski. On the "dangerous" list were Harold Varmus, David Baltimore, George Todaro, and Jim Watson, whom Gallo blamed for having inspired the editorial supporting the OSI investigation in the *Boston Globe*.[23]

Gallo considered Watson "sort of a friend," but one who "for complex political-psychological-historical reasons cannot help pushing and getting involved in these things. In short, he is a loose cannon. . . ."[24] To Gallo it seemed that Watson wanted "every special or great scientist to purge and be purged of their guilt as he did in his book when he admitted to taking Dr. Rosey Franklin's results in a matter that was, let us say, not without extreme aggressiveness.[d] Therefore, we must all have one or two skeletons in the closet; or like [sic] perhaps two or three scientists who gain by me going down and by certain forces that stand to make *much money* if the U.S. patent dies."[25]

Sam Broder professed to be worried less about the patent than the impact of the OSI investigation on Gallo's research. "Bob is being tied up in knots," Broder told Larry Kramer, the playwright turned columnist for the gay magazine *Out Week*.[26] "I can't talk science with him," Broder said. "His mind is distracted and he can't focus on it. Enough is enough already." The day Kramer's article appeared, Gallo was attempting to regain his focus at the Wailea Beach Resort in Maui, where he had been invited to deliver a "special lecture" to the Third Annual Conference on Retrovirology.[27]

When Gallo resurfaced it was at Fordham University in the Bronx, where he announced a breakthrough discovery — a cure for Kaposi's sarcoma, the malignant lesions that account for about one in five deaths among AIDS patients.

"We have compounds from a company in Japan," Gallo told his audience, "that wipe out the Kaposi's sarcoma in a way I have never seen before. That is, no toxicity and the tumor's gone, and never reappears."[28] Gallo hadn't published any such results, and he hadn't presented any data at Fordham to back up his claims. But when the news of a "cure for KS" was reported in the media, AIDS patients demanding the drug chained themselves together in the New Jersey offices of the Japanese pharmaceutical company that owned the rights to the compound Gallo mentioned.[29]

Thinking someone would surely give him the name of the miracle compound, a Chicago Kaposi's patient named Jerry Stevens simply picked up the phone and called Gallo's lab. "You have probably forgotten our conversation," Stevens wrote Gallo's administrative assistant, Howard Streicher, the following day, "but I have not and I will not forget it in a long time. I have never in my life been talked to in such a demeaning, condescending, rude and abrupt manner by anyone let alone an alleged health care professional on the public payroll.[30]

"I am dying from AIDS and in particular Kaposi's sarcoma," Stevens went on, "which is what motivated me to call Dr. Gallo's office in the first place. My call was not intended to harass you as you attempted to make it sound. It was only a call of a man who wants very much to live. I want to know the name of the compound referenced by Dr. Gallo in his presentation of February 22, 1990, and I don't think this is an unreasonable request. I am still at a loss as to why you refused to give me that information. How cruel it is to publicly talk about a cure and then refuse the information to the public."

When Stevens got no reply from Streicher he wrote directly to Sam Broder,[31] which was the first Broder had heard about a breakthrough in Gallo's lab. When Broder learned that Gallo's remarks at Fordham had been based entirely on experiments in mice, not AIDS patients, he ordered Gallo to apologize to Stevens and to explain that he didn't have a cure for Kaposi's sarcoma after all. "I would be grateful," Broder added, "if all parties took the legitimate feelings and sensitivities of these patients into account. Patients' sensitivities on this kind of an issue can understandably be quite fragile."[e]

It had been early January when Suzanne Hadley requested the originals of the Gallo lab's notebooks, but by mid-March she still didn't have them.[32] When Hadley reminded Sam Broder of the urgent need to secure the notebooks before they could be tampered with, Broder assured her that Howard Streicher was working overtime to assemble them. But when Hadley called Dick Adamson to check on Streicher's progress, she learned that Gallo, who was in California, had left instructions not to release any notebooks until he had "reviewed them and approved the release."

The day ended with a call from Gallo's personal lawyer, Joseph Onek, who promised that Hadley would have the notebooks by Monday. When they didn't materialize, Hadley told Onek that if the notebooks weren't in her hands by six o'clock she was coming to get them. If Hadley did that, Onek said, everybody would read about it on the front page of the next day's *Washington Post.* Since then another week had passed, and Hadley still didn't have any explanation of why the notebooks hadn't been delivered. "I am deeply concerned," she told Bill Raub, "about the *appearance* this may create as to the inquiry process."

John Maddox, still hoping to publish replies by Gallo and Montagnier to the *Tribune,* assured Gallo of "the sympathy I have for the torrid time that evidently lies ahead of you. In the light of everything, I'm more than ever convinced that the best course of action is to publish your own account of what happened before the NIH committee gets down to work. Obviously the committee would take offence if you were to do this after the inquiry had begun. But naturally, anything that you were to publish would have to be 100 percent true, and beyond challenge."[33]

Maddox didn't think it was necessary for Gallo to answer every one of the *Tribune*'s points. "The main charge," he said, "is simply that you KNOWINGLY misappropriated LAV.[f] If you could prove that LAV and 3B are different, that would of course be a strong riposte. It's obviously less satisfactory to be able to say only that you didn't do so knowingly, and that there might have been an accident, but that's much better than saying nothing at all."

When Gallo didn't respond, Maddox telephoned for an answer. "And Bob said, 'I've got four drafts here,'" Maddox recalled. "'It's very difficult to know which is the best.' And I said, 'Well, send any one or all of them and we'll talk about it.'" When nothing arrived in the mail, Maddox called again, saying "'Look, this is getting embarrassing because Montagnier's done his stuff.' So I met Bob in Washington, and we had dinner and he showed me a draft of a reply that he had. It was too long, but never mind that. It included the significant phrase, 'I cannot rule out the possibility of laboratory contamination.' And I said, 'Well, that's OK. Why don't you let me have it?' He said, 'Well, I'll get it retyped.'"

Maddox never got Gallo's response, and he returned Montagnier's unpublished letter. But Maddox's patience had limits. When Gallo abruptly canceled a Frankfurt news conference where he had promised to present his version of the discovery of HIV, *Nature* criticized him in print.[34]

"*Nature* and *Science* have great power," Gallo complained to Maddox. "They influence many scientists in a way that a reporter in a newspaper cannot hope to. Consequently, they also bear greater responsibility. As the editor of *Nature*, as a scientist and as a friend, why did you feel it necessary to rehash all of the most vicious innuendoes or assertions in the recent editorial pages concerning my simple decline of a press interview? This editorial has hurt me very badly — enough so to initiate the worst form of gossip against me at a place like Johns Hopkins. The situation is hard and depressing enough. I need some patience and understanding until the interviews are completed. Above anyone I looked to you for both."[35]

After a follow-up article in the *Chicago Tribune* suggesting that a number of the government's assertions in court and before the patent office had been untrue, Suzanne Hadley was sufficiently unnerved to call a friend in the Justice Department.[36] Already, senior NIH officials had expressed concern that the OSI investigation might "turn up something that could overturn" the Gallo blood-test patent.[37] "I asked him, 'Have you seen this story?'" Hadley recalled. "And his reaction was, 'My God, this will blow the roof off the place'— that Justice not just was misled, but might have actively been a part of it. Or at least assented without protesting to something they knew, or should have known, was not true."

The French, who thought the Gallo affair had ended three years before, were suddenly reading and hearing about "SIDAGATE," SIDA being the French acronym for AIDS.[38] Montagnier, who had remained quiet since the settlement, admitted to *Le Monde* that the possibility that Gallo had stolen LAV "did cross our minds." But he was careful to note that "the possibility of accidental contamination must first be considered before accusing someone. I think that if this turns out to be the case there is no reason to accuse Dr. Gallo of theft."[39]

Reading the news from Paris, the NIH's international liaison office warned Bill Raub that a "reawakening of the controversy between Dr. Gallo and Dr. Montagnier could threaten the HHS-Pasteur settlement."[40] When Gallo learned Montagnier had called on him publicly to acknowledge that HTLV-3B was LAV, he became livid.[41] It was "completely shameful to hear such things," Gallo told *Liberation*. "If the Pasteur Institute and Professor Luc Montagnier want to have all the glory from the first day, I would be happy to accept that and to have done all the work. There is no investigation by the NIH. There is a probe that followed from that of the journalist. Why don't you wait for the results?"

Moving to secure the public relations front, Gallo had provided senior editors at *Newsweek* and the *Washington Post* with his version of history.[42] Now he urged HHS to launch its own public relations offensive against "the barrage of material being circulated regarding our work, the blood test patent, and the history of HIV." Many "important pieces of information" had come into his hands, Gallo said, and should be "shared and discussed so there can be a planned action or lack of it."[43] But when Gallo asked for a meeting with Sam

Broder, Bill Raub, and the HHS lawyers, he was refused; Jim Mason suggested Gallo simply give his new information, whatever it was, to Suzanne Hadley. After looking over Gallo's material, Hadley concluded that "Dr. Gallo does not have significant information about this matter other than what he is providing to the inquiry team."[44]

If HHS was no longer behind him, Gallo would launch a private offensive of his own. "Welcome back," Gallo wrote Joe Onek, just back from a late-winter vacation and selected by Gallo to lead the charge.[45] "You will be tanned, happy, rested and at the peak of your mental prowess when you read this." Onek, a quintessential Washington insider, had clerked for Supreme Court Justice William Brennan after graduating from Harvard and Yale Law School, then worked for Senator Edward M. Kennedy. He had served during the Carter administration in the Office of the White House Counsel, then opened a successful practice with two other former Supreme Court clerks, Joel Klein and Bart Farr. According to the *Washington Post*, Onek, Klein and Farr had become "the hottest law firm" in town.[g]

For good measure, Gallo also enlisted Bob Charrow, the former deputy HHS general counsel, who had been deeply involved in the government's defense of Gallo against Pasteur. Another addition to the pick-up team was Robert Keith Gray, a prominent Republican who headed the Washington office of the powerhouse public relations firm Hill & Knowlton.[46] Gray, who billed his regular clients $400 an hour, had met Gallo at an awards ceremony attended by Robert Maxwell and volunteered his *pro bono* assistance along with that of Frank Mankiewicz, a former press secretary to Senator Robert F. Kennedy who had landed at Hill & Knowlton after resigning as head of National Public Radio.[47]

Gallo was brimming with plans for how to manage the OSI inquiry. But he cautioned his staff that "It should not be obvious that we are using a PR firm or a lawyer."[48] Despite Gallo's attempts to influence the makeup of the Academy panel, when the members were announced they didn't include Ludwik Gross or Hilary Koprowski. It was an impressive group nonetheless: Stanley Falkow from Stanford,[49] Alfred Gilman and Joseph Sambrook from the University of Texas, Mary Jane Osborne from the University of Connecticut, Arnold Levine from Princeton, John Stobo from Johns Hopkins, Robert Wagner from the University of Virginia, and Judith Areen, the dean of the law school at Georgetown University, a non-Academy member chosen for her legal acumen.[50]

With the exception of Areen, the panel members were scientific heavyweights, and several were potential Nobel Prize winners. "Anybody who thinks this is a wash job doesn't know the members of this committee," remarked Mary Jane Osborne. Despite her initial reservations, Suzanne Hadley was forced to agree. "There was nobody on the panel who was going to give Gallo a break he didn't deserve," Hadley said.

Bill Raub's charge to the panelists was to review the OSI's strategy and the major pieces of evidence in the case, "and advise us about the issues requiring further attention." Farther down the road, the panel would be asked to consider the inquiry's findings "and advise us if the matter can be closed or if a formal investigation of possible scientific misconduct is warranted." Raub hoped the panel's "expertise, independence, and objectivity" would ensure "a thorough and fair review."[51]

It wasn't the way the panel members would have chosen to spend their time. "It's hard," sympathized Jim Watson, who had escaped service on the panel, "partly because no one really wants to be involved in this sort of thing. But when charges are made, it's in everyone's interest that it be done swiftly."[52]

In Watson's view, the major problem facing science wasn't deliberate dishonesty or the outright faking of data, which was what OSI had been set up to investigate. Fabrication happened rarely, because it was too obvious and too easily found out. "Corruption comes in priority over ideas," Watson said, "of giving credits. That's where people can be disillusioned, in stealing something which should be shared, or which they don't deserve at all. There are seldom penalties for that. That's more often taken as part of normal life. That becomes much worse now with money being scarce for science."

Gallo spent the days before his first OSI appearance at one of the UCLA ski meetings, which had moved to Keystone, Colorado, from their former venue in Park City.[53] Perhaps as a signal to the OSI that Gallo was still a leader in his field, the meeting's organizers, Sam Broder and Flossie Wong-Staal, selected him to deliver the keynote address.

Gallo's talk on "Human Retroviruses, The First Decade," which lasted ninety minutes and was accompanied by more than 100 slides, amounted to an excruciatingly detailed history of Gallo's own research.

Several who heard Gallo speak remembered thinking he was throwing the gantlet before Suzanne Hadley and the OSI.

"He went back to about 1970 or so," Paul Luciw said, "the early days of retrovirology, and all that. He didn't show the titles of the papers, and he didn't accurately in many cases describe the contents. The little phrase or title in each slide in many cases was a distortion of what the paper was about, an incredible reinterpretation. It was almost like a legal defense in a way. Someone that's a leader in a field would never give a seminar like this, with just constant citations to his own work. It's just so out of place. What's the purpose — to call attention to himself and all his discoveries?"

Nearly everyone working on HIV and AIDS was at Keystone, including Bill Haseltine, Robin Weiss, Mika Popovic, Jay Levy, Simon Wain-Hobson, Beatrice Hahn, Gerry Myers, and Jim Mullins. But it was one of the lesser-known presenters, Mario Stevenson from the University of Nebraska, from whom Gallo at last heard some welcome news.

From a hemophiliac living in Omaha, Stevenson had isolated an AIDS virus that was a *dead ringer* for LAV — a discovery, in the opinion of the *Washington Post,* that "could help vindicate Robert Gallo's controversial claim to have discovered the AIDS virus independently of a rival French group."[54]

Stevenson already had submitted a paper on his LAV-like virus to the *Journal of Virology.*[55] The only problem was that he couldn't identify the patient in whom the virus had been discovered. "We were getting a number of blood samples from the clinic at the University of Nebraska medical center, where they have a large hemophiliac population," Stevenson explained. "We were taking samples from the freezer. There was no code number with those samples, because I was very aware that if people were able to get code numbers from samples then the patient could be identified, and I didn't want that to happen."

There were only forty-three nucleotide differences between LAV and the virus Stevenson called MFA, roughly half as many as between LAV and HTLV-3B, which made it critically important to learn when and where the source of MFA had become infected. Not surprisingly, the cancer institute offered to help, and Stevenson reported that "we've narrowed it down to about a three-month time span when we got the blood. We're now trying to identify which patients were coming in and getting blood at that time. I think we've identified about twenty-five possible individuals. The problem is, we don't know if this individual is still alive."

Whatever the provenance of MFA, Stevenson was certain of one thing. It couldn't be a laboratory contaminant of HTLV-3B or LAV, because "we didn't *have* any HTLV-3B growing in the laboratory, or LAV."

Buoyed by Stevenson's discovery, on April 8, 1990, Gallo made his premier appearance before the Office of Scientific Integrity, to which he presented a twenty-page review of his research. "I am confident," Gallo began, "that this review body will learn that my coworkers and I have been wrongly treated, that there has been no wrongdoing in my laboratory, that there has been substantial misrepresentation in select press, and we hope that these evaluations will be able to help us rectify these misconceptions. We are justifiably proud of our work."

What followed was a compendium of the government's erroneous assertions during the dispute with the Pasteur[h] plus some new ones, including Gallo's mistaken contention that he had announced the discovery of HTLV-3B at the Pasteur in January 1984 — a month before Chermann's presentation at Park City, and three months before the actual date of the meeting in Paris. But Gallo did acknowledge that LAV *had* grown in his lab — not just "transiently," but continuously, and in a permanent cell line.

As for Gallo's claims that he had identified the AIDS virus before Françoise Barré, to OSI he admitted that he had been unable to culture *any* material from AIDS patients during late 1982 and 1983. Perhaps most significant was Gallo's admission, for the first time, that Mika Popovic had cultivated an AIDS isolate called MOV. But Gallo cautioned that, in light of Mario Stevenson's Nebraska isolate, it was "premature to make a definitive conclusion that 3B and LAV were derived from the same sample."

Within hours of his presentation copies of Gallo's statement had begun making the rounds of the NIH campus. To those unfamiliar with Gallo's previous statements, or the details and chronology of his research, it must have looked impressive and sounded convincing. "What the smart money is saying around here," Mal Martin said, "is that he's going to get out of this thing. They're going to say that no wrongdoing was found, and the whole thing was just something that was made up."

. . .

Aided by the General Accounting Office, the investigative arm of Congress, John Dingell's staff had continued to sift the financial records of Gallo's laboratory. Among the documents it unearthed was a lucrative purchasing agreement with a small local company, Pan-Data Systems, which had been transformed from a startup operating out of a post office box to a million-dollar-a-year supplier of scientific services to the government.

Among the researchers in Gallo's lab who had purchased hundreds of thousands of dollars' worth of scientific materials from Pan-Data was Zaki Salahuddin. As the GAO had now learned, Salahuddin was also Pan-Data's director of corporate development, and his wife its founding chairman. "A gross conflict of interest," John Dingell thundered, "on the part of a prominent AIDS researcher at the National Institutes of Health," who had hidden his "improper financial interest in a biomedical firm doing substantial business with his own laboratory at the NIH."[56]

Gallo told the GAO he hadn't known until three months before that Salahuddin had been involved with the company.[57] To the *Washington Post*, however, Gallo said he first learned of the Salahuddin–Pan-Data connection a year before. He had "screamed about it" to Zaki Salahuddin, and "the next day his wife was out of the company."[58] But there was more to the story than that.

Among the products advertised for sale in Pan-Data's catalog were several items from Gallo's lab: HBLV, HTLV-1, HTLV-2, T-Cell Growth Factor, even H-9 cells producing HTLV-3B. Pan-Data's lawyer, Julian Greenspun, explained that the company had isolated its own strain of HBLV, and that the HTLV-1 and HTLV-2 being sold by the company had come from a "proprietary source. They're not selling stuff that they're not supposed to from NIH." But a new isolation of HTLV-2 by Pan-Data would have been worthy of reporting in the scientific literature, and the GAO had found records showing that the same "H-9/HTLV-3" sold by Pan-Data to Georgetown University, Johns Hopkins, and Harvard had been purchased by Gallo's lab from Electronucleonics — which was producing it under contract to Gallo. The purchaser had been Zaki Salahuddin.[i]

After an unpleasant morning listening to Dingell's excoriations about the NIH's "lax atmosphere for personal gain," Bill Raub conceded there was "no condoning the kind of activity described here this morning." Henceforth, Raub assured Dingell, all NIH employees involved in recommending or granting subcontracts would be required to sign statements affirming that they had no financial interest in any of the candidate companies.

Gallo blamed Salahuddin for having "brought Mr. Dingell into our lives."[59] But Salahuddin thought he was being made a sacrificial lamb by NCI higher-ups, who hoped the subcommittee's investigation of Gallo would stop there. "I have not committed a murder," Salahuddin said. "I have not run away with somebody's wife. I have made probably mistakes. I have lost my friends, my health, my diabetes is running wild, my ulcer is beginning to bleed. I'm in such a situation that I don't know what to do. Maybe walk off the sixth-floor window of my laboratory."[j]

Within a few weeks, Salahuddin was facing a criminal grand jury investigation. "I wish they have used the same yardstick they do with many of their other people," Salahuddin said. "Here's Gallo, they provide him double coverage, internal investigation and so forth, all this moral turpitude he is accused of for such a long period of time. No one ever talks of suspending him. In my case they go immediately for the knife and throw me to the wolves."

In far-off New Mexico, Mika Popovic was also feeling some heat. At New Mexico State University, Popovic had been struggling to establish what the administration hoped would be a "world-class" retroviral research unit. But Popovic had resigned his new job after just eighteen months, after the university's president saw an article in *Science* quoting an unnamed colleague describing Popovic's pool experiment as "really crazy."[60]

Since the onset of the OSI investigation, Popovic had let Gallo do the talking. Finally summoned by the inquiry panel, Popovic made his entrance with much exaggerated bowing and Old World formality, to the point that Suzanne Hadley half-expected him to kiss her hand. But when Popovic began to speak about the fate that had befallen "my best work of my life," Hadley remembered thinking that Popovic intended to save himself at Gallo's expense.[61]

About Gallo's frequent claims to have isolated HIV before the French,[62] Popovic recalled that in late 1982 and early 1983 a handful of AIDS patient cultures had displayed "some RT positivity." When all the cultures had died without yielding any virus, there had been "not immediate excitement about it. Obviously we didn't think, 'Aha, here is a cytopathic [cell-killing] virus, let's go after it,' and so on. I have probably talked too much."

Popovic kept talking anyway. No one, he said, had recognized in 1983 that Claude Chardon was infected with HIV in addition to HTLV-1, as Gallo now claimed — only that there was something unusual about the Chardon culture, "that there is something killing the cells." As for the electron micrograph of what Gallo had claimed in *Nature* was an AIDS virus growing in Chardon's cells, Popovic admitted that no one had seen the AIDS virus in those pictures in 1983.

Apologizing for the state of his notebooks, Popovic explained that in Czechoslovakia experimental records were kept by technicians and junior scientists, not senior researchers. "To be honest," he said, "I didn't write detailed notes for six years in my native language. When I came here nobody gave me whatsoever any instructions how we should write our notes or anything else. And when the litigation started, suddenly I was asked for notes."

Popovic was well aware he had been "criticized strongly" for the pool experiment, with what he now admitted was some justification. "I know it wasn't a bona fide experiment," he said. "If I take speci-mens from several virus-positive individuals, then the probability is higher that I can catch an isolate which would be sufficiently infec-tious and replicative than if I would have done single, one by one. If you have to do single, one by one, it would take a long time."

"You will never be able to trace it to its source," Suzanne Hadley said. "The one that grew. Will you?"

"I fully agree with you," Popovic replied. "I am not questioning."

One of the enduring mysteries around the pool, apart from its exis-tence, was why it had been necessary to add material from additional patients after the first six weeks. The reason, Popovic explained, was that he had been trying to keep the pool from dying. "I was afraid that I would lose the culture," Popovic said. "Therefore, I told myself, 'Oh, good God, I won't have it.' So I again collected, how many, seven samples concentrated, and I exposed them to concentrated culture fluids. There was also a lot of contamination started to develop. I mean mold, not virus contamination."

In his *Science* article, Popovic had described HTLV-3B, though not by name, as having been isolated from "patients with AIDS or pre-AIDS," whose virus cultures "were first shown to contain particle-associated RT." But Popovic's notes showed that most of the pool patients hadn't tested positive for RT, and Popovic admitted to OSI he hadn't had any RT data at all on most of those samples. "The cells were grown up," Popovic said, "then they were sent out for further analysis. The data came back later. This was the usual pattern in almost all cases. Obviously, it was more or less a blind experiment."

Hadley pointed out that when the RT data had arrived later, it showed that most of the pooled samples had been negative.

"There can be questioned many things," Popovic replied.

In Suzanne Hadley's view, the "$64,000 question" was whether LAV had been deliberately transformed into HTLV-3B, either by adding LAV to the pool or simply renaming the French virus and claiming it as Popovic's own discovery.

"Of course not," Popovic replied.

On the other hand, he went on, suppose he *had* added LAV to the pool. Wouldn't that have been a legitimate use of a virus that had been sent to Gallo's lab for the express purpose of being grown and studied? There wasn't anything in the collaborative agreement with the French that precluded Popovic's combining LAV with material from American AIDS patients, only its commercial use.

"If I have a cell line which is virus positive," Popovic explained, "and I take another virus-positive cell line and mix together and put together LAV, it is bona fide experiment. What is difference, if I take from one of these flasks, I have two different and mix together, and then I put in one cell line? Or I have cell line which is positive and I take the virus and put it there? What is difference between these two?"

Popovic wasn't saying he had done such a thing — in fact, he was denying having done it. He was only saying it would have been all right if he had. When Hadley wondered whether LAV might have gotten into the pool by accident, Popovic replied that "it could happen. There is a possibility it could occur. I won't rule that out."

Hadley's final line of questioning concerned MOV, the mystery virus that had made its first appearance in Popovic's notes a few days after the purported creation of the pool, and that had been used by Sarngadharan to make the Gallo ELISA. Since the ELISA was a test for AIDS-virus antibodies, MOV must have been an AIDS virus. But neither Popovic's notes, nor those from Betsy Read and Ersell Richardson, contained the faintest clue to its origin.

Popovic couldn't resolve the mystery, explaining that he didn't know for sure where MOV had come from. It might have been an

African patient named Moweni, whose cells he had picked up in Switzerland on the way home from the family reunion in Basel.

"What is the basis for your thinking it might be Moweni?" Hadley asked. "Just because of the name and the MO?"

"I don't have experimental data," Popovic replied, "but extensively I co-cultured that Moweni sample with cell lines. That would be my recollection." But it was also possible that MOV had come from another patient named Hector Millian.

After listening to Popovic's testimony, Paul Parkman, the FDA virologist on the inquiry panel, wondered why Gallo and Popovic hadn't tried to sort out all the confusion earlier, by testing the original pool samples for a virus with a genetic identity to LAV.

"At that time it didn't matter too much," Popovic said. "It is easy later to be smart."

"What are the odds of running into somebody you're avoiding in a crowd of 12,000 people?"[63] the *San Francisco Examiner* asked on the eve of the Sixth International AIDS Conference. "Conference-watchers," the *Examiner* reported, "wonder whether there'll be a tête-à-tête between Dr. Robert Gallo of the United States, and Dr. Luc Montagnier of the Pasteur Institute in Paris."

Montagnier made news on the first night, announcing that he had solved the riddle of why some HIV-infected individuals quickly developed AIDS while a handful lived without symptoms for ten or fifteen years. The culprit, Montagnier explained, was mycoplasma, a tiny organism that inhabits human cells, and whose presence explained why a slow-growing virus like HIV was deadly in most patients but seemingly benign in others.

Montagnier seemed to be suggesting that, in the absence of mycoplasma, people with HIV might not get AIDS at all — an improbable theory at best — and many in the audience thought it an embarrassing performance as well. "He's really hyping it up," Paul Luciw said. "He's making it much more important and exotic than it deserves. The Frenchmen at the meeting, these are some of the junior people, they were pretty frank about that. They said what he's doing now is embarrassing the French scientific community. He could stop all his work now and get an awful lot of credit, but he's really moving backwards."

Montagnier, who had been scheduled to chair a panel later in the conference, beat a hasty retreat to France. There wouldn't be any tête-à-tête with Gallo, who still hadn't arrived in San Francisco, and whose presence was missed by Randy Shilts. At each of the earlier AIDS conferences, Shilts observed in the *San Francisco Chronicle*, there had been "one dominant figure from the world of science: Dr. Robert Gallo of the National Cancer Institute. You could always pick him out in the hallways, surrounded by an entourage of admiring scientists. He delivered keynote addresses and pontificated to devoted journalists who religiously recorded his every observation."[64]

Gallo wasn't accustomed to negative press, but suddenly there seemed to be a surfeit of it. A long and flattering account of Gallo's career, written for *The New Yorker*,[k] had been abruptly canceled by the magazine's editor, Robert Gottlieb, after the OSI investigation was announced. Now *Spy*, an irreverent monthly modeled on the British magazine *Private Eye*, had published a less-than-flattering portrait of Gallo.

The author of "Lab Rat" was a Berkeley psychology professor, Seth Roberts, who first encountered Gallo giving a talk on "viruses of late 20th century man."[65] After Gallo finished speaking, Roberts approached him with a question. "I asked him how people could die of AIDS when there was so little detectable virus," Roberts recalled. "He said, 'OK, let's take the brain.' The virus attacks glial cells, and thus it destroys the architecture of the brain. I'll send you a reprint.'"

Gallo tried to move away, but Roberts persisted. "I asked him, 'How much AIDS virus is in the glial cells?' He said, 'Neurologists at NIMH say a lot.' I said, 'How much is a lot? What percent of the glial cells are infected?' Then he started shouting at me. 'Do you know what lymphadenopathy is? Can you pronounce it?' I said, 'I'm a professor of psychology at Berkeley. The brain is my subject.' He told me I should go to medical school."

Roberts's article was the longest *Spy* had ever published, and if the magazine hadn't been a few days late reaching the West Coast it would have been an instant sell-out among the conference attendees.[66] But Abraham Karpas had purchased several copies while changing planes in New York, and within hours of Karpas's arrival multigeneration photocopies were being passed around.

"In Tyson's Corner, Virginia, in 1985," the article began, "a woman was buying a car. When she mentioned to the salesman that she was a scientist, he told her a story about a neighbor of his, a scientist as well, who had recently complained at a cocktail party that he had been cheated out of a Nobel Prize in Medicine. A few years later the same woman was chatting with a man who did landscaping for her. He happened to say that one of his clients had said he'd been cheated out of two Nobel Prizes."

Roberts continued in the same vein, repeating gossip from anonymous sources, much of which focused on Gallo's quest for the Nobel: "In the early 1980s his good friend George Klein, a virologist, was on the Nobel committee. At a conference that year, Gallo made sure to have dinner with Klein every night; then someone told Gallo that Klein had been replaced on the committee by the immunologist Hans Wigzell. Gallo dined with Wigzell the very next night."

Throughout most of the conference, rumors of Gallo's arrival or nonarrival dominated conversations in the Chinese restaurants and quaint cafés of North Beach. "Gallo was supposed to cochair a session at 1:30 on Saturday," Paul Luciw recalled. "About eleven or twelve o'clock, Jay Levy came up to me and said, 'It looks like Gallo isn't going to be here. Can you be cochair of this session?'"

The news that Gallo wasn't coming arrived in a short note, faxed to one of the conference organizers, explaining that he had decided to extend his visit to the Soviet Union. "For some time now," Gallo said, "I have had plans to be in Leningrad and Moscow associated with a leukemia meeting in Germany. In part because of a recent meeting with President Gorbachev during his visit to Washington, I have also agreed to give additional lectures on HIV while there."[l]

Despite Gallo's regret at missing the San Francisco conference, it was "important to me that my absence will not be misinterpreted or regarded in any way other than my commitment to improving international scientific relationships toward those goals we all share."[m]

When Abraham Karpas got the word that Gallo wasn't coming, he was dining with Michael Koch and Seth Roberts at The Hunan Restaurant on Sansome Street. Tapping his glass with a fork, Karpas proposed a toast: "To Bob — wherever he is hiding."

"Of Course We *Did* Grow LAV"

As the San Francisco AIDS conference neared an end, United Press International announced Robert Gallo's deliverance. According to UPI, the government's investigation of Gallo "apparently has failed to find any proof that a U.S. researcher stole credit for discovering the AIDS virus from a French scientist."[1]

The story, which appeared on the front page of the *San Francisco Examiner,* was prompted by a seven-page article in that week's issue of *Science,* which had examined Gallo's laboratory notebooks "as well as documents obtained by the well-known mechanism of the Washington leak," and had "spoken to a number of persons close to the AIDS discovery — those who are on the 'Gallo team' and those who are not."[2]

Science had asked "a small number of senior scientists with no direct involvement in the issues to review the documents we have obtained. They agreed to do so off the record." While acknowledging that those documents represented only part of the record available to the Office of Scientific Integrity, *Science* nonetheless quoted one of its anonymous reviewers as concluding that "there's just no evidence of fraud here."

As Jim Swire and Suzanne Hadley could have testified, sorting out the discrepancies and anomalies in the Gallo laboratory's notes required far more than a casual reading. It also required having *all* the notes. Whoever *Science*'s reviewers were, the article's author, Barbara

Culliton, hadn't explained what they made of the redacted Gonda letter, or *"HUT78/v; Ti7.4/v = MOV,"* or "Cloning of HT cells ~ HUT 78," or the replacement of LAV and MOV with HTLV-3B, in Sasha Arya's notebooks — assuming they had even been given the relevant documents.

It didn't matter, because the OSI's investigation of Gallo was still many months from reaching a conclusion. According to UPI, its reporter had mistakenly thought the "no evidence of fraud" quote had come from a member of the National Academy panel and represented a final verdict in the Gallo case. The reporter's editor had passed the story because of his own misimpression that *Science* was the official publication of the National Academy.[a]

That the *Science* article amounted to a public exposition of Gallo's OSI defense hadn't surprised some of Culliton's colleagues at *Science,* who had long considered her a Gallo partisan and who were troubled by Culliton's membership in the Institute of Medicine — the group of distinguished physicians within the National Academy that had selected the panel members to oversee the investigation about which Culliton was now writing. Culliton wasn't a doctor, or even a scientist. She was a journalist, and in any other province of journalism, such a relationship would have been perceived as a flagrant conflict of interest.[3]

Science writers like Omar Sattaur, Colin Norman, Steve Connor, and *Nature*'s Declan Butler — all of them British, as it happened — brought a healthy degree of journalistic skepticism to their coverage of a field increasingly fraught with vested interests. Too many of their American counterparts fit the description offered by Natalie Angier of the *New York Times,* who acknowledged that "we science journalists, perhaps more than any other class of reporters, too often serve as perky cheerleaders for our subject and our sources. Maybe that is because most of us really do love science; or maybe we are so worried that the rest of the world does not that we feel obliged to bring out all the bells, whistles and bullhorns. But in any case we sometimes end up writing copy that sounds like an unvarnished press release."[4]

It wasn't a bad description of Culliton's article, which failed to point out that many of Gallo's statements to *Science* contradicted the assurances he had given Colin Norman five years earlier.[b] Nor did Culliton mention that, in a series of OSI interviews during the previous two months, Gallo admitted not having told the truth about many things.[5]

"Not to go into this now," Gallo had said. "But for example, 'Oh, we never grew LAV,' and of course we *did* grow LAV." The lies, Gallo explained, had tumbled out during "my passionate period." There was "a point," Gallo said, "where I say I didn't grow LAV. And of course, LAV was grown. But the point is not commercial, not mass-produced. . . . I was just anguished as to what was coming out of the newspaper. At that moment bombs were going off."[6] His emotions had simply gotten the best of him, Gallo explained, as when he wrote the memos to Peter Fischinger, filled with insupportable claims, that formed the basis for the government's defense in court.

Behind the OSI's closed doors, Gallo demolished the defense that had been raised in his behalf by the government during the Pasteur dispute. His pre-LAV AIDS virus isolates, Gallo said, had never existed. "I never made a claim in the literature for the December '82 samples," Gallo said.[7] "I never made any claim for the February '83 samples," though of course he had, many times.[8] "I wasn't sure that they were going to play any role in AIDS whatsoever," Gallo went on, "and what their characteristics were, and whether they were all one and the same virus type. The data is there that we detected non-HTLV retroviruses on and off again all along, but they weren't characterized, they weren't linked to disease, they weren't found regularly. Sometimes they weren't grown or grown well. Many times, most times that is the story."

It was a far different story from the one Gallo had told in *Science,* the *New England Journal of Medicine, Scientific American,*[9] the "official history" in *Nature,* and his sworn affidavit in the patent case — and different as well from the story the Justice Department had told the patent office and the courts. Gallo confessed that he hadn't had anything like forty-eight AIDS virus isolates when the four *Science* papers were published, another claim he had made dozens of times, including in the official history.

"There was about ten," Gallo said — two fewer than the French, who had had theirs first.[10] As Berge Hampar suspected, Gallo's other "isolates" were merely AIDS patients' frozen blood samples that had been unthawed and tested for viral antibodies — and there were only eighteen of those.[c] Asked why he had claimed forty-eight isolates when he had really had fewer than a quarter of that number, Gallo told OSI "to be quite frank, I was nervous . . ."[11]

Except for HTLV-3B, the only AIDS virus isolate in Gallo's lab worthy of the name had been R.F. But Gallo conceded that it hadn't been necessary for Popovic, having succeeded in growing LAV, to search for his own isolates. "Retrospectively," Gallo said, "we could have simply used LAV and solved the problem." If that wasn't enough candor, Gallo abandoned his insistence that LAV couldn't possibly have contaminated Popovic's cultures. "Let me say," Gallo told OSI, "that it is extremely likely that at least once there was cross-contamination from what is 3B or MOV or LAV."[12]

Had Gallo been half as forthcoming during the interference, the Pasteur would have gone back to France with the blood-test patent in hand.

In asking the question "Is 3B really LAV?" *Science* had cited the Nebraska isolate as new evidence that HTLV-3B might *not* be LAV. A few days before Culliton's article appeared, Gerry Myers got a call from Jules Hallum, a retired virologist who had been recruited, after what Bill Raub described as "a very long search," as the new permanent director of the Office of Scientific Integrity.

Though he had once chaired the microbiology department at the Oregon Health Sciences University, Hallum wasn't coming to OSI from the front lines of science. During the previous eight years, he had published only a single scientific article.[13] *Science* described him as "pleasantly rambling in the style of a beloved college professor." Suzanne Hadley thought Hallum lacked the determination and instincts for his new job, and Hallum admitted it was "much more pleasant to find no misconduct" than to judge a fellow scientist guilty. "Everyone in the office gets depressed when we find misconduct," Hallum said.[14] "It's surprising to find out that scientists are just like other people."

Hadley, who hadn't been a candidate for the permanent directorship because her doctorate was in psychology rather than the biological sciences, had been appointed Hallum's deputy, but it was not destined to be a happy marriage. "Jules is intellectually slow," Hadley said. "He has no energy. Personally, he's weak. I could run rings around him. He's just not very bright. I can forgive almost anything but that."

Based on his conversation with Hallum, Gerry Myers thought the

OSI was mainly interested in assembling evidence that would get Gallo off the hook, particularly the homology of the Nebraska isolate with LAV.

"He had been in touch with the Nebraska people," Myers said, "so I guess Gallo or somebody got him going in that direction. The Nebraska people told him that I had done some analysis, and he asked if he could have that by fax. So of course I sent it to him, and I sent him eight other pages of trees. I cautioned them that they need to spend some time in interpreting those trees, and understanding how they were constructed and what they mean."

But the OSI hadn't wanted any explanations from the man who created the trees. "Apparently there was never any suggestion that they wanted to talk to me," Myers said. "They only wanted me to send data. They want to do this very, very quickly."

The Academy panel hadn't been present during the OSI's initial interviews with Gallo and Popovic, but the panel members had read their statements and examined the supporting evidence. As the San Francisco AIDS meeting was drawing to a close, the Academy panel voted, unanimously, to recommend that the OSI's preliminary inquiry be replaced with a formal misconduct investigation of Gallo and Mika Popovic.

Its decision, the panel told Bill Raub, was based on missing data in Popovic's notes, and "a possibility of selection and/or misrepresentation of data" in Gallo's *Science* articles. In the panel's opinion, "this situation fits the stated requirements to proceed from the Inquiry Phase to a Formal Investigation." Al Gilman, a psychopharmacologist from the University of Texas, saw the panel's role as akin to a grand jury. "Our job," Gilman said, "is to decide whether there's sufficient evidence of schmucky behavior for people to go on and do an investigation."

Bill Raub had wanted the Academy panel to lend the NIH's investigation the imprimatur of objectivity, but Raub hadn't meant for the crew to take control of the ship. "I have given considerable thought to the recommendation," Raub told the panel, "both because of my high regard for the Panelists and because of their uniquely important role toward ensuring the efficacy and objectivity of our process. Moreover, I recognize the sincerity and positive intent behind the proposal. Nevertheless, I conclude that redesignation now would be premature, although I plan to discuss this matter when we next convene the Panel. At that time, we also can discuss the Panel's role."[15]

"Raub and NIH didn't want a real inquiry," Princeton's Arnie Levine said later. "They wanted to save face for NIH and Gallo." But the Academy panelists were accustomed to being in charge of things, and they were undeterred. "I'm willing to listen to Raub and what he wants to do," said Howard Morgan, a distinguished physiocardiologist from Pennsylvania's Geisinger Clinic. "But I think ultimately, for the good of U.S. science, we've got to be sure that this is done properly. I think what concerned a fair number of people on the panel is that it could appear that they were trying *not* to do a thorough investigation, when in fact I think they're trying very hard to do it exactly right. And yet it may not be perceived that way in the community in general."

What mainly concerned Morgan and the other panelists was the same thing that had struck Jim Swire and Myron Weinberg — the apparent lack of supporting data for Popovic's key experiments. "Some of the notebooks are not complete," Morgan said, "and then it becomes more difficult to know for sure whether the data that have been reported represent exactly what was observed. It may not be that you will ever be able to find a written record of all the data that are in print."

But the central question, described by Morgan as "that obvious thing about which virus is which," still could be resolved, by examining the viruses from the ten patients that Popovic said had comprised the pool. To OSI, Popovic had seemed to hint that some such effort was already under way in Gallo's lab. But if it was, Gallo hadn't said anything about it. Either way, the Academy panel thought it was time.[16] "We're going to do some science," said Levine.

The examination would be done by Roche Diagnostic Systems, a California subsidiary of Hoffman–La Roche, the Swiss pharmaceutical behemoth that owned the rights to a new and extremely powerful technology known as polymerase chain reaction. PCR, which would shortly win a Nobel Prize for its inventor, the surfing biochemist Kary Mullis,[17] was brilliant in its simplicity, described by one scientist as "one of those ideas where you say, 'Why didn't *I* think of that?'"

With PCR, it was possible to seek out a particular strand of DNA, including viral DNA, from among many competing strands, then quickly amplify the target strand millions of times. No longer was it necessary to spend weeks isolating, culturing, and cloning virus from the pool patients' T-cells. If any HIV DNA had been integrated into those cells, it would become evident within a few hours.

Designed by Cornell's Volker Vogt, the Roche experiments would first compare any DNA in the pool samples with HTLV-3B and LAV.

Other single-patient isolates, including MOV, would also be compared with LAV. Finally, samples of the original LAV_{Bru} virus from Paris would be compared with HTLV-3B.[18] If LAV-like DNA existed in even one of the pooled samples, it would seem that Gallo was in the clear. If not, Vogt said, the only verdicts could be "contamination" or "mischief."[19]

On a Tuesday morning in early July 1990, Suzanne Hadley informed the NCI that she would arrive at Gallo's laboratory later in the day to collect whatever material from the pool patients remained in the lab's freezers. Besides the ten pool samples and MOV, Hadley's shopping list included R.F. and blood cells from Hector Millian, one of the patients from whom Mika Popovic thought MOV might have been isolated.[20] When Gallo learned his frozen samples were about to be requisitioned by the OSI, he called Hadley in a rage.[21]

The seizing of his samples represented his "loss of involvement" in the investigation, Gallo declared, nothing less than an "impoundment." Hadley explained that she was running the investigation, not Gallo, and that the extent of his involvement was to supply the OSI with information. "I said, 'We're coming over to get them at six o'clock today,'" Hadley recalled. "It was like, 'How can you do this — Gestapo.' It was hard for him to understand."

Hadley arrived promptly at six, accompanied by the NIH legal adviser, Bob Lanman, and an NCI scientist, Gregory Curt, wheeling a portable liquid nitrogen freezer. The invaders were met by Gallo, who protested their presence as an offense to his lab and his integrity. While Curt sealed the requested samples in white Styrofoam boxes and wheeled the freezer away, Gallo continued to fume.[d] Hadley felt like the vampire surrounded by angry villagers carrying torches.

"His whole lab," she said later, "they just worship Gallo and will not challenge him. Anybody who gets a bunch of people around him, who get in a mind-set that he can do no wrong and that everybody else is wrong and is out to get him, you know that's a prescription for disaster. Because nobody is asking the tough questions on the inside."

"Former top AIDS researcher at NCI charged," announced the *Baltimore Sun,* reporting that Zaki Salahuddin had been formally accused of violating conflict-of-interest statutes and accepting illegal gratuities in the Pan-Data case.[22] Salahuddin had offered to talk, but the federal prosecutor assigned to his case hadn't been interested in testimony about other goings-on in Gallo's lab. "He's a very tough guy," Salahuddin said. "He could have made some deal with me. From the beginning he has been thinking of just putting me into jail, that's all. I look at my children and cry. My daughter is nineteen. My boys are fifteen and sixteen. My daughter will have to break her education and start working. My boys are already taking jobs."

Like Mal Martin, Salahuddin was convinced Gallo would walk away from the OSI investigation, while Mika Popovic took the fall. "Nobody could tell you that Gallo was dumb," Salahuddin said. "If Gallo is so bright, why didn't he ask the question 'Now let's see. You got a virus, and we got a virus from France?' That's the first question Gallo normally asks. I have gone through it. You're trying to tell me Bob is dumb? No, he's not dumb. He's one of the brightest persons I know. If I am sitting on the commission, it should not wash under any circumstances that it was Mika's fault."

But Salahuddin was also sure that "nothing will come out of it. No one wants America to go down. They just rally around the flag. NIH and Gallo are inseparable right now. If he goes down, NIH goes down." Still, Salahuddin had five questions he hoped the OSI investigators would ask.

"The first one," he said, "is what did Gallo do when he first saw Mal Martin's paper showing gross similarities between 3B and LAV?[23] The second one, did he take steps at that time to learn whether there had been a contamination? Third one: where is the data showing that Mika's [LAV] cultures were terminated in January 1984? Fourth one: why was Gallo so strong against anyone who suggests that LAV and 3B are the same virus? And the fifth one, what has become of the New Jersey Pair?"

The New Jersey Pair, now consigned by Gerry Myers to the never-never land of laboratory contaminations, was soon to be joined by the Nebraska isolate. As events unfolded, it developed that the discoverer of the Nebraska virus, Mario Stevenson, once had worked in the lab of another Nebraska researcher, a former Israeli tank-driver named David Volsky. Volsky, who had moved on to Columbia University, didn't remember ever having used HTLV-3B or LAV in his Omaha lab. Volsky did, however, recall having asked the Pasteur for a sample of the CEM cell line the French were using to grow LAV. But when Montagnier checked his records, he found that what Volsky had really asked for — and what he got — was *LAV-infected* CEM.[24]

Confronted with the receipt for CEM/LAV bearing his own signature, Volsky conceded it was "technically possible" that the Nebraska isolate was a contaminant of LAV. To Mario Stevenson, it came as "a big surprise" that LAV had previously been grown in the same laboratory where he had isolated the Nebraska virus. But Stevenson was "quite willing to accept the possibility that what we described is simply a reisolation from a strain we were already carrying." When Gerry Myers examined the DNA sequences from Nebraska, he had no doubt. "It's a contamination," said Myers, who sent off a letter reporting the same to *Nature.*[25]

A few days after his letter appeared, Myers got a curious telephone call. From his laboratory in Madison, Howard Temin had been watching the contretemps between Gallo and Pasteur, and Myers remembered being puzzled by what sounded like a cryptic warning. "Howard told me," Myers said, "that everybody should be careful not to conclude that 3B was LAV — and that anyone who did would end up with egg on his face."

With more than his usual grumpiness, Mal Martin had agreed to be interviewed by OSI as an interested witness in the Gallo case.[26] "Mal says, 'What's in this for me?'" Gerry Myers said. "'Why should I care about this? Don't give me this truth and beauty line.' But I think down deep Mal does care, for precisely that reason. It's personally offensive to him. It really offends him deeply."

Martin had been predictably unimpressed with Suzanne Hadley and Jules Hallum. "The committee is incompetent," Martin said. "Totally incompetent. Hallum is very weak, and Hadley has taken the lead. It's a little depressing, seeing how inept they are. The interested scientific public had been under the impression that the Academy committee was involved. But they haven't been involved to any extent I've been aware of. They're chomping at the bit to *get* involved. I'm sending them a memo describing my conversations with Gerry Myers about his tree analysis."[27]

The OSI had seemed to Martin primarily concerned with the question of whether HTLV-3B and LAV might be independent discoveries. "I showed them a lot of restriction enzyme digestions," Martin recalled.

"I said, 'Any card-carrying virologist you talk to today will say that both of these isolates came out of the same person. They are one and the same.' They said, 'Well, how can we get to the bottom of this?' I said, 'You've got to go to the notebooks.'"

But Martin had left OSI with the impression that there was some problem with the Gallo lab's notebooks. "I had a feeling," he recalled, "from something Gallo was saying to one of his colleagues in the cancer institute: 'Can you imagine if somebody asked you about some experiments you did eight years ago? Would you be able to reconstruct them?' He was complaining, like he was being picked on. On the other hand, if you think you're going to get a Nobel Prize or if you have a patent that's bringing you $400,000, you better be damn sure you have all the records. I think he trashed stuff."

Gallo thought Mal Martin had done the same.[28] The pool-sample comparisons outlined by the Academy panel required a sample of the original LAV_{Bru} for use as a control, and requests to the Pasteur Institute had been unavailing. The OSI had hoped to use instead the LAV Martin had brought back from Paris. But Martin couldn't find either his LAV sample or the records of his lab's experiments with the French virus, which he suspected had been lost when the researcher who had performed them transferred to the CDC.[e]

When Gallo's lawyer, Joe Onek, got wind that Martin's LAV notebooks were missing, he promptly filed a Freedom of Information Act request for all correspondence between Martin and the Pasteur Institute, Don Francis, Berge Hampar, George Todaro, Jim Swire, and Bob Nowinski.[29] Onek also wanted "copies of all files in Dr. Martin's office labeled or listed under 'Laboratory of Tumor Cell Biology' or 'Gallo.'"

Gallo accused Martin of either destroying his LAV data or removing it from his office, telling the NIH's office of internal investigations that one of Martin's secretaries "could provide more information about these issues."[30] But when the woman was questioned, she didn't know anything about records or documents having been destroyed or removed. Martin's sample of LAV, along with notebooks showing its use in subsequent experiments, was eventually located and turned over to the OSI.

The federal government often releases bad news on Friday afternoon, when it is likely to be seen and heard by the smallest possible number of newspaper readers and television viewers, and when officials will be unavailable for comment. Thus it was that late on the afternoon of Friday, October 5, 1990, Bill Raub announced that the OSI's Gallo/Popovic inquiry had been upgraded to a formal investigation.[31]

The preliminary inquiry, Raub said, had "resolved certain of the publicized allegations and issues" regarding Gallo's research, and had shown others "to be without substance." In particular, the inquiry team had concluded "that Dr. Gallo had a substantial number of HIV detections and isolations from several different sources at the critical time that HTLV-3B (the principal virus isolated by the Gallo laboratory) and LAV (the virus isolated by the Pasteur Institute) were being grown in Gallo's laboratory."

At the same time, "certain issues" had been identified during the inquiry that warranted a formal investigation, mainly those involving Popovic's *Science* article. The targets of the investigation would be the article's two primary authors, Gallo and Popovic, and it would include the "testing of a number of biological samples in an effort to determine the origins of HTLV-3B, the virus that Dr. Gallo and his colleagues used to develop the blood test for human immunodeficiency virus (HIV)."

The die had been cast the previous weekend, when the Academy panel met with Raub and Hadley to review the progress of the inquiry. After listening to Hadley's presentation, the panel members had agreed, once again, there was sufficient reason to believe scientific misconduct had occurred in Gallo's lab. Hadley remembered Bill Raub, who had mostly listened through the day-long session, suddenly slapping the table with his hand. "He said, 'That's my threshold,'" Hadley recalled. The moment was also remembered by Princeton's Arnie Levine. "It was at that point," Levine said, "that Raub understood the way to save NIH was not to cover up the truth, but to let the truth come out."

Minutes after Raub's statement was on the wire, Gallo was on the phone. "Dr. Gallo urgent. Line 5" read the message from Hadley's secretary. "Wants me to interrupt Dr. Hadley, it's urgent." The news that he had become the target of an official misconduct investigation, Gallo said, was "all over the campus." The NIH had "crossed the Rubicon."[32] As Hadley scribbled feverishly, Gallo continued to talk. "Nobody believes Mika has any notebook . . . only scraps. . . . I insulted Raub. I'm running out of gas. If I did wrong let me be punished . . . speed at which paper was written. I didn't think a thing about it. Knew MP had crisis with LAV . . . I think I wrote that statement . . . wrote as fast as could. . . . [T]his is trivial. It is not ethics. I'll win in the end. I couldn't care less what I said about LAV."

Hadley's next call was from a livid Joe Onek. His client already had "answered every question a hundred times," Onek said. His advice to Gallo would be to "talk to OSI one more time," but that was it. In fact, Onek intended to give OSI a deadline for completing the investigation. If the deadline wasn't met, Gallo would "go public," although it was hard to imagine Gallo going any more public than he already had. By the time Suzanne Hadley left her office, she was wrung out. "A wrenching afternoon and evening," she said later. "Howard Streicher was as close to tears as I've ever heard him."

The next day's headlines did nothing to assuage any tears. "The National Institutes of Health," began the front-page story in the *New York Times,* "will open a full-scale investigation of possible misconduct in the laboratory of Dr. Robert Gallo, one of America's most prominent researchers. A statement from the institutes said a preliminary inquiry into research on the AIDS virus at the laboratory had exonerated Dr. Gallo in some respects. But a spokesman, Donald M. Ralbovsky, said the beginning of a formal investigation meant that 'evidence has been found of possible misconduct' in Dr. Gallo's laboratory."[33]

Howard Streicher described Gallo as "flabbergasted" by Raub's decision. But when Gallo called Hadley that evening at home, Hadley thought he sounded suicidal. "He asked me, 'Why is this so sudden?'" Hadley recalled. "He said, 'I may have harmed Mika and myself by pushing too hard. I am lost. Maybe I should just jump out the window. Maybe I should just shoot myself.'"[34]

According to John Maddox's editorial in *Nature,* the OSI had found "no evidence to support earlier allegations that Gallo's HIV was from the outset, and knowingly, identical with that supplied to his laboratory by Dr. Luc Montagnier at the Pasteur Institute and called 'LAV.'"[35] But Raub's statement hadn't said anything of the kind, and Maddox, who often wrote his "leaders" at the last minute while smoking furiously and drinking red wine, evidently hadn't read the statement carefully.

Privately, Maddox thought Gallo was finished, whatever the investigation's outcome. Over a Saturday lunch at the Old Ebbitt Grill, his favorite Washington watering hole, Maddox predicted that the sequencing experiments would find HTLV-3B and LAV to be the same virus, but that there would be no way to say for sure how the one had become the other. Maddox imagined Gallo announcing that he had been vindicated, "while everyone else will say 'He's guilty.' And that will be the end of it." Gallo would resign from NIH and go somewhere else — Maddox's suggestion was Italy. Gallo might yet discover something really important, Maddox said, "if he were less concerned with succeeding at science."

Bill Raub's statement that Gallo had had "a substantial number of HIV detections and isolations from several different sources" sounded exculpatory on its face: if Mika Popovic had even one viable and productive HIV isolate of his own before LAV arrived from Paris, what motive could there have been for stealing LAV? But Gallo had admitted his "pre-LAV isolates" were bunkum. The only HIV-producing culture besides HTLV-3B had been the Haitian, R.F., which had come too late and which even Popovic conceded hadn't been a viable candidate for the AIDS blood test.

When Onek demanded that Raub issue a new statement declaring that the NIH inquiry had cleared Gallo of stealing the French virus, Raub told Onek to forget it. "It is possible," Raub informed Onek, "that the results of the planned biological testing or other aspects of the investigation could indicate the possibility that misappropriation occurred. If so, the issue of misappropriation would become a focus of the investigation."[36]

Suzanne Hadley, who had spent days explaining to the media that Raub's statement didn't mean the possible "misappropriation" of LAV was no longer an issue, conceded that Raub's language had been "purposely obfuscatory," and she regretted not insisting that the statement be more precise. "The clear implication," Hadley said later, "was that because Gallo had much to choose from, he had no need to misappropriate LAV. The fact is, of course, that Gallo had nothing but LAV."

Raub agreed, too late, that his statement should have been phrased differently. "We didn't rule out misappropriation," he said a few days after the announcement. "There were detections and there were isolations. The statement is more careful about that than some of the news reports. They were attempting to get growth, and had varying degrees of difficulty, of viruses from different sources. I think the critical questions at the moment are around that first paper, which reports the detection, the isolation and the continuous growth of the thing that came to be labeled as HTLV-3B. At the moment, what I want to do is resolve this matter on that paper. Because it goes to the heart of an awful lot of things."

Berge Hampar had had dinner with Gallo, and Hampar had come away thinking OSI was in for a fight. "You can't talk sense to him," Hampar said. "He's going to do what he wants to do and he's going to take the lumps. He says, 'I've admitted it's possible the viruses were mixed. What else can I admit?' I think, underlying all of this, he feels the French are such crappy scientists and 'I,' being him, did all of this stuff and why are we getting involved in this crap? That's his nature, unfortunately."

Five days after Raub's announcement, Hampar himself was in front of the OSI, a seventeen-page statement in his hands.[37] "I knew that if I didn't make a good presentation this whole thing could be lost," Hampar said later. "I spent two weeks going through all the stuff, putting arguments together, not making any statements without some support of facts." But Hampar's OSI experience was reminiscent of Mal Martin's. "It was obvious after I finished that they didn't really understand what I was saying," Hampar recalled. "I felt that I had presented enough information to question not the issue of whether he stole the virus, because I don't know that, but the point of did he really have [his own] isolates? The only conclusion you can draw is, he didn't have anything."

When John Dingell's staff, its attention briefly diverted from the Baltimore case, invited Jules Hallum and Suzanne Hadley to Capitol Hill for a briefing, Hadley explained that the OSI had found numerous discrepancies and unsupported statements in several of Gallo's papers. To keep the investigation manageable, the OSI had decided to focus on the four articles published in *Science* in May 1984, which it now designated Papers A through D.

There were major problems, Hadley said, with Paper A, Popovic's paper on the isolation of HTLV-3 and the discovery of the HT and H-9 cell lines. Paper B, the Gallo-Salahuddin paper claiming the "detection and isolation" of HTLV-3 in forty-eight patients with

AIDS and pre-AIDS, was less a case of misconduct than overarching hyperbole.

The data for Paper C, Jorg Schupbach's article reporting genetic similarities between HTLV-1, HTLV-2 and HTLV-3, had gone missing; Schupbach claimed to have tossed it out before going home to Zurich. The Schupbach paper was wrong — the genetic similarities reported by Schupbach among HIV, HTLV-1, and HTLV-2 simply didn't exist, as the DNA sequences of HTLV-3B and LAV had since made clear. But the nonexistent homologies appeared to be the product of bad science, and there was no OSI penalty for bad science.

Of the four papers, Paper D, Sarngadharan's report of his ELISA testing, seemed the most straightforward. There wasn't any reason to doubt Sarngadharan had gotten the results he reported, since they paralleled those he had obtained using the CDC's independent blood samples. The only question was whose virus Sarngadharan had used to make his ELISA.

When Onek heard Dingell's staff had been briefed by the OSI, he was on the phone to the subcommittee's chief investigator, Peter D. H. Stockton. A magazine writer once likened Stockton to Indiana Jones, but Stockton hardly qualified as dashing.[38] With his baseball cap, sneakers, graying beard, and knapsack, on some days Stockton could have passed for a homeless person, rather than a scratch-handicap golfer or an expert on nineteenth-century French painting, both of which he was.

"If you closed your eyes," Stockton said later, "you'd think this is Baltimore telling us about Imanishi — 'Popovic is a foreigner, he doesn't speak English well, and these guys are going after him.' He said that all this stuff is just a bunch of horseshit that they're investigating now. He says the OSI is paralyzed by Dingell — they know they're going to get a new asshole from Dingell unless they deliver Gallo's head on a platter."

In fact it was the Academy panel that had pushed for a formal investigation. Judy Areen, the dean of Georgetown Law, thought it silly to suggest that she and the other panelists gave a fig what John Dingell thought. "I don't want to argue with Joe," Areen said. "What I do is say that the panel's participation was not shaped by posturing or speculation about what Dingell would or wouldn't do. That's one of the advantages of having a panel of people who are not NIH employees."

As with other major OSI investigations, the newly constituted Gallo investigative team would include three nongovernment scientists, the OSI's traditional way of involving the larger scientific community in its deliberations, and also spreading the responsibility for its verdicts. But searching for three respected, and no doubt busy, university researchers willing to spend what promised to be months as coinvestigators in the Gallo case was like looking for shuffleboard partners on the deck of a sinking ship.

While the NIH searched, Gallo was en route to Los Angeles for the annual meeting of the American Association of Blood Banks, where he and Montagnier were to share an award for what was now the joint discovery of the AIDS blood test. As he packed for the trip, Gallo had the radio tuned to a popular public-affairs program, which that morning featured an interview with a *Business Week* reporter, Bruce Nussbaum, who had authored a book purporting to show that Wall Street and the NIH had conspired to slow the approval of potential AIDS drugs.[39]

Midway through the program, a female caller brought up Gallo's name. "I don't really think it's fair," the woman said, "for Mr. Nussbaum to base his case on Bob Gallo, who happens to be an arrogant megalomaniac. My parents are both cancer researchers, who have been dedicated for the past thirty years, and have worked also with the NIH, and have for many years said that it's wrong for society in general to have put doctors as gods. I think Bob Gallo has done a disservice to research in general."

"I don't disagree with you," Nussbaum replied. "The people who cover medical and scientific issues for the newspapers, for the *Washington Post*, for the *New York Times*, where are they on these issues? Most science writers like the gee-whiz of science, and they like the scientists, and they treat them as if they were God."

"You're saying there's too close a relationship?" asked the program's host, Diane Rehm.

"Yes, indeed," Nussbaum replied, "there's too close a relationship. They are not penetrating. They're not doing the political reporting of these institutions that other reporters do for every other institution. We're not getting the right information from our newspapers."

"All right," said Rehm, interrupting her guest. "I understand that Dr. Gallo himself is on the line with us this morning. Dr. Gallo, good morning to you."

"Yes, good morning," Gallo replied. "I'm a little bit shocked at the kind of things that are coming on the radio program. I don't know Mr. Nussbaum. I've never met him."

"Have you had a chance to look at his book?" Rehm asked.

"No," Gallo said, "but I read the review and I heard enough about it from others. But I heard that the book in fact doesn't really deal significantly with me."

"You're absolutely right," Nussbaum said. "The book deals only tangentially with Dr. Gallo."

"I'll have a book," Gallo said, "that will be out in early 1991 that will deal with the scientific process and what I saw firsthand. The laboratories that attacked this problem, without megalomania, as I listened to on your program, and without the desire of profit, which we didn't know we could make a dime from, who risked their lives daily working on a virus they didn't know how infectious it was, at a time when the bulk of the country, the scientists in this country, the institutes, didn't have material going into their institutes because of the fear of the problem. The people risked their lives on a daily basis, made the opening that allowed the virus to be cultured, proved the cause of the disease, developed a blood test allowing the epidemic to be studied and saved tens of thousands of lives, are the people you're slandering."

"Dr. Gallo," said Rehm, "I think that one of the points that Mr. Nussbaum has made repeatedly here this morning is that the system itself is so geared toward big science and big drug companies —"

But Gallo wasn't finished. "I work in a laboratory," Gallo said, his voice now shaking with anger. "It's one individual laboratory with six senior people and visiting scientists from all over the world — from Africa, Asia, Iran, Europe. About seventy-five percent of the people with me are from foreign countries, their salaries are twenty to thirty thousand dollars, they're M.D.–Ph.D.s, they work day and night, they work seven days a week. So do I. People who surmise that they know better, without a depth of understanding of science, who listen to every malcontent —"

"I think you're expressing the type of attitude which is part of the problem," Nussbaum shot back. "You simply dismiss anyone who is criticizing the NIH in any way."

"No," Gallo retorted, "I don't dismiss anyone."

"Your attitude is one of incredible arrogance," Nussbaum said.

"*You* write a book about a bunch of — a variety of scientists," Gallo said. "I haven't read the book. I've read the excerpts only. And you tell me *I'm* arrogant. I work hard on a problem that causes human death, both cancer and AIDS. I'm not reviewing anybody's funding in this world. I'm not against anybody's laboratory being funded. That's not arrogant."

"I think you're really expressing the type of attitude that is really at the core problem of the NIH," Nussbaum said. "There's absolutely no accountability at the NIH."

"No accountability!" Gallo retorted. "There's a, there's a . . ."

"And you're not open to any criticism," Nussbaum said, "even if that criticism is valid. You simply dismiss all criticism as invalid."

"A lot of wild statements are being made," Gallo went on, "instigated in part by media, by things I don't understand. I don't do anything different but go to my lab and work with my colleagues in the lab. I don't sit on review bodies. You say there's no accountability at NIH. These are things maybe you don't know. I have a site visit. Every three years my laboratory, and any laboratory I know of at NIH, gets reviewed by an outside group of a dozen people, or eight people, or ten people. In detail. In addition, every year we have to make presentations to another independent body, a board."

"I hate to disappoint you," Nussbaum said, "but you do not play a major role in my book."

"I'm glad to hear it," Gallo replied.

"Dr. Gallo," said Rehm, "I want to thank you for calling in this morning."

On a chilly Saturday morning in December of 1990, a forlorn Mikulas Popovic made his first appearance before the OSI's newly assembled investigative team.[40] In addition to Suzanne Hadley and Jules Hallum, Popovic was greeted by the three members of the OSI's "expert panel" charged with considering "all available pertinent evidence" and counseling the OSI on whether fabrication, falsification, plagiarism, or "any other serious deviations" had occurred in the reporting of Popovic's research.[41]

Five years before, Mika Popovic had been the envy of his friends and colleagues back in Czechoslovakia. Not only had he escaped the Eastern Bloc for America, he had landed in the biggest and best-known laboratory at the National Cancer Institute, the center of the oncological universe. There, he had proceeded to discover the cause of AIDS and to enter the lexicon as one of the most cited scientists of all time — an impossible dream for a one-time physician in the Czech Air Force.

"As you can imagine," Popovic told the OSI, reading from a statement prepared by his lawyer, Barbara Mishkin, "I am deeply troubled and disappointed that what I consider my best contribution to science has been called into question. In addition, my professional and personal integrity have been attacked, and I have been discredited before my scientific peers and the general public."

What had once given him "great satisfaction," Popovic went on, "has become the source of endless misery and frustration. I want you to know that I never did anything in connection with HIV research (or any other research) with intent to fabricate, falsify, plagiarize, deceive, or mislead, and the only possible errors of which I am aware, in my opinion, are minor and technical in nature. Moreover, any errors were unintentional and can only be considered 'honest errors.'"

For those errors Popovic had many explanations. During his work with LAV and HTLV-3B, Popovic had been distracted by personal problems, including his worry about receiving political asylum following his brother's defection to Switzerland. In December of 1983, at a critical moment in Popovic's search for the AIDS virus, his small lab had been moved on short notice to another room, an event that had been "especially disruptive from an intellectual and productivity standpoint, particularly because it resulted in the loss of many cell cultures."

Popovic had been "working under a great deal of pressure, under very difficult conditions, and without technical support." He had been surprised to discover that the equipment in Gallo's lab was of "poor quality," especially his centrifuge and his laminar flow hood. Not only was Popovic uncomfortable writing in English, the preparation of his *Science* article had been "further compromised" when Gallo had given him only a few days to finish the manuscript. Because of the accelerated publication, the paper had had "to focus on HTLV-3B as a prototype, instead of the R.F. isolate whose origin was more certain."

The OSI had expressed concern about what looked like falsification in Popovic's article. The R.F. isolate, for example, was listed as "N.D." for electron microscopy, and the paper included the standard definition for "N.D." as "Not Done." But Matt Gonda had tried three times to find virus in R.F.'s cells, and he had failed every time, which meant R.F. had been *negative* for electron microscopy — something Popovic had admitted to Gallo and Peter Fischinger.[f]

To the OSI, reporting negative experiments as "Not Done" was fraud, an attempt to cover up an unfavorable result by pretending it didn't exist. Now Popovic explained that by "Not Done" he hadn't meant that the experiments hadn't been *attempted.* He didn't "fully appreciate," Popovic said, "the distinction among 'not detected,' 'not determined,' or 'not done.'"

As for why his article had described the pool culture as "continuous" despite two reinfections with patient material and an unknown number of infusions with HUT-78 cells — or, rather, "HT" cells — Popovic claimed to have seen no evidence that, however much it faltered and sputtered, the pool had ever stopped producing virus. "I now understand," he told the investigators, "that 'continuous' apparently can be understood in this context to mean 'self-perpetuating.'"

Popovic's description of the pooled samples as "first shown" to be RT positive also seemed deceptive to OSI, since Ersell Richardson's lab notes recorded all but one sample as RT *negative.* Popovic explained that he hadn't meant to imply that *each* of the samples had been RT positive *before* it was pooled — only that the pooled culture fluids had been RT positive afterward.

Cornell's Kenneth Berns, one of the OSI's expert advisers, wanted to know how Popovic could have been sure there was AIDS virus in the pool samples if they hadn't been tested for reverse transcriptase before they were pooled.

"We didn't know," Popovic replied, raising an unanswered question about why those patients had been pooled in the first place.

Another adviser, Priscilla Schaffer from Harvard, wondered whether Popovic had been concerned that, by pooling so many isolates in the same culture, "if you got something there was no way that you could figure out which one it was."

Popovic admitted that he had, raising an unanswered question about whether the pool had been his idea or somebody else's.

"Did you ever think," asked Jules Hallum, "you should go back and find out which isolate was the one that had these properties that made it go? It seems to me that is the other half of the experiment."

Popovic agreed, but observed that "it is very difficult experiment to do."

Popovic had gone back over his records, but he still wasn't sure of the source of MOV. The one thing of which he was sure, Popovic said, was that MOV was not another name for LAV. When he had scrawled "HUT 78/V; Ti7.4/V = MOV" in his lab notes, he had merely meant to indicate that LAV and MOV were the same *kind* of virus — a new human retrovirus that probably caused AIDS.

The third OSI expert, a University of California AIDS researcher named Mike McGrath,[g] thought it odd that Popovic's *Science* paper included data from MOV and HTLV-3B, but didn't identify either virus. "I feel," McGrath said, "that is, you know, misleading. . . ."

One of the points for which Popovic offered no explanation was the declaration in his *Science* paper that LAV hadn't been grown in a continuous culture. "I did not write the questioned sentence," Popovic said, "so I do not know what its author intended." Popovic didn't say who the author was, but there weren't many possibilities.

"Can I just go back to one point that I am still a little confused about?" interrupted Ken Berns. "That is, that you started off with a section by talking about the fact that LAV — you had great difficulty in infecting a continuous cell line later on. But what you are describing to us now is really your experience with having infected a continuous cell line with LAV."

"Can we go off the record?" Popovic asked.

"I'm not sure you want to," interjected Barbara Mishkin.

"That's right," Suzanne Hadley said, picking up one of the early drafts of Popovic's manuscript. "I want to stay on the record. What I wanted to ask you about, Dr. Popovic, is if you are able to look at this section in the paper where it states that LAV was never put in a permanently growing cell line. That is noticeably different from what is in this manuscript. That passage about its not being in a permanently growing cell line is not in this manuscript."

"Yes," Popovic replied.

"What I wanted to ask you is," Hadley said, "if on page nine, you could look at this and tell us if you wrote what is in here, if you are able to answer that now?"

"I am sorry?" Popovic replied.

"Take your time," Hadley said.

"I think," Popovic began, "I am sure, that originally I had referenced the LAV in my very rough draft. I think so. Even I think I insisted on it. I thought that we should include the LAV data in the paper. I think I was right, because all my paper is suspicious because those LAV data are not included."

"Then it was changed during the editing," Popovic said. "LAV was put to the end of the manuscript, in the end, and I think it was Dr. Gallo's decision not to include LAV data."

Popovic recalled having disagreed with Gallo. "I told him in those times," Popovic said, "and I am telling it now, that it would be better to refer to the French work and present the LAV data, what we had. That has been my opinion all along. I talked to him about it two weeks ago, and he told me that he is taking full responsibility for this."

A few days after Popovic's OSI appearance, Peter Stockton and another Dingell investigator, Bruce Chafin, summoned the General Accounting Office for an update on the Baltimore case. It was the GAO's Baltimore team that had put together the case against Zaki Salahuddin, and in the interim the investigators had unearthed a new problem for Gallo. "Prem Sarin's going to get his shortly," Stockton said after the meeting broke up.

As Gallo's deputy lab chief, Sarin had continued to dabble in science between administrative tasks, mainly testing compounds that various companies thought might represent an effective treatment for AIDS. One such company was Praxis Pharmaceuticals, whose potential product was a foul-smelling extract of egg yolks called AL-721.[h]

Praxis had turned to Gallo, who had handed the task to Prem Sarin, who had concluded that, at least in the laboratory, AL-721 appeared to prevent the infection of T-cells by HIV. Gallo had published Sarin's results in the *New England Journal of Medicine* to considerable fanfare,[42] and told the *Wall Street Journal* he found Sarin's results "encouraging."[43] The *Journal* story doubled the price of Praxis's stock and launched AL-721 as the latest fad "cure" among people with AIDS.

Despite the fanfare, AL-721 hadn't worked in AIDS patients. The following year, Sarin had become involved with a German company, Homburg Degussa Pharma, which also had a drug, D-penicillamine, it hoped might be effective against HIV. Over dinner at La Ferme, Nancy Reagan's favorite restaurant, Sarin told representatives of Degussa it would cost them $50,000 to carry out a study of D-Pen in Gallo's lab.

The Reagan administration's push to "privatize" NIH had led to a number of collaborative agreements in which government laboratory research was partly funded by the corporate interests that stood to benefit from it. When Degussa agreed to pay half the $50,000 in advance, Sarin asked that the check be made out to "FAES," the acronym of the Foundation for Advanced Education in the Sciences, a private organization that channels research funding to NIH laboratories.

D-Pen hadn't worked any better than AL-721. But the $25,000 check from Degussa had gone into a personal bank account opened by Prem Sarin in the name of "FAES"— the "Family Account for the Education of the Sarin Children." Now Sarin was in the soup, and for advice he turned to Zaki Salahuddin, who had gotten off with three years of probation. "He wanted to know how I managed to avoid going to jail," Salahuddin recalled, "and what should he do? I suggested he should offer to talk about 'Sahib,'" the Indians' private name for Gallo. "He told me, 'But that would hurt Sahib very much.' I said, 'OK, you made your decision. I'll send you a postcard in jail.'"

Sarin's defense at his trial was that he had merely been holding the $25,000 until Degussa produced the second $25,000 payment, at which time Sarin planned to turn the entire sum over to NIH.[44] Unfortunately, the government's evidence showed that Sarin had used the first $25,000 to pay off several personal lines of credit. That, and using one of his sons' Social Security numbers to open the bank account, Sarin admitted, had been "the worst mistake of my life."

After deliberating less than four hours, the jury convicted Sarin of embezzlement and making false statements to the NIH.[i] The prosecution asked for six months' incarceration, but Sarin got two months in a halfway house in Baltimore, the court evidently having been swayed by the seventy-five letters it received from other scientists, many of whom expressed the opinion that Sarin had been the victim of some bureaucratic mix-up.

Questions about Sarin's consulting activities had been raised at the Dingell subcommittee's hearing on Pan-Data months before, and John Dingell found it "discouraging" that NIH hadn't pursued the Sarin matter then. "It is not the business of the subcommittee to supervise the daily workings of the NIH," Dingell said. "But if we have to do it, we will."[45]

Bill Raub, who sat stonefaced in Dingell's hearing room while the GAO investigators laid out the case against Sarin, agreed with the

Chairman that "in hindsight, the level of trust was too high. One of the things we need to develop across NIH is a greater talent for selective suspicion."[j]

"How the hell does Gallo dodge these bullets?" Peter Stockton asked later. "Being there and not knowing that these things are going on? Gallo told us, 'Hey, come on, it's not my job to be doing that kind of thing. Goddammit, I'm a scientist and I'm trying to cure AIDS, and I can't be bothered with this kind of crap.' And we say, 'Somebody's got to be concerned about this. You just don't turn laboratories over to felons to run wild. You've got to keep some control over what's going on.'

"It's just a circle jerk," Stockton said. "I've never seen anything quite like it."

"If Chance Will Have Me King"

For months Robert Gallo and Joe Onek had been dropping hints that the mystery of HTLV-3B and LAV would soon be resolved in Gallo's favor. Anyone who persisted in believing that HTLV-3B was LAV by another name, Onek declared ominously, was "living in a world of his own imagining. Forewarned is forearmed."[1]

The first clue to what was up had come a few months before, when Gallo wrote Jean-Claude Chermann in Marseille seeking information about the various shipments of LAV to Bethesda in 1983.[2] Then Mika Popovic, having resigned his job in New Mexico, suddenly reappeared in Gallo's lab, hired by NCI under contract to consult on "scientific misconduct issues."[3] Not long afterward, one of Gallo's assistants, Marvin Reitz, sent Gerry Myers a new AIDS virus sequence, "J61," that didn't resemble any of the others in Myers's HIV Sequence Database. Around the same time, someone from Gallo's lab called Jim Mullins at Stanford to ask if he would help analyze an "early sample" of HTLV-3. Wanting nothing more to do with Gallo's intrigues, Mullins declined.

On a sultry night in August of 1990, Gallo, Dani Bolognesi, and Daniel Zagury, in Bethesda for Gallo's annual AIDS meeting, called Suzanne Hadley at home, "in their cups." As Hadley understood their message, the OSI, which was coordinating the analysis of Popovic's pool patients, should *not* ask the Pasteur for samples of LAV_{Bru} to use in those experiments. Baffled, Hadley said good night and hung up the phone.[a]

Attempting to obtain a LAV_{Bru} sample of his own, Gallo turned again to Chermann, by then on extremely bad terms with Luc Montagnier. But in moving to Marseille, Chermann had left all his LAV_{Bru} samples at the Pasteur.[4] When Chermann asked Françoise Barré to help, she replied that the Pasteur's new director, Maxime Schwartz, "wishes not to give this kind of sample" to Gallo.[5] Gallo's next move had been an official request to the French National Collection of Micro-organisms, which was headquartered at Pasteur, for a certified sample of the same LAV virus "that was originally sent to us in 1983."[b] But Gallo hadn't included an import license and other necessary documents, and his request went unprocessed.

What Gallo, Joe Onek, and Howard Temin had been hinting at became clear in February 1991, when a short report from Gallo appeared in *Nature*. According to Gallo, HTLV-3B was *not* LAV_{Bru}.[6] More to the point, LAV_{Bru} was not LAV_{Bru}. Or at least the LAV_{Bru} in Gallo's freezer didn't match Simon Wain-Hobson's DNA sequence in *Cell*.

A few months before, Mika Popovic had unthawed and cultured a tiny remnant of the original LAV_{Bru} brought to Gallo's house by Montagnier nearly eight years before. The virus had been sequenced, and the sequence published by Gallo differed from HTLV-3B by a good 10 percent. "These data," Gallo wrote, "clearly show that none of the LAV samples received in July and September 1983, which are still available for analysis (and which have never been in continuous cell-culture), was the source of HTLV-3B. Nor could the materials of which these are samples have been the origin of the published LAV-1 sequence. From the information available, it seems most likely that the single virus species (here called JBB/LAV) found in these samples is that derived from the patient BRU."

Everything was back to square one. HTLV-3B still had an identical twin, the AIDS virus Simon Wain-Hobson had sequenced. But as Gallo had just shown, that virus wasn't LAV_{Bru}, which meant *HTLV-3B* wasn't LAV_{Bru}. Something had happened in Paris, but solving that mystery was Wain-Hobson's problem. "The issue of how two HIV-1 isolates that are so similar appeared in two different parts of the world has been distracting and divisive," Gallo's paper concluded. "We hope that our analyses will put the issue on a more factual basis."

"Paper may vindicate Gallo team's claim to have beaten French," declared an excited *Washington Post*, announcing that the American scientist "dogged for years by charges that he stole the credit for discovering the AIDS virus may have been vindicated by dramatic new findings." Should Gallo's findings be confirmed, said the *Post*, they "would appear to lift the cloud of suspicion that for six years has shrouded the accomplishments of Gallo's laboratory."[7]

Montagnier was described as "angered and shaken" by the *Nature* paper. "I don't think this solves the case," he said. "It adds more confusion. The implication is that our virus was a contamination from his virus. I think that is completely wrong. We cannot accept that." But Gallo was magnanimous in victory. "This report gives no encouragement," he said, "to anyone who would like to believe that science is more about personalities and secrets than about solving problems."

Howard Temin hoped Gallo's bombshell at least would put an end to suggestions "that there was some kind of chicanery involved in the initial isolation of what is now known as HIV." But the *Post* nevertheless dusted off Gallo's old reverse-contamination hypothesis, speculating that "at some point between late 1983 and 1985," LAV_{Bru} had been "contaminated by Gallo's 3B."

The fact that one of its nine co-authors was Jean-Claude Chermann lent the *Nature* paper extra credibility. But Chermann said he hadn't agreed with the paper's conclusions. Chermann still thought the original LAV_{Bru} sequenced by Gallo *might* have come from the same patient as HTLV-3B, and that the 10 percent difference had arisen because LAV_{Bru} had been grown in cord blood cells, whereas HTLV-3B had first been grown in a permanent cell line. But when Chermann asked Gallo to insert a sentence to that effect, Gallo had refused. "I don't know who's trying to make polemics," Chermann said. "For me, it is a scientific paper. I am not a polemical man."

Françoise Barré had pleaded with Chermann not to cosign the paper. "She told me," said Simon Wain-Hobson, "that Gallo got Chermann to sign the paper by telling him it was a good way to screw Montagnier." According to Barré, when Chermann stopped in Bethesda at the end of January, just as the paper was going to press, he had received the royal treatment from Gallo — lunches, dinners, lots of wine and good fellowship. "I think he is easily manipulated by Gallo," Barré said. "Also naïve. I know very well for a long time the effect that Gallo has on Jean-Claude. Many times in the past I thought I had convinced him about something. And then he has a beer with Gallo and he is saying the opposite."

When Gerry Myers saw the partial sequence in *Nature* of what was now being called "new Bru," he recognized it as the mysterious J61 he had been given by Marv Reitz a few months before. But when the full J61 sequence reached Los Alamos on a diskette, Myers noticed something that hadn't been apparent from Gallo's article.

The relatively short DNA fragments of LAV_{Bru} and HTLV-3B shown in *Nature* were the ones that were furthest apart genetically. When the full sequences were compared, the difference between the two viruses was only 5 percent, not 10. "It's not nearly as black and white as what's being depicted in the press," Myers said. "With Gallo's lab things are never quite what they seem."

No sooner had Myers reported his conclusion to Marv Reitz than he had a call from Gallo. "He was all over the map," Myers recalled. "He went on for forty-five minutes, rambling and shouting about his enemies and his past history, accusing me of not helping him, claiming everyone was against him, and so on. He sounded about as paranoid and desperate as I've ever heard him. He was talking about conducting his own investigation of the people who were conspiring against him."

In addition to the misalignments, Myers had also found fifteen or twenty typographical errors in the *Nature* sequence. Gallo conceded the sequence alignments in *Nature* were "sloppy" and "simple-minded," and explained that Marv Reitz had "just put them in the computer and pushed a button." When Reitz told Myers a letter correcting the typos would soon be on its way to *Nature,* Myers suggested it should also acknowledge the real 5 percent difference between "new Bru" and HTLV-3B. When no acknowledgment was forthcoming, Myers and Mal Martin sent *Science* a letter of their own.[8]

"I finally read the *Nature* thing," Wain-Hobson said on the Monday morning after the article had come out. "And I got so angry with it that I didn't even finish it. I mean, 'Perhaps it is time for the French to come forward with their own records and early isolates.' Those isolates have been accessible for seven years. As simple as that. It's remarkable. It's like acupuncture. You've got a headache somewhere so you put a needle elsewhere and you forget the headache. It's quite incredible."

Wain-Hobson understood that a reverse contamination in Paris was impossible, simply on the strength of Murray Gardner's and Mal Martin's LAV samples, both of which had left France a month before the arrival of Sarngadharan bearing HTLV-3B. And therein lay what must be an important clue: how could it be that the LAV_{Bru} given to Gardner and Martin in April 1984 didn't match the LAV_{Bru} Montagnier had taken to Gallo in July 1983?

Later that morning, Wain-Hobson paid a visit to Françoise Barré. After checking her records, Barré confirmed that no LAV samples except those from Frédéric Brugière had ever been provided to Gallo's lab.

The first shipment had been in April 1983, when Jacqueline Gruest had taken Gallo viral DNA from the culture called JBB/LAV, so-called because the T-cells in which the virus was grown had come from a researcher named Jean-Baptiste Brunet. In July, Montagnier had taken Gallo a frozen vial of fluid containing JBB/LAV. In September, Barré herself had packed up the third and last shipment to Gallo: more JBB/LAV, plus a second LAV_{Bru} sample labeled *M2T-/B*, a designation that that virus had been grown in bone marrow cells. It was *M2T-/B* that Betsy Read had used to infect HUT-78, Ti7.4, and the other cell lines, and it was the Ti7.4, culture Flossie Wong-Staal had shown to be indistinguishable from HTLV-3B.[c]

Gallo had stated in *Nature* that none of the LAV JBB/LAV samples received in July and September 1983 were a match for new Bru. But that didn't include M2T-/B, the only LAV sample Gallo hadn't been able to locate in his lab. When Wain-Hobson asked Barré, she said she thought she had some tubes of M2T-/B in one of her freezers. "She's hunting," Wain-Hobson reported. "She says, 'I must have them somewhere.' The thing is just finding them."

While Barré hunted, Wain-Hobson pored over her lab notes. The entries from early September 1983 showed that Barré had had three AIDS virus cultures growing in her lab: $LAV_{Bru,}$ IDAV-1 from Christophe Lailler, and IDAV-2 from the hemophiliac Eric Loiseau.[d] The Lailler virus "grew very well, right from the outset," Wain-Hobson said. "They were growing up Lailler in big quantities, to try and get good Western Blots and ELISAs."

Wain-Hobson already had determined that the protein sequences of the Brugière, Lailler, and Loiseau viruses bore a few tiny genetic differences. One, unique to Lailler, was a short string of amino acids:

Q-R-G-P-G. The original Bru virus didn't have the Lailler signature. But the LAV sequence Wain-Hobson had published in 1985 in *Cell*, and which until now everyone had thought was LAV_{Bru}, *did* have it. So did Montagnier's B-LAV, which had begun growing in November of 1983. And so did Lee Ratner's sequence of HTLV-3B. Had Gallo's lab taken the trouble to compare amino acid sequences it would have discovered that there was much more to the story, and that $QRGPG$ was the key that unlocked the door. But it was a door Gallo hadn't wanted to go through.

An accomplished flautist from a picturesque village on the Brittany coast, Christophe Lailler had won a music scholarship to Beloit College in Wisconsin. He later told his doctors his first homosexual contact had been during his freshman year, which probably meant he had become infected with HIV in the Midwest, perhaps during a weekend visit to Chicago.

After graduation Lailler had returned to France, intending to read law at the Sorbonne, but the first symptoms of AIDS put an end to his studies. In February 1981, four months before the first AIDS cases were recognized in the United States, Lailler had complained to his doctor of fever and lymphadenopathy. According to Lailler's mother, the puzzled doctor asked if Lailler had recently visited a tropical country. By March of 1983 Lailler had begun losing weight, and in June he had gone to see the "AIDS doctor," Willy Rozenbaum. By then his lymph nodes were distended; it was one of those nodes, biopsied and delivered to the Pasteur, which had yielded LAV_{Lai}.

As he lay dying, Lailler played his flute for the other patients on his ward. "So courageous," his mother recalled. "The doctors, they were astonished." Then she mentioned something that had worried her for years. "I have often thought," she said, "that he was the one who brought the virus to France." Told that what were now seen, in retrospect, as the very first AIDS cases in France had occurred while her son was still in America, Sophie Lailler seemed visibly relieved.

An eight-year-old vial of M2T-/B had finally turned up in the back of Barré's freezer, and a little after ten o'clock on the morning of Tuesday, March 20, 1991, Wain-Hobson carried a sheaf of sequencing films from his lab to a basement darkroom in the Pasteur's retrovirology complex. Working in the glow of a dim red bulb, Wain-Hobson placed the films into a developer. Two minutes later the machine ejected the first negative, then a second and a third.

The first sheet contained the sequence of IDAV-2, the virus from Eric Loiseau. Holding it to the light, Wain-Hobson saw the nucleotides that coded for the amino acids GPG but not Q and R — which was fine, since the Loiseau virus wasn't supposed to have *QRGPG*. The second negative out of the developer was IDAV-1, the Lailler virus, which *was* supposed to have it. As Wain-Hobson read off the amino acids — I-R-I-Q-R-G-P-G — he let out a whoop and slapped the machine. Sensing something historic was happening, postdocs and technicians began gathering around.

The third sheet to emerge was M2T-/B from Barré's freezer. It, too, had *QRGPG*. The M2T-/B Françoise Barré had sent Gallo as an AIDS virus isolated from Frédéric Brugière had actually been the virus isolated from Christophe Lailler. The only thing wrong had been the label on the tube — *Bru* instead of *Lai*. But LAV_{Lai} was every bit as much a French discovery as LAV_{Bru} — and so was Gallo's HTLV-3B, which was simply LAV_{Lai} by another name. All Wain-Hobson could think to say was a quote from *Macbeth:* "If chance will have me King. . . ."[e]

Françoise Barré's response to the news that she had suffered a contamination was *"merde"*— the same comment, Wain-Hobson observed, made by General Cambronne upon learning Napoleon had been defeated at Waterloo. To cheer her up, Wain-Hobson pointed out that whether it was called LAV_{Lai}, LAV_{Bru}, or HTLV-3B, the reference strain of HIV used by virtually every AIDS research laboratory on the globe was still a Pasteur discovery. "Finally we can just close the book on the origins of the virus," he said. "*Bru* got carded out."

In retrospect, Barré thought she must have been the victim of an aerosol contamination, in which virus particles are wafted from one flask to another, and which easily could have occurred under the hood in the cramped room where she and Chermann had cultured their early HIV isolates. Christophe Lailler's lymph node had been biopsied on June 6, 1983, and put in culture three days later. On July 20, the day Montagnier had arrived home from Gallo's task force meeting, Barré had infected the M2T-/B cells with "true Bru," and fresh JBB cells with Lailler. That was when Barré thought the contamination had happened.

Wain-Hobson didn't agree. On July 20 the M2T-/B culture had given a low RT reading, whereas the Lailler culture was quite high, which suggested that M2T-/B was still *Bru*. Wain-Hobson's choice for a contamination date was August 3, the day Barré concentrated supernatants from *Bru, Lai,* and *Loi* for Françoise Brun's ELISA. It must have been then, Wain-Hobson thought, that LAV_{Lai} had overgrown the LAV_{Bru} virus cultured in the M2T-/B cells.

Montagnier, having heard the news, rushed to Wain-Hobson's lab. He wasn't smiling. At least, Wain-Hobson said, there had been a contamination of one Pasteur virus with another — not like what had happened to Gallo, a contamination by somebody else's virus. "Yes," Montagnier said, "at least there is that." When the discussion turned to how quickly Pasteur could publish, Wain-Hobson thought he could have a paper ready in two weeks. Montagnier thought it important that Suzanne Hadley know what Wain-Hobson had just discovered. But he was reluctant to inform NIH directly, for fear that Gallo would find out and thwart Pasteur's efforts to publish.

For months Bill Raub had been corresponding with Maxime Schwartz, the molecular biologist who had replaced Raymond Dedonder as the director of the Pasteur, asking for early samples of LAV for the OSI's sequencing studies.[9] Initially distrustful of the American investigation, Schwartz eventually had agreed, but the samples hadn't yet been sent. Wain-Hobson pointed out that if the sequencing studies included only LAV_{Bru} and the B-LAV cell line, the OSI's verdict on the genesis of HTLV-3B might be inconclusive.

"What if we send them M2T-/B as well," Wain-Hobson suggested, "and simply say that since this is one of the samples that Gallo acknowledges having received in *Nature,* we think no survey would be complete without it." As for where to publish, Wain-Hobson thought *Nature* was out, considering that John Maddox hadn't alerted anyone at Pasteur about Gallo's impending paper on LAV_{Bru}. Beyond that, Wain-Hobson predicted that "any paper we send to *Nature* would be in Gallo's hands within twenty-four hours."

Wain-Hobson's choice was *Cell,* which unlike *Nature* and *Science* didn't have a news department that could leak the article before publication. There also seemed a certain symmetry to publishing the dénouement of a very long story in the journal where the original LAV sequence had appeared. In the meantime, however, Montagnier had gotten a call from John Maddox, apologizing for not informing the Pasteur of the Gallo paper, and for the rhetorical excesses in the accompanying news article by Barbara Culliton, who had taken the Gallo beat with her upon leaving *Science* for *Nature*.

When Maddox expressed interest in publishing any data that might shed light on "this most interesting question," Montagnier replied that he would think about it. But when Wain-Hobson learned Montagnier was seriously considering publishing in *Nature,* he shook his head. "How many times does he have to be screwed," Wain-Hobson said, "before he realizes he's been raped?"

Raymond Dedonder, now quite elderly and not very well, represented the end of an era at the Institut Pasteur, and in French science as well. Dedonder was a biochemist trained in France, who spoke English poorly and for whom Britain and the United States were alien cultures not entirely to be trusted. Dedonder's successor, Maxime Schwartz, spoke flawless English and was thoroughly Americanized, having been a postdoc in Jim Watson's lab at Harvard in the late 1960s, where he had participated in antiwar demonstrations and campus politics.

When Wain-Hobson, Montagnier, Barré, and Dedonder assembled in Schwartz's office for a formal presentation of Wain-Hobson's data, Schwartz agreed that the Pasteur should send Suzanne Hadley M2T-/B.[f] It was Dedonder who pointed out that Wain-Hobson's data was bound to have repercussions for the 1987 agreement, since it represented proof positive that the American AIDS test was being manufactured with a virus discovered at the Pasteur. The agreement, Dedonder said, might have to be rescinded unilaterally. Maxime Schwartz, who deferred to Dedonder in most things, didn't disagree, but Schwartz thought patent questions were premature. "Maxime said, 'Let's just do the science now,'" Wain-Hobson recalled. "'We can deal with the patent issue later.'"

The Pasteur manuscript was completed in eleven days, with Wain-Hobson the first author, Montagnier last. Everyone agreed that Chermann not be asked to sign the paper, lest he leak the story to Gallo. When Wain-Hobson called *Science*'s editor, Daniel Koshland, to alert him that the Pasteur had an important paper ready for submission, Koshland wanted to know what it was about. "I told him, 'Just let me send it to you,'" Wain-Hobson recalled. "He promised to move very quickly and very discreetly."[10]

The news that HTLV-3B was LAV after all[11] warranted an entire page in *Le Monde,* which declared the 1987 agreement with the Americans now "in question."[12] The *Washington Post* wasn't prepared to abandon hope, implying that perhaps it had been Christophe Lailler, rather than Frédéric Brugière, who had had sex with someone in the Popovic pool.[13]

Taken by surprise, Gallo responded that "the history of the discovery is not the simple report of one virus."[14] But inside his lab, the mood was reported to be glum. "I had a call from Marv Reitz," Wain-Hobson said a few days after the *Science* paper appeared. "He's convinced 3B is LAV. He said, 'We had a contamination.' He's trying to convince Gallo to accept the inevitable. I asked him why it's taken Gallo so long to admit the obvious. His answer was, 'Politics and ego.' It's that simple."

If Gallo's lab had done what Wain-Hobson's had just done — compared HTLV-3B not just with LAV_{Bru} but also with M2T-/B — there wouldn't have been a *Nature* paper to begin with. Gallo claimed that particular comparison hadn't been performed because no sample of M2T-/B remained in Gallo's lab, but Wain-Hobson had heard differently.

"I know from Marvin Reitz," Wain-Hobson wrote Gallo, "that Howard Streicher in your own lab said that a sample of Ti7.4 LAV [M2T-/B] from July 84 *was* available. . . . You now see why we had a hard time believing that statement. In fact it is untrue. Why did you choose not to analyse the Ti7.4 sample?"[15]

Gallo was "surprised and disturbed" by Wain-Hobson's question, which he dismissed as "your greatest misunderstanding. . . . We could not find any freezes of cultures of Ti7.4 despite a very extensive search through our freezers. It was apparently long ago thrown out by Mika. I sincerely hope that this letter convinces you that I have acted in better faith than you seem to believe."

What Gallo didn't say was that, a year before, Reitz had written to ask Jean-Claude Chermann for help in identifying four LAV samples he had located in the Gallo lab. According to Reitz's letter, one of those was M2T-/B. When Reitz said he didn't know what the designation meant, Chermann explained that the "M" stood for *moelle* — French for bone marrow which had been depleted of T-cells and B-cells.[16]

Gallo also didn't say that, months before, he had obtained from Murray Gardner a sample of the LAV Gardner had taken back to California following the tripartite meeting at the Pasteur — the same isolate Marty Bryant had used in showing that LAV was indistinguishable from HTLV-3B. "They just asked me for it, and I gave it to them," Gardner said. "They didn't say why they wanted it." Had Gallo compared Gardner's LAV — really LAV_{Lai} — with HTLV-3B, he would have seen they were one and the same — incontrovertible evidence that HTLV-3B had its origins in France. But if Gallo had done that experiment, he hadn't mentioned it in *Nature*.

Howard Temin had been suggesting that whoever thought HTLV-3B was LAV should prepare to be embarrassed. Now Temin was embarrassed, and Simon Wain-Hobson felt badly. "Clearly, he is a great scientist," Wain-Hobson said, "but he's over his head politically. He wanted the 3B-LAV issue to just go away, and like the Palestinian question it didn't go away. Now he's beginning to awaken to the fact that he's gone too far. Perhaps it's true what Gerry says, that Temin's real concern is not saving Gallo but saving NCI. That he thinks if Gallo goes down they will both go down together."

Newsweek quoted Temin as calling the HTLV-3B affair "an enormous distraction" for science.[17] But Temin assured Gerry Myers he thought the issue was important, especially "in the midst of an epidemic." Then more than ever, Temin said, "we really need reliable information because it has an enormous impact and mistakes have large consequences in the real world. If anything standards must be higher in the midst of an epidemic because the consequences are so great."[18] Although accepting that Gallo "will always be in one or the other controversy" Temin was determined to seek closure on this one, drafting a statement to be signed by Gallo and Montagnier and intended for *Science* or *Nature*.[19]

"The nucleotide sequence similarity of LAV_{Bru} and HTLV-3B," it began, "the two major early isolates of HIV, has been a subject of much controversy. Recent work has done much to clarify the origins of this similarity." But when the statement appeared in *Nature*,[g] it bore only Gallo's signature, and it contained a sentence Temin hadn't written: "I note that both laboratories had other isolates in 1983–84 and, in short, none of this affects the history of the important events written for *Nature* in 1987 and *Scientific American* in 1988 by L. Montagnier and myself."

As received by *Nature*, Gallo's statement also contained an expression of regret that "if during this period anything I said shed more heat than light." According to John Maddox, it was he, Maddox, who had deleted the apology "for reasons of space." Gallo confused matters utterly by telling the *Washington Times* that he, Gallo, had removed the apology, on the advice of friends who feared it would be misinterpreted. In any event, Gallo said, he only meant to say that "I regretted having been mad."[20]

Gallo's statement, the *Wall Street Journal* observed, "provided a terse closure to a bitter trans-Atlantic dispute over who discovered the AIDS virus — a dispute that clouded much of the past decade's work on the epidemic."[21] To reporters in Paris, Montagnier expressed "relief at the end of this seven-year quarrel," adding that "I think that at a certain moment there was a lie."[22] As for whether Gallo's concession would lead the Pasteur to reopen the 1987 agreement, Montagnier replied that "the terms of the accord could eventually be put up for question."

Gallo claimed to be surprised by all the "bombs going off" in Europe as a result of his acknowledgment, after seven years, that HTLV-3B was LAV. "They had one patient, one isolate," Gallo said. "They had no antibody or blood-test data to link that patient's problems to the virus. We had many isolates. I don't know what Montagnier's motives are. I find his statements bizarre for a colleague and a scientist. I find them obviously outrageous." Suggestions that Montagnier had discovered the cause of AIDS were "horse manure."[23]

In the nearly two years since Jim Wyngaarden's exit from the National Institutes of Health, Bill Raub had done a more than competent job of managing a federal agency with what was now a $9 billion annual budget. But Raub, a research scientist with a Ph.D., hadn't been a candidate for the permanent NIH directorship, reserved by tradition for a medical doctor. In searching for Wyngaarden's permanent successor, the Bush administration sought a rare combination, a physician-scientist who shared the president's opposition to abortion and the use of human fetal tissue in medical research.

Although Bernadine Healy had once served on an NIH panel that voted to permit limited research with fetal tissue, the forty-seven-year-old Harvard Medical School graduate had managed to pass the administration's litmus test.

Healy wasn't the president's first choice, but she was a cardiologist, a conservative Republican, *and* a woman. The daughter of a New York City perfume manufacturer, Healy was described by people who knew her as "smart," "very traditional," "strong-willed," and a "tough bird."[24]

Eager to begin her tenure as what the *Boston Globe* called "the chief executive officer of American science,"[25] Healy had left her daughters, aged five and twelve, in Cleveland with her husband, Floyd Loop, a cardiac surgeon who headed the renowned Cleveland Clinic, where Healy had been director of research. As she was moving into the director's residence on the NIH campus, Healy downplayed the difficulties of commuting between her new job in Bethesda and her family in Cleveland. "I'm a passionate mommy," she told the *Baltimore Sun*. "I love my children dearly and I'm very devoted to the family. I've always done a lot of traveling in my career."[26]

Among Healy's first official acts was a written reprimand to Gallo, not for anything to do with the OSI investigation but for "specific instances where you and employees supervised by you failed to comply with HHS Regulations for the Protection of Human Subjects."[27] The reprimand stemmed from a separate probe, by the Office of Protection from Research Risks, a quasi-independent part of NIH responsible for ensuring that human experimentation by NIH researchers, or those funded by NIH, was conducted according to federal ethics regulations.

A few months before, the OPRR had shut down a long-running collaboration between Gallo and his French friend Daniel Zagury to develop the world's first vaccine for AIDS. There hadn't been any Nobel prizes for the discovery of the AIDS virus, and Gallo had become convinced that "it will wait until there's success in therapy or vaccine." Vowing that he would "be the first" with an AIDS vaccine,[28] Gallo had organized a small group of collaborators, among them Zagury, Hilary Koprowski, and Dani Bolognesi, to join him in the search for a vaccine.[29] Gallo had named his team HIVAC, for HIV VACcine. When HIVAC didn't produce anything of interest, other NIH researchers began calling it "LOVAC."

Thanks to stringent FDA regulations born of the thalidomide debacle, testing a vaccine, or any new medicine, in the United States takes an average of seven years. Beyond that, the pool of HIV-negative men and women at risk for AIDS, the group in whom any candidate vaccine would have to be tested, is not large enough to permit many such trials.

In Africa, the number of prospective test subjects was infinitely larger, and there were no bothersome regulatory agencies to worry about. Zagury had served as a French Army surgeon, and he still had military contacts in the central African nation of Zaire, the former Belgian Congo, where there was more AIDS per capita than almost anywhere else on earth. In looking for a venue to test a possible AIDS vaccine, Zagury said later, "we decide, after a tennis party with Bob, that it would be important to go in a place where there is a major problem with AIDS."[30]

The Gallo-Zagury collaboration traced back to December 1984, when Gallo had begun sending Zagury cells, viruses, and other AIDS-related biologics that might be useful in preparing a vaccine for HIV.[31] In the intervening six years, the two had co-authored a dozen articles, including several reports of Zagury's ensuing vaccine studies.[32] Around the time of the Pasteur settlement, Zagury had created a media sensation with the disclosure that he was the first researcher in the world to have tested a candidate vaccine for AIDS — on himself. Gallo called Zagury's self-experimentation "an important first step,"[33] and other scientists thought it "daring" and "exciting work."[34]

But as the OPRR subsequently learned, several months before his self-inoculation Zagury had tested a rudimentary candidate vaccine on a half-dozen Zairian AIDS patients. Their immune systems hadn't responded, and during one of his frequent visits to Bethesda Gallo had introduced Zagury to another NIH scientist, Bernard Moss, who had succeeded in inserting a piece of HTLV-3B into a virus called vaccinia. Gallo arranged for Zagury to take a quantity of the Moss vaccinia recombinant to Africa.

Vaccinia, which causes cowpox in cows, has been used since the days of Edward Jenner as a vaccine against smallpox in humans.[35] But the Moss recombinant had been made with a strain of vaccine never tested in humans, and Moss made Zagury promise to use it only for experiments in monkeys. As the OPRR had learned, Zagury had given the Moss recombinant to dozens of HIV-negative Zairians — including at least two-dozen infants and children, in violation of both NIH and World Health Organization regulations.[36]

Ethical guidelines for medical experiments involving children are unequivocal: They can be used as test subjects only if children are the potential beneficiaries of the unproven treatment or if, for scientific or ethical reasons, adults cannot be used in their place. In the case of an AIDS vaccine, neither was true. Children in Zaire weren't at risk for AIDS, and there were plenty of adults who were. Zagury didn't pretend otherwise. He had used the children, he explained later, because "their immune systems are the best."[37]

For Gallo, the immediate problem was that none of Zagury's experiments had been approved by the National Cancer Institute's medical ethics committee, or by the OPRR itself. When NCI officials questioned Gallo, he admitted Zagury had told him children were subjects in the Zairian experiments, but that "they were children who were HIV infected" and whose mothers had been "begging for the therapy."[38] Apart from the fact that inoculating HIV-infected children with a vaccinia virus would have exposed them to a serious risk of fatal disease, the OPRR observed that if the mothers' concern for their children's safety had been the basis for their requests, "then the information presented to them and the consent process appear to have been seriously flawed."

When the Moss recombinant didn't generate the hoped-for HIV antibodies in his Zairian subjects, Zagury had shifted his experiments to the Hôpital Saint-Antoine in Paris, where he began administering a similar vaccine to AIDS patients in hopes it would slow the course of their disease. It hadn't, and two months after OPRR shut down the Gallo-Zagury collaboration over the African violations, the *Chicago Tribune* reported that three French AIDS patients in the Saint-Antoine trial had died — not of AIDS, but of vaccinia disease caused by incompletely inactivated virus.[39]

The previous summer Gallo and Zagury had co-authored a *Lancet* article on the vaccine tests at Saint-Antoine.[40] But the article hadn't mentioned the three deaths, and Gallo hadn't reported them to the OPRR, although two of the deaths had been mentioned in a presentation by a Zagury collaborator at Gallo's most recent AIDS meeting. Gallo said he hadn't heard the presentation,[41] but admitted learning about the Saint-Antoine's deaths at least three months before the OPRR learned about them from the newspapers. Gallo hadn't reported the deaths to OPRR, he said, because he didn't know the dead patients had been subjects in the vaccine experiments. He thought they had died of AIDS.[h] "If this wasn't so serious," Gallo remarked, "it would be worthy of a comedy."[42]

Despite the *Lancet* article and Gallo's co-inventorship with Zagury on a pending NIH patent for a "peptide cocktail" vaccine Zagury was also testing in Paris,[43] Gallo assured the OPRR that his involvement in

Zagury's vaccine experiments had been "zero."[i] But federal regulations had been violated, and the OPRR had sanctioned Gallo and Zagury for "a continuing lack of understanding" of those regulations. It also cited Zagury, but not Gallo, for having failed to inform it of the three deaths at Saint-Antoine.

The OPRR also blamed itself. The NIH's efforts to protect the subjects of medical experiments by its own scientists, the OPRR acknowledged, had been a failure.[j] Following an investigation, the French government banned any further use of vaccinia in people with AIDS,[44] prompting demands from AIDS patients and others to know why Zagury's research had been shut down. To mollify public concern, the Ministry of Health agreed to test Zagury's vaccinia vaccine in a properly controlled, randomized clinical trial. When the trial results were finally in, the vaccine proved to be worthless.[45]

During her confirmation hearings, Bernadine Healy had hinted at her own feelings about scientific misconduct, and possibly the Gallo case, observing that there was "a lesson for science in the play *Amadeus.*"[46] Although Mozart had been "magical and brilliant," Healy said, he also had been "difficult, childish, nasty and unconventional," while his rival, Salieri, had been "talented in a workmanlike way and popular at court." In Healy's opinion, if medical research were to advance "the Mozarts must be allowed to flourish."

Healy's remarks didn't provide much encouragement for the Office of Scientific Integrity, struggling to bring its investigation of Gallo and Popovic to a close. Over the past eighteen months, the OSI had interviewed Gallo nineteen times and Popovic on four occasions,[k] and there had been interviews with many others — although not with Prem Sarin, "Kaly" Kalyanaraman, Don Francis, or Zaki Salahuddin, each of whom might have shed important light on the questions under investigation. The French wondered why Jean-Claude Chermann had been invited to testify, but not Françoise Barré or Luc Montagnier. "Another screw-up," Suzanne Hadley said later.

After a few months of being outmaneuvered by his deputy, Jules Hallum had demanded that Hadley be transferred somewhere else — anywhere else — in the NIH. As she departed for a new job in the Office of Science Policy and Legislation, the NIH's congressional liaison, Hadley heard that "Jules is telling a lot of people that I had completely emasculated him. If it's true, it was the easiest job I ever had." Rather than struggling to absorb the details of the Gallo case, Hallum was happy to let Hadley continue running the Gallo investigation from afar. Just as news was breaking that the OPRR had halted the Gallo-Zagury vaccine experiments, Hadley summoned the OSI's three scientific advisers for an all-day session at the National Library of Medicine on the NIH campus.

Popovic's lawyer, Barbara Mishkin, had tried to separate her client from Gallo in the minds of the OSI, and to engender the investigative panel's sympathy by portraying him as a victim of Gallo's power and ambition. "Bob Gallo is a fairly important man in the field," Mishkin said, "and if Mika were to do anything that could be even interpreted as abandoning ship, he might never work in this field again."[47]

When Popovic addressed the investigators for the last time, he petitioned for clemency on the ground that he had been punished enough. *He* was the one who had isolated HTLV-3B and discovered the H-9 cell line, Popovic said, but *he* had never been considered a codiscoverer of the AIDS virus. *Time* magazine had described him merely as "one of the East European tissue culture experts in Dr. Gallo's lab." Seven years later, he was "currently unemployed and unemployable," though he didn't mention the half-million dollars he had collected from the patent on the Gallo ELISA, with another million yet to come.[1]

The OSI investigation, Popovic said, reminded him of nothing more than his former life in Eastern Europe. "From the outset of this investigation," he said, "I feel I have been presumed guilty and forced to prove my innocence. I had thought that in this country, the approach was the reverse. Worse, there seems to be no end to the investigation. At some point, prolonged exile from the laboratory will destroy my ability to function as a productive scientist. Such ostracism is not new for Czechoslovaks; after all, Franz Kafka lived in Prague. I came to this country to escape such unfairness. Please do not prove me wrong."

On that desperate note Popovic departed the room, leaving the investigative team to assess the evidence against him and consider his fate. The verdict, unanimous, was that Popovic had falsified some of the most important data in his 1984 *Science* paper, and had therefore committed scientific misconduct as defined by HHS regulations. The more difficult question was whether Gallo was also guilty.

As far as anyone knew, Gallo hadn't performed any of the questioned experiments with LAV or HTLV-3B. All the data under scrutiny had been produced by Popovic or Sarngadharan. But Gallo had done much more than stand by and watch. Not only had he directed and guided Popovic's research, he had revised Popovic's *Science* paper extensively and written significant portions of it, including the now-discredited conclusion that LAV and HTLV-3B might be different viruses. Even if Popovic hadn't understood the definitions of terms like "not done" and "continuous culture," Gallo certainly had, and Gallo was the paper's senior author.

There remained the separate question of what Gallo *hadn't* done. Priscilla Schaffer, one of the first women to receive tenure at Harvard Medical School, thought Gallo's major failing was his "refusal, flatly, on several occasions, to look at the notebooks or peruse the primary data of the people working for him. The buck's gotta stop somewhere," Schaffer said. The other advisers, Ken Berns and Mike McGrath, weren't as certain that Gallo should take the fall along with Popovic. "Ken didn't like that idea," Schaffer said later, "because that makes everybody culpable. He and Mike both felt that if you really want to interpret misconduct very strictly, it's the guy who falsifies or fabricates or changes the data."

Unlike previous meetings of the investigative team, this session was tape-recorded. It had been Suzanne Hadley's intention to send Popovic the tape of his own remarks, and to use the recording of the panel's subsequent discussion as a guide in drafting the OSI's report. When an OSI secretary confused the tapes and sent Popovic the tape of the panel discussion, Popovic discovered that he, but not Gallo, was about to be found guilty of scientific misconduct.

Popovic's lawyer, Barbara Mishkin, informed the OSI that her client wished to submit some additional evidence for its consideration. During the investigation, Popovic had said nothing about having secreted the early drafts of the *Science* article with his sister in Czechoslovakia. Now it looked like the time had come to play his ace. Most of the drafts weren't dated or numbered, and it took Suzanne Hadley days to sort them out. Once they were in sequential order, Hadley could see precisely how references to LAV in Popovic's handwritten originals had been eviscerated by Gallo with comments like "Mika you are crazy."

"Did I give my sister copies of all of the papers I wrote?" Popovic asked in his covering letter to Hadley.[48] "The answer is no, this was not a usual behavior for me. But I did it in this case because I believed that sometime in the future, I might need them as evidence to prove that I gave fair credit to Dr. Montagnier's group." Popovic pointedly reminded the OSI that "I did not agree with Dr. Gallo that the references to the work we did with the French virus should be omitted or even significantly minimized. I thought it was wrong not to credit Dr. Montagnier's group's contributions more clearly."

Apart from whether Gallo had committed scientific misconduct in his capacity as Popovic's superior, the hidden manuscripts suggested that Gallo might be guilty for his rewriting of Popovic's paper. Hadley thought Gallo was guilty on both counts, but that the former finding would be harder to defend, considering that the OSI had never extended the definition of scientific misconduct to include someone's failure to oversee the work of a subordinate who had committed misconduct.

According to Hadley, Jules Hallum thought Gallo was guilty in his role as Popovic's lab chief, but wasn't sure about Gallo's culpability for the manuscript revisions. Bill Raub, who as Bernadine Healy's deputy had continued to participate in the OSI investigation, thought Gallo was guilty for the revisions, but wasn't sure about his accountability as lab chief. After listening to arguments on both sides, Raub asked Hadley to draft a report concluding that both Popovic and Gallo had committed scientific misconduct, and be guided by the reactions of the OSI's advisers to the report.

Hadley's report began with the observation that "science, for a laboratory chief, subsumes more than direct work at the bench."[49]

> It includes setting standards for scientific rigor; it includes serving as a role model for responsible scientific conduct; and it includes appropriate scientific oversight of subordinate scientists to ensure that all work originating in the laboratory is authentic and accurate. . . . Beyond his misconduct as laboratory chief, and more specifically related to the Popovic *et al.* paper, are Dr. Gallo's own actions of direct falsification of statements about the French virus, LAV, and his complicity in the fabrications and other falsifications that were perpetrated by Dr. Popovic. Dr. Gallo bears sole responsibility for the statements about LAV, which are demonstrably false. Moreover, as senior author of the paper, as one who knew or should have known about the quality and extent of Dr. Popovic's

data, Dr. Gallo must be held accountable for his failure to ensure the integrity of those data. Dr. Gallo has claimed credit for the Popovic *et al.* paper and the other 1984 *Science* papers; so must he bear responsibility for the falsehoods in the Popovic *et al.* paper. Accordingly, the OSI finds that Dr. Robert Gallo engaged in scientific misconduct.

As Simon Wain-Hobson's paper identifying Christophe Lailler as the source of HTLV-3B was going to press in *Science,* Hadley's draft report was in the mail to Priscilla Schaffer, Ken Berns, and Mike McGrath. Having pushed Bill Raub to formalize the investigation of Gallo, the Academy panel was also eager to see the report, and to learn the outcome of the experiments comparing Popovic's pool patients with LAV. Without informing Bernadine Healy, Raub had scheduled a two-day meeting with the Academy panel members, reserving a block of rooms at the Hyatt-Regency in Bethesda.[50] When Joe Onek learned the Academy panel would see the OSI report before his client, he sent Healy what Hadley described as "a typically nasty Onek letter."

"Bill decided he better tell Bernadine what was going on," Hadley said. "Then *she* went ballistic. She didn't care for the Academy panel at all. She thought they were leaking all over the place, which was partly true, but I think she more resented the fact that she wasn't a member of the Academy. I was the one who had to call up Fred Richards and tell him, 'Guess what, the meeting's off.'"

Richards, the Sterling Professor of Biochemistry at Yale University, hadn't been happy about being asked by the Academy to replace Stanley Falkow, who had pleaded the press of business, as the panel's chairman. "I'm certainly not eager to do it," Richards said when his appointment was announced. "But when the Academy calls up and asks for help, there's a citizenship component. Then you do it, whether you like it or not."

Now, Hadley said, Richards was "dumbfounded, and furious, and I don't blame him." So was Al Gilman, who had assumed the role of Richards's *consigliere.* "I think this sucks," Gilman said. "The committee has two choices. We can resign, or we can hang in there and hope to get our shot in. While there'd be some pleasure in resigning, personally I'd just as soon not. We were asked to do a job and I'd just as soon finish it."

The panel had been scheduled to hear an update on the pool virus comparisons. In its absence Hadley arranged for Tom White, the scientist overseeing the PCR experiments at Roche, to present his data to the OSI investigative team. To rule out the slightest possibility of laboratory contamination, of which there already had been plenty, White's five-person team had avoided working in any of the company's labs where any strain of HIV had ever been used. In addition to remnants of the ten pool samples and other relevant cultures stored in Gallo's freezers for nearly a decade, the OSI had provided White with a battery of LAV samples for comparison: the now-recovered Mal Martin virus; "true Bru" and LAV_{Lai} from the official French depository in Paris; and a certified sample of Montagnier's B-LAV cell line.[51]

None of the ten pool samples, White told the OSI, had contained an AIDS virus that looked remotely like HTLV-3B or LAV. In White's opinion, it was "essentially impossible" that HTLV-3B had grown out of the Popovic pool — or, for that matter, that HTLV-3B and LAV had come from different patients.[52] In fact, four of the ten samples had contained *no AIDS virus at all*.[m] Not only that, the vial produced by Gallo's lab in response to the OSI's request for the earliest frozen sample of the pool was also virus-negative.[n]

Next White had examined MOV, the mystery virus used in the most critical experiments conducted by Popovic and Sarngadharan, but whose source Popovic had never identified.[o] So secretive had Popovic been about the genesis of MOV, even Sarngadharan hadn't known which patient it had come from.[53] Neither had Beatrice Hahn or George Shaw. "I would ask Mika point-blank — 'What is MOV?'" Shaw recalled. "And he just simply wouldn't answer."[54]

Tom White had the answer. MOV hadn't come from Moweni, the African AIDS patient. It hadn't come from Hector Millian, another of the possible sources suggested by Popovic; in fact, the sample of Millian's blood in Gallo's freezer hadn't contained any AIDS virus.[55] But the MOV sample from Gallo's lab did contain an AIDS virus, and that virus was LAV_{Lai}. "I'll never forget that moment," Suzanne Hadley recalled, "when Tom said, 'MOV is LAV.' I went to tell Bill Raub, and Bill looked like somebody had stuck him with a hypodermic."

· 20 ·

"I Know I Don't Lie"

The report of "Case 89-67: Activities in the Laboratory of Tumor Cell Biology, NCI," ran to more than 21,000 words, and it deconstructed what the Office of Scientific Integrity considered multiple false statements in one of the most cited scientific articles of the decade.[a] On the strength of those statements Mikulas Popovic had been found guilty of scientific misconduct, but the same was no longer true for Robert Gallo.

As instructed by Bill Raub, Suzanne Hadley had drafted a report that found both Gallo and Popovic guilty, a conclusion with which one of the OSI's scientific advisers, Priscilla Schaffer, had agreed. But the two other advisers, Ken Berns and Mike McGrath, had balked when they read Hadley's draft. "I was really surprised to hear this on the phone from Suzanne," Schaffer recalled. "She said 'Well, Ken is really unhappy with that, and Mike doesn't like it either.' And she said, 'I've had reason to stop and think seriously about this, and so has Jules. And so we've changed it.' I was blown out of the water. It was clear that they had also had some meetings with some higher-ups and that's when it all fell apart."

With Gallo's guilty verdict erased, Berns had "no problems with anything" in the report. Neither did McGrath, who thought it "gut-wrenching."[1] Gallo had argued that what the OSI viewed as false statements were merely errors of haste, an unavoidable consequence of the rush to save the blood supply. But the OSI observed that "the process of 'saving the blood supply' was proceeding apace, quite independently of the *Science* papers." The report went on to distinguish between fraudulent misrepresentations and what the OSI considered lesser untruths, such as Gallo's repeated claims to forty-eight AIDS virus isolates — a "troublesome" misrepresentation, but not one that rose to the level of scientific misconduct.

One misrepresentation that did cross the threshold was *Figure 2A,* a graph purporting to show that HTLV-3B had been in "continuous production" for "over five months" before the paper was published.[b] Considering that the manuscript had been sent to *Science* at the end of March 1984, Figure 2A could only be interpreted as meaning that Popovic had been growing the AIDS virus nonstop since late October of 1983. But according to Popovic's notes, the only AIDS virus growing in Gallo's lab in October of 1983 was LAV.

If Figure 2A were really a depiction of Popovic's success with LAV, given Gallo's subsequent denials it could have amounted to a colossal falsification. But when the OSI asked for the data to support Figure 2A, Gallo couldn't locate it. Sarngadharan had done the actual assays and read the data to Popovic over the phone, and he said he no longer had those notebooks.[2] In OSI's opinion, even if the data had once existed, spiking the pool culture with material from more patients and more fresh T-cells, as Popovic admitted having done, had rendered Figure 2A "meaningless" and made false the claim of continuous production.

Another falsification, in the OSI's view, was the paper's description of the creation of the Popovic pool from individual AIDS patient cultures "first shown" to be positive for reverse transcriptase.[c] Although the paper didn't mention the word *pool,* Popovic assured OSI that the questioned sentence described the creation of the pool from which HTLV-3B had emerged.

Thanks to the drafts of Popovic's manuscript, it was possible to see that the passage in question hadn't been written until version seven, and that the "first shown" part of the statement hadn't appeared until version eight. Gallo wouldn't admit writing that sentence either. But it paralleled Gallo's later assurance to Peter Fischinger that HTLV-3B had been isolated by Popovic from material "pooled from several patients who showed high R.T. activity in primary culture."[3]

To OSI, Popovic admitted he hadn't known whether the individual culture samples were RT-positive or not. Asked what, then, had led him to think they might contain the AIDS virus, Popovic said he had looked for visual evidence in primary culture that the cells were being killed by a virus. But Tom White's discovery that four of the pool samples contained no AIDS virus not only meant they couldn't have been RT-positive. It also meant there couldn't have been any visual evidence of a T-cell-killing virus in those four cultures, and the OSI had concluded that the "first shown" sentence was not only untrue but intentionally misleading.

Even allowing for Gallo's *"post-hoc* interpretation"— that the "first shown" passage referred to the *pooled* culture fluids and not the individual cultures — "the fact remains," said the OSI, "that the fluids were not 'first shown to contain particle associated RT,' as stated in the paper."

As predicted by Mal Martin and Berge Hampar, the OSI had avoided the large questions. Had there been a pool at all? Or was the "Popovic pool" an after-the-fact attempt to cover up the renaming of LAV as HTLV-3B? Or, as Jim Swire had suspected, was it MOV that had been renamed HTLV-3B? But a misconduct verdict stemming from any of those questions might have threatened the patent and the settlement. So might the OSI's verdict on Gallo's renaming of Adi Gazdar's HUT-78 as a newly discovered cell line, "HT."

The HUT-78 affair had come under scrutiny via a paper by Gallo and Popovic in *The Lancet,* listing HUT-78 and H-9 as independent entities and suggesting they had been established from different patients.[d] Gallo and Popovic argued that when the *Lancet* paper was published, in December 1984, they hadn't had any reason to think HT and H-9 were HUT-78.

The OSI countered that, six months before, Popovic had asked another NCI scientist, Dean Mann, to compare H-9 with HUT-78 from Gallo's lab.[4] According to Mann, the two cell lines had been genetically identical. Mann said he had informed Popovic of all his findings, and even written them down for him. Popovic denied ever having seen Mann's results. But the OSI concluded that, "well before the letter to *The Lancet* was prepared and submitted, Dr. Popovic knew that H-9 was identical to at least one strain of HUT-78."

The principal issue raised by the *Lancet* letter was whether Gallo and Popovic had committed misconduct with respect to HUT-78 or merely "very bad science." The OSI opted for bad science. Had Adi

Gazdar been interviewed by the OSI, he might have pointed to the early drafts of the *Science* paper, including one in Popovic's handwriting, identifying the source of the HT cell line as a patient with Sezary syndrome — the same diagnosis of the patient from whom Gazdar had established HUT-78 — rather than "an adult with lymphoid leukemia," the diagnosis in the published version.

There were still larger questions, about why the evidence of Popovic's experiments with LAV had been withheld from the Pasteur lawyers, whether some of the lab notes had been tampered with, whether false statements had been made under oath, and whether Vince DeVita, Peter Fischinger, Ed Brandt, Jim Mason, and the government's lawyers had been lied to during the dispute with Pasteur. But such questions involved federal statutes, and they were light-years beyond the scope of any investigation the OSI had ever attempted, not to mention its authority. Rather than prying open those heavy doors, the OSI devoted the remainder of its report to dissecting a half-dozen otherwise inconsequential experiments it believed had been falsely reported by Popovic in *Science*.

One was Popovic's description of the S.N. isolate as "Not Done" for electron microscopy, an experiment which had been done and was negative (an identical entry in Gallo's May 8, 1996, letter to *Nature* evidently escaped the OSI's notice). Unmoved by Popovic's explanation that he had intended "N.D." to mean "not determinable"— especially when his own paper defined it as "Not Done"— the OSI concluded that the description of the S.N. EM, and several negative experiments as "N.D." amounted to falsification of data. Another falsification, the OSI said, was the reporting of an immunofluorescence experiment as 10 percent positive, whereas the experiment had been entered in Betsy Read's notebook as "very few" cells positive, without assigning a numerical value to the number of positive cells.

The report concluded with a slap at Popovic for his failure to keep adequate experimental notes, observing that "the poor quality and scant extent of his laboratory records was striking," while those notes which did exist were "overwhelmingly cryptic and obscure, lacking even minimal detail necessary to understand what was done, what methods were used, and what results were obtained." But the OSI hadn't explored the question of *why* so much key data was missing.

The issue that dwarfed all others was Gallo's replacement of Popovic's essentially truthful, if incomplete, account of his use of LAV with the double fiction that LAV and HTLV-3 might not be the same kind of virus and that LAV had "not yet been transmitted to a permanently growing cell line for true isolation." Gallo admitted writing the "not yet been transmitted" sentence. But he denied that it meant what it said, reminding OSI that "I am the only person who knows what I meant." All he had meant, Gallo explained, was that LAV hadn't been successfully grown in Paris — which of course it had been. For his excising of Popovic's data on LAV, Gallo blamed Luc Montagnier, who "made it clear to me in July 1983 that the work on LAV was not collaborative any more . . . that we had approval only to study LAV, not to publish any results with it."

Montagnier denied making such a statement, pointing out that he had continued to send Gallo the requested shipments of LAV, *Bru* serum, anti-interferon and other materials — odd behavior for a non-collaborating scientist.[5] Gallo was inconsistent at best, telling OSI on another occasion that he had had "full freedom to do anything we wanted with LAV and publish on our own and solve the problem."[6] Gallo admitted disagreeing with Popovic over the excisions of LAV, but not that he had lied about it later. "Never once," Gallo declared, "did anybody say to me, 'Did you ever put LAV in a cell line permanently?' and I say, 'No, we never did.' I mean, I know I don't lie."[e]

The OSI found Gallo's explanations "at odds with Dr. Popovic's account," and particularly with Popovic's actions "in securing some of the draft manuscripts overseas specifically because of his concerns about what he viewed as a failure to adequately report the work on LAV." Moreover, the OSI said, it was "difficult to credit Dr. Gallo's professed reticence to describe in the paper his own laboratory's work with LAV, since in draft 4 Dr. Gallo wrote in his own hand that his laboratory had successfully grown LAV in a continuous cell line (H-4)." But in the end, the OSI took Gallo at his word about the questioned sentence.[f]

There would be no verdict of misconduct. Even so, the OSI said, Gallo's behavior had "fallen well short of the conduct required of a responsible senior scientist and laboratory chief." Gallo had "acquiesced in Dr. Popovic's wrongdoing." He "may even have tacitly encouraged, and at a minimum, he did not discourage, the conditions that fostered the misconduct," and he would have to share responsibility for Popovic's conduct, "for what it was and what it was not. . . . The investigative team believed that even though Dr. Gallo's actions do not meet the formal definition of scientific misconduct, they warrant significant censure."

Suzanne Hadley didn't think it mattered whether Gallo was officially guilty or not. "The report is severely critical of Gallo," she said. "It almost doesn't make a difference what you call it. Could he be fired? He could be fired for sure. Personnel action could be taken on the basis of this report."

Gallo wasn't the one whose job was in jeopardy. As the OSI report was being put in final form, Suzanne Hadley had begun comparing the information the OSI had unearthed with the government's representations in the Gallo patent applications and during the dispute with Pasteur. Hadley was no longer a part of the OSI, and while she had had the major hand in the report's preparation, it was only toward the end that she had begun to see how the pieces fit together. "If the data are false in a paper, they're false in a patent application," Hadley said.

Early on, Bill Raub had included questions about who had invented the HIV blood test as among the issues to be addressed by the OSI. Having read the record of the Justice Department's defense in the patent case, Hadley saw numerous instances where facts assembled by OSI contradicted claims by the government's lawyers, and by Gallo himself under oath. "Somebody lied," Hadley said. "What eventually ended up in the Department of Justice was not the truth. And I think had that been known, had a truthful report been given in 1987, I don't think we would be sitting here today talking about this."

Much of the data in Popovic's *Science* paper which the OSI now deemed to be false had been reproduced verbatim in the government's patent application for the HT cell line. That application, in turn, had been "incorporated" into the separate application for the blood test. Scientific misconduct aside, if Popovic and Gallo had known that HT was HUT-78 before the patent was issued, it could be a problem for the government.

So could Gallo's sworn declaration in the patent interference claiming that Popovic had "discovered" the permanent T-cell lines in which the AIDS virus had grown continuously. "Not true," Hadley said. "Popovic *used* cell lines previously discovered by others. I told Bob Lanman and I told Bill Raub, 'I've looked at the patents and I think there's some serious problems. I'm going to write something.'"[8]

On a Monday morning in early June of 1991 Hadley sent her "patent memo" to Lanman. A few hours later, walking past Bernadine Healy's office, she was flagged down by Healy's secretary with a message that the director was calling from her limousine. Healy had read the OSI report the night before, and she didn't like what she saw. "She said, 'It reads like a novel,'" recalled Hadley, who stepped into Healy's office to take the call.[7] "She said, 'I want it to read like a scientific report: introduction, charge to panel, methods, results, discussion. The results should not have any evaluative comments.' She also said, 'The OSI will not look good with this report.'"

Hadley remembered being "kind of speechless. I've never had an NIH director tell me to rewrite a report. I told her, 'That could really set us back.'" Hadley explained that Mika Popovic was leaving the country in less than a month, and that she had promised him a chance to give OSI his written response before the report became public. Beyond that, the OSI's scientific advisers had approved the report, and they would have to sign off on any changes. "I asked her, 'Can I think about this?'" Hadley recalled. "She said, 'You can do it in two days.'"

When Healy hung up, Hadley walked around the corner to Bill Raub's office. "I said, 'Do you believe this?' He was astounded. He said, 'I was with her at eight o'clock last night and she said, "This report is wonderful, it gives me exactly what I need to deal with Gallo."'" Raub promised to check with Healy and call Hadley back, but the news wasn't good. "He said, 'Bernadine will not talk about the Gallo report. She wants it rewritten, period.'"

Hadley went upstairs to her office and wrote Healy a memo, requesting that the director order the revision in writing and warning that such a request had the potential for "significantly vitiating" the Gallo report, as well as fatally compromising the OSI's independence from NIH. Her concerns were especially grave, Hadley said, because NIH scientists were involved.[8] Given their strained relationship, Hadley hadn't expected Jules Hallum to back her up. But Hallum warned Healy that any revisions would leave OSI open to charges that it had "produced a 'whitewash' of Dr. Gallo, regardless of what your intention might be."

"Thus," Hallum told Healy, "I cannot in all conscience accept your order for a re-write of the Gallo report, a report accepted by our advisory panel, without further discussion and negotiation with you. . . .

[I]n the Gallo case I was specifically told by Dr. Raub as Acting Director to prepare the report as the evidence directed and to 'Let the chips fall where they may!' That is exactly what OSI has done and I stand by the report. . . ."[9]

Rather than risk accusations that she had compromised OSI's independence, Healy let the report stand.[10] The letter that accompanied Popovic's copy was terse. "The results of the investigation," it said, "indicate that you falsified, fabricated, and misrepresented data in the *Popovic et al. Science* paper, and therefore, that you engaged in scientific misconduct, as defined by the Public Health Service."[11]

Gallo's letter was only slightly better. "The results of the formal investigation indicate that you did not engage in scientific misconduct as defined by the Public Health Service," it began. "At the same time, as set forth in the draft report, the OSI, with the unanimous and strong concurrence of the scientific advisory panel, found that your conduct had in numerous respects fallen well short of the conduct required of a responsible senior scientist and laboratory chief. . . ."[12]

For Gallo, the most troubling aspect of the report was a single paragraph. Tom White hadn't finished his final experiments with the pool patients, and the report noted that a final chapter on the genetic comparisons with LAV and HTLV-3B would be added later. "The issue of contamination/misappropriation," the report said, "has not been resolved, and may not be, even with the results of the OSI-commissioned sequencing now underway. However, there is reason to believe the results of the sequencing will shed additional light on the matter."

Suzanne Hadley had won her battle with Bernadine Healy, but it wasn't possible to face down the director and survive. The day the report went to Gallo and Popovic, Jules Hallum ordered the Gallo case files transferred from Hadley's new office in the legislative division back to OSI, where Hadley could complete the final stages of the investigation under Hallum's close supervision.[13] Hadley was still in shock from the Healy contretemps when Hallum called to say he had to see her right away. "He told me I was being 'reined in,'" Hadley said, "that I was to make no more decisions in the Gallo case. He said, 'You understand I don't like this, but I have to obey orders.' Jules was embarrassed."

Hadley admitted to feeling relieved. "I just have been so harassed," she said. "The hell with it, I just want to get rid of it, I don't need this shit anymore. I fought as long and hard as I could. It was getting harder and harder, and finally with this asinine order it was patently impossible. And even if it were possible, I don't need this."

Hadley had been one of NIH's rising stars, a GS-15 with an Inspector General's Merit Award, a sheaf of rave performance reviews, and a shoo-in candidate for the government's elite Senior Executive Service. Recognizing that her upward mobility at NIH had just come to an abrupt halt, Hadley told Hallum that rather than move back to OSI, she was withdrawing from the Gallo case altogether.[14]

"I never wanted anything out of this," Hadley said later, "except to do it right. But I certainly never wanted to get just absolutely destroyed. I would have been demolished by Bernadine. She absolutely would have destroyed me. I think by that time her malevolence was at such a height that any excuse at all she would have seized upon."

As news of Hadley's withdrawal spread, one of her first calls was from Ken Berns. "He was very upset," Hadley recalled, "saying, 'This is going to be a disaster.'" Priscilla Schaffer saw Hadley's reining-in as a fatal blow to Raub's authority. "Bill got thrown aside," Schaffer said. "That man is a saint. He epitomizes what the NIH is all about — honesty, integrity, a bit of a polyester double-knit, but a great man. And now look at this. It turns my stomach."

Less than a week after the OSI report reached Gallo's lawyer, the Associated Press declared Gallo's vindication. "No evidence of misconduct," the AP said, quoting an unnamed government official, "has been uncovered in a National Institutes of Health investigation of the laboratory of Robert C. Gallo, the NIH researcher credited with co-discovery of the AIDS virus."[15]

The AP reporter evidently hadn't seen the report, which contained a misconduct verdict against Mika Popovic, and Hadley thought the rest of the AP's story was wrong as well. "That just burns me up," Hadley said. "The unnamed source goes on to say the investigation did not discover anything that calls into question the 1987 French-American agreement. The report concludes by saying the specific issue of misappropriation versus contamination 'has not been resolved.' The report raises questions that would make a Pasteur lawyer sit up and start wondering about coming to Washington and having some meetings."

However much Bernadine Healy might admire Mozart, Gallo was an employee of the United States government, charged with overseeing fifty-odd NIH scientists and a $12 million annual budget. The OSI report had nothing good to say about Gallo, and on Healy's desk there was an even thicker report from the OPRR, sanctioning Gallo for violating human subject regulations. Considering what the OSI and OPRR investigators had uncovered, not to mention the Sarin and Salahuddin affairs, Healy might have had difficulty explaining to John Dingell and her HHS superiors why she hadn't taken steps to clean up Gallo's operation.

When Healy brought the hammer down, it was in the form of a military-sounding memorandum, signed by Healy and Sam Broder, addressed to "CAPT Robert C. Gallo," his commissioned rank in the Public Health Service.[16]

"In accordance with Public Health Service (PHS) regulations prescribed in the Commissioned Corps Personnel Manual, Subchapter 46.4, Instruction 1," the memo began, "you must comply with the lawful orders of your official superiors." There was "reason to believe" that Gallo "may not have diligently exercised your management and control responsibilities as a NIH Laboratory Chief. Several serious issues related to misconduct by government employees under your supervision have recently been identified, including acts leading to criminal charges under Title 18, United States Code. To correct the identified deficiencies and to focus your full attention on your primary responsibilities as a NIH Laboratory Chief, you are hereby directed to follow the requirements set forth in the accompanying memorandum."

Gallo was directed to "familiarize" himself with all HHS and NIH regulations relevant to his job, including standards of conduct for federal employees and the rules governing medical experiments on human subjects. He was to "terminate" his outside activities and committee memberships, and devote the extra time to running his lab. No longer could Gallo accept travel paid for by universities or private companies, which meant that at least for the moment, his globe-trotting days were over.

Manuscripts Gallo submitted for publication would have to be approved in advance by NIH. So would speeches, appearances, or interviews, "whether in person, by telephone, or by other communications device, with a representative of the press or other communications media if such interview pertains to your official duties, whether past or present." Finally, Gallo would be required to review "all primary data" produced by any scientist under his supervision before that data was submitted for publication, and to ensure that his assistants maintained "written laboratory notebooks and records sufficient to permit scientific peers and supervisors to adequately interpret and duplicate the work."

Healy and Broder reminded Gallo that "several investigations involving you or other individuals assigned to the Laboratory of Tumor Cell Biology have not been completed. Thus, neither this memorandum nor the memorandum attached should be interpreted as foreclosing other appropriate actions that may be necessary upon conclusion of these ongoing investigations."[17]

Gallo promised to "do my best to comply," although in his opinion his "past administrative failures" were only two: "I trusted some people too much, and I did not know about the need for approval before analyses of human blood samples. Dr. Broder would add at least two more: I have traveled too much and had a penchant for speaking too much to the press. I cannot disagree."[18]

Neither could the auditors in the NIH's Division of Management Survey and Review. During one two-year stretch, the auditors found, Gallo had visited Austria (four times), Canada, Costa Rica, Denmark, France (four times), Germany (five times), Great Britain (three times), Hawaii, Hong Kong, India, Israel (twice), Italy (seven times), San Marino, Spain (four times), Sweden (twice), Switzerland (three times), Taiwan, and Trinidad. And those were just his foreign destinations. "The amount of travel is unbelievable," said the DMSR's chief, a former FBI agent named Howard Hyatt. When the DMSR questioned how Gallo could manage a complex research program and supervise more than fifty employees while spending so much time out of the country, Dick Adamson replied that Gallo's travel had not had "any impact on his responsibilities or his accomplishments as a laboratory chief," and reminded the investigators that "Dr. Gallo is a preeminent scientist of Nobel Laureaut [sic] potential."[19]

On a Saturday morning in late July, Suzanne Hadley's telephone rang at home. The caller was Gallo, evidently the last person in Bethesda to learn that she had withdrawn from the Gallo case. "At the beginning of the conversation he was not coherent," Hadley said, "more like he was into just a stream of consciousness. It's like he pushed the button and the tape starts going. Unstoppable, rapid, jumping, completely illogical. Finally, about halfway through the conversation, he sort of came down. If you've ever heard rapid cyclers, it was like that, a manic disorder."

While Hadley took dictation on a legal pad, Gallo said he wanted her to know he had tried his best to cooperate with OSI. His passions had simply gotten the better of him. "I didn't know the truth about the people in the pool until later," Gallo said. "I now understand I should have looked at Mika's notebooks. Did I know to do this at the time? No. Harmison and Fischinger were on my neck every day — 'Hurry up.'"[20]

"I think it's fair to say that he was really shaken by the report," Hadley said afterward. "He thinks that if we could just sit down face to face and talk it out, that he would be persuasive. If he could just sit down with me for a day or so, he could explain a lot of this. As if we hadn't interviewed him umpteen times over the last year." Gallo didn't seem to understand that he had been the subject of an official investigation. "He said, 'But why did you have to go and write it all down and put it into a report?'" Hadley recalled. "I said, 'Because that's the way the office operates.' He said, 'Yeah, but why did you have to give it to Healy and Broder?'"

Having taken action against Gallo on her own terms, Bernadine Healy had even less use for the Office of Scientific Integrity — "a bunch of Keystone Kops," is how she described the OSI. An internal NIH review, initiated by Healy, was already under way to examine the OSI's "structure" and "function," including how it kept its records and whether it adhered to its published procedures. "We are also looking," Healy warned, "at matters of tone."[21]

John Dingell heard Healy's remarks as a prelude to dismantling the OSI, which happened to have an ongoing investigation involving a scientist at the Cleveland Clinic, the institution from which Bernadine Healy had come. The target of that investigation, one Rameshwar K. Sharma, was suspected of citing research data that didn't exist and experiments that never took place in applying for a million-dollar NIH grant.[22]

The Sharma case might never have attracted Dingell's notice except that Healy, as the clinic's research director, had played a key role in an internal inquiry, which concluded that Sharma hadn't intentionally misrepresented his work.[h] As required by HHS regulations, a report on the clinic's inquiry had been forwarded to the OSI, which had reached the opposite conclusion: Whatever Sharma's intentions, he had violated federal law. The OSI also criticized the Healy panel on several counts, including its failure to examine previous drafts of the application in question and the inclusion of a scientist who was a Sharma collaborator. But the OSI's strongest criticism had been leveled at Healy's use of euphemisms like "anticipatory writing" to justify Sharma's conduct.

Dingell's staff was convinced the Sharma case had predisposed the NIH director against the OSI from the start. Healy protested such insinuations as "patently untrue," but she thought it prudent to honor the chairman's concerns by recusing herself from any involvement with the OSI until the Sharma case had been resolved.[23] Healy's recusal notwithstanding, Dingell was determined to shine a light on the NIH director's treatment of Suzanne Hadley, and the Sharma case would be his lantern.[24]

Dingell's sympathy toward Hadley was evident from the outset of the hearing, despite Peter Stockton's worry that the chairman might attack Hadley by mistake. "My greatest fear," Stockton said, "which he's done in the past, is that he would start drilling the wrong one. So we kept saying, 'Now this Suzanne Hadley, the one with the fuzzy hair, now she's the good one.'"

The bloodletting began with the second panel of witnesses, which included Bernadine Healy and Jim Mason, once again back in the assistant HHS secretary's job as Robert Windom's replacement. "I thought we did beautifully with Bernadine," Stockton said. "We pretty much humiliated her. She said, 'Well, I had these sleepless nights and maybe I didn't do really well with that and maybe I made a mistake and that's why I empaneled the second one. Bullshit. That had nothing to do with it. It was because Sharma was pissed off that he wasn't going to get promoted. I mean, come on."

The biggest surprise was the alacrity with which the Republican members of the subcommittee had grilled a Republican presidential appointee, and the acrimony with which Healy responded to their questions. According to the *Cleveland Plain Dealer*, Healy ignored efforts by her aides to tone down her statement.[25] "The bottom line," said Stockton's sidekick, Bruce Chafin, "is she's got her mind made up when it comes to Hallum and Hadley and these cases, and the only way to deal with this woman is a collision course. Some people you can threaten, or cajole, and you can influence them. I'm convinced we're not going to be able to influence this woman until she fears us. She's going to have to start listening to her aides, or there'll be another train wreck, and another, and sooner or later she'll be carried out in a body bag."

"Intellectual Recklessness
of a High Degree"

"Censure is urged for AIDS scientist," announced the *New York Times,* which had obtained a leaked copy of the OSI's still-secret report.[1] "Professor Gallo is accused of having censored the article on the discovery of the AIDS virus," exclaimed *Le Monde,*[2] which somehow got the same report, and whose story focused on Mika Popovic's revelation that Robert Gallo had rewritten his *Science* paper to hide the crucial experiments with LAV.

"If Popovic had said at the outset what he has said now," declared Luc Montagnier, "it could have saved a lot of time. And, more important, the outcome of the 1987 agreement would have been different."[3] Even Daniel Zagury, Gallo's most vociferous French supporter, had questions for Gallo. There had been *"no* differences" between him and Mika Popovic, Gallo assured Zagury. Popovic hadn't taken the draft manuscripts to his sister to conceal evidence of Gallo's wrongdoing, but merely "for posterity."[4]

Relations between Gallo and Montagnier appeared to have smoothed three years before, in anticipation of a shared Nobel Prize, but the OSI investigation had put Gallo under a cloud, and also more distance between the two men. In hopes of restoring at least the appearance of comity, Gallo had invited Montagnier to speak at his next AIDS meeting.[a] Montagnier declined, citing "the multiple untrue or uncorrect accounts of our past relationship" in Gallo's just-published memoirs.[5]

Gallo's book, *Virus Hunting,* was drawn mainly from his own recollections and those of his staff.[6] Perhaps for that reason, it frequently left the impression that some insight or discovery occurred sooner than it actually did. A number of noteworthy events were missing altogether, including the tripartite meeting in Montagnier's office. The many errors of fact ranged from trivial — Zaki Salahuddin, who still didn't have a Ph.D., had become "Dr. Salahuddin"— to significant misstatements about the history of research on AIDS,[b] larded with gratuitous shots at Michael Koch and others who had questioned Gallo's veracity.[c]

Pasteur's early isolations of HIV were described as "detections," while Gallo's previously acknowledged detections had once again become "isolations."[d] But Montagnier found himself most offended by Gallo's assertion that the French had learned from Gallo how to grow LAV in cord blood cells. "This is *untrue,*" he informed Gallo, "and I already told you that before."[e] Montagnier also objected, once again, to Gallo's assertion that he, Montagnier, had broken off the Pasteur-Gallo collaboration in July 1983.[f] Unless Gallo retracted the falsehoods, Montagnier declared, "I do not feel like resuming any kind of good relationship with you. P.S. My first name is *Luc,* not *Jean-Luc.*"

Gallo agreed to correct four of the five errors raised by Montagnier in the upcoming French edition of his book.[7] But when the book appeared in the Paris bookstores, only one of the changes had been made,[8] and something new had been added: a preface by Jean-Claude Chermann recounting the discovery of LAV that read as though Chermann had done it single-handedly. If Gallo was attempting "to introduce division between Chermann and myself," Montagnier said, "congratulations, you have succeeded! But I repeat my warning: the preface of Chermann to your book will not be helpful for you and him. On the history of LAV discovery in my laboratory, you know nothing about it."[9]

The misconception was abroad, promoted by Gallo, that the 1987 agreement had resolved the question of who discovered the AIDS virus by settling equal credit on Gallo and Montagnier. But the agreement hadn't touched the question of discovery — or what Maxime Schwartz called "the problem of knowing how Gallo isolated his virus. It was left out. This is an essential point. There was the discovery of

Montagnier published in May 1983. No one asked to know if the virus came from the same patient as that of Professor Montagnier. Today it's different."

With the leak of the OSI report and the attendant publicity in Paris, French government officials "no longer excluded" the possibility that the 1987 agreement would have to be renegotiated.[10] Neither did Schwartz, who was certain that if Mika Popovic's paper had been published as Popovic had written it, "there would not have been any litigation."[11] But it hadn't, and there had been, and nearly all the American royalties the Pasteur had received as a result of the settlement with the Reagan administration had gone to pay the institute's lawyers.

In light of what had since become public, and what the American government appeared to have known at the time but kept from the French, Pasteur now wanted reimbursement for its legal fees plus back royalties, interest, and a greater share of future royalties. Rounded off, the Pasteur's bill added up to some $25 million. Four years after Ronald Reagan and Jacques Chirac declared the dispute settled forever, the ball was again in play.

Lowell Harmison, Peter Fischinger, and the other HHS and NIH officials who had run defense the first time around were gone from the government. Gallo, not certain where to turn for help, had sent Jim Mason an impassioned letter.[12] "Le Monde has orchestrated a mass media campaign within the last two days," Gallo complained. "I received three telephone calls today. Now it has spread to all of France, and they state that the report concluded I stole the virus from France, blocked Popovic from discussing it, etc., etc. I need your help — desperately, and I think NIH and the government are also being slandered in the worst way." Mason, who hadn't forgotten the trouble Gallo had caused over his interview with Larry Altman, let Gallo twist in the wind.

The patent dispute and the settlement were beyond the OSI's purview. But nothing was beyond the purview of John Dingell, whose staff defined its mandate as "everything that moves, burns or is sold." Hoping that a congressional committee which handled 40 percent of the nation's legislation[13] could get the attention of a Republican administration, Rob Odle, a partner in the Washington office of Weil, Gotshal & Manges, invited Peter Stockton to dinner.

Odle's principal value was his Republican connections, which went back twenty years — to Watergate, in fact, when Odle, as staff direc-

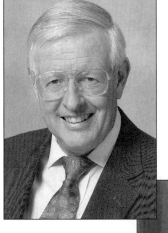

Murray Gardner *(Courtesy University of California, Davis, Health System)*

HHS Secretary Margaret Heckler and Robert Gallo at the April 23, 1984, news conference where Heckler announced Gallo's discovery of the cause of AIDS *(AP/Wide World Photos)*

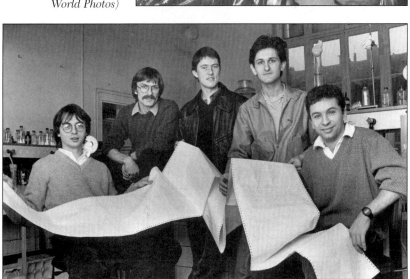

The Pasteur sequencing group, with a printout of the first DNA sequence of the AIDS virus (LAV-1) in November 1984. LEFT TO RIGHT: Marc Alizon, Simon Wain-Hobson, Stewart Cole, Olivier Danos, and Pierre Sonigo *(Michael Philippont/Sygma/CORBIS)*

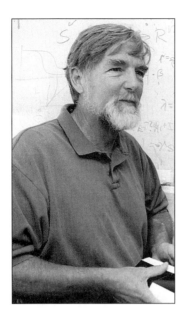

Gerald Myers
(Los Alamos National Laboratory)

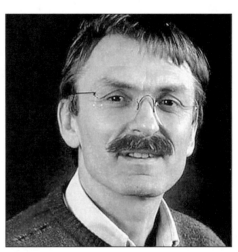

Simon Wain-Hobson
(Institut Pasteur)

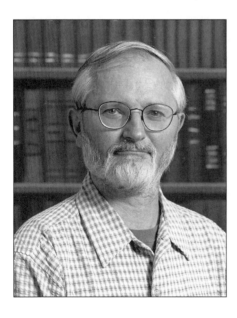

Paul Luciw
(Courtesy University of California, Davis, Health System)

Malcolm Martin *(NIH)*

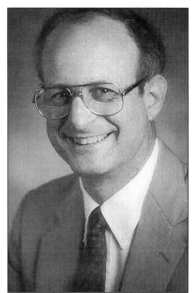

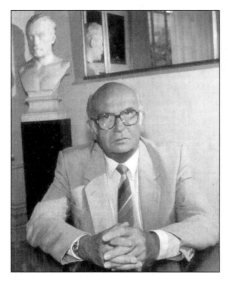

Raymond Dedonder *(Institut Pasteur)*

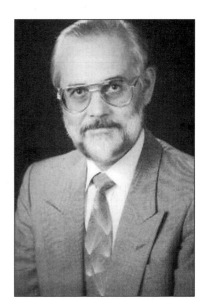

Peter Fischinger
(National Cancer Insitute)

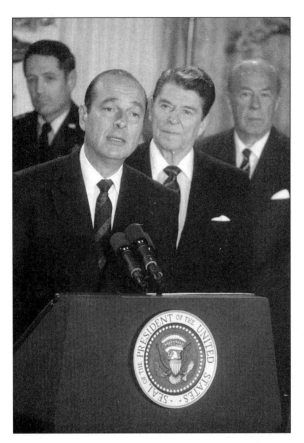

French Premier Jacques Chirac and President Reagan, announcing the first settlement of the Gallo Pasteur dispute, March 31, 1987 *(AP/Wide World Photos)*

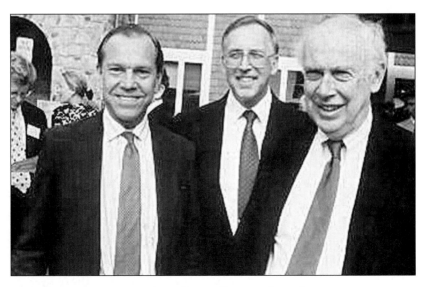

LEFT TO RIGHT: James Wyngaarden, William Raub, and James Watson *(NIH)*

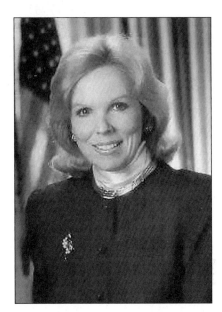

Bernadine Healy *(NIH)*

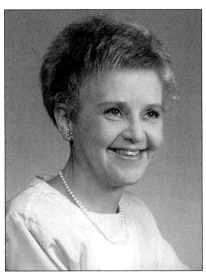

Suzanne Hadley *(Olan Mills)*

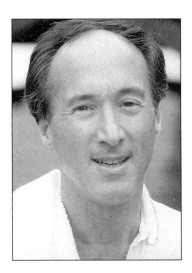

James Swire *(Elizabeth Swire Falker)*

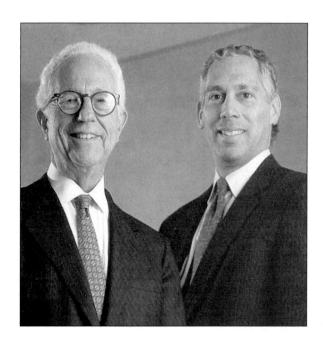

Ira Millstein and
Michael Epstein
(Douglas Levere)

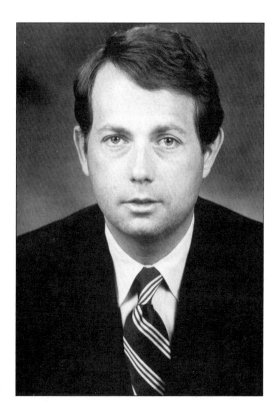

Rob Odle
(Courtesy R. Odle)

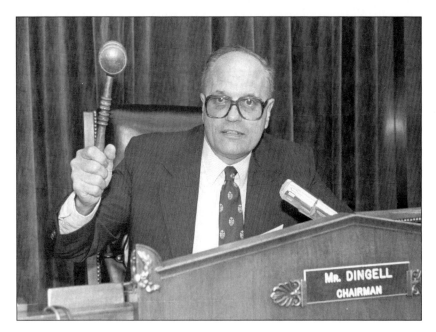

John Dingell

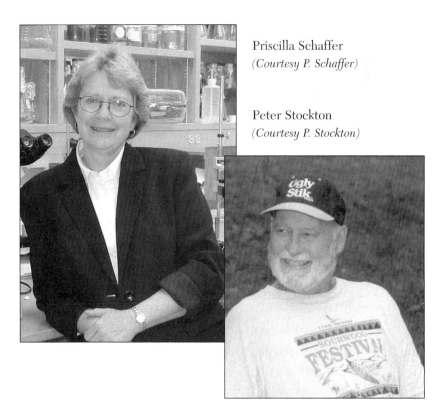

Priscilla Schaffer
(Courtesy P. Schaffer)

Peter Stockton
(Courtesy P. Stockton)

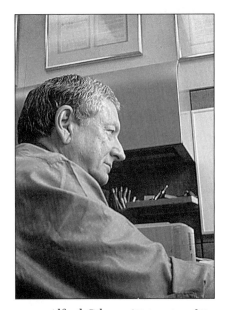 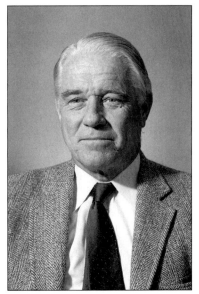

LEFT: Alfred Gilman *(University of Texas Southwestern Medical Center at Dallas)*, RIGHT: Frederic Richards *(Courtesy F. Richards)*

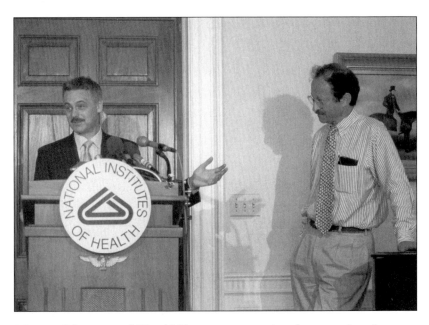

Maxime Schwartz and Harold Varmus, announcing the second settlement with the Institut Pasteur, July 11, 1994 *(AP/Wide World Photos)*

tor of Richard Nixon's 1972 reelection campaign, had removed certain sensitive files from the reelection committee's headquarters following the Watergate break-in.[14] As the lead-off witness before the Senate Watergate Committee, Odle had acknowledged that the files contained "things which have no place in a political campaign."

Having escaped indictment for obstruction of justice, Odle had served as an assistant secretary of energy in the Reagan administration, then joined Weil, Gotshal. In a city where convicted felons become talk-show hosts and after-dinner speakers, Odle's status as a Watergate survivor gave him some cachet. "I know about the kind of dirty business that can go on in the White House," he would say earnestly. "The wiretaps, all the dirty tricks — I know how that works."

"Odle has a strange sort of simplicity," said Suzanne Hadley, who had been invited to dinner as an observer. "I'm not sure if its real or not. Like, 'These people really want to do the right thing,' and 'I've been in the Nixon White House so I know how bad not doing the right thing can be.' Have you ever had dinner with a blind person who keeps talking about being blind? It's really embarrassing. It was like that, only 'I was in the Nixon White House, I know what it's like.'"

Odle must have made an impression, because within days of the dinner John Dingell was demanding that HHS hand over a copy of Suzanne Hadley's memo on the blood-test patent. "There may have been repeated instances of false and misleading statements in the patent application and in the November 1986 sworn declaration of Dr. Gallo," Dingell warned the new HHS general counsel, Michael Astrue.[15] The chairman also wanted to know "whether, after November 8, 1991, the statute of limitations would bar any possible perjury charges in connection with Dr. Gallo's declaration."[16]

Within the Executive Branch such letters were known as "Dingell-grams." The Environmental Protection Agency received 150 of them a year, an average of three a week, and it had an employee, known as "Mrs. Dingell," who spent most of her time keeping track of the chairman's queries and demands. After the EPA came the FDA, followed by the Defense Department, the Securities and Exchange Commission, and the Department of Transportation.[17]

The NIH and HHS were far down Dingell's list. But Mike Astrue assured Dingell that the moment the OSI report was final, he would seek the Justice Department's advice on whether the AIDS test patent should be amended or withdrawn.[18] As for prosecuting Gallo, Astrue had alerted the HHS Inspector General that the federal five-year statute of limitations on Gallo's declaration was about to run out. After November 8, 1991, it would be extremely difficult, though not impossible, to bring charges for any false statements the declaration might contain.

In the summer of 1991, the fifteen or so attorneys who comprised Onek, Klein and Farr had closed their door and gone their separate ways.[19] Among the rumors buzzing around the downtown legal community, one suggested that Onek's colleagues had grown impatient with the number of hours their senior partner was devoting to the Gallo case, which kept Onek's name in the papers but didn't add much to the firm's annual income.

Onek, who admitted that his representation of Gallo was "a labor of love," landed at one of Washington's more obscure firms, Crowell and Moring, known among lawyers as "Cruel and Boring" because of its mind-numbing focus on representing corporate clients before federal regulatory agencies. Suzanne Hadley had concluded that, despite his increasingly tortuous efforts to craft a defense from what had become a cascade of damaging facts, Onek was convinced of Gallo's innocence. "Oh, passionately," Hadley said. "I don't think it's good that he believes so passionately. I think a lawyer needs to keep some distance to really serve his client well."

Onek did display flashes of exasperation, as on one occasion when he was asked to explain several of Gallo's contradictory statements. "Oh," Onek had sighed, "Gallo will say anything"— not the highest testimonial that could have been paid to someone under investigation for scientific fraud.[20] When it came to Gallo's sworn declaration, Onek hadn't had any choice but to admit that the statement contained misstatements of fact.[21] What mattered, Onek said, was that Gallo hadn't *intended* to mislead the patent office.

When Gallo swore in his declaration to have had between twenty-five and thirty *isolates* of the AIDS virus before Mika Popovic began growing LAV in Bethesda, Onek explained, he had meant to say *detections*. The fact that there hadn't been any reagents with which to detect the AIDS virus was beside the point. Gallo's assertions that "nothing could be done" with the July 1983 LAV sample, and that Popovic's growth of LAV was "only temporary," might be untrue, but that wasn't Gallo's fault. Gallo's statements had been "based on conversations with members of his laboratory." Harder to explain was Gallo's affirmation that he had had an electron micrograph in February 1983 of "the virus which would later be called HTLV-3." According to Onek, Gallo's statement wasn't false; it simply didn't mean what it said.

"They're sitting down," Suzanne Hadley said, "and trying to decide, 'How can we come up with an innocent explanation for these things?'" But Onek didn't even try to explain Gallo's claim under oath to have seen "no evidence" that LAV was the cause of AIDS before the blood-test patent was issued.

The Office of the HHS Inspector General spent most of its time tracking Medicare cheats and others who committed financial fraud against the government, and its investigators routinely recovered tens of millions of taxpayer dollars each year. But when it came to electron micrographs and reverse transcriptase assays, the OIG's investigators were lost at sea.

Hadley's meeting with the OIG agent assigned to determine whether Gallo had committed perjury in the sworn declaration hadn't gone well. "She said, 'But didn't Gallo have other isolates?'" Hadley recalled. "'And didn't the French have trouble growing the virus? Gallo was the first one to really be able to grow it, wasn't he?'" Hadley had tried to set the woman straight. "I said, 'In the first place he didn't have any isolates until after he'd grown LAV. And even if he did, what does that have to do with whether he lied in his sworn declaration?'"

Armed with what Peter Stockton described as "their carefully nurtured ignorance of the facts," the inspector general's investigators had asked the Justice Department whether it had any interest in prosecuting the government's star AIDS researcher for perjury over statements he had made during a complex scientific dispute with a French research institute nearly five years before. "Not surprisingly," Stockton informed Dingell, Justice had "found the matter confusing" and "was dubious about its prosecution."[22]

Suzanne Hadley, still on the NIH payroll, had been reassigned from the congressional liaison office to one of the agency's backwaters, an obscure unit whose mission was to promote science education in the public schools. With little to do except rethink the events of the past eighteen months, Hadley had begun to comprehend "how badly I missed the boat." What dismayed Hadley most was her failure to get an early handle on the full compass of the case — to see how some of the entries in Mika Popovic's notes, or some of the phrases in his *Science* article, while seemingly disconnected, might have implications in a larger context for the patent, the blood test, the veracity of the Reagan administration, and the settlement with the French.

"I just didn't get it," Hadley said, "and that's really bad for somebody who prides herself on being a hot-shot investigator. I thought I had hold of the case. I didn't have hold of all but a teeny corner of it. Boy, did I get bamboozled. We were just overwhelmed. We didn't know what was important. We didn't know what questions to ask. We didn't know for sure that 3B was LAV, and we certainly didn't know that MOV was LAV. We had the chance, and we blew it. *I* did. It was so much bigger than we imagined. Once I began to get my wits together, it was too late."

So broad was the scope of the Gallo case that it seemed ludicrous, in retrospect, to have attempted to fit it into the narrow framework of a scientific misconduct investigation, which typically focused on the misreporting of an experiment in a published article. Even more than whatever had happened in Gallo's lab, Hadley was appalled by the government's behavior, in and out of court.

"Whatever one thinks about Gallo," Hadley said, "he had support all the way up the line. They had data back in 1984 showing they were the same virus," a reference to Flossie Wong-Staal's unpublished data. "I mean, *the same isolate.* And it's taken until now? You know what I'm saying? The data have been there all along. There never was an iota of a chance that HHS would do an honest thing. Before anything had even happened the die was cast, the decision was made. After that it was simply a matter of crafting a litigation strategy."

Hadley's choices were between keeping her head down until retirement or finding a forum in which she could finish the investigation she had started. But keeping her head down wasn't Hadley's style, and Dingell's subcommittee offered such a forum. Other federal "whistle-blowers" could testify that casting one's lot with John Dingell was a career-suicide move, but Hadley professed not to care. "When your government does the wrong thing," she said, "you have to do what you can to set it right."

With Hadley's arrival on Capitol Hill, the Dingellgrams arriving at HHS and NIH suddenly assumed a more informed tone. According to one letter that landed on Bernadine Healy's desk in late November of 1991, following Hadley's departure from OSI a number of disturbing events had occurred.[23]

Priscilla Schaffer, Ken Berns, and Mike McGrath had been "entirely eliminated from any meaningful participation" in the finalization of the Gallo report, Dingell told Healy. Dingell also understood — from whom he didn't say — that the OSI's findings against Gallo and Popovic were being softened, and that there was a "surprising lack of interest" in pursuing the implications of the Roche report, which remained under lock and key.

None of the principals in the case — Gallo, Popovic, Sarngadharan, or Betsy Read — had been questioned by OSI since the Roche study cast doubt on the veracity of the Popovic pool, and a reopened Gallo investigation was the last thing the NIH wanted. When Dingell's staff asked Jules Hallum whether OSI intended to pursue the "possible misappropriation" of LAV in view of the Roche findings, Hallum shook his head. If it did, Hallum said, the Gallo case could go on forever.

When the Roche study inevitably leaked to the press,[24] Hubert Curien, the French minister of research and technology, lost no time in calling for a reopening of the 1987 settlement. A redivision of royalties between HHS and the Pasteur, Curien said, was now "imperative." The Americans themselves had proven that HTLV-3B was LAV, another of those "successive bits of evidence which have come to light concerning what really happened in Robert Gallo's laboratory, and which we had all suspected."[25]

On a Saturday morning in early December of 1991, Priscilla Schaffer, Ken Berns, and Mike McGrath assembled in Bethesda for what they expected would be the last time, to read the final draft of OSI report 89-67. Mika Popovic was still guilty of scientific misconduct, but the report had been through more revisions at the hands of Jules Hallum's new deputy, an agronomist named Clyde Watkins. Most of the report's criticisms of Gallo were gone, including his censure. "We were told in no uncertain terms," Schaffer said, "that all the report dealt with was the Popovic paper, and that's it."

The Roche DNA sequence studies were listed in the report's index as "Appendix X."[g] But there wasn't any "Appendix X," and the question of how LAV_{Lai} had become HTLV-3B was relegated to a single sentence in the middle of the 119-page report. "Even with the results of the OSI commissioned study," it read, "the issue of contamination or misappropriation has not been resolved definitely." When Gerry Myers heard that Gallo still wasn't prepared to admit that HTLV-3B was LAV_{Lai},[26] Myers decided the only model for Gallo was the elder Karamazov. "Dostoyevsky really got him right," Myers said.

Also missing was any hint that the OSI had obtained the CDC blood-test data at the core of the patent dispute. At Hallum's request, Don Francis had sent OSI "the very printout that I carried to Paris to meet with Bob Gallo and the group at the Institut Pasteur the first week in April in 1984."[27] The data on the CDC printout had been analyzed by the OSI's resident statistician, who concluded that the results of the Gallo and Pasteur ELISAs were "remarkably concordant," which Francis and the French had been saying for years.[28] But there was no mention of the statistician's conclusion in the report, or even that the CDC data had been obtained and analyzed.

Bernadine Healy was delighted with the revisions. "Congratulations!" she told Hallum. "Professional. Beautiful. Proud of it. Excellent format. All of it is impeccable. Magnificent. Knew it would be better, but hadn't expected such a vast improvement. Learned from it."[29]

Before it could become official, the report would have to undergo a final administrative review by HHS. But it nonetheless leaked to the *Washington Post*, which declared that the OSI finding "vindicates Gallo, one of the world's foremost AIDS researchers, who has maintained his innocence over the past eight years against a plethora of accusations that ranged from having stolen the AIDS virus from his French counterparts to having falsified scientific data to further his own reputation."[30]

"After all of this money and all of this time," Bernadine Healy complained, "the issues came down to things like whether 10 percent or 'very few' was a fabrication.[h] These are not the big issues that everyone thought this was all about." Healy, who had done her best to vitiate the report, now explained that it was the "big questions" to which she had wanted an answer: "Was this virus somehow stolen by the Gallo laboratory? Was credit stolen? Did the Gallo laboratory really develop the blood test for AIDS — did they really save the blood supply? Did they give appropriate credit for those cell lines, and were they generous with those cell lines? These are the questions that the

American public wants to know, and I believe that we have an obligation, one way or the other, to make sure that the answers to at least
those questions are answered."[31]

The National Academy of Sciences thought the same. The Academy
had answered Bill Raub's call for help, and it hadn't been pleased by
Bernadine Healy's efforts to minimize the Academy panel's role.
When Academy officials made their displeasure known in high places,
Healy had reconvened the Richards panel — not as a free-standing
committee this time, but a group of individual "consultants."[32]

On a blustery Wednesday at the end of January 1992, six members
of the panel[i] assembled in the Little Theater of the NIH Clinical Center for a two-day discussion of "the most bizarre case" in which the
panel's chairman, Fred Richards, had ever participated.[33]

The OSI's increasing paranoia over leaks had resulted in security
so tight that, before the Richards committee was given the Gallo
report, each member had been required to sign a statement likened
by Al Gilman to "what you have to sign before you go to work for the
CIA." Anyone who violated the pledge risked losing his NIH grants,
and whatever notes the panel members took would have to be surren-
dered upon leaving the room. Moreover, each member was required
to agree "to cooperate fully with any Government investigation of any
unauthorized disclosure" of the report's contents. "It was pretty hysterical," Gilman said later. "They wouldn't even allow us to take our
briefcases in the room."

The OSI report the panelists were finally handed was almost completely changed from the Suzanne Hadley version. "There are some
comments in there about Gallo that aren't very complimentary,"
Gilman said later, "but it isn't nearly as strong as it used to be." Bernadine Healy, her recusal from OSI matters rescinded by Jim Mason,[j]
reminded the panel that the question before it was whether the OSI
had arrived at its conclusions "in the proper fashion," not whether the
panel agreed with those conclusions.

The Richards committee had a number of disagreements
anyway, among them the OSI's verdict that Gallo's "alternative interpretations" of the "not yet been transmitted" sentence were reasonable. The committee members had been reading, writing, and
peer-reviewing scientific papers for decades, and they had seen

it all. "It's a priority claim," one member scoffed. "He knew it was in continuous culture, and stated that it was not. That's evidence of misconduct."

Gallo met with the committee for more than an hour, in Al Gilman's words "burning to make a presentation." But Gilman didn't think Gallo had helped himself. "He don't get it," Gilman said afterward. "He doesn't understand what he did wrong." Before the meeting concluded, Healy engaged the panel members in an informal discussion. "What she wanted to know," Gilman said, "is, does Gallo have no redeeming qualities at all? Is this guy the scum of the earth? Or is there a spark of genius there that ought to be nourished? Or is he mentally ill?"

Hoping to preclude a "National Academy panel report," Healy had asked each of her "consultants" to provide her with an individual opinion. Not to be outdone, the panelists drafted a consensus statement and each sent Healy a copy.[34] Their collective opinion was unvarnished. Gallo and Popovic "went to school" with LAV, "yet they later failed to mention the fact that they had propagated the French virus. In fact, they denied propagation of the French virus and stated (in the Popovic *et al.* manuscript) that the French virus had never been transmitted to a permanent cell line"— a statement, the panel observed, that "is simply false, and was known to be false at the time the paper was written."

The Academy panel couldn't say whether LAV had been stolen and renamed HTLV-3B, but it didn't matter. "Given the quality of the information derived from propagation of the French virus," the panel declared, "we believe that this constitutes intellectual recklessness of a high degree — in essence, intellectual appropriation of the French viral isolate." Gallo's "failure to distribute uninfected H-9 cells freely" the panel found "essentially immoral in view of the growing seriousness of the AIDS epidemic."

The panel was also troubled by what it saw as a yawning discrepancy in the OSI's treatment of Gallo and Popovic, to whom "different standards appear to have been applied." Neither Gallo nor Popovic, the panel noted, had admitted writing the RT sentence, and "with no way to identify the actual source, the blame could be distributed among all the authors. Yet the blame has been specifically placed on Dr. Popovic."

"We did our best," Al Gilman said later. "I have no idea whether we will have an impact. We made very strong statements. Whether Healy will take them to heart or not, I do not know. She can ignore us. I don't think she wants Gallo at NIH. He's an embarrassment. But I don't know exactly how she'll handle it. I think they're behaving very politically at the moment. Get this goddamn thing out of their office with minimal damage to themselves."

A few days after the first news reports of the Richards committee's conclusions, a letter arrived at the Academy's imposing headquarters on Constitution Avenue, five blocks from the White House. Addressed to its governing body, referred to simply as the Council, the letter was signed by an Academy member named Serge Lang.

As he read the Richards Committee's rebuke, Lang, a Yale mathematician, founder of the field of Diophantine geometry and a recipient of the Cole Prize, the top American award for mathematics, thought it warranted a reconsideration of Gallo's own election to the National Academy.[35] "Gallo's nomination," Lang reminded the Council, had been "based in large part on his purported contributions to discoveries concerning the AIDS virus," which now appeared not to have been Gallo's discoveries.[36]

Lang's challenge provoked the predictable telephone call from Gallo, who suggested in a follow-up letter that as "the most cited scientist in the world for the decade of the 1980's"[37] he deserved Academy membership, and that Lang's "continued references to me regarding matters about which you have no facts and certainly no understanding of are deeply disturbing and shocking."[38] Gallo cited as an example the excisions he had made in Popovic's *Science* paper. "What I meant by the question 'are you crazy' and the comment 'this is incredible,'" he told Lang, was simply that Popovic's statements about his work with LAV were "bizarre without more data."

"How can one respond to a madman?" Lang asked.

"I don't know if there's ever been an example of somebody who's been removed from the Academy," observed Fred Richards. "There are lots of cases of people who are not elected who probably should be, or vice versa. People have resigned from the Academy. But I don't recall anybody ever being thrown out. Once you're in, you're a member of the club." Although Lang's appeal for a reconsideration of Gallo's election prompted expressions of support from a number of Academy members, including at least one Nobel laureate, the matter was tabled by the Academy without further action.[39]

.   .   .

Following Bernadine Healy's rancorous appearance before John Dingell's subcommittee, the consensus was that Healy's NIH tenure was growing shorter. "Witnessing this spectacle," concluded *Science & Government Report*, "it was difficult to avoid the aroma of a cesspool of bureaucratic paranoia in Bethesda. Though Bernadine Healy has been head of NIH for only a few months, an increasingly heard speculation in Washington biomedical circles is that she and the office are not a happy match, and that she's not destined for a long tour of duty. A deft administrator does not leave fingerprints in executing dire deeds."[40]

Healy had tried not to leave any fingerprints in assembling an antidote to the Richards committee, her own advisory panel on the Gallo case drawn from the top rank of NIH researchers: Edward Korn from the Heart Institute, Richard Klausner from Childhood Diseases, Robert Chanock from NIAID, Gilbert Ashwell from the Kidney Institute, and Arthur Levine, the former chief of the NCI's pediatrics branch.

At Healy's request, Jules Hallum had drawn up a list of deficiencies uncovered by the OSI investigation that were "traceable in substantial measure to Dr. Gallo's hands-off approach to management of his laboratory."[41] From the "Wise Men," as Healy called her little group, she now wanted advice on what administrative action she should take against Gallo: fire him, take away his laboratory, impose further administrative sanctions — or do nothing.

Healy instructed the Wise Men to read the OSI report and the Richards committee's recommendations, and let her know their reactions to both. But after the now-standard signing of confidentiality agreements and Healy's imprecations not to mention the group's existence to outsiders, Rick Klausner was astonished to learn that the Wise Men were expected to listen to a presentation by Gallo and Onek. "I was floored," Klausner recalled. "It was the worst violation of confidences. I said I wasn't going to come."[42]

On the morning of the presentation Klausner got an urgent message from Healy's office directing him to attend, and he reluctantly made his way to the NIH's Building One. Gallo was "incredibly disarming," Klausner said later, "eloquent and convincing. What he said, if true, was convincing, and I had no way to judge. Gallo explained what he meant, and we didn't challenge it. He clearly felt a sense of vindication from all of us. My own feeling was we just wanted out, that there was no point to this. I can't convey how inappropriate this whole thing felt."

After Gallo's departure, "some of us held our views tenaciously," Art Levine recalled. "Some changed views. Some never articulated a view. I don't remember a lot of discussion." But Klausner recalled the general feeling among the Wise Men as "not particularly flattering to Gallo . . . pretty critical," and also that Healy had orchestrated the entire exercise to justify taking no further action. "She had decided long before what she was going to do," agreed Klausner, "and this was to get a prominent group of scientists to give their imprimatur. The reality is, we didn't agree to anything."

Of the five Wise Men, only John Gallin and Ed Korn sent Healy their written assessments of the Gallo case.[k] Gallin claimed later to have destroyed his memo and all of his notes. But Korn had kept a copy of his, and if Healy had been hoping for a more agreeable opinion to counter the Richards committee, she was disappointed. The Richards committee's report, Korn wrote, was "entirely consistent with my own view."[43] If Popovic was to be found guilty of misconduct, so should Gallo be. But whether Gallo was guilty or not, it was Korn's recommendation "that you remove Dr. Gallo from his position as Chief of the Laboratory, explicitly for failing to fulfill the responsibilities of scientific leadership."[l]

Following the Wise Men's last meeting, Healy implored Jim Mason that "[r]easonable attempts must be made to clear Dr. Gallo's reputation with regard to accusations of misconduct — and also to accusations that he knowingly and willfully misappropriated a French virus, for which there is no apparent evidence."[44] When Mason didn't seem interested in vindicating Gallo, Healy went public, telling the *Washington Post* she had given Gallo an opportunity to defend himself against the Richards committee's charges and had "found many of Gallo's answers convincing."[45] When Klausner and Levine discovered that Healy was talking to the press about what had transpired behind supposedly locked doors, they shared the same reaction.

"I think I was used," Levine said. "I was 'had,' completely," Klausner said.[46]

"It Can't Be the Money"

"It may be the greatest scientific fraud of the twentieth century," Sam Donaldson intoned on a Thursday evening in April 1992, as Robert Gallo's face flashed across the screen. "Eight years ago, this man was hailed as the genius who discovered the AIDS virus."

Donaldson cast his *Prime Time Live* report on "the rise and fall of Dr. Robert C. Gallo" as a detective story, the tale "of how one of America's most renowned medical research scientists almost got away with taking credit for something he hadn't done." Even now, Donaldson exclaimed, his eyebrows dancing, "important elements of the United States government seem reluctant to have all the facts revealed."[1] But Donaldson saw the Gallo case, and the investigations it had spawned, as emblematic of something larger, a story "of how a fight for wealth and glory can interfere with the desperate effort to conquer a deadly disease."

Gallo hadn't wanted to talk to ABC. "So," Donaldson explained, "one morning last week we went out to NIH to speak to him on his way to work." The picture switched to Donaldson, microphone in hand, on an interception course as Gallo walked briskly toward Building 37. "Can you tell us, Doctor," Donaldson asked, "why you originally claimed credit for discovery of the AIDS virus?"

"Mr. Donaldson," Gallo replied, picking up his pace, "do you really stoop this low?"

Donaldson, who had made his reputation shouting questions at Ronald Reagan from the White House lawn, kept up the pace.

"In a patent application," Donaldson hollered as Gallo scurried through the door, "you swore under oath that you discovered the AIDS virus."

"Mr. Donaldson," Gallo replied, "you're a creep."

"Do you have anything to hide, Dr. Gallo?" Donaldson persisted as Gallo slipped into an open elevator.

"I said, 'Mr. Donaldson, you're a creep.'"

"That may be," Donaldson said, "but we're asking you whether you were the original discoverer of the AIDS virus or not."

"Ask yourself," Gallo shot back as the elevator doors slammed shut.

Donaldson had been more successful with Don Francis, who recounted in detail the April 1984 tripartite meeting in Montagnier's office. "The isolates that we had in the United States looked identical to what the French had described the year before," Francis said.

"So when you left that meeting," Donaldson said, "you, the French, and Dr. Gallo were agreed that the French should be credited with having discovered the AIDS virus?"

"That was the understanding," Francis said.

The night before *Prime Time* aired, Gallo called Francis in a conciliatory mood, the threats he had made to Francis over the Shilts book evidently a thing of the past. "He said, 'No matter what happens on the broadcast, we're still friends,'" Francis recalled. "He was as rational as I've ever heard him. He said, 'I've made some big mistakes. Some of it was my fault, and some of it was the administration's fault. I recognize that.' Then he said, 'CDC should have gotten more credit.' I said, 'It's really an issue between you and what you did to the French, with whom we were collaborating.' He said, 'I understand that.'"

Within days of the broadcast the tide had turned again, with Gallo's lawyer, Joe Onek, demanding that Francis "promptly write a letter to Dr. Gallo retracting your previous statements and setting the record straight." If Francis refused, Onek threatened to "take appropriate legal action to determine whether your erroneous statements were the result of faulty memory or deliberate misrepresentation."[2]

There was one person *Prime Time* had missed: Mac Haddow, Margaret Heckler's former chief-of-staff, now reincarnated as a health-care consultant after serving part of a one-year prison sentence for violating federal conflict-of-interest laws. According to Haddow, interviewed a month later on the BBC program *Horizon,*[3] the HHS lawyers had had "great concerns about the credibility of the documentation" provided to them by Gallo's lab during the Pasteur dispute.

"There was a point," Haddow said, "where it became very clear to me that the NIH people were not being truthful. The further we looked into it, the more scrutiny we gave to it, the clearer it became that the original position of the NIH, which was that we had a hands-down winnable case, was not true."

Haddow recalled Gallo as "incensed that there would be a question about his scientific integrity," and "furious with the French. As he sat in my office, he told me the French were trying to steal away the Nobel Prize from him, and that even though there may be questions raised about the chain of custody of the virus and the procedures used, that those were all lies, and that he could attest to the fact that there was nothing done with the French virus. *Nothing*, and he pounded the table when he said it."

Haddow admitted that HHS had tried to bluff Pasteur in hopes the French would go away. "The determination we finally came to," Haddow said, "was that Bob Gallo, as strong as he was on his views, couldn't support the claims he was making from a legal standpoint. And so our attorneys recommended that we play it out until we saw how strong the French were, play it out as strong as we could, but if we got to the point where we knew we were going to court that we should roll over and accept a reconciliation and settlement of this problem. The French attorneys didn't know how weak our case was and they never discovered it. So we were able to craft an agreement that probably disadvantaged the French, but it was because we hid our weakness fairly effectively. We felt in a political sense that it was important for President Reagan to show that he had an interest in the AIDS problem."

The BBC program wasn't aired in the United States, but Haddow's declaration was reported in the press. "Had we known then what we know today," Haddow told the *New York Times*, "we would have had a moral obligation to allow the French to have all the royalties. We have no right to them."[4] Complaining about the Haddow interview to Max Frankel, the editor of the *Times*, Joe Onek charged that the story was "just one of several articles which we believe to have been unfair to Dr. Gallo."[5] Like certain other publications, Onek said, the *Times* had given far too much coverage to the Gallo case, and not nearly enough to what Onek termed "a French AIDS scandal" brewing in Paris.

The focus of the French scandal was the CNTS, a semiofficial agency of the French government that collected blood for transfusions and blood products, including the blood-clotting factors most hemophiliacs require to keep from bleeding to death. In Paris, a criminal trial had just gotten under way in which four senior officials of the CNTS, including its former director, Michel Garretta, stood accused of knowingly distributing HIV-contaminated clotting factors in the summer of 1985.

The essence of the charge was that the blood from which the clotting factors were produced either should have been discarded, or subjected to a heating treatment that would have inactivated the HIV it contained. Barring that, heat-treated clotting factors could have been imported from abroad. But Garretta, who admitted knowing that some of the blood from which the factors were being made contained HIV, had nonetheless ordered that the untreated blood be used "until all the stocks are gone."[6] Garretta's motive appeared to have been nothing more complicated than sparing his agency the extra expense involved.

The highly politicized case had been brought on charges filed by a French hemophiliac represented by the lawyer for the National Front, the far-right-wing political party headed by Jean-Marie Le Pen. Another political layer had been added by the fact that the government in power at the time of Garretta's decision was that of Socialist prime minister Laurent Fabius, since replaced by his conservative rival Jacques Chirac. The *New Yorker* was not alone in observing that French socialism was also on trial.[7]

About a thousand of the five thousand or so hemophiliacs in France were then positive for HIV, but Garretta argued that many of those, perhaps most, had become infected before the HIV blood test became available in 1985. Many obviously had.[8] But an unknown number — estimates ranged between five and fifty — had needlessly become infected before heat-treating was begun by the CNTS in October 1985. Convicted under an ancient law intended to punish merchants who sold adulterated products, Garretta got four years in jail. He was freed after thirty months, only to face new charges under an even older law of "poisoning." The former CNTS research chief, Jean-Pierre Allain, whom prosecutors conceded had tried to warn Garretta of the dangers of contaminated blood, got four years, two of them suspended. Allain was also reindicted on poisoning charges, something *Nature* called "an offence against the civility for which France is distinguished."[9]

The jailing of Garretta and Allain — especially Allain, who had accepted a Cambridge professorship a few months before his indictment, and whose wife, Helen Lee, worked for Abbott Laboratories in Chicago — roiled the international scientific community, including Allain's Cambridge colleagues and a number of prominent Americans.[10] The prevailing opinion, expressed by one French scientist, was that the convictions had been "unavoidable, in order to satisfy public opinion."[11] But John Maddox warned in *Nature* that "nobody should be surprised if observers now conclude that the French judicial system will go on finding defendants for AIDS-related trials until the understandable anger of the relatives of those infected with HIV is stilled."

In the months that followed, the list of those charged in *L'affaire du sang contaminé* grew longer, eventually including Georgina Dufoix, the former minister for social affairs in the government of Prime Minister Laurent Fabius, Edmond Hervé, Fabius's minister of health, and ultimately, Fabius himself.[12] Most of the articles beneath the front-page headlines across Europe failed to mention that the same fate had befallen the hemophiliacs of several other countries, including Germany, Canada, Japan, and the United States, where more than three thousand hemophiliacs had died of AIDS[13] — and where non-heat-treated clotting factor was still being sold, with the FDA's approval, at the time of Garretta's decision to use up the untreated stocks in France.[a]

Hoping to somehow twine the fate of the French hemophiliacs with the Gallo-Pasteur dispute, Gallo's supporters in France, principally Jacques Leibowitch and Bernard Seytre, a freelance journalist who had translated the French edition of Gallo's memoirs,[14] tried to focus public attention on the history of HIV antibody testing in France.

Seytre claimed French officials had blocked the introduction of the Abbott ELISA, which could have been used to screen blood destined for the hemophiliacs, in order to protect the French blood-testing market for Pasteur.[15] Appearing on American television,[16] Jacques Leibowitch, now employed as a consultant to Abbott,[17] accused the French government of attempting to preserve the country's economic interests by refusing to begin using the Abbott test until after the Pasteur test became available.

Seeking to turn the scandal to Gallo's advantage, Joe Onek declared that the trouble in Paris "demonstrates which country was first in developing a workable blood test; it also highlights the ironies involved in the French government's current efforts to secure more patent royalties from the blood test."[18]

The real story began on February 11, 1985, when Abbott Laboratories, whose ELISA was still undergoing prelicensing tests by the American Red Cross, asked the French government to approve the test in France. Seventeen days later, on February 28, Diagnostics Pasteur, in which Institut Pasteur owned a minority interest and the French government held the majority, filed a similar application in behalf of the Pasteur's LAV-based ELISA, then undergoing field tests in Paris and other French cities.

The data submitted by Abbott to support its French application, including the fact that 86 percent of HIV-positive samples were likely to be false, caused concerns in Paris similar to those that were delaying the introduction of the Abbott ELISA in the United States.[b] "It seems indisputable," concluded Robert Netter, the chief of the National Health Laboratory, the French equivalent of the FDA, "that [the Abbott] test must be the subject of a thorough study in France, the same as that being made by Diagnostics Pasteur for its own test."[19]

Two days after Netter's note, the FDA, under pressure from HHS and the Reagan White House, put aside its concerns about accuracy and licensed the Abbott ELISA.[20] Eighteen days later, Diagnostics Pasteur informed the French Ministry of Health that it could begin supplying tests at the rate of 125,000 a month by April 15.[21]

When the French government compared the field tests of the Pasteur and Abbott ELISAs, it learned what the FDA and the American Red Cross already knew — that the Pasteur ELISA was twice as accurate in terms of false positives.[22] Even Jean-Pierre Allain, who had worked for Abbott during the 1970s and returned to the company after resigning from the CNTS to work on a second-generation HIV blood test, admitted that "the specificity of the Abbott test during the first six months to a year was not very good."

In mid-June, the French national health laboratory was alerted to a new problem with the Abbott test. Because of problems with virus production and other components, the performance of some Abbott tests was significantly worse than others. That revelation was followed by a report in *The Lancet* that the Abbott test produced not only repeated false positives but false negatives.[23] The national health laboratory had been prepared to approve the Pasteur test on April 25 and the Abbott test three weeks later, on May 13, or as soon as the company submitted the additional data requested by the French government.[24]

On May 9, however, the prime minister's science adviser, François Gros, recommended that Abbott's application be tabled until the Pasteur test had been licensed.[25] At the time, Gros was also director of the council of trustees of the Institut Pasteur. Even so, the Pasteur test was approved for use in France on June 21, and the Abbott test on July 24 — a lapse of thirty-three days, compared with the ten months the FDA had waited to approve the Pasteur ELISA in the United States.

In the opinion of Jacques Leibowitch and Bernard Seytre, the French had had an ethical obligation to put the flawed Abbott test into service immediately following its approval in the United States, thereby preventing the infection during those thirty-three days of at least a few hemophiliacs and transfusion recipients. The rancorous public debate over which course should have been taken might have been avoided, had it been known that Abbott didn't have enough blood tests to supply the American market, much less France.[c]

By the beginning of April 1985, the American Red Cross was only testing half the new blood it collected, and the independent blood banks were farther behind.[26] A month before its French application was approved, Abbott was still experiencing major production problems and test-kit shortages because of its inability to increase virus yields from the H-9 cell line. "Inventory levels continue at 1–2 days best case and cannot be increased . . . until antigen inventory increases," the company's senior researchers were informed in mid-June of 1985. "Critically need scaled up antigen purification process and higher producing cell line."[27]

Nine days later, Abbott notified the FDA of its need to change its method of cloning H-9 "in order to supply the growing number of customers desiring to screen their blood supply." Not until mid-July, a week before Abbott finally began selling AIDS tests in France, was the new purification procedure deemed to be producing enough virus to enable the company to prepare a shipment of 300,000 tests "exclusively for France."[28]

Laurent Fabius and his former social affairs minister, Georgina Dufoix, were acquitted of all charges after François Gros testified that "the entire responsibility" for delaying approval of the Abbott ELISA was his alone (Edmond Hervé, Fabius's minister of health, was convicted but not sentenced to prison). Gros acknowledged that "a secondary objective" in his decision had been the commercial success of the Pasteur ELISA. "We tried to do what it took," Gros said in a 1994 television interview, "so that the French test would not be forgotten relative to the American test."[29]

With the documents reflecting Abbott's production problems still locked in the company's files, Gallo claimed the French government's "refusal to use our test" had allowed "thousands of French citizens to become infected" with HIV — a preposterous charge.[d] Joe Onek demanded to know why the United States "owes the French anything, when they barred the U.S. blood test from the French markets for narrow commercial reasons, killing their own citizens."[30]

Ignoring the fact that the Institut Pasteur had had nothing to do with the manufacturing or licensing of the French blood test, Onek warned the new HHS secretary, Louis W. Sullivan, that "officials of the Pasteur Institute may well be implicated in this scandal." It would be "extraordinary indeed," Onek told Sullivan, for the Bush administration "to provide additional blood test royalties to institutions that were willing to jeopardize the lives of French citizens in order to give the French blood test a competitive advantage over the American blood test."[31]

Pressing the attack, Onek began circulating a March 1985 letter to Gallo in which Montagnier had observed that LAV didn't appear to cause AIDS in every infected patient. According to Onek, the letter proved that "in March 1985 Dr. Montagnier had little understanding of the relationship between the HIV virus and AIDS, which may help explain why the French government was willing to delay approval of the American blood test."[32] Gallo copied the letter to Daniel Zagury, with the suggestion that Montagnier's comment "should become publicly available" in France.[33]

What neither Gallo nor Onek mentioned was that, in the spring of 1985, Margaret Heckler and the United States government had held precisely the same view.[e] Maxime Schwartz thought efforts to blame Montagnier were doubly unfair, since it was Montagnier who had begun urging, in the summer of 1983, that the French government begin testing stored blood for LAV antibodies with the Pasteur's prototype ELISA. "This story was started by friends of Gallo," said Schwartz, "this story about the delay of the test. I think Leibowitch is at the center. It has been used by Gallo and Joe Onek. Gallo bears a big responsibility for that."

In the wake of *Prime Time,* Gallo weighed his options for how to respond to Sam Donaldson. "I remain confused," he confided to Peter Biberfeld in Stockholm.[34] "A few friends feel: (1) I should not go to the press (2) that the T.V. show was obvious to do harm and unfair; (3) that we should take a low profile and long term strategy and let others help over the next two years. Some others believe I must answer in the public arena and soon."

The solution was presented by the National Cancer Advisory Board, the NCI's civilian overseers, which expressed outrage at Donaldson's "unwarranted and scurrilous attack on the integrity of Dr. Robert Gallo." The board's subcommittee on AIDS, chaired by Howard Temin, would hold a public meeting at which Gallo would be free to respond "to charges that have been widely made about your behavior with respect to the discovery of HIV-1, a response that you have not yet had a chance to make in public."[35]

Temin, who despite never having smoked would soon be diagnosed with terminal lung cancer — "just bad luck," Temin said — hadn't worked much on AIDS, having spent the years following his Nobel Prize turning out a steady stream of solid papers on oncogenes and animal retroviruses from the McArdle Laboratory at the University of Wisconsin. But Temin had noted with satisfaction the crucial role played by reverse transcriptase in the discovery of the AIDS virus — "an illustration to the public," Temin said, "that you can't tell what's going to happen with basic research. Here is something which started out to be about as obscure as anything could be, and all of this came out from it."

Temin was bothered by the increase in what he called "sharp practices" among the new generation of researchers, things "that others call uncollegial behavior, unethical behavior, unprofessional behavior, other types of misconduct, and rudeness." But he thought the OSI's investigation of Gallo hadn't been well advised — not because of its impact on Gallo's lab, which had "continued to be productive," or on the NCI's budget, which scarcely noticed the $56,000 the investigation had cost the cancer institute, but because it had done incalculable harm to the public image of science.[36]

In hopes of redressing that image, and his own, Gallo would be permitted to offer the cancer advisory board his response to the *Chicago Tribune*, Sam Donaldson, the OSI, and the Academy panel. When Mika Popovic heard what was being planned, he wanted to make a presentation of his own. "I realize that I am no longer employed by NIH and that I am not as prestigious a scientist as Dr. Gallo," Popovic said, reminding Temin that it was he, not Gallo, who had been found guilty of scientific misconduct.[37] But Temin declined Popovic's request. The NCAB meeting was to be Gallo's moment.[38]

Gallo's statement would be followed by two hours of questions, not extemporaneous questions from the floor, but questions carefully culled from those submitted in writing beforehand. "How much valuable research time," one questioner wanted to know, "was lost by Dr. Gallo and his associates while they were obliged to be occupied with matters unrelated to research activities during the past five or six years?" Another wondered how Gallo could "possibly continue to make important advances in AIDS research if you are forever 'hounded' by clearly never-ending investigations?"

In addition to *CNN*, *ABC News*, *USA Today*, *People* magazine, and *The Economist*, the organizations requesting seats at the meeting included the State Department and the government of France. But the media wouldn't have a chance to question Gallo afterwards. Concerned about the "potential for disruption," the organizers planned to whisk Gallo down a back stairwell to an elevator and thence a waiting car that would speed him off the NIH campus.

Mike Astrue, the HHS general counsel, thought the cancer board's plan sounded half-baked, a "blatant" and "one-sided" proceeding well outside the NCAB's mission, which was "to provide general advice and guidance to the National Cancer Institute." Lou Sullivan, the HHS secretary, agreed with Astrue. But when Sullivan's deputy, Kevin Moley, ordered Bernadine Healy to pull the plug on the Gallo show, Healy refused.

"She hung up," recalled a disbelieving Astrue. "She made it quite clear she wasn't going to cooperate." Astrue replied with a blistering memo to Healy, predicting that the event would turn into "a guaranteed circus" and "undermine years of effort to ensure public confidence in the fairness of this Department's review of the Gallo matter." If the meeting went ahead, Astrue warned, Healy and the other NIH officials responsible should "consult [their] private attorneys regarding [their] potential personal liability." Astrue's next call was to Howard Temin. "I told him he had to cancel the meeting," Astrue said. "He said he'd think about it. He wasn't sure whether he would or he wouldn't. He wanted to see it in writing. I explained that the meeting was illegal. He said basically that he didn't care."

Temin was already in Washington, where that same morning he had received the National Science Medal from President Bush in the White House Rose Garden. A few minutes after the ceremony, Temin was handed a letter from Astrue.[39] "The meeting that you have scheduled for tomorrow," it read, "exceeds the statutory authority of your committee and therefore must be cancelled. If you have any questions about this advice, I would be happy to review the matter with you. You need to be aware that unauthorized expenditure of federal funds may expose you and others to various types of liability."

To Astrue's relief, Temin backed down. "What I care about," Astrue said later, "is trying to maintain a fair process. Bernadine may consider it irrelevant that anyone else has an opinion on this. She's arrogant, she's egotistical, she's totally out of control. She doesn't listen to anybody but herself. The fact is, it's a very sensitive matter, and it makes no sense at all to have NIH sponsoring meetings that are invariably going to be interpreted as promoting one side of the controversy."

To the reporters who showed up for the nonmeeting, Temin described Astrue's letter as "threatening. I took it to be threatening, and I was threatened by it. If I wasn't threatened by it, I wouldn't have canceled the meeting."[40] For the cancellation Joe Onek blamed the Pasteur's "venal" lawyers at Weil, Gotshal, who had somehow prevented — Onek didn't say how — an "extraordinarily disappointed" Gallo from delivering "an extremely powerful statement" in his defense. Had Gallo been allowed to go ahead, Onek said, he would have made public "documents that were never seen before."[41] When the Pasteur lawyers, curious to know what important information Gallo had withheld from Jim Swire and the OSI, filed a Freedom of Information Act request for the new documents,[42] Gallo admitted that no such documents existed.[43]

Despite the best efforts of Gallo, Onek, Bernadine Healy, and the NCI, the world's view of the discovery of HIV was gradually being altered in the Pasteur's favor. When *Time* reported on the 1992 International AIDS Conference in Amsterdam, it put Montagnier on the cover, alone, identifying him as the "Master Detective" of AIDS research.[44] "In a field that is filled with prickly egos," *Time* said, "the 59-year-old Parisian is a rarity: an unassuming professional who has faced controversy and emerged with his reputation enhanced." *Time* described Gallo as "one of the world's most famous — and ambitious — scientists," who "grabbed the spotlight and tried to deny the significance of the French achievement — until the facts came out and Montagnier got the credit he deserved."

Nature also seemed to be steering a more moderate course, declaring that if the French believed they could "make a fair case for an increased share of the royalties, they should not hesitate to do so," while if the United States "believes that Gallo rightly earned 50 percent of the credit for developing the patented blood test, it should not be reluctant to defend itself."[45] Even the *Washington Post,* perhaps chastened by Rob Odle's documentation of nearly a dozen "indisputably false statements" in the paper's coverage of the Gallo case,[46] had become more sympathetic toward the French.

"For years," the *Post* observed in an editorial, "Dr. Gallo was coy about the scientific value of the Pasteur samples, saying they were not the origin of his discovery. He steadfastly refused to acknowledge fully the French contribution. Then last year he made an admission in the journal *Nature:* The virus "discovered" in his laboratory was indeed the virus isolated and identified by Dr. Montagnier. This belated admission changes everything, the French claim. . . . The U.S. government apparently hesitates to renegotiate the settlement agreement — in part because of the continuing investigations, civil and criminal, surrounding Dr. Gallo's conduct at the time of the patent application and later on." Echoing the question that had hung over Richard Nixon during Watergate, the *Post* asked, "What did Dr. Gallo and U.S. representatives know, and when did they know it?"[47]

Mike Astrue, who had been the White House ethics officer before moving to HHS, hadn't been involved in the original settlement, and he had no personal investment in its preservation. Neither did Astrue want to see the Bush administration pay reparations to the French that weren't warranted, despite what seemed to be an evidentiary shift in favor of Pasteur. "Clearly they feel the tide is swinging their way on the facts," Astrue said. "But if you look at the media reporting on this in the last couple of years, it seems like every three months some newspaper claims that either Gallo or the French is vindicated."

On the question of whether the Pasteur could force a reopening of the 1987 accord in court, Astrue was doubtful. "As a legal matter," he said, "it is very, very rare for an American court to undo a settlement between parties. In this particular settlement, the French view of the facts hasn't changed a great deal. They just feel vindicated. At the time they settled they knew there was some risk that history would bear them out, or some risk that history would undercut them. There was always the possibility of subsequent facts coming out."f

That didn't mean HHS might not agree to a voluntary rewriting of the settlement. "I have never said that we would only adhere to whatever we were legally entitled to, and not consider anything else," Astrue said. "You get out of the range of legal choice and into international comity, and 'do-the-right-thing.'"

The 1987 agreement had created a new body, the French and American AIDS Foundation, to administer the division of royalties from the blood test, and each side held four seats on the foundation's board: Montagnier, Schwartz, Dedonder, and Alain Gallochat, the Pasteur's general counsel, for the French; Gallo, Jim Mason, Bernadine Healy, and Mike Astrue for the Americans. With a majority vote, the board had the power to alter the royalty stream from the patent in any way it liked. "All I need is somebody to make a resolution at the next meeting," Rob Odle said, "and then five people to vote for it. It's a very simple thing. You don't need to make findings of fact on guilt or innocence, intentional or accidental, or this or that."

Since the accord, the AIDS test had generated more than $20 million in patent royalties.[48] If the French proposal were adopted, the Pasteur would receive the entire amount — a cost to HHS of some $25 million over the remaining ten-year lifetime of the patent. The

French demand for another $25 million, to cover back royalties and expenses incurred during the original litigation against HHS, would be put off until later. "This way, we get half of what we want," Odle said, "and really all of what we want, symbolically."

Odle had all four of the French votes, but he needed one from the American side. Gallo and Healy were out of the question, but Odle thought it conceivable that Mike Astrue, or even Jim Mason, might vote with the French. Despite the increasing amount of time he was spending on the case, Astrue had avoided taking a position on its merits. Now, in an "Eyes Only" memo to Sullivan, Astrue offered the secretary his opinion.[49] The patent dispute was "severable" from the misconduct case, Astrue said, and HHS ought to sever the two issues. It would be "in the public interest" for the United States to relinquish future royalties to the Institut Pasteur. Unless this were done, the Gallo affair would continue to be a considerable distraction for NIH and a strain on American relations with the French.

"For two million dollars a year for ten years," Astrue concluded, "HHS is buying more positives than negatives." Astrue's memo was followed by a last-minute appeal from Jonas Salk, asking Sullivan to accept the Pasteur's request for a reallocation of royalties so that "the spirit of accord reached in 1987 will be maintained"[50] — and by an eight-page "privileged and confidential" memo from Gallo, asking Sullivan to "give serious consideration to the impact of any concessions to the French on my reputation."[51]

Shortly before nine o'clock on the morning of September 16, 1992, Raymond Dedonder, accompanied by Maxime Schwartz, Alain Gallochat, and a Weil, Gotshal lawyer named Mike Epstein, arrived at Stone House, an imposing hilltop mansion on the NIH campus and site of the foundation board's meeting.

More than seven years had passed since Dedonder had led the Pasteur delegation to Washington to meet with Lowell Harmison and Peter Fischinger. Having recently lain near death in a Paris hospital, Dedonder had gathered himself for what he hoped would be the final chapter in a dispute that had gone on far too long. The unusually heavy security around Stone House made Mike Epstein, who was sitting in for Ira Millstein, wonder what NIH was expecting from the French delegation.

When Epstein asked where Astrue was, Bernadine Healy replied that the meeting should begin without him. Perhaps, Healy said vaguely, Astrue would be along later. Jim Mason was also missing — Healy didn't mention that Astrue and Mason had been ordered by Sullivan not to attend — and Epstein took their absence as a signal that the outcome of the meeting was a *fait accompli*. As the board members settled themselves around the conference table, Epstein noticed that Gallo stayed close to Healy's side. "She was very protective of Gallo," Epstein said later, "based on her body language."

The first order of business, the approval of the minutes of the last meeting, was disposed of summarily. So were the second and third items on the agenda, a budget matter and a tax question. The fourth order of business was the Pasteur's motion for a reallocation of royalties, and as Epstein read the language into the record Healy's attention remained focused on the stack of papers in front of her. When Epstein paused to glance up, he saw that Healy was editing a speech. The four French members voted in favor of the proposal, Montagnier having sent his proxy with Maxime Schwartz. Only after Gallo and Healy voted "No" did Healy announce that she also had proxies from Astrue and Jim Mason. On Secretary Sullivan's instructions, they had voted "No" as well.

During the rest of the meeting, Healy never met Schwartz's glance. "I sat right across the table from her," Schwartz said, "and for two hours she never once looked me in the eye." Declining a tepid invitation to stay for lunch, the French took the next flight back to Paris. Once their plane was in the air, HHS issued a hard-line statement. "If the French believe that intentional wrongdoing occurred," it said, "it is best that those concerns be aired and resolved publicly, and not evaded by an arrangement between the two countries." The vote of the American delegates, an HHS spokesman said, should be interpreted as "an official statement that we believe the French don't have a case."[52]

Ira Millstein, who had engineered the 1987 settlement on behalf of the Pasteur and had considered it one of the jewels of his career, had been in touch with Epstein and Odle from his aerie in the General Motors Building, and he was dumbfounded by the American response. "Honest to God," Millstein said later, "I have no idea why they're doing this. It can't be the money."

Millstein had urged the Pasteur to settle in 1987, telling his client that a settlement made sense because "no one will ever know what happened" in Gallo's lab, and that "this literally could go on forever." It would be a settlement with honor for both sides, Millstein argued at the time, because the American government had assured the Pasteur that HTLV-3B was not LAV.

With the OSI investigation the settlement had been "totally discredited," and Millstein felt betrayed by his own government. "They take the position that a settlement is a settlement," Millstein said. "But that isn't what you expect of the United States government. The U.S. side knows we urged Pasteur to settle on the basis that there may have been honest confusion about the viruses. We were all misled, because I was told it was not Montagnier's virus."

"Slander Is the Worst Crime"

A *dozen blocks from Ira Millstein's office, on the twenty-fourth floor of* the Chrysler Building, Jim Swire was putting the finishing touches on a new lawsuit. Once again the plaintiff was the Institut Pasteur of Paris, the defendants Robert Gallo and the United States of America.

Maxime Schwartz had warned the Bush administration that the government's failure "to even consider our proposal will necessarily force us to examine other forums."[1] The administration hadn't listened, and the French were girding to go back to court, this time with a demand for $200 million in damages.

Swire had reentered the case at the behest of SANOFI, the French conglomerate that held a majority interest in Diagnostics Pasteur. The government of France was interested in national honor, the Institut Pasteur in scientific credit and a greater share of patent royalties. But SANOFI was all business, and it wanted the American patent for itself. Swire's advice had been to "go straight to the White House with a draft complaint, saying here's what we're going to do to you if you don't give us the patent."

A week after Rob Odle's royalty reallocation plan was scuttled by the foundation board, Jim Swire was in Paris, a draft of the new lawsuit in his briefcase. But Washington's attention was focused on the presidential election, now six weeks away, and Swire counseled patience. With Bill Clinton in the White House, Swire said, the matter might be resolved without going back to court. Even if George

Bush were reelected, it was certain that Bernadine Healy would be replaced.

The odds of Healy's replacement had improved the day before, when she was summoned to Capitol Hill to explain why NIH had wasted time and money applying for patents on still-undiscovered portions of the human genome, only to see its applications rebuffed by the patent office. Healy's HHS overseers had cut out the bulk of her prepared testimony, some of which ran counter to administration policy. But Healy had delivered it anyway, and Mike Astrue was now one of many determined to make sure her days in Washington were numbered. "She's ticked off everybody," Astrue said. "She's ticked off a lot of people at the White House. She's going around playing lawyer and she doesn't know what she's talking about."

Science & Government Report was calling Healy "the short-tempered diva of biomedical research,"[2] and it was true that she hadn't endeared herself to many who worked for her. Healy had raised eyebrows by ordering an expensive redecoration of the NIH director's mansion and by hiring a personal press secretary, the first in NIH history, whose responsibilities were said to include making sure the director's weak chin was not evident in news photographs. Some of her subordinates recalled the time Healy refused to continue a meeting of senior NIH executives until a carpenter could be summoned to fix a nail in her chair that had snagged her pantyhose.

But the telegenic Healy had become a media celebrity, whose name and face were so recognizable that Ross Perot had invited her to become his vice-presidential running-mate.[a] Declining Perot's offer, Healy began instead trying to cut a deal with the Clinton camp that would allow her to stay on after the election. "It would be exciting," Healy said, "to be part of a new administration — and I don't mean that in a disloyal way."[3]

The Bush administration didn't agree. A scheduled briefing by Healy on "health issues" for the Democratic vice-presidential candidate, Al Gore, was canceled minutes after the Bush White House learned about it. Any hopes Healy might have harbored for staying on in a Clinton administration were dashed during a postelection dinner party at the Georgetown home of Pamela Harriman, who was about to become Clinton's ambassador to Paris, and who had invited the president-elect to meet a few of her friends. Over lamb chops and spinach, John Dingell explained to Clinton that there were two Republicans at HHS who warranted his personal attention. One was David Kessler, the head of the FDA, who should be allowed to stay on. The other was Bernadine Healy, the director of the NIH, who should not.

For the better part of a year, Dingell and Healy had been grappling over the OSI's files on the Gallo case. In exercising its oversight responsibilities, Dingell reminded Healy that his subcommittee needed to see the evidence on which the Office of Scientific Integrity had concluded that Mika Popovic, but not Gallo, was guilty of scientific misconduct.[4]

Turning the OSI's files over to Dingell meant turning them over to Suzanne Hadley, and the last thing Healy wished for was a Hadley-inspired subcommittee report lambasting the NIH's exculpation of Gallo. But the HHS lawyers had overruled the OSI, and presently boxes of jumbled documents had begun arriving at the subcommittee's office. One especially sensitive shipment was delivered by the NIH police, who were stopped by their Capitol counterparts in the lobby of the Rayburn House Office Building and told to leave their weapons at the security station before proceeding upstairs. The NIH police replied that they didn't leave their weapons anywhere. In that case, said the Capitol Police, they couldn't come in. The stalemate was broken when a subcommittee secretary appeared with a hand truck, loaded it with boxes, and wheeled it into the elevator.

When some of the OSI documents found their way to reporters, Jules Hallum solicited security advice from the Pentagon and the CIA, which suggested coding documents destined for the subcommittee with odd v-shaped markings that resembled distant seagulls flying between the lines of text. When the leaks continued, Army counter-espionage experts with black boxes appeared to sweep the OSI's conference room for hidden microphones and check the telephone lines for taps. OSI staffers, observing the sweepers in action, wondered who Jules Hallum thought was bugging his phones, Gallo or John Dingell.

It wasn't Dingell. But Dingell's staff did have sources inside the OSI, one of whom reported that Hallum, rather than surrender the steno books in which he had taken notes during the OSI's interviews of Gallo and Popovic, had ordered them shredded.[5] Healy assured Dingell that nothing at OSI had been destroyed — one OSI official had *wanted* to destroy some interview tapes, Healy said, but the person he ordered to do it had refused. To reassure the subcommittee, all OSI personnel were providing signed statements affirming that they hadn't destroyed any sensitive materials. When further investigation revealed that Hallum's notebooks had indeed been shredded, rather than investigate the shredding the NIH began looking for the subcommittee's informant.[6]

On an early March morning in 1992, Suzanne Hadley, culling the OSI files in her warren at the subcommittee's office, got a phone call from her nominal supervisor at NIH. Hadley was still on the NIH payroll, and the woman asked her to return immediately to the NIH campus, where an urgent task awaited her attention.

Arriving after a forty-minute subway ride from Capitol Hill, Hadley was handed the draft of a speech to edit — hardly an urgent task. As Hadley browsed through the text, she noticed someone hovering outside her office door. The man didn't seem to want to come in, but neither was he going away. When Hadley got up from her desk and walked into the corridor, the man held out his hand. In it was a black leather case containing an identification card and a small gold badge that bore the words "Federal Bureau of Investigation."

"It took me a minute to hear what he was talking about," Hadley recalled. "He said, 'Hallum and Watkins have been very concerned about documents getting out of the office. And documents getting to you.' He said, 'NIH is very concerned about this. They have said that it has completely made the OSI dysfunctional because these documents made their way to the press.' A couple of times he mentioned going to the U.S. attorney in Baltimore."

Hadley's first call was to Peter Stockton. Within minutes Stockton and the rest of Dingell's staff were on the phones: to FBI headquarters, to Justice Department headquarters, to the United States attorney, to NIH and HHS. Before the afternoon was over, the story had been pieced together.

A few days earlier, Bernadine Healy had called Richard Kusserow, the HHS inspector general, to report that one or more OSI employees had been copying documents and passing them to Suzanne Hadley. Healy wanted the culprits caught. But Kusserow, a former CIA and FBI agent, had been around Washington long enough to know that leak investigations rarely accomplished anything except to embarrass the officials who ordered them. Nor was Kusserow particularly eager to open an investigation of someone to whom he had recently given the Inspector General's Integrity Award. When Healy explained that a leak investigation was her chance to get Hadley — "those were the words she used," Kusserow said later, "'get Hadley'"— Kusserow told Healy to call the FBI and hung up the phone.[b]

John Dingell had gone apoplectic upon learning that Healy had called in the FBI to investigate someone "who had consistently, and at great personal sacrifice, cooperated with Congressional and law enforcement investigation"— especially since Healy had made "no serious effort . . . to deal with the now admitted destruction of documents" requested by the subcommittee.

"Let me be blunt, Dr. Healy," Dingell's letter concluded. "There is no public interest in covering up mismanagement, let alone possible criminal acts involving fraud, false statement [sic] and document destruction. And there is no damage to the public interest in revealing such things. On the contrary, reporting such possible corruption in a government agency is surely one of the highest duties of a career civil servant."[7]

In short order, the Special Agent in Charge of the Baltimore FBI office and the United States Attorney for Maryland found themselves in the subcommittee's chamber. "They didn't understand any of the backdrop to it," recalled Bruce Chafin. "They didn't know about the destruction of documents, they didn't know about the August hearing, the whole history of Dr. Healy versus Dr. Hadley, or Dr. Healy versus the OSI. The FBI agent got Healy doing a Chicken Little routine on him, and so he goes roaring off like I guess he's supposed to. They're only now filling in the picture, and I don't think they're too thrilled about it."

The OSI wasn't a law-enforcement agency or an intelligence agency. It didn't have authority to classify official documents, and "leaking" OSI files to a congressional oversight committee was hardly a crime. Informing Healy that her "leak investigation" was being closed for lack of basis, the United States attorney, Richard D. Bennett, pointed out that whatever documents had been provided to the subcommittee informally were the same documents Dingell had been "seeking through appropriate channels."[8]

Peter Stockton took advantage of Bennett's visit to Capitol Hill to reiterate Dingell's growing concern that the Justice Department hadn't yet opened an investigation of possible perjury and obstruction of justice by Gallo during the patent dispute.[c] More than five years had elapsed since Gallo had signed the declaration, but it was still possible to bring charges outside the statute of limitations, for example by alleging the existence of a continuing conspiracy to conceal the original crime.

Bennett explained that such prosecutorial tactics were normally reserved for organized crime figures, and that even under the best of circumstances perjury was difficult to prove. Beyond that, Bennett thought scientific misconduct cases were next to impossible for juries to understand; even prosecutors and investigators had to struggle with the details. Bennett's office had negotiated a guilty plea from Zaki Salahuddin and won a jury verdict against Prem Sarin, but those cases had involved money, not viruses, and prosecutors knew how to explain money to juries.

Stockton still thought a jury could comprehend the false statements in Gallo's declaration if the evidence was presented in the right way. "You say, 'Here are the following fifteen statements,'" Stockton explained. "We're going to focus on seven critical statements in this goddamn thing, and here's the evidence to show they're not true, and Gallo was aware at the time they're not true. We gotta put this goddamn thing together. We'll just tell them, 'We've got this case for you. It's all worked out. We've got the false statements identified, we've got the evidence listed here for you, we've got the witnesses.'"

The forty-five-page, single-spaced document that shortly emerged from Suzanne Hadley's word processor was more than a precis for a potential perjury case against Gallo. It was an epitaph for a misguided OSI investigation, one for which Hadley herself took most of the blame.[9] The subcommittee's critique stopped short of accusing anyone of stealing LAV. But it did accuse the OSI of deliberately suppressing evidence that a motive had at least existed for such a theft, and of having failed to investigate discrepancies in Gallo's laboratory records that could have established whether a theft had occurred.

Persuaded by Bennett that a criminal prosecution wasn't on the Justice Department's menu, Stockton decided the critique might be used instead to form the basis for a civil fraud case. According to Stockton's theory, refined with *pro bono* help from some expensive downtown lawyers who owed Dingell a favor, the defrauded party would be the People of the United States. Even though the federal government was cashing the royalty checks generated by the patent, the theory went, those royalties had been fraudulently obtained, since the government had misled the courts and the patent office about its right to the proceeds of the patent — and had itself been misled by the scientists who claimed to have invented the blood test.

The OSI's Gallo report had been signed by Jules Hallum and sealed by Bernadine Healy. But it wouldn't become absolutely, positively final until it had been approved by the Office of Scientific Integrity Review, an obscure HHS agency whose principal function was to ensure that the OSI's findings of scientific misconduct were sufficiently supported by the evidence to avoid future lawsuits against the government.

The OSIR's chief, a former National Institutes of Mental Health psychologist named Lyle Bivens, had promised Jim Mason that he would have the Gallo report out the door by June of 1992. But May had come and gone, and the OSIR was still grappling with the twists and tangles of the case. When Bivens heard Dingell's staff had prepared a critique of the report, he thought he better find out what the subcommittee knew before rendering an opinion of his own.

After briefing Bivens, Bivens's deputy, Larry Rhoades, and the OSIR's lawyer, Chris Pascal, Stockton concluded that the OSIR was "a lost ball in the tall weeds. They don't know shit. They know absolutely nothing. They know less than I do. They've got terrible problems with the thing. I mean, the isolates — I know twice as much about the isolates as they know. We gave them the long critique that Suzanne did, and let them sit out here in the lobby and read it. Lyle asked me about three times, 'Can't we take this with us? We'll assure you that our security is terrific, we'll never let it out.' No way are we gonna let them have it."

Hadley had known Lyle Bivens since her own days at NIMH, and Hadley thought he was "looking really worried. We spent most of the time just going through the chronology of LAV and HTLV-3B. And that's when Lyle started looking more worried than when he came in looking worried. The first question is, 'Was it willfully misappropriated?' And the second question is, 'Did Gallo know it was willfully misappropriated?' They were asking, 'What is the evidence that MOV is only another name for LAV?' So we had to go all the way back to the beginning of LAV in the cell lines in October, and MOV appearing out of nowhere in November in the very same cell lines."

What Bivens, Rhoades, and Pascal had made of all this, Hadley wasn't sure. "Their eyes are always empty," she said. "You want to knock on their forehead and see if anybody answers. The problem with this whole case has been knowing what questions to ask. I was flummoxed for a long time. I didn't understand the difference between a detection and an isolation, or that Mika hadn't been able to grow out any virus from all those patient samples. That's why I think the Richards committee focused on the *Science* papers. It was an easy out for them. They saw something that looked like fraud and 'That's it, go after it.' Not that they were wrong, but everybody forgot about the really important stuff. Like, did he steal the virus or didn't he?"

The OSIR had the authority, at least on paper, to change the OSI's verdict in a case. But of the hundred or so misconduct cases investigated by OSI during its three years of existence, no one could recall an OSI finding ever having been reversed. "From a structural standpoint, it's really very interesting," Stockton said. "We asked Lyle the question 'Can you buck Bernadine?' It's very clear he can't. We said, 'What the hell are you talking about? You outrank her. You're up in the fucking department.' He just laughed."

A week after the briefing, Larry Rhoades was back to reread the critique and take extensive notes. A week after that, Lyle Bivens was telling Jim Mason that the OSIR's review of the Gallo case wouldn't be finished anytime soon. The OSIR, Bivens explained, had "identified several specific issues or questions that we want to follow up."[10]

Nobody had been happy with the way OSI had discharged its responsibilities: not John Dingell, at whose behest the agency was created, not Bernadine Healy, who had inherited it, and certainly not the scientific community, which had shuddered as it watched a government agency pass judgment on the veracity of complicated biomedical research.

Many of those found guilty of scientific misconduct were clearly guilty. A number had confessed. But that didn't change the fact that OSI's investigations were occasionally wrongheaded, often bumbling and cumbersome, and frequently took months or years when they might have been completed in weeks or months. The disputes and debates over the Gallo case, and the concerns it raised about the NIH investigating itself, had only underscored the need for a better system.

With few defenders and many detractors, the OSI's days were numbered, and in the early summer of 1992 it ceased by exist. Henceforth, scientific misconduct investigations would be conducted by a new agency, the Office of Research Integrity, headquartered not within the NIH but at HHS. Unlike the old OSI, the new ORI would no longer combine the functions of investigator, prosecutor, judge, jury, and executioner. The ORI would investigate, draw conclusions, and render findings, but scientists found guilty of misconduct could appeal their verdicts to a quasijudicial board of administrative judges, before whom their lawyers could cross-examine accusers and present rebuttal witnesses, much as in a court of law.

That news that the NIH would no longer be responsible for investigating suspected misconduct pleased many who worked there. "Investigating folks is not NIH's bag," one NIH official said. "This just doesn't sit well with the scientific constituency that NIH has to work with 365 days a year." Nor would the NIH ever again be placed in the position of having to investigate its own scientists. "This will no longer be a procedure," Jim Mason said, "in which an agency may appear to be judging itself, or its own people."

Despite a last-minute attempt by Bernadine Healy to create a new Research Integrity Policy Board headed by herself, the NIH director would no longer play a role in the scientific misconduct process. Named as the ORI's acting chief was one of Jim Mason's deputies, a respected physician-administrator, J. Michael McGinnis. Lyle Bivens would head the ORI's Division of Policy, and Jules Hallum its Division of Research Integrity Assurance. But Hallum, who had lost the fight to remain as director of the new agency and to keep it within the NIH, thought it a "convenient" time to resign from public service. "I used to have a reputation before I worked for the government," Hallum said on his way out of town.[11]

On a Saturday afternoon at the beginning of November, Gallo called Peter Stockton at home and got his message machine. "I was down painting somebody's apartment," Stockton said. "So I called him later, and he goes through all this horseshit. He keeps saying, 'Have I ever done anything wrong to you? Have I ever pissed you guys off? I'm really sorry, you know.'"

Stockton had been quoted in the *Nouvel Observateur* as saying "everybody knows that Gallo stole the virus,"[12] and Gallo had mailed Stockton a translation of what Gallo considered "an extraordinary defamation," remarking that "I have always been taught that slander is the worst crime a man can commit short of physical murder. I believe it."[13] On the phone with Gallo, Stockton explained that he had been repeating what he had been told, that "very prominent scientists in this country have come up to me and said, 'You're wasting your time on this thing. Everybody knows that Bob Gallo stole the virus.' Then he shoots right back, 'That's Watson, that's Watson.'"

Stockton thought Gallo sounded worried, and when Gallo asked to come talk to the subcommittee staff Stockton was sure something was up. "It might be kinda fun," Stockton said later. "The trick is going to be to push him, but not panic him so that he flies out the door, either literally or figuratively. If he just goes crazy then nothing is accomplished." From their telephone conversation, Stockton had gotten an impression that Gallo might be ready to point a finger at Mika Popovic, "and point it strongly enough, and in front of enough people, so that we then could go to Mika directly and say, 'Here's what Bob told us.' That's our only hope, to get Mika to crack. Because otherwise I don't think we'll ever prove this."

The first clue to what was troubling Gallo came when Lyle Bivens reappeared in the subcommittee's office, accompanied by Mike McGinnis and a half-dozen ORI staff members. "McGinnis started out by saying, 'We're not prepared to discuss Gallo,'" Suzanne Hadley recalled. "'It's still very much in the active-process phase. We have not reached a final decision.' Then Lyle made some passing remark about waiting for comment."

"I said, 'Wait a minute — did you just say that Gallo has something from you and you're waiting for comment?' Their response to that was 'We just can't talk about it right now.' But after that they began saying things like 'substantive departures, we can make the hard calls, we can support that we came to an independent finding here.' Under further questioning, they made it clear Popovic did not get this thing, whatever it is, but Gallo did.

"And then their lawyer jumped in, Chris Pascal, and he said, 'Look, I'm going to be honest with you here. Partly what we're trying to do is protect you guys from any accusation that this has been driven by the subcommittee.' He said, 'I am very confident that our decision has been independent.'

"I said, 'Have you rewritten the OSI report?' Lyle said, 'No, we have prepared an addendum to it.'"

"You could have blown me over," Stockton said later.

At the end of December 1992, Gallo assured his French colleague Guy de Thé, who had recently left Lyon for a new job at the Pasteur Institute, that "Everything is O.K." Gallo couldn't resist adding a P.S.: "Your boss is a turd."[14] But everything was not O.K. "This is to notify you," began the letter addressed to Gallo that arrived at Joe Onek's office, "that the United States Department of Health and Human Services' Office of Research Integrity has made findings of scientific misconduct against you."[15]

It had been nearly ten years since the French had discovered the AIDS virus. Seven years had passed since the Institut Pasteur had filed its lawsuits, five years since the settlement was celebrated in Paris, three years since Bill Raub's assurance to John Dingell that NIH was prepared to "resolve the unanswered questions about Gallo's research" raised by the *Chicago Tribune*. The White House had twice changed hands, wars had been fought, the Berlin Wall had fallen. Gallo had been provisionally guilty of misconduct, then not guilty. Now he was guilty again, for "falsely reporting that LAV had not been transmitted to a permanently growing cell line."[d]

Lyle Bivens and Mike McGinnis owed nothing to Gallo, Bernadine Healy, the NIH, or the National Cancer Institute. The ORI hadn't labored to put the best possible face on a series of unfortunate facts. Indeed, Jim Mason had let it be known that he wished to let the facts speak for themselves. The way the ORI saw those facts, Gallo's explanations of why he had written the "not yet been transmitted" sentence contradicted Gallo's own testimony to NIH investigators and common sense as well.

It was indisputable, the ORI said, that LAV *had* been successfully transmitted to a permanent cell line before the *Science* papers were published, in Gallo's own lab as well as at the Pasteur.[e] Even if Gallo's excuses about intending the sentence to refer only to the Pasteur were true, that wouldn't justify the inclusion of a false statement in the Popovic paper.

Nor, said the ORI, was there any evidence to support Gallo's argument that he hadn't had permission to publish data derived from LAV, since the written agreement signed by Mika Popovic didn't preclude Gallo "from conducting all research with LAV, publishing data on LAV, or referring to LAV in a published paper." Gallo's claim that reporting Popovic's growth of LAV in a cell line would have "embarrassed" the French prompted the ORI to point out that Gallo had shown "no compunction in embarrassing the French" at Cold Spring Harbor, and had "denigrated the French techniques and findings on numerous occasions."

As for Gallo's contention that reporting Popovic's research with LAV would have forced him to include the French as co-authors of the *Science* paper, the ORI noted that Gallo was contradicted by his own testimony. Of Gallo's insistence that he hadn't intended to conceal the growth of LAV in his own laboratory, the ORI wondered why, in that case, Gallo had spent years denying to colleagues and the media that LAV had grown in his lab.

"ORI does not believe," the addendum concluded, "that the reasons proffered by Dr. Gallo for the deletion of the reference to LAV's infection of a permanent cell line are valid." Joe Onek's argument, that Gallo hadn't mentioned Popovic's growth of LAV because he had known so little about Popovic's experiments, was dismissed by the ORI as beyond credulous: "Dr. Gallo must have realized the significant role of LAV in the LTCB's research before the Popovic paper was submitted based on his review of Dr. Popovic's drafts of the manuscript."

In the ORI's view, Gallo wasn't merely guilty of falsifying a sentence in a scientific paper. Gallo had failed in his "strong moral obligation to facilitate scientific progress," impeding research on AIDS while enhancing his own influence through his control of HTLV-3B and H-9.

> ORI notes that Dr. Gallo's failure to reveal the utility of LAV effectively ensured that most researchers would use HTLV-3B in AIDS research because they would have thought it to be the only HIV isolate grown in a permanent cell line. Consequently, this virtually ensured HTLV-3B's preeminence in AIDS research. Clearly, other laboratories could have

substantially accelerated their research with LAV if Dr. Gallo had informed them that LAV was grown in a permanent cell line and in which cell line this had been accomplished. Dr. Gallo's failure to do so impeded potential AIDS research progress with LAV. . . . ORI believes that the evolution of the Popovic paper, Dr. Gallo's repeated denials that the LTCB grew LAV in a permanent cell line or that LAV played a role in the LTCB's research, and Dr. Gallo's failure to reveal LAV's growth to others, including the French, indicate that Dr. Gallo wanted to hide the LTCB's growth of LAV in a permanent cell line and the role LAV played in the LTCB's experiments. ORI believes that the disputed statement was intended to further that goal. . . . ORI believes that Dr. Gallo knew that LAV was grown in a permanent cell line and understood the significant role that LAV played in the seminal experiments. . . . ORI believes that the statement falsely reports the status of LAV research, was knowingly false when written, and concealed important information on LTCB's research on LAV.

The misconduct finding against Mika Popovic would stand, and the ORI blamed Popovic for kindling the suspicions that had swirled around his research for more than eight years. It was Popovic's "inability to identify the origin of MOV, his inadequate description of the creation and maintenance of the 'pool,' and his failure to develop adequate records and retain critical data" that represented "the foundations upon which the misappropriation/contamination allegation rests."

Popovic's claim that he had selected the pool samples by looking for the cell-killing effects of the AIDS virus was "questionable" at best. The absence of laboratory records reflecting the origins of MOV was "disturbing." But the ORI, like the OSI before it, wasn't able to say whether there had been an accident, or whether someone had simply renamed LAV and claimed it as Gallo's own discovery. "ORI supports the OSI finding," the addendum concluded, "that it is not possible to resolve the question of misappropriation versus contamination."

"It's pretty tough on Gallo," Mal Martin observed after reading the entire addendum. "But it's also clear to me that nobody at ORI knows very much about HIV." Otherwise, Martin said, the report never would have suggested that R.F. could have been used for the blood test in place of HTLV-3B with "modest delays" of a few weeks. "Nobody" Martin said, "can grow the damn thing."[f] Luc Montagnier's advice to Gallo was to not appeal the misconduct finding, but to "accept the report" and get on with his work. According to Montagnier, Gallo replied that Howard Temin had made the same recommendation, but that it was easy for someone with terminal cancer to give such advice.

Montagnier had tendered his advice over dinner at La Ferme, where Gallo had arranged a discreet meeting. The restaurant's owner, Marcel Montagnier, no relation to the French scientist, recalled being warned by Gallo that the dinner was "very secret," and that "I should pretend it didn't happen." It remained secret until the *Washington Post* reported that two noted scientists "often depicted as enemies" had met over dinner to discuss joining in a 'Manhattan Project' for AIDS."[16] Only when Montagnier saw the *Post,* Simon Wain-Hobson said later, "did he realize he'd been hornswoggled again by Gallo." Any future collaborations were in Gallo's imagination. "I'm not saying I will collaborate with *him,*" Montagnier said. "I will collaborate with *NIH,* but I will not forget completely about the past. It's more easy for him to forget about the past than for me."

Rumors had again begun circulating that Gallo was about to depart NIH, not for Yale or Johns Hopkins but for his alma mater, Philadelphia's Jefferson Medical College. But Montagnier had come away from dinner with the impression that Gallo wouldn't be going soon. "If he was going to leave NIH now, it would be like feeling guilty," Montagnier said. "And Gallo will never accept to consider himself as guilty. He's not able to see the true face of him. He's trying to minimize — 'Just one sentence which was wrong.' I'm not going to talk about that with him anymore. For the scientific community, for many people, it's clear."

It wasn't clear to Gallo, who dismissed the ORI report as the product of an "endless and incompetent" investigation.[17] To a man who had read about the misconduct finding in *Time,*[18] Gallo replied that "my colleagues and I isolated the AIDS virus in 1984. Actually, we made many isolates (a total of 48) between 1983 and early 1984. This has been acknowledged by everyone as has been the fact that it is my colleagues and myself who showed that HIV is the cause of AIDS and who also developed the life saving blood test which has protected our blood supply since 1984."

"It is like a nightmare," Gallo told another well-wisher. "ORI is comprised of only bureaucrats (not one scientist), and they are under Dingell's thumb.[g] I will probably appeal and I will probably win. But the damage is done forever and the cost will also be heavy and permanent."[19]

Gallo was quick to reply when Peter Piot recalled his excitement upon learning, two months before Margaret Heckler's news conference, that the Pasteur ELISA had achieved an almost perfect score in detecting LAV antibodies in Piot's Zairian patients.[20] "I read with interest and wonder your interview in *Global AIDS News*," Gallo wrote Piot, "regarding how Montagnier gave you such accurate blood test results in February 1984. It is nice to see how everything is so simple. Montagnier alone discovers the virus, and in the new version is now the one who shows it is the AIDS virus."[21]

One of Gallo's letters was from the organizers of an international colloquium, rescinding an invitation tendered months before for Gallo to speak in Jerusalem the following July. The reason for the withdrawal, the organization explained, was "the recent highly publicized controversy concerning your AIDS research."[22] Although the colloquium was a minor meeting, Gallo confessed to an Israeli researcher that the cancellation of his appearance "hurt me more than anything."[23]

In hopes of clearing the air in Israel, Gallo tried to explain the history of his predicament. The original OSI investigation, he said, had been initiated by the acting NIH director, Bill Raub, who "had zero credentials, but thought he had a chance to become permanent." It had been directed by "Ms. Suzanne Hadley . . . a 'social-psychologist,' (whatever that means). Hadley is now on Dingell's staff and continues her pursuit of me aimed at the patent. It is clear to most that all along she had been working with and for Dingell's staff, but paid by NIH (quite unbelievable)."

For help, Gallo turned to Jim Watson, to whom he had previously afforded a large part of the blame for his troubles.[24] "I have heard it said," Gallo told Watson, "that some, even perhaps you, believe LAV was 'swiped' by me. I assume this means I directed Popovic to do it since I did not do the experiment myself. For numerous reasons this is ridiculous, and obviously unfounded. But how should one prove a negative? And why should one have to do it?

"Jim, please pay greater attention to our lack of due process; take note of what is happening in France with the blood test scandal and their failure to use our test; note also the amount of money involved in the patent; and note how long and how many investigations I have gone through, my work incredibly interrupted and my name smashed, and ask what has been objectively found? Why was this done?"

Watson, who had been tapped by Bernadine Healy to head a $3 billion NIH project to sequence the entire human genome, had been enlisted previously by Gallo to intercede with Healy "about the need to bring the OSI investigation to a quick conclusion."[25] At Healy's suggestion, Watson also had gone to plead for a reprieve with John Dingell's staff. "His message was, 'This is very bad for NIH,'" Peter Stockton recalled. According to Stockton, Watson's "big point was that Gallo is a manic depressive. He thinks the subcommittee should back down because Gallo's crazy. He thinks we should talk to Gallo's shrink."

Stockton had concluded that Watson himself was "as nutty as a fruitcake. He sounds like one of these flaky guys who has these flights of ideas and doesn't make a lot of sense.[h] We said, 'Do you want to read the critique, so you'd know what this Gallo thing is all about?' He says, 'Oh, no, being an NIH person, I better not do that.' We say, 'Why not?' He says, 'Well, Bernadine might start wondering where I'd seen it.' We asked him, 'Did Bernadine send you?' He says, 'No, Bernadine didn't send me. I did tell Bernadine that I could talk to these Dingell people, and she said, "Well, give it a try." Watson claims he doesn't get along with Bernadine terribly well.'"

Having resigned from NIH under what he described as pressure from Healy,[i] Watson was back at Cold Spring Harbor full-time, and it was there that Gallo's latest letter reached him. "If you are in the D.C. area within the next month or so, I would like very much to see you," Gallo wrote. "As you know, I have always felt I needed a few people, like you, to know the truth of these events which have impacted on so much of my life." Watson replied that he planned to attend an upcoming testimonial dinner in Washington for Kay Jamison, an authority on manic-depressive and bipolar disorders, who had just published a bestselling book, *Touched with Fire*, that explored the link between those illnesses and artistic temperament. "Will you be there?" Watson asked Gallo. "I hope so, since then we could talk."[26]

Gallo sent Jamison his regrets, explaining that on the day of the dinner he would be in Rome.[27] He returned home to discover that

Bernadine Healy was no longer his boss. Proclaiming her "fierce belief in the mission of the NIH" in such diverse forums as *Good Morning America* and *Glamour* magazine, Healy had continued her campaign to join the Clinton administration.[28] Gallo had tried to help, arranging an honorary degree from the University of Brescia in Italy, in recognition of Healy's "most extraordinary courage and leadership in a very difficult period in the history of the NIH."[29]

But even honors from Italian universities couldn't undo Healy's terminal alienation of John Dingell and other powerful House Democrats, including Patricia Schroeder of Colorado, the cochair of the Congressional Caucus for Women's Issues, who was incensed by Healy's accusation that Congress was trying to "micromanage" health research issues. Nor was Healy's standing improved when the ORI concluded that Rameshwar K. Sharma, the Cleveland Clinic researcher whose case had originally been heard by a panel Healy chaired, had committed scientific misconduct.

When a glum-looking Healy, wearing an Armani suit, announced her resignation, she told the reporters gathered at Stone House that "before I went to bed last night, I looked out the window and hoped I'd see enough snow that work would be called off today." Asked why she was leaving NIH, Healy replied, "I don't really know. I'd tell you if I truly knew, but it doesn't really matter."[30]

Healy confessed she was "heartbroken" not to have been asked to stay, but few of the NIH's institute directors were sorry to see her go. "At her good-bye party, they wouldn't stand next to her," Florence Haseltine, a former Healy speechwriter, told the *Washington Post*. "I guess they got tired of being yelled at by her."

"The Steaks Are Not Done"

The replacement of the Office of Scientific Integrity by the Office of Research Integrity included a procedural innovation intended to satisfy scientists who had likened the OSI to a star chamber. Henceforth, anyone found guilty of misconduct by the ORI, including Robert Gallo and Mika Popovic, could appeal his or her case to a quasijudicial entity within the Department of Health and Human Services to be known as the Research Integrity Adjudications Panel.

The adjudications panel was new, but the creature from which it sprang, the HHS Departmental Appeals Board, had been around since 1973. A university that hadn't received its full disbursement of research funding, or a health-care provider to which the government owed Medicare payments, was required to plead the case before the appeals board before taking the government to court. When Gallo and Popovic filed notice of their intention to appeal the misconduct findings against them, three HHS lawyers who specialized in contract disputes and the recovery of federal funds became their final arbiters.[1]

The strategy adopted by Joe Onek was to stretch the case against his client to the breaking point, then let it snap back in ORI's face. Onek argued that ORI shouldn't be permitted to render *any* criticisms of Gallo, including those that fell short of formal scientific misconduct, without being forced to defend those accusations with the same rigor as a formal finding of misconduct.

In addition to the misconduct charge for the "not transmitted" sentence, the ORI had censured Gallo on four counts, the most serious being his "imposition of restrictive conditions" on the distribution of HTLV-3B and the H-9 cell line. In preparation for Gallo's appeal, his laboratory staff had begun mailing, at government expense, a form letter to dozens of researchers with whom Gallo thought he might have shared HTLV-3B, H-9, or both.

"As you are probably aware," the letter began, "the accusation has been made against Dr. Robert C. Gallo and the Laboratory of Tumor Cell Biology (LTCB) of the National Cancer Institute that we may have delayed progress in the field of AIDS research because we did not distribute reagents, particularly following the discovery of HIV (after May 1984)."[2]

Nobody had accused Gallo of not distributing *any* viruses or cell lines for AIDS research, only of withholding HTLV-3B and H-9 from his enemies or potential competitors and restricting the experiments that some friendly collaborators could perform. But most of the scientists who received the letter weren't likely to have read the ORI report, and many found themselves dismayed to hear that Gallo was being accused of having withheld AIDS reagents from everybody.

The ORI scientists who had found Gallo guilty of misconduct would play no role in defending their conclusions against Gallo's appeal. That task fell to the ORI's new litigation branch, whose lawyers had a very short time to grasp the intricacies of retroviral isolation and reverse transcriptase assays. On an unseasonably warm afternoon in early April 1993, the ORI lawyers gathered around a witness table in the Dingell subcommittee's main hearing room, piled with sandwiches and Diet Cokes. Suzanne Hadley was impressed with the litigation branch chief, a hulking former prosecutor named Marcus Christ, whose idea of fun was sailing small boats single-handedly across the Atlantic. But Christ's young assistants, Debbie Parrish and Nancy O'Connor, reminded Hadley of a pair of Hostess Twinkies —"sweet, fluffy, not a lot of substance."

"They're still operating with little bits of things," Hadley said after several hours of fielding questions from Christ and his team, "and they don't understand what anything has to do with anything else. They're off on tangents. Debbie started off with what did I know about the review of the Popovic paper? Was it really sent off for review, and did I know who the reviewers were? I said 'Who cares?

So what?' She said, 'Well, Gallo is all the time saying this paper was written in a big hurry and *Science* should have caught this stuff.'" Hadley remembered thinking that was the first time Gallo had blamed *Science*'s reviewers; she wondered if the journal's cleaning staff would be next.

For Christ, Parrish, and O'Connor, Hadley recounted her own struggle to fit the pieces of the Gallo case — MOV, the EMs, the pool, Claude Chardon, the blood-test comparisons, the government's defense of the Pasteur lawsuit — around Popovic's use, or misuse, of LAV. "I told them I missed the big picture in the initial OSI report," Hadley said. "I reminded them about the existence of the patent report — pathetic little document that it is, it's a symbol of the transition between not understanding the big picture and understanding the big picture."

Hadley brought with her the subcommittee's newest critique of the investigation that Christ and his team were being called upon to defend. "I told them, 'Here's what we think of the ORI report,'" Hadley said, "'the good parts and the bad parts, and you better hear it from us because it's going to come out at some point. Mistakes were made.' I told them the part about LAV was mostly pretty damn good. It was well written, well reasoned. But the part about misappropriation was not only factually wrong, it was misleading."

The next stop for the ORI lawyers was Manhattan, where their request for a meeting had left Jim Swire slightly nonplussed by the fact that the United States government, which only a few years before had been defending Gallo against the Pasteur's claims for reparations, was now asking for Swire's help in proving that Gallo had deliberately concealed Popovic's use of the French virus.

After several hours of conversation, Swire concluded that Christ and his team had at least a tenuous grasp of the central facts. "But I have no idea what their trial skills are," he said later. "You can have all the stuff assembled and in your head, and then Gallo goes into his duck, feint, bob and weave, and what're you going to do? Can you control him? It's not going to be an easy thing. Even with all the information I have in my head, and all the knowledge of what documents are where and so forth, it would take me a tremendous amount of time to put it together."

Worried about sending its untested lawyers up against Joe Onek and Barbara Mishkin, the ORI had asked the Justice Department to lend it a couple of experienced prosecutors to manage the Gallo and Popovic appeals. Justice had declined, on the ground that the department's role in the defense of the blood-test patent posed a potential conflict of interest — an excuse Swire found ludicrous. "The government is going to lose their butts," Swire said. "You're talking about a major league outside counsel like Joe Onek against a couple of kids. These people are going to get up to speed against Onek in two and a half months?"

The challenge facing the ORI lawyers was compounded by the separation of the cases against Gallo and Popovic. Although the Gallo case was far more important, in many ways the case against Popovic was more complex, since several of the Popovic findings involved the interpretation of relatively arcane laboratory data and techniques.

To help with the Popovic appeal, the ORI had hired a fourth counsel, Steve Godek, who was happy to leave a Washington law firm after five years as a junior associate for something more exciting than insurance regulation. But Godek's learning curve was also a steep one. "I just spent all afternoon with him," Hadley reported after a mid-April meeting. "Godek wanted to know if I thought Max Essex would be a good witness for them to call. He said, 'Well, we've heard he's really not as good a friend of Gallo's as everybody thinks.' I said, 'He's good enough. Forget that one.'"

The federal misconduct regulations hadn't required the OSI or the ORI to produce evidence of intent to deceive on the part of Gallo or Popovic, only that they had published fabricated data or statements. But as the date for the Popovic hearing approached, the appeals board abruptly raised the bar. No longer would it be enough to demonstrate that the questioned items in Popovic's paper were false. Unless the ORI could prove Popovic *intended* to mislead his readers — and, moreover, that his intentional deceptions had had adverse consequences for the scientific community — the appeals board would dismiss all the misconduct findings against him.

The board had already dealt the ORI one body blow, with a prehearing decision that it wouldn't be allowed to show a "pattern of conduct" on Popovic's part by introducing discrepancies in his research beyond those mentioned in the ORI report. Now it would have to prove what had been in Popovic's mind, something real-world prosecutors found next to impossible. "It places a very heavy burden on ORI," Marcus Christ said, "a burden that we were not aware of when we started."[3] But there was no way to reopen the Gallo investigation to assemble evidence of intent, and the ORI would have to play an old game by new rules.

The news that greeted the ten thousand researchers attending the Ninth International Conference on AIDS in Berlin, in early June of 1993, was mostly not good. The Concorde trial, an Anglo-French study of AZT, had demonstrated what many AIDS patients already knew, that the drug was ultimately ineffective in slowing the progression of AIDS.[4] Jonas Salk's efforts, with assistance from Don Francis, to make a polio-style vaccine for AIDS also appeared less than promising. Following Salk's presentation of his preliminary data, the stock price of the California company that planned to market the vaccine dropped from twenty-four dollars to fourteen. According to Robert Bazell of *NBC News*, "many researchers in the audience declared the data to be nearly meaningless."[5]

The only encouraging news seemed to come from Gallo, who had been chosen to deliver the Frederick Deinhardt Memorial Lecture, named in honor of a departed scientist who had been among the first German researchers to receive HTLV-3B and H-9. According to Gallo, he had discovered that a protein from the newest human herpesvirus, HHV-7, might behave as a vaccine against HIV, by blocking the CD-4 receptor on the surface of T-4 cells.[a] Gallo didn't present any evidence that an HHV-7 vaccine would actually work. But he nevertheless planned to test it in patients soon, and "I hope to have progress for you the next time I talk to such a meeting."[b]

"Gallo didn't present much data on anything," Don Francis said later. "It was a very strange talk. He mentioned everyone in his lab, the people he'd worked with, what we're going to do, and this and that." The scene grew stranger when a member of the audience rose to address the conference organizers. "This guy stood up," Francis said. "I have no idea who he was — and said, 'I have a question. Was the invitation to Dr. Gallo sent *before* his conviction for scientific misconduct or after?'"

Mal Martin had agreed to testify against Popovic and Gallo. But before leaving for Berlin he had begun to waver, explaining that he didn't want to come off as "another Don Francis." Many scientists were counting on Martin, the ORI lawyers replied, and would be disappointed if he backed out. Then why weren't *those* people testifying, Martin had asked. Jay Levy had declined to testify about his unsuccessful efforts to obtain HTLV-3B and H-9, on the grounds that censuring Gallo for not sharing reagents was "like getting Al Capone for tax evasion." In Berlin, Martin had urged Levy to change his mind. "He said, '*I'm* going to do it,'" Levy recalled. "'Why aren't *you*?'" But Levy remained convinced that testifying was "a no-win situation. People will say if I do testify, it's all sour grapes. If the guy wins, my grants are dead. Gallo carries a very big stick."

Leaving his hotel for the conference center, Martin turned when he heard Gallo call his name. "I saw him there talking to somebody," Martin recalled, "and he sort of followed me out. He said why am I picking on him? 'I mean, after all, we work at the same institution.' Then he went on the offense. He said, 'Look, you're not free of any wrongdoing.' If I go to his hearing and testify against him, he's going to put me under oath and he's going to spill the beans.

"I said, 'What beans?' I said, 'Bob, are you threatening me?' He said, 'No, I'm just discussing it.' I said, 'Bob, did I write a letter to you requesting that cell line?' He said, 'Yeah.' I said, 'Did you write an answer back to me with requirements that were a little ridiculous?' He said, 'But it wasn't my fault.' I said, 'What do you mean it wasn't your fault.' He said, 'DeVita made me do it.'"[c]

Martin replied that "If I'm asked at a hearing whether I requested the cell line and you refused it, I'm going to say the facts are the facts. He said, 'I understand, I understand.' The guy is so dysfunctional. He had a bodyguard about fifteen feet away. Because he's such a high-profile and important person, every year when he goes to the AIDS meeting they always give him a security person to take care of him. It was a couple of guys with walkie-talkies. I remember I shrugged my shoulders as he was telling me this story. He said, 'Don't shrug your shoulders, it's my career here.' I didn't say it, but 'Bob, you made your own bed.'"[6]

Gallo's confrontation with Martin wasn't the only contact about which the ORI had become concerned. While Gallo was in Europe, Joe Onek had telephoned a number of NIH scientists and officials, including Stu Aaronson, Bill Blattner, Sam Broder, Tony Fauci, and Bernadine Healy, to solicit them as prospective witnesses in Gallo's behalf. The calls stopped when the ORI's chief counsel, Chris Pascal, reminded Onek that federal regulations prohibited him from communicating with HHS employees without the ORI's consent.[7]

The most troubling incident involved Mike McGrath, who had served on the OSI advisory panel with Priscilla Schaffer and Ken Berns. Schaffer and Berns had agreed to testify at both appeal hearings, and McGrath had been expected to appear as well in his continuing role as a consultant to the ORI. But at the last moment, McGrath had abruptly resigned his consultancy.[8] According to Steve Godek, the explanation from McGrath's lawyer was that his client's decision had followed statements from Gallo and Onek "which Dr. McGrath considers threats."[9] When Godek asked what kind of threats, McGrath's lawyer replied only that "if Dr. McGrath were to testify, that Joseph Onek, counsel for Dr. Gallo, would use cross-examination to make it 'personal' against Dr. McGrath."

On the morning of Monday, June 7, 1993, only one member of the three-member Research Integrity Adjudications Panel, an HHS lawyer named Cecilia Sparks Ford, was present in panel's chamber on the sixth floor of the Hubert H. Humphrey Building to hear the opening argument by Mika Popovic's lawyer.

Barbara Mishkin didn't dispute that some things in the *Science* paper weren't true. But, Mishkin said, either Popovic wasn't responsible for those things, or else they didn't represent conscious attempts on his part to deceive. Mishkin also demanded to know why ORI had afforded Popovic all the blame for the purported misstatements on which his misconduct finding was based, since Popovic had "lost control" of the paper to Gallo. Taking advantage of the appeals board's ruling on intent, Mishkin explained that Popovic's defense would be one of "honest error," and let the ORI try to prove otherwise. Even if every one of the questioned items cited by the ORI were actually false, Mishkin said, they would amount to nothing more than "harmless errors."

Mishkin conceded that the "first shown" sentence regarding the RT testing of the pool samples, on which the most significant count of misconduct was based, was "not precise." But then, her client hadn't written that sentence. As for the S.N. micrograph and other negative experiments that had been reported as "N.D.," Mishkin explained that Popovic hadn't meant to suggest that the experiments hadn't been done. When Popovic used "N.D.," he had meant "Not Determined" or "Not Determinable," the definitions he learned in Europe — though Mishkin didn't say whether the Czechoslovakian equivalent of "Not Determinable" also bore the initials "N.D."

Finally, Mishkin pointed out that even if Popovic *had* meant to say "Not Done"— which he hadn't — that phrase could also mean incomplete or unfinished, "as in 'the steaks are not done.'" Lost in Mishkin's rhetoric was the fact that the only "Not Done" that mattered, the electron micrograph of R.F., which Gallo still claimed could have been used for the blood test, had been "done" by Matt Gonda three times and been negative each time.

The ORI lawyers hadn't had time to go back through the mountains of paper with which Gallo and his assistants had deluged the OSI, sheaves of lab notes and lengthy written responses to each of OSI's questions. Although filled with artful omissions and misinformation — Betsy Read claimed Gallo had made changes in several of her submissions that she told him were incorrect[10] — the OSI documents contained some critical pieces to the puzzle, including one that bore on the charge against Popovic. Responding to a question about the electron micrograph results for the five isolates reported in Popovic's paper, Gallo had explained that one of the five, W.T., was "never sent for EM analysis, so the paper should state 'not done.'"[11]

The ORI had asked Priscilla Schaffer to suggest an expert witness who could explain retrovirology to the appeals board, and Schaffer had given Steve Godek two names: Irvin Chen, a respected researcher who had worked with David Golde on HTLV-2 at UCLA; and one of Schaffer's Harvard colleagues, Joseph Sodroski, a member of Bill Haseltine's lab who had played a key role in the ill-fated sequencing of HTLV-3B, and for whom Gallo had written a glowing tenure recommendation the year before.[12]

There was animosity of longstanding between Gallo and Golde, who had given Gallo the cell line in which Kalyanaraman had discovered HTLV-2.[d] To avoid any suggestion of anti-Gallo bias, the ORI had chosen Sodroski, who waved and smiled at Popovic as he took the stand. Once there, Sodroski dismissed the Pasteur's research as "sporadic examples of virus isolation" and proclaimed the blood test work by Sarngadharan and Popovic as "seminal" in establishing the diagnostic assay that was used to protect the blood supply.

"I told Steve he was going to do that," Schaffer said later. "I told him, 'If you want him to inform the board about HIV, he's perfect for that. But don't get him involved in this case, because he is sympathetic.'"

The ORI lawyers hadn't helped their case by persisting in mispronouncing Popovic's name as *Pop*-o-vic, while Barbara Mishkin made a point of pronouncing it correctly (Po-po-*vich*), and Hadley didn't know what to make of Popovic's demeanor. "He kept acting like he wanted to talk to me," she said. "He kept getting up close to me during the break. I had run out of water, and he jumped up and filled my water glass from a pitcher — bowing to me. Every time I would get up he would jump up out of his chair, and move his chair for me and bow."

Having overcome his ambivalence, Mal Martin spent much of his time on the stand dissecting the "first shown" sentence. In Martin's opinion, the description in Popovic's paper of how the pool had been developed — or what Popovic now said was a description of the pool — was "unacceptable and useless." But the ORI's lawyers hadn't given Martin an opportunity to say what he really thought, "that the pooling experiment was never done," because "I wasn't asked the right question."

Martin was followed by Roche's Tom White, who arrived in a rush from the airport. No sooner had White taken the stand than Mishkin objected to Godek's submission of the Roche report, even though it was "Appendix X" of the ORI report that formed the basis for Popovic's appeal. Without waiting for Ford to rule, Godek offered Mishkin a deal: if Popovic were willing to stipulate that the report showed that four of the ten pool samples contained no virus, he would withdraw the report itself. When Mishkin quickly accepted, Godek seemed pleased with himself. "The deal of the century," he said later. Suzanne Hadley held her head. The fact that the Roche report wasn't in evidence meant no questions could be asked about White's other findings, such as the determination that MOV was LAV.

Tom White might have been the ORI's best witness, but his testimony was a qualified disaster. After several minutes of answering Godek's questions in words of many syllables, Godek asked for a recess and led White out into the hall. When White explained that he couldn't answer the questions the way Godek was phrasing them, Godek said he would try to be more precise. But the testimony that followed wasn't much better, and Godek dismissed White after only an hour.

Godek conceded that Ken Berns had "ended up looking like an idiot," after Mishkin produced an old article in which Berns himself had mistakenly described an experiment which hadn't been done. But on the evening of the seventh day, an ebullient Godek called Hadley at home. "He said, 'If we win this case, it'll be because of Priscilla Schaffer,'" Hadley said. "Apparently she was great, with a couple of exceptions," one of which was Schaffer's lament that "we may never know" the source of HTLV-3B.

"Of course we know," Hadley said. "It's LAV."

During her prehearing interview with the ORI lawyers, Popovic's former technician, Betsy Read, had recounted the key events of late 1983, beginning with her attempts to grow LAV during Popovic's visit to Switzerland. When Read was asked whether she had ever actually *seen* the Popovic pool, she said she hadn't.[13] Now, on the witness stand, Read said she had.

"Did you ever see this pool?" Marcus Christ asked.

"Yes," Read replied. "I mean, I saw it as some centrifuge tubes filled with cell culture supernatant."

"How was it labeled?"

"I have no idea and don't remember what it was labeled as. It was in a cold room in an ice bucket."

"How do you know it was a pool?"

"Because Mika told me it was."

Had Christ been given time to learn more of the science, he might have realized that Read wasn't describing an active virus culture, but vials of culture fluid Popovic told her had *come from* a pool. Among the questions not asked was *where* the pool culture had been maintained, or *why* Popovic had tended it himself rather than delegating that routine task to his technician.

Read *was* asked, however, about her testing of Popovic's cultures for the presence of the AIDS virus. The French had used Frédéric Brugière's sera to type their LAV cultures, a technique Gallo criticized as "ridiculous and bad virology," although for months Mika Popovic had done the same thing.[e]

That had changed by February 1984, when Sarngadharan had come up with a highly specific antibody produced by inoculating laboratory rabbits with MOV, a reagent Gallo later claimed as among his most important contributions. "It wasn't until the rabbit antibody," Gallo said later, "that we knew the cause of AIDS."

According to Read's notes, that would have been nearly three weeks after Park City, on February 24, 1984, the day she first used the rabbit antibody to test eleven of Popovic's cultures. Nine hadn't reacted, suggesting that they hadn't contained any live virus. The two that did react, and strongly, were identified in Read's notes as "H/L" and "H/Ti/L."

Read's notes showed that she had been using "H" as shorthand for HUT-78,[f] and Suzanne Hadley thought "H/L" and "H/Ti/L" looked suspiciously reminiscent of "HUT-78/LAV" and "Ti7.4/LAV"— the two LAV cultures that, according to Gallo, had been purposely "discontinued" the previous January, locked away in Popovic's freezer.

On the witness stand, Read insisted the rabbit antiserum had been made with HTLV-3B. Hadley passed Christ a reminder that the rabbits had been inoculated with MOV.

"It wasn't MOV?" asked Christ.

"Mika had made the pool," an exasperated Read replied. "He had some cells and some cell culture supernatant that were all sent over to Sarang to develop this reagent for us."

Tom White had established that MOV and HTLV-3B were both LAV, and Popovic's notes suggested to Suzanne Hadley and Jim Swire that LAV had been renamed MOV. Now Read seemed to be saying that MOV and the pool were synonymous. "Betsy's eyes definitely crossed," Hadley said. "She kept looking madly at Mika for help, who was slumping down in his chair, getting redder and redder." But the appeals board hadn't permitted Christ to pursue the "misappropriation" of LAV, and after a few more questions Read was excused.[g]

Priscilla Schaffer left the hearing room with Lyle Bivens in search of a cab, and she was troubled by Bivens's demeanor. "Lyle was very quiet," she said later. "I really don't know what's going on in his head. There's something deeper than I can see. He was very polite, but I think there's a whole lot more to this than meets the eye."

Suzanne Hadley's appraisal was more succinct. "Lyle looks like he's been hit by a train," Hadley said.

Having returned from Berlin by way of Paris and Reykjavik,[14] on the tenth day of the hearing Gallo took the stand on Popovic's behalf. Hadley thought Gallo seemed to make a point of looking at the ceiling while Christ was addressing the appeals board.

Gallo admitted editing Popovic's *Science* paper, but he refused to answer questions about what parts of the paper he had, or hadn't, changed. "Things got pretty hostile," said Todd Betke, a young lawyer from Weil, Gotshal whom Rob Odle had dispatched to take notes.

"The ORI counsel was saying, 'Dr. Gallo, if you could just listen to the question, respond to the question.' Gallo was not comfortable being in a legal proceeding where he's not supposed to talk at certain times. He preferred to just argue back and forth, and the judge had to keep telling him to shut up."

When Christ asked Gallo what he meant by writing "Mika you are crazy" on Popovic's draft article, the board wouldn't allow Gallo to answer. "The basis of the objection," Betke said, "was that it wasn't relevant to this proceeding, it was the subject of a later proceeding. Then they asked him, 'Is your handwriting on this page?' And he said, 'To the best of my knowledge, no.'"

Rather than pointing out that Gallo had admitted writing the comments to Serge Lang,[h] Christ pursued the question of why Gallo had hastened the publication of the *Science* articles, a haste which Popovic blamed for the large number of errors in his own paper. "He said, 'Well, there were leaks — and we were seeing all this positive serology,'" Hadley recalled. "So I said to Marcus, 'Just ask him the question: What positive serology was he seeing, and did that include the serology from the CDC, from Pasteur?'"

"I would say it would contribute to it, I suppose," Gallo replied.

Christ: "And what about the Pasteur sera, was that one of the things, were you seeing anything from Pasteur?"

Gallo: "We didn't get any sera from Pasteur other than the one single one for the patient."

"Did you see any *data*," Christ asked, "when you were at the Pasteur Institute in April of 1984?"

Before Gallo could answer, Mishkin's cocounsel, Bill Bradford, leaped up to object on Popovic's behalf. "We're now getting into events that occurred after the submission of this paper for publication," Bradford said.

Ford sustained the objection, and after a few more futile attempts to extract information on other topics, Christ gave up.

"No further questions," he said.

"I can go to work now?" Gallo asked.

No one who attended the Popovic hearing expected the ORI to win, and that included Marcus Christ. "By nature I'm a pessimistic individual," Christ said. "This has done nothing to change that." Christ agreed with Lyle Bivens and Priscilla Schaffer that the appeals board lawyers were over their heads scientifically. "I think that's a real problem," Christ said. "I think that a lot of the arguments that were thrown out, in particular by one of Popovic's expert witnesses, would have been seen through quite clearly by a scientist. And maybe they were by this board. But I don't know."

Christ thought Cecilia Ford "a very bright person, and we did what we could to try to teach her. But I think these cases need scientists on the panel. To be perfectly honest, I think it's somewhat insulting not to have a scientist on the panel. Because, let's face it, there was the Richards committee — all scientists. They said Popovic was dirty. The OSI had a scientific group of advisers. They said Popovic's dirty. The ORI itself is comprised of scientists. They say he's dirty. Now you've got a nonscientist that's going to sit there and potentially say, 'Oh, no, he's not.'"

"We Did It to Ourselves"

A week before Mika Popovic's appeal hearing, a Mayflower moving van backed up to the director's mansion on the grounds of the National Institutes of Health. Nobody was surprised when Bernadine Healy's last day in office began with an interview on CBS and ended with another on CNN; Healy's staff joked that the director's frenetic press secretary, Johanna Schneider, would also be driving the van to Ohio, where Healy was preparing to announce her candidacy for the Senate.[1]

As Healy was packing, word leaked that Bill Clinton was expected to nominate "a Nobel-prize-winning molecular biologist from the University of California," to head the National Institutes of Health.[2] The cheers from the NIH campus could be heard for miles around. Harold Varmus wasn't a career bureaucrat. He was a real scientist who had participated in fundamental discoveries about the nature of cancer. From his own late nights in the lab, Varmus understood the concerns and frustrations of the hundreds of researchers who labored in the NIH's laboratories, and the thousands of university scientists whose work it funded.

Eschewing the NIH director's mansion as "not my style," Varmus bought a house in the trendy Cleveland Park section of Washington, D.C. The space where Healy had parked her Mercedes remained empty. Harold Varmus, knapsack over his shoulder, rode a bicycle to work, didn't wear a tie, and insisted that everybody call him "Harold."

Varmus's first appearance in the NIH cafeteria, where he stood in line to order a turkey sandwich, prompted Joanne Belk to observe that Bernadine Healy had never been known to set foot in the cafeteria, let alone heard to say, "Please call me Bernie."

If Varmus's nomination was a dream come true for NIH, it was Robert Gallo's nightmare. A decade before, Gallo had shared the Lasker Prize with Varmus and Mike Bishop, an experience remembered by Varmus's wife, the journalist Connie Casey, for Gallo's complaints that no limousine had been made available to chauffeur the Lasker winners around New York City.

There once had been high hopes at NIH that Gallo would someday share the Nobel Prize with Bishop and Varmus. But when a Nobel was awarded for cancer research in 1989, it had gone to Bishop and Varmus alone. Gallo wasn't the only one depressed by the news. MIT's Bob Weinberg was described by Arnie Levine as "devastated," and Levine, who had discovered an important cancer gene called p53, wasn't terribly happy.

But the enmity between Gallo and Varmus was legendary. Gallo referred to Varmus and Bishop as "the Pope and his Bishop."[a] Varmus dismissed Gallo as "a thug," and delivered the ultimate scientific coup de grâce: "He'd be great in industry."[3] Of all the scientists Gallo might have chosen to head the NIH, the only one who ranked below Varmus was Abraham Karpas.

On an early September evening in 1993, eight hundred scientists, AIDS activists, and journalists, not including Harold Varmus, filed into Washington's Kennedy Center for the world premiere of *And the Band Played On*, the HBO movie based on Randy Shilts's book. The *Washington Post* called the film, whose cast included Richard Gere, Glenne Headly, Sir Ian McKellen (as Max Essex), Anjelica Huston, Steve Martin, Lily Tomlin, and Swoosie Kurtz, "predictably loud, earnest, sad and moving . . . largely an indictment of corporate greed, homophobia and the Reagan-Bush years."[4]

Peter Stockton, attending a wedding on Martha's Vineyard, hadn't made the premiere. But Suzanne Hadley, now working full-time on the subcommittee's final report of its investigation of the Gallo case, took Stockton's ticket, put on a yellow formal, and slipped in just before the doors closed. As she sat in the darkened theater, Hadley thought it bizarre to watch the events of 1983–1984 she was reconstructing on paper being played out on the screen by Alan Alda as Gallo, Matthew Modine as Don Francis, and Alex Courtney as a hapless Mika Popovic who quailed at Gallo's shadow.

Stopping in New York on his way home from Bogotá a few days later, Luc Montagnier watched the television premiere — according to HBO, the most-watched movie of the year — from his Manhattan hotel room. "I thought the casting was rather good," Montagnier said later. "Especially for Gallo." Portrayed by the French actor Patrick Bauchau, Montagnier had his most dramatic moment at a fictional news conference, when he announced that the DNA sequences of HTLV-3B and LAV "are identical to a degree that would not be anticipated from any two isolates from the same family."

In the film, a reporter covering the news conference turns to a scientist in the audience and whispers, "I'm not quite sure what he was saying — the virus Gallo has is the same kind the French have?"

"Not the same *kind*," the scientist answers. "It's the same virus *exactly* — from the same *patient*."

It hadn't been quite that easy. But Randy Shilts, less than six months away from dying of AIDS, thought the movie "substantially accurate in how it portrayed the conflicts between the French and the Americans." Don Francis, who reportedly had turned down an offer from the Clinton White House to head the CDC,[5] admitted that parts of the movie had been fictionalized, by reordering events in time and, in some cases, inventing whole scenes to compress elements of the story into a dramatic narrative.

In one scene later changed by HBO, Gallo finishes a lecture with a platitude about "the smile of healthy children" as the driving force behind his work — then observes privately to Francis that "the line about the kids gets them every time." After Gallo protested the slur, HBO redubbed the film to have Gallo's character say, "I've used that line fifty times and I still believe it."

"That was the lowest point for me," Gallo told the London *Observer.* "I had to sit with my wife and watch that stinking thing . . . there is not a single scene in that film in which I appear that is remotely true. I could have sued for $15 million and I would have won — but only after five or six years of lawyers going over my life. I had had enough of that sort of thing, so I said, 'Damn it, I can't do it,' and dropped the case."[b]

Gallo denounced the movie to Jim Curran as the "most vicious, slanderous, and ludicrous piece of garbage I have ever seen. The part that concerns me regarding your comments occurs roughly two hours into the film. You are jogging. Don Francis is driving a car slowly along your side. You say 'Good news — bad news. Good news, Gallo has the virus and a blood test. Bad news, he (Gallo) wants all the credit and all the patent.' I wish to know — did you say that to Don Francis? Thanks. Best regards."[6]

Curran replied that the quoted conversation, like others in the movie, had never taken place.[7] But he reminded Gallo that he and others at CDC had been persuaded that LAV was the cause of AIDS by Chermann's presentation at Park City, and that the CDC had felt an obligation to help the French make their data public.

"I did not previously know of your activities," Gallo fired back, "within the U.S. and HHS to give proper credit to the French group for the primacy of their discovery."[8]

It was *Nature,* after nearly a year's delay, which assured the primacy of the Pasteur's discovery by publishing Tom White's paper on the origins of HTLV-3B and the fate of the Popovic pool — the first time anyone outside HHS had seen the data in the Roche report, of whose existence most scientists weren't even aware.[9] "We conclude," White wrote, "that the pool, and probably another LTCB culture, MoV, were contaminated between October 1983 and early 1984 by variants of $HIV-1_{Lai}$. Therefore, the origin of the HIV-1 LAV/3B isolate also was patient LAI."

White's paper included a table which showed, after some deciphering, that four of the seven samples added by Popovic at the last minute to "save" the pool hadn't contained any AIDS virus. More remarkable, three of the four patients in question never even had AIDS. The paper didn't contain the word "misappropriation," but noted delicately that the possible "replacement" of MOV with LAV couldn't be ruled out. "I wish they could have put the statement about 'no sample of the pool is known to exist' in bold letters," said Gerry Myers, who had peer-reviewed the paper for *Nature* with Simon Wain-Hobson.

Appearing for the interview he had requested with John Dingell's staff, Gallo insisted he hadn't read White's *Nature* paper, which contained "nothing new — it was already published in that paper from the Midwest." But not having read the paper hadn't stopped Gallo from sending White a two-page letter of complaint,[10] or insisting to Dingell's staff that "the Roche analysis proves [the existence of] the pool."[11] Challenged by Suzanne Hadley to identify anything in the paper that proved the pool had ever existed, Gallo admitted there wasn't.

When the questioning turned to Flossie Wong-Staal's comparisons of LAV and HTLV-3B in the summer of 1984, Hadley observed that "this is the issue that clearly pulls Bob's chain big-time. It is the issue around which he experienced a true cognitive meltdown, seeming to completely fail to understand what the questions were about. His attorneys got the drift of the questions very well, and insisted on a lunch break."

According to Hadley's interview notes, after composing himself at lunch "Gallo now admits — on the record — that he knew, in the summer of '84, that it was quite possible there had been a contamination in *his* laboratory. Yet Gallo called Montagnier and accused *him* of the contamination." As for his years-long insistence that LAV and HTLV-3B had come from different patients, Gallo told Dingell's staff that "maybe I hung on longer than I should have." But, he said, "there is something subjective about being human."

Tom White's paper was among the four hundred exhibits assembled by the Office of Research Integrity for Gallo's appeal hearing, a proceeding whose scope had been vastly broadened by the appeals board's ruling that ORI would have to defend its four "censures" of Gallo as well as its finding of scientific misconduct.[12]

The alleged "censurable conduct," the board said, might be more damaging to Gallo's reputation than the formal misconduct finding itself. Now the board had gone farther, demanding that ORI present it with an "offer of proof" stating precisely what the ORI intended to prove at the hearing, and how.[13] If Marcus Christ and his lawyers couldn't show enough evidence beforehand to suggest that misconduct had occurred, the board would dismiss all the findings without a hearing.[14]

The first "censurable finding" held that Gallo had abused his authority as a peer-reviewer by making "gratuitous and self-serving" changes to the Pasteur's first *Science* paper, changes that "misstated [its] findings and observations" and "promoted Dr. Gallo's own hypothesis." The second censure argued that, in his role as senior author of Popovic's *Science* paper, Gallo must bear "substantial responsibility for the numerous discrepancies in the Popovic paper, including the four instances of scientific misconduct attributed to Dr. Popovic." Third, as laboratory chief Gallo had "failed to instruct, supervise and manage the scientists under his supervision . . . particularly Dr. Popovic, in order to ensure that their practices and methodologies conformed to those which were acceptable within the NIH and the scientific community at large."

The ORI admitted it couldn't prove Gallo's editing of the Pasteur's paper amounted, by itself, to scientific misconduct. If it could have, it would have charged Gallo with misconduct on that count as well. What it could show was that Popovic's paper contained "numerous demonstrably false and incorrect statements, and that Dr. Gallo breached his responsibility as senior author by introducing them or by failing to correct them." But under the board's new rules, the ORI couldn't prove Gallo deserved to be found guilty of misconduct on the basis of those misrepresentations alone.

Nor was ORI prepared to argue that Gallo's responsibility for the veracity of Popovic's research and administrative failures as Popovic's supervisor rose to the level of scientific misconduct; it had included them in the addendum merely because it thought they warranted comment. As expected, the appeals board dismissed the first three censures as failing to meet the misconduct threshold, though with the caveat that Gallo's editing of the Pasteur paper might be admissible if the ORI could prove "intent to deceive, misrepresent, suppress, or distort data" in a way that enhanced Gallo's own "claims to priority or primacy."

But the board agreed with ORI that the fourth censurable finding, Gallo's failure to acknowledge that the H-9 cell line was HUT-78 and to make it available to everyone who wanted it, *might* reach the level of formal scientific misconduct.[15] The H-9 censure embodied a potentially more serious offense than even the formal misconduct charge of covering up Popovic's work with LAV. In essence, the ORI was accusing Gallo of putting his scientific ambition ahead of patients who were dying of AIDS. "By obscuring the identity and restricting the availability of the cell line in which he successfully mass-produced the AIDS virus," the ORI lawyers declared, "Dr. Gallo seriously hindered progress in AIDS research."[16]

The original OSI investigation hadn't dealt with the sharing of H-9, only its renaming. But the evidence assembled by ORI included dozens of documents attesting to what it termed the "obnoxious" conditions Gallo placed on some of his principal competitors. A recently retired Jim Mason was prepared to testify that Gallo's refusal to provide H-9 to the CDC was "so egregious" that Mason had been "forced to intercede on behalf of CDC researchers whose requests for the cell line and other reagents had not been honored by Dr. Gallo."

The Gallo hearing, scheduled for early November 1993, would go ahead. But just as it had for Popovic, the ORI would be required to show that Gallo had *intended* to commit what now amounted to two counts of scientific misconduct.

A few weeks before, the board had invoked its intent standard for the first time in reversing the misconduct finding against Rameshwar K. Sharma, the Cleveland Clinic researcher whose case had entangled Bernadine Healy. Sharma, who had been represented by none other than Joe Onek —"if scientists are in trouble," said Onek, "they call me up"— admitted the questioned statements in his grant applications weren't true. But, Onek said, Sharma hadn't *intended* to deceive the NIH. The appeals board had agreed, ruling that Sharma's conduct amounted to simple negligence rather than fabrication.[17]

"They say we lost Sharma, and so the office is down the toilet," Lyle Bivens said. "Well, it's not."[18] But the ORI lawyers were privately convinced that the obstacle raised by the intent ruling was nearly insurmountable. In theory, under that ruling a scientist could publish falsified or fabricated results, then wait to see if he got caught. If he did, he could simply claim he hadn't *intended* to deceive anybody. It would be up to the ORI to prove otherwise. In Steve Godek's opinion, proving intent in misconduct cases was "impossible, unless you get a confession. The board doesn't know what it's doing."

Lyle Bivens regretted the day he agreed to let the appeals board adjudicate the ORI's findings. "We chose the board," Bivens said. "We could have gone to the American Arbitration Association. We did it to ourselves." For reasons Bivens couldn't fathom, the appeals board seemed to be going farther out of its way than necessary to make things difficult for the ORI. In their offer of proof, Christ and Godek had argued that five years' worth of public declarations by Gallo that

Popovic hadn't grown LAV was more than enough evidence of Gallo's intent to deceive the scientific community. The board had dismissed the evidence as "unconvincing" and excluded it from the hearing. Also excluded would be any effort by ORI to show that Gallo had deliberately obscured the identity of H-9 as HUT-78. Nor did the board want to hear about the "misappropriation" of LAV.

Seeking to establish motive, Godek and Christ argued that the "not yet been transmitted" statement, as written by Gallo, was not only deliberately misleading but part of an "underlying current of secrecy" that included Popovic's experiments with MOV. "The evidence," they declared, "reveals that MOV is simply LAV, renamed."

Having raised the intent standard in the first place, the appeals board now decreed that MOV couldn't be invoked to show intent because it went beyond the conclusions of the OSI's original investigation. "Evidence offered to show the alleged identity of MOV and HTLV-3B as in fact LAV/LAI," the board said, "will not be admitted in this proceeding."

In compiling their witness roster, the ORI lawyers had interviewed nearly a hundred people. Mal Martin, Don Francis, Ed Brandt, Al Gilman, Priscilla Schaffer, and Fred Richards had put their names on the list. So had Bernie Poiesz, who was prepared to recount a conversation in which he had asked Gallo whether H-9 and HUT-78 were the same and been told to mind his own business. Montagnier, reluctant to testify in person, had agreed to swear an affidavit recounting the telephone conversation a month before the Heckler news conference in which he told Gallo of his success in growing LAV in a B-cell line.

In Bethesda for Gallo's annual AIDS meeting, Jean-Claude Chermann and Françoise Barré had taken a couple of hours to meet secretly with Marcus Christ and Nancy O'Connor. Chermann, who complained that Gallo had been ignoring him, promised to send the ORI some documents when he got home. When Christ and O'Connor had finished asking about the Pasteur's shipments of LAV to Bethesda and the development of the Pasteur ELISA, they asked the standard lawyer's question: Was there anything else they ought to know?

Well, said Barré, perhaps one thing.

At Gallo's AIDS meeting the year before, Barré had been surprised to encounter Mika Popovic waiting to board a bus that would take the conferees to dinner at a Chinese restaurant. When Barré asked Popovic how he was, she recalled that he replied "How do you think I can be, with this thing going on?"[19]

When the conversation turned to Popovic's *Science* paper, Popovic wanted Barré to know that he had tried to give the Pasteur credit for the discovery of the AIDS virus, but that Gallo had removed all mention of LAV from the manuscript. Barré thought Popovic seemed to be in a confessional mood, and she listened while he continued to talk.

He hadn't been responsible for most of the things that were done in Gallo's lab, Popovic went on, but suggestions that there hadn't been a Popovic pool were baseless. There had indeed been such a pool. In fact, Popovic had pooled *all* the single-patient cultures in his lab, including R.F. and LAV. When Barré asked why he had mixed the other cultures with LAV, she remembered Popovic replying, "To enhance its capacity to grow."[20]

Barré recalled remarking that Popovic must have known the only virus to grow out of such a mélange would be LAV, which had been around the longest and was far better adapted than any of Popovic's own isolates to growth in continuous culture. Popovic answered that he hadn't necessarily assumed the out-grower would be LAV, because R.F. was also "a strong virus." But he didn't think it would matter which virus grew out of the pool, or that there would never be any way to tell. In those days, Popovic reminded Barré, no one could have guessed there would be so much genetic variation among individual isolates of HIV. Or so Barré now said.

When Suzanne Hadley heard what Barré had told the ORI lawyers, her hair stood on end. "I asked Marcus," Hadley recalled, "'are you telling me that she did not disclose this to anybody at Pasteur in all this time?' He said no, that she didn't really think this was such a big deal. That she had just believed all along that Mika knew that he was using LAV. I said, 'Marcus, do you think there was any misunderstanding?' He said, 'Oh, no, there couldn't have been.'"

Popovic conceded the conversation had take place, though not as described by Barré, and he denied "unequivocally" that he had "knowingly" added LAV to the pool.[21] But set against the facts that had emerged during the investigations, if Barré's account of the conversation was accurate, it resolved the mystery of what had happened in Gallo's lab.

• On November 1, 1983, while he was working with LAV and MOV, Popovic claimed to have initiated a new AIDS virus culture by pooling T-cells from three patients — a carpet salesman, a hemophiliac, and a Jamaican immigrant — in HUT-78. It was Gallo, seeking an AIDS virus he could call his own, who had conceived the idea of a patient pool. "I selected three," Gallo recalled. "I said, 'Who cares if it comes from a single patient or you put it in a pool? I don't care if we can trace the lineage.'"[22]

Gallo's admission — ten years after the fact — that *he*, not Popovic, was responsible for the pool, came during a 1993 interview with the Discovery Channel, and it had gone unnoticed by the ORI. But it was consistent with the reservations Popovic had expressed to the OSI, and it reprised what Omar Sattaur claimed to have heard from Kalyanaraman, that "Popovic was instructed by Gallo to mix up the viruses — the Pasteur isolate and their own isolates," in hopes of obtaining "some synergistic effect."

• The pooled culture hadn't taken off. A week later, Popovic added more material from the same three patients and continued his work with MOV. Still the pool had sputtered and faltered, and six weeks later it was nearly dead. On January 2, 1984, Popovic claimed to have launched a last-ditch effort to "save" the pool by tossing in material from seven new patients. But as Tom White had discovered, four of the seven cultures hadn't contained any AIDS virus. The other three cultures had been negative for reverse transcriptase, meaning those cells, although infected with HIV, weren't producing any virus either.[c]

• What never had made sense was why Popovic had chosen seven nonproductive cultures to "save" the pool when he had four virus-producing cultures in his lab: the highly productive MOV (really LAV), HUT-78/LAV and Ti7.4/LAV, and the feeble R.F., which Betsy Read had transmitted to HUT-78 only days before in an effort to keep it alive.[23]

It would have made the most sense to use LAV to save the pool, and in theory Gallo and Popovic both agreed there hadn't been any reason not to. The agreement with the Pasteur precluded only the *commercial* use of LAV, and in early January of 1984 Popovic wasn't thinking about an AIDS blood test. Popovic told OSI, "If I have a cell line which is virus positive, and I take another virus-positive cell line and mix together and put together LAV, is bona fide experiment." Popovic's focus had been on finding the right virus, not the patient in whom it was found; an AIDS virus was an AIDS virus. As Gallo put it, "If I use HTLV-1 in a paper, I can use multiple sources of HTLV-1. It is the same virus to me then. It is all the same, like measles, you know. That is the way we were thinking. Didn't matter what strain we were using or what the original parental lineage was of that."[24]

- Following Gallo's return from the tripartite meeting in early April 1984, it had become necessary to send a virus to Frederick for scaled-up production in anticipation of the commercial AIDS test. There hadn't been so much urgency before Gallo left for Paris, but it was there he learned the French were about to begin commercial production of LAV for their ELISA. By his own account, and Gallo's, Popovic had wanted to use R.F. for the blood test. But the R.F. micrographs were negative, it wasn't growing that well, and Gallo had insisted on the more prolific pool virus, HTLV-3B.

- June 5, 1984, was the day Beatrice Hahn produced the restriction map of R.F. If Popovic had put R.F. in the pool, as Barré claimed, he had no doubt been hoping that HTLV-3B, the virus which emerged, was R.F. But R.F. was so different from HTLV-3B that what had grown out of the pool had to be something else; if LAV had gone into the pool, it was most likely LAV that had grown out. Unfortunately, Gallo and Popovic had just published a paper in *Science* in which Gallo claimed that LAV hadn't been successfully grown in a continuous culture, even suggesting the French virus might not be the same kind of virus as HTLV-3B. With no way to undo Gallo's statements, Popovic had taken his sister the drafts of his *Science* paper showing his success in growing LAV, figuring that "sometime in the future I might need them as evidence."[25]

- The final piece to the puzzle was Popovic's explanation, after nearly ten years, of why his *Science* paper, most of whose data had come from experiments with the pool virus, hadn't mentioned a pool or identified that virus as HTLV-3B. The reason, Popovic said, was that he had "planned to use the isolate R.F. as the prototype in the paper, rather than the pool," a plan never implemented because "the publication date for the paper was accelerated and work with the RF was 2–3 weeks behind that of the pool."[26]

That scenario not only answered the question of why the *Science* paper hadn't mentioned a pool, it explained all the angst over the "first shown" passage, which stated that "Continuous production of HTLV-3 was obtained after repeated exposure of parental HT cells to concentrated culture fluids harvested from short-term cultures of T cells obtained from patients with AIDS or pre-AIDS. The concentrated fluids were first shown to contain particle-associated RT."

Whoever wrote those words hadn't been describing a pool experiment at all. He had been describing the coculturing of "HT" with the five isolates identified in the *Science* article: R.F., S.N., L.S., B.K., and W.T.[27] Following Gallo's substitution of HTLV-3B for R.F. in making the blood test, the need had arisen to identify the source of HTLV-3B. Although it didn't quite fit, the passage in *Science* had been put forward as a *post hoc* description of the "Popovic pool."

Marcus Christ and Nancy O'Connor questioned Françoise Barré by telephone after her return to Paris, and her story remained consistent with the one she told in Bethesda.[28] The ORI lawyers had planned to have Barré testify at the hearing, but only about Gallo's editing of the Pasteur's *Science* paper. Even with the board's prohibition of any testimony about misappropriation, once Barré was on the stand Christ thought he could find a way to get the Popovic conversation on the record.[d]

The ORI's concern, in the meantime, was whether Barré would remain firm in her resolve to testify. After her name turned up on the ORI witness list, Gallo had invited her to lunch in Paris. "When he began to speak," Barré recalled, "I realized that he wanted to talk about the upcoming appeals board hearing. Dr. Gallo asked if it was true that I would testify at the hearing as a witness for ORI. I said it was true, and he asked why I would do this. I told Dr. Gallo that both the French embassy and IP [Institut Pasteur] officials had encouraged me to testify. I also told him that both Drs. Montagnier and Chermann had agreed to testify for ORI, and with those two testifying, I felt I could not myself refuse."[29]

"Dr. Gallo told me that if I testified it might not turn out well for me. He said that some of the ORI witnesses in the earlier appeal hearing of Dr. Popovic had been made to look ridiculous. I told Dr. Gallo I am not an aggressive person, that I wanted this matter to be over, and that while I intended to answer truthfully any questions that were put to me, I did not intend to go beyond those questions in making my responses."[e]

Three days before Gallo's appeal hearing was set to begin, the Research Integrity Adjudications Panel handed down its ruling in the case of Mikulas Popovic: not guilty of scientific misconduct on all counts.[30]

Gallo had dismissed the ORI investigation as the product of an investigation by bureaucrats who didn't understand science.[31] The appeals panel was entirely composed of nonscientists, but Gallo welcomed their verdict in the Popovic case. So did many others, but not for the same reasons. "I think that will be a pretty popular decision," said John Moore, a New York University AIDS researcher who had been a postdoc under Robin Weiss. "Certainly around the grapevine people have said, 'Oh, well, that was right. The big man is the one to get.' If Gallo had gotten the Nobel Prize he wouldn't have shared it with Popovic. Whatever Popovic is guilty of, the man in charge is the one who carries the can. It's traditional. With power comes responsibility, and Gallo had the power. Just go for the top, leave the smaller fry alone."

At the Office of Research Integrity, the response was less roseate. "My initial reaction is one of outrage," said Lyle Bivens after reading the seventy-nine-page Popovic opinion. "The board is way off the mark." The source of Bivens's outrage wasn't so much the not-guilty verdict as the way the appeals board had reached its conclusion, and what that seemed to portend for the Gallo case. "We're going to ask for a one-week delay this afternoon," Bivens said. "If we get it, we'll have a week in which to consider all the possibilities, ranging from simply rearranging our strategy and our witness sequence to withdrawing the case. If we don't get it, it's going to be hard to make a snap decision just to drop the case. We may be committed just to starting on Monday."

Marcus Christ needed the extra week "to figure out what the Popovic decision does to the Gallo case. What are the standards that have now been set out by the board? Is it possible to satisfy those standards and go forward with this case? We could simply say, 'OK, you've made it impossible, you've set up these standards that are absurd and don't apply, and we're not going to go forward.'"

In reversing Popovic's misconduct finding, the board hadn't disputed the facts unearthed by the OSI's investigation. Rather, the board said, the passages and phrases the ORI had deemed deliberate falsifications also could be read in ways that made them true — or at least not false. At most, the ORI had established that the Popovic paper contained ambiguities. "It took the most benign interpretation of every false statement, however implausible, and accepted that," Bivens said.

The ORI's reading of the "first shown" sentence, the board said, was "not the only reasonable reading." It wasn't "unambiguously clear" that whoever had written the sentence meant the samples had been tested for RT *before* pooling, and it wouldn't have been "illogical" to have tested them after pooling.

The fact that nearly all of the samples had tested RT-negative didn't appear to have registered with the board, and the ORI lawyers hadn't gone back and looked at Gallo's written submissions to OSI, including one where he admitted that the pooled culture fluids had been put into HUT-78 *before* a portion of those fluids could be tested for RT at one of his contract laboratories. "So technically," Gallo had said, "the fluid was not first shown" to be RT positive.[32]

The appeals board lawyers also found credible Popovic's testimony that he had used "N.D." to convey that the data was "inconclusive, unquantifiable, or not determinable," even though the *Science* paper itself defined "N.D." as "Not Done." To the board that didn't seem to have mattered. "If Dr. Popovic had truly intended to mislead the reader into thinking that the experiments in question here had not been even attempted," it said, "we think it more likely that he would have used 'NT-not tested,' rather than the more ambiguous 'N.D., not done.'"

That kind of logic had led Mal Martin to conclude that lawyers had no business adjudicating science; there wasn't a scientist on earth who didn't know what "Not Done" was supposed to mean. "*What* is going on?" Martin asked after reading the board's opinion, which dismissed Martin's own testimony as coming from a witness who "simply cannot be considered disinterested."

Martin admitted that "I'm not unbiased. There's no question. Because I'm outraged by what happened. But that doesn't mean I can't tell the truth. Who picked this board? In a legal dispute, the truth really doesn't matter. It's how it's portrayed, and what kind of spin you put on it. In science, truth is the most important thing. It's heartbreaking to see what happened to those guys at ORI. They really tried their hardest. It was out of their hands, though."

The board's assessment of the other experts who testified for the government was almost as harsh. None of the ORI's witnesses, the board observed, "had direct experience isolating a novel retrovirus." Neither, of course, had Mika Popovic, or for that matter any of

Popovic's witnesses. In the history of the world, only four scientists had isolated a "novel" human retrovirus: Bernie Poiesz, "Kaly" Kalyanaraman, Françoise Barré, and François Clavel. All the ORI's experts had done, said the board, was find fault with Popovic "simply for doing things differently from how they would have done things." The only government witness the board found persuasive was Joe Sodroski, whose testimony had "supported Dr. Popovic's case more than ORI's case."

"They found Mika's demeanor to be credible," said Suzanne Hadley. "Fred's not credible because he didn't do the investigation. Priscilla's not credible because she *did* do it. Mal's not credible because he's got a hard-on for Bob. Sodroski alone is credible, even though he was a collaborator on the Gallo sequence paper." In twenty years of science, Priscilla Schaffer had never heard her credentials questioned. Now three government lawyers were suggesting that Schaffer didn't know what she was talking about.

"I will put my own expertise against any scientist in the world," Schaffer said. "I wouldn't be a full professor at Harvard if I didn't know what I was doing. I have to ask myself, aside from their scientific incompetence, which comes through glaringly, what is the reason for this incredible bias? And my conclusion is that they're under pressure. Within this same building, a couple of floors apart, there's a pile of lawyers who are working to protect the patent."

"There's much more behind this than I can imagine," Fred Richards said a few hours after a Federal Express truck delivered the board's opinion to his home in New Haven. "These damned people on that panel, they have just behaved atrociously. For the kind of things we're dealing with in this Gallo business, the lawyers have no business being in here at all. They're never going to contribute anything to it except exacerbation. The scientific community is perfectly capable of handling these things themselves. They've done so for years."

Early Sunday morning found Steve Godek in his office at ORI headquarters, a few miles up the Rockville Pike from NIH. "There was nothing impartial about that decision," Godek said. "How can you say that every witness ORI put up was irrelevant, unreasonable, or incredible? And not find incredible or unreasonable testimony from Popovic's witnesses, who were all his friends and colleagues and mentors?"[f]

Only the day before, Godek had learned about the August 1985 memo to Peter Fischinger in which Gallo maintained that HTLV-3B had been "pooled from several patients who showed high R.T. activity in *primary* culture"— precisely what Popovic and Gallo had testified the "first shown" sentence didn't mean. Even though a copy of the memo had rested for seven years in the files of the HHS general counsel, Godek had never seen it until after the verdict was in. "This is a bomb," Godek said. "How can Dr. Popovic say this isn't what he meant?" But the bomb had gone off too late.

Godek spent the weekend parsing the board's opinion, and he compiled a list of "mistakes, just factual mistakes and internally inconsistent statements," that covered three pages.[g] "I think we all know there's certain implications for the patent," Godek said. "The entire opinion goes much farther than it has to. The stuff about 'sound and fury signifying nothing'? Total horseshit. We've tried to figure out why the board has been hostile."

A related mystery was why the board had seen fit to include in its opinion its own history of the discovery of the AIDS virus, a recounting of events that had no bearing on the case against Popovic, wasn't relevant to the charges against him, and which seemed to cancel any claim by the board to impartiality.

According to the board's chronology, it was Gallo's *Science* papers that established that a retrovirus was the cause of AIDS, and "Dr. Popovic's success" with the H-9 cell line that had made possible "the blood test needed to ensure the safety of donated blood supplies." In fact, Popovic's paper was "a seminal work, possibly the most important paper in virology in the 20th century." When Fred Richards saw that, he laughed. "I'm going to ask my virological friends for all the ones that they would have put ahead of it," Richards said. "The work of John Enders comes to mind."

It hadn't escaped Suzanne Hadley that the board's version of history parroted the government's arguments in defense of the blood-test patent. "Where did that stuff come from?" Hadley wondered. "That stuff isn't on the record. It wasn't part of the hearing. The board doesn't know the first thing about the history of the Pasteur ELISA. There's too much pseudoscience in this opinion. They got it from somewhere."

What troubled Hadley even more was the board's addressing of issues it hadn't allowed the ORI to raise at the hearing, and on which it hadn't heard any testimony. Having forbidden the ORI to introduce evidence of misappropriation, the board had nevertheless concluded that an "accidental contamination" of the Popovic pool was "at least as likely a possibility as deliberate contamination."

"On the basis of what?" Hadley asked. "How the hell would they know what happened?" But there was more. The ORI, the board said, had failed to "establish any motive for Dr. Popovic to deliberately substitute the French isolate for the results of his pooling experiment, and we see no apparent reason why he would have done so, given the number of other isolates which he successfully grew on T-cell lines."

Shaking his head in wonderment, Steve Godek pointed out that the ORI hadn't established a motive for misappropriation because it had been explicitly prohibited from doing so. Nor had ORI been able to give the board any information about Popovic's "other isolates" on which to base such an opinion. "Misappropriation was never an issue in the hearing," Godek said. "They wouldn't let us put it in. Whenever I attempted to ask Popovic about LAV in the lab I was slammed by the board."

Christ, Godek, and the other ORI lawyers had spent nearly nine months preparing for the Gallo and Popovic hearings, assembling hundreds of exhibits and interviewing dozens of prospective witnesses. Without challenging the ORI's facts, the appeals board had told ORI it believed statements in scientific articles could be read in ways other than the obvious. Then it had begun rendering opinions in Popovic's favor about matters that hadn't been in evidence.

Godek thought the ORI could still win the Gallo appeal. "Because there's evidence of intent," Godek said. "All we have to show is that Gallo's explanation is not reasonable or likely under the circumstances. The way that we show that, is that he was specifically deleting references to the French and the use of LAV in the laboratory."

Lyle Bivens thought it didn't matter what evidence the ORI presented. "I don't think we have a chance in the Gallo hearing," Bivens said on Tuesday afternoon, "based on what I see in the Popovic case. And the question is, what's more damaging? A report coming out like this at the end of the hearing process? Or for us to get out of it and say, 'Look, the board has created a situation and imposed standards which make it impossible for us to in good conscience proceed?'"

Nine days after the board's ruling in the Popovic hearing, the Office of Research Integrity withdrew its eleven-month-old determination that Gallo had committed scientific misconduct.[33] It was taking that action, the ORI said, "in light of recent Research Integrity Adjudications Panel decisions, including the related Popovic decision issued on the eve of the Gallo hearing. These decisions established a new definition of scientific misconduct as well as a new and extremely difficult standard for proving misconduct.[h]

"ORI maintains that the standards applied by the panel reflect a fundamental disagreement with ORI as to the importance of clarity, accuracy and honesty in science. However, because ORI is bound by the panel's decisions, it will not continue its proceeding against Dr. Gallo. As a practical matter, the panel's recent decisions have made it extraordinarily difficult for ORI to defend its legal determination of scientific misconduct regarding Dr. Gallo."

"Our reputation has always been one of independence and integrity," said the board's counsel, Andrea Selzer. "We have no motivation for or against one party or another. We're bound by what the law is and what parties argue to us." Selzer emphasized that the board didn't "have information about cases unless it's submitted to us by the parties in the court, so we probably know less about all of these cases than all the people who are involved. It's up to the attorneys before us to make their arguments and to present the evidence."

Which only made Suzanne Hadley wonder, once again, where the board had gotten the information in its ersatz history of AIDS research.

Gallo, somewhere in Canada, was "delighted that O.R.I. has dismissed the case against me, and that I have been completely vindicated. I will now be able to redouble my efforts in the fight against AIDS and cancer. There are several hopeful new avenues of AIDS research that my laboratory is pursuing."[34] To Nicholas Wade, the science editor of the *New York Times,* Gallo was "the one scientific hero who has yet emerged in the fight against AIDS."[i] Abraham Karpas had no choice but to agree.

"Bob for Pope," Karpas said.

"Dr. Gallo Is No Longer Here"

Science & Government Report *compared the case of Robert Gallo to* "an underground fire that won't go out."[1] With the ORI's withdrawal, the flames had died down but the embers continued to smolder, fanned by John Dingell. At Dingell's suggestion, the HHS inspector general had spent months gathering evidence on the larger issues not addressed by the Office of Scientific Integrity — the invention of the HIV blood test, the defense of the blood-test patent, and the veracity of Gallo's sworn declaration in the patent case.

Federal prosecutors, citing the ongoing misconduct inquiry, had twice declined to consider bringing charges against Gallo for perjury. But the inspector general's office had plodded ahead, crisscrossing the country to interview Jay Levy, Marty Bryant, Lee Ratner, Ed Brandt, and others never interviewed by OSI. The inspector general had even obtained the original Mika Popovic–Betsy Read notebooks sequestered by Suzanne Hadley at the outset of the OSI investigation, which it delivered to the United States Secret Service.

Part of the Secret Service's job is tracing anonymous letters that threaten the president's life. For this the agency has a "questioned documents" section that operates a machine called an Electrostatic Detection Apparatus, or ESDA, which can "read" otherwise invisible indentations on a sheet of paper left by something written on the sheet above, or many sheets above — addresses, telephone numbers, and other pieces of information that frequently offer clues to the identity of an anonymous letter-writer.

Popovic had remarked to OSI that some of his purportedly contemporaneous lab notes were "put together a little bit later, I would say."[2] It had been Suzanne Hadley's idea to run the Popovic and Read notepages through the ESDA, not because she had any particular reason to suspect the ESDA would see something interesting. What the ESDA saw cast serious doubt on what the government had claimed were contemporaneous records of the research that had been done in Gallo's laboratory.[3]

An example was the page dated January 2, 1984, on which Popovic recorded what purported to be the third and final infection of the pool. The ESDA had seen a "ghost" of that page indented on another page dated January 19 — but not on any of the pages dated in between. Even if Popovic had been keeping notes on a tablet and tearing the pages off day by day, it was hard to see how the pages between January 2 and January 19 had escaped indentation. According to the Secret Service, the entire January 2 page had been created at a single sitting. But Popovic had testified that some of the information on that page, including the negative RT readings for the seven samples Popovic claimed to have added that day, hadn't been available until several days after January 2.

Another questioned page was the sheet on which Betsy Read recorded her initial "Lav transmission" to HUT-78, Ti7.4, and three other cell lines, with the notation to "test at 9 days against *Bru* Sera." Read told Dingell's staff she had written "test at 9 days" at the same time as the other entries on that page. But the Secret Service's vast ink library determined that "test at 9 days" had been written with a different pen, and the ESDA had revealed an indentation of "test at 9 days" on an unrelated notepage dated twenty-three days later — long after the nine days in question had passed.

More curious, two copies of the "Lav transmission" page existed, one provided to the Pasteur lawyers in 1985, the second given to OSI five years later. Each was identical, except that the OSI page was dated October 21, 1983. On the page given to the French, the date had been altered to read October 24, 1983. When Read was shown the two pages by the Dingell staff, she said she had never seen the one dated October 24.[4]

The Popovic note pages had been delivered to the OSI in binders, enclosed in clear plastic sleeves. Where the sleeves had come from wasn't clear. Like Popovic, Betsy Read had photocopied all her notes for the Pasteur lawyers, and she hadn't been given any plastic protectors to put them in.[5] When the Secret Service put the page protectors through the ESDA, it found that several bore indentations of note pages — but not necessarily the same pages they were protecting — as though the pages had been placed on top of the protectors while they were being composed.

On one protector, the ESDA had seen two indentations overlaid: one of the October 20, 1983, page on which Popovic had written his protocol for infecting HUT-78 and Ti7.4 with LAV before leaving for Switzerland, and another reflecting data from late February and early March of 1984 that had appeared in Popovic's *Science* paper.

According to the dates they bore, the two pages had been created some five months apart. But it was difficult to imagine Popovic, with his self-admitted deficiencies in keeping experimental records, scribbling down his laboratory results as they occurred and immediately preserving each sheet of paper in a plastic protector — and harder still to imagine Popovic creating an October 1983 notepage on top of a protector, then creating another page five months later on top of the *same* protector.

It was easier to imagine someone creating the pages shortly before they were presented to the Pasteur lawyers in plastic protectors, hastily trying to reconstruct experiments from more than two years before. That might explain the curious misdatings in Popovic's notes, such as the use of "1984" for "1983," and why Popovic designated a culture as "LAV" in a letter to Matt Gonda and something else in his own notebook.

There were a number of similar anomalies. But the smoking notepage appeared to be the one on which Betsy Read had recorded the immunofluorescence experiments she conducted December 14, 1983, when Read had used Frédéric Brugière's serum to check Popovic's various cultures for the presence of the AIDS virus. Among the cultures Read tested that day were two, both strongly positive, identified as "HUT78/HIV" and "Ti7.4/HIV."[a] The only problem was that the experiment had been done three years before the term "HIV" was coined by the Varmus committee. According to the Secret Service, someone had written "HIV" over the letters "LAV."

At the time the "HIV" page was given to the Pasteur lawyers, Popovic and Gallo were still insisting that Popovic hadn't succeeded in growing LAV. Now the Secret Service had come up with *prima facie* evidence of what Jim Swire had suspected from the start: somebody in

Gallo's lab had retrospectively created, altered, and suppressed documents to conceal Popovic's success in growing LAV, replacing "HUT-78/LAV" with "HUT-78/inf" or "HUT-78/v"— or "HUT78/HIV."

Betsy Read told John Dingell's staff she had "no clue" who had overwritten her notes, and that the page in question "may not always have been in my possession."[6] Whoever had done it, the revelation that the existence of two productive LAV cultures in December 1983 had been purposely obscured to keep that information from the Pasteur lawyers, the patent office, and the courts would have irrevocably altered the outcome of the OSI investigation, changed the course of the legal proceedings — and, not incidentally, made it impossible for Gallo to claim at an appeal hearing that there hadn't been any intention to conceal Popovic's work with LAV.

The lawsuits, the interference, and the OSI investigation were over, and now there wouldn't be an appeal hearing. But the ESDA results could still be used in a prosecution for providing false evidence and testimony in an official investigation. A few weeks after the ORI withdrawal Suzanne Hadley and Peter Stockton were in Baltimore to see Dale Kelberman, the assistant United States attorney who had prosecuted Prem Sarin and Zaki Salahuddin.

"We were with him two hours and fifteen minutes, nonstop," Hadley said later. "I started out telling him that while science fraud was not his primary responsibility, this case was about lying under oath and obstructing. And I concluded with the point that the whole U.S. government got misled here and it got lied to, and the government turned around and lied. At the end he said, 'Yeah, that's what I think is really important about this whole case. We don't like to be lied to.'"

Kelberman had been reading the newspapers, and Hadley recalled that "One of the first questions he asked was the predictable one: 'Well, wasn't all this settled in '87?' He asked me what I thought of the appeals board ruling in Popovic, and what I thought that said about the merits of this case. He was particularly concerned about ORI's dropping the Gallo thing. Why did I think that happened? He said several times that gave him concern."

In Peter Stockton's opinion, the principal bar to any prosecution of Gallo was Gallo himself. "Gallo can go round and round and confuse it, you know," Stockton said. "'Justice did this, and I told them that, and that's not what I meant, and besides we were trying to do this quickly.' He gets up before a jury and he says, 'For Christ's sake, I'm trying to solve the AIDS epidemic and all this happened in a matter of hours, and we did our best, and they fired these statements in front of me, and I barely had time to look at them.'"

Kelberman agreed to look at the documents Stockton and Hadley had provided, including the ESDAs, but the clock had run itself out. In mid-January 1994 the United States attorney for Maryland concluded that "no matter what we might think of the relative merits of such a prosecution," the procedural rules governing criminal prosecutions "prohibit us from prosecuting many of the alleged false statements and other conduct by Drs. Gallo and Popovic."[7]

Several of the allegedly false statements had been made in the District of Columbia, outside Maryland's jurisdiction, where Gallo had signed the patent application in the hours before Margaret Heckler's news conference. No matter, because for most of the alleged offenses, "which includes almost all the statements at the core of this case," the statute of limitations had expired.[8]

The prosecutors were careful, however, to note that "our decision not to seek prosecution of Drs. Gallo or Popovic does not mean that we believe they should continue to receive their annual royalty payments. On this issue we express no opinion other than to observe that Dr. Gallo, as of approximately May 1991, has acknowledged that it was the French Institut Pasteur sample sent to his lab that formed the basis for the AIDS test." Whether Gallo and Popovic should continue to receive royalties, or whether the government should make any effort to recoup the royalties already paid them, were "matters which are more appropriately addressed by the Department of Health and Human Services."

Less than a week after the prosecutors' declination, Maxime Schwartz was back in Washington, asking John Dingell's staff for help in opening the doors at HHS. Reid Stuntz, the subcommittee's chief counsel, thought lobbying Congress was "the kind of stuff they should have been doing a long time ago, frankly. They should have been doing this on both sides of the aisle. At least they're doing it now, because you've got a whole new administration with whole new players."

Mike Astrue, the HHS general counsel, had been receptive to the Pasteur's position, but Astrue had left town with George Bush. "Now they've got to train somebody else," Stuntz said. "And everybody else is going, 'Shit, I've got a zillion things on my plate, why do I want to take over this old turd from the Bush days? From the Reagan days?" But somebody over there's going to have to learn it, to deal with it. It's kind of like, who's going to draw the short straw?"

To help the Clinton administration learn, the Pasteur lawyers compiled an affidavit attesting to the ways in which the French had been misled by HHS into signing the 1987 accord.[b] Rob Odle arranged for Peter Stockton to deliver the document to Astrue's replacement, a Columbia University law professor named Harriet Rabb, who evidently had drawn the short straw. "I think she's been told by the powers that be that it's better to get into this now rather than wait for it to blow up," Odle said. "I think everybody knows there are other swords."

Rabb impressed Suzanne Hadley as "a tough cookie," high praise coming from Hadley. But Rabb evidently hadn't been briefed by Astrue before he departed. "She clearly knows nothing about the facts," Hadley said. "She said, 'Why don't you tell us what you know?' Peter turned to me, so I started with the patent and what Gallo knew at the time. Bruce interrupted and she said, 'No, I want to hear this.' So I just talked for about fifteen minutes. She and her deputy were taking notes, saying 'Can you elaborate on that? Tell us more about that. What's the evidence?' and all that stuff."

Maxime Schwartz had been in touch with Harold Varmus almost from the moment of Varmus's confirmation, and following his visit with Dingell's staff Schwartz had stopped by NIH to say hello. Varmus had been polite, if not cordial, and had asked Schwartz for a memorandum explaining the Pasteur's position. By mid-February the memo was in the mail.

Much had happened since the 1987 settlement, Schwartz explained, "and many facts and documents have surfaced despite significant resistance and roadblocks imposed by the two prior Administrations."[9] Of the two issues at the focus of the original dispute, only one had been resolved, the question of "the credit for the discovery of the virus that causes AIDS. There is no longer any disagreement within the scientific community regarding the discovery of the AIDS virus. Dr. Gallo's 1991 *Nature* publication admits that he did not discover a new virus."

On the remaining issue — the allocation of royalties from the HIV blood-test patent — Schwartz felt that action was now "imperative."

The government's position hadn't changed since the Reagan days, Schwarz said, and it "wholly ignores Dr. Gallo's 1991 admission, and continues to be based on the now universally abandoned premise that Dr. Gallo independently discovered an AIDS virus different than Pasteur's."

Mike Astrue had determined that reimbursing the Pasteur for past royalties would require an Act of Congress and a special budget appropriation, and the French had scaled back their demand to 75 percent of future royalties, with the remaining 25 percent going to AIDS research. But Schwartz's appeal was about more than money.

"The Clinton Administration," he told Varmus, "need not perpetuate a lie. Failure to act on the part of the U.S. sends a frightful message to the international scientific community: don't cooperate and don't collaborate. By sharing one's discoveries, one runs the risk of appropriation. If one's adversary is a powerful government or scientist, there may be absolutely nothing one can do about it, even if one can prove one's work was appropriated either deliberately or unintentionally. If left uncorrected, the effect this will have is more than just 'chilling'— it will cost lives."[10]

John Dingell's staff had arranged to provide Varmus the same background briefing it gave Harriet Rabb. But when Varmus asked Dingell whether he really needed to meet with Stockton and Hadley, Dingell said he didn't think it was necessary. Varmus promptly canceled the briefing, launching Reid Stuntz into Dingell's office to find out why the chairman had let the NIH director off the hook. Apologizing that he hadn't understood the significance of the briefing, Dingell dialed Varmus on his speakerphone. He was sending his people to NIH after all, Dingell said, and he expected Varmus to receive them.

On a mid-February afternoon in 1994, Peter Stockton, Bruce Chafin, Janina Jaruzelski, Dennis Wilson, and Suzanne Hadley walked into the NIH's Building 1 to find an annoyed-looking Varmus waiting with Harriet Rabb. Stockton began by asking for Varmus's opinion of the appeal board's decision in the Popovic case. "So Varmus immediately said, 'Well, I think it's just fine,'" Hadley said. "'I'm satisfied with the recent decisions. I've read the documents.' Somebody said, 'Just exactly what documents have you read?' 'Well, the Popovic decision.' And it turns out that's the *only* document he's read.

Hasn't read the Richards committee report, hasn't read the offer of proof, absolutely zero. So at this point he begins to preach: 'Well, you have to distinguish between jerks and crooks.'"

"Now he's edging toward the door," Hadley said. "So as he's headed out with his notebook in his hand, Bruce says, 'Look, I want to tell you something. This is in the way of a "heads-up" to you. The subcommittee's doing a report on Gallo, and a decision has been made at the top levels that the current administration's actions will be dealt with in the context of that report. You people have been on board long enough now that your actions or inactions are fair game, and they will be a part of that report.'"

Years before, Varmus himself had spoken to Popovic, "in confidence," about how LAV had become HTLV-3B, and had come away convinced that Popovic "knows what happened." Whatever explanation Popovic had given then, Varmus hadn't passed it on to Dingell's staff, who departed mystified by their icy reception. When Suzanne Hadley called Sam Broder to report on the meeting, Broder offered an explanation:

"'Harold Varmus really hates Gallo,'" Hadley said, quoting Broder. "'And he hates me, too. And he hates you, Hadley, too.' Sam said, 'Harold is a darling of HHS. He's revered. And the way HHS treats the rest of us is like the sisters that have to clean up after the darling sister.' He asked me, 'You know about medieval history?' I said, 'Not very much.' He said, 'Well, they had these ecclesiastical courts, and when one of the priests did a bad thing the other priests would take care of it. And if the secular authorities moved in, they got a lot of gas from the ecclesiastical types. That's what it's like with Harold. Varmus hates Bob Gallo, but he will punish him in his own way, in his own time.'"

Maxime Schwartz and Harold Varmus were about the same age. Both were molecular biologists, and both had been educated at Harvard. Under different circumstances, they might have become close friends. By the end of March Varmus hadn't answered Schwartz's memo of the month before, and Schwartz sent him a copy of Françoise Barré's affidavit recounting her conversation with Popovic.[11]

A few weeks later the French government fired a shot across the Atlantic, consecrating the discovery of the AIDS virus at the Institut Pasteur by issuing a commemorative postage stamp. Schwartz put one on his next letter, reminding Varmus that the trustees of the Franco-American foundation were scheduled to meet again in July. "I would much prefer to see the royalty issue resolved prior to that date," Schwartz said. "I wonder whether we could meet in Washington at one of the dates listed hereafter to discuss this issue further."[12]

When Varmus replied six weeks later, he told Schwartz it was his "considered judgment that no alteration of our shared royalty arrangement is warranted."[13]

"I couldn't believe it," Schwartz said later. "He has taken so long, and now he takes the same position as the previous administration. The next day we talked by phone, and I explained to him why I was utterly shocked by his letter. We had a long discussion. He did not feel at ease. My impression was that he agreed with me, but there was something that prevented him from reacting the way he would like to react. And I explained to him that we can't stay there."

Since replacing Vince DeVita, Sam Broder had defended and protected Gallo. Now there were indications Broder, like DeVita before him, was growing disillusioned. Reportedly horrified by Daniel Zagury's use of Zairian children in his AIDS vaccine research, Broder had ordered Gallo's name removed from the pending HHS patent on Zagury's vaccine. When Suzanne Hadley showed Broder Gallo's statement that the patent had been initiated by Broder himself, Broder exploded. "He said, 'That's bullshit!'" Hadley recalled.[14]

Hadley took advantage of what looked like an opening to remark that while the OSI investigation had focused narrowly on the four *Science* articles, it had turned up evidence that several of Gallo's subsequent articles also contained false statements, including the since-discredited claims to have isolated the AIDS virus in November 1982 and to have had five HIV isolates, including R.F., by February 1983.[15] But the most outlandish claim was in a 1985 *PNAS* paper by Gallo and Zaki Salahuddin, published as the dispute with the Pasteur was beginning to heat up, in which Gallo claimed to have obtained more than a *hundred* AIDS virus isolates "since the fall of 1982."[16]

The paper didn't describe the patients from whom those viruses had come, or give the dates of the isolations. It did, however, state that the "minimum conditions" for calling something an AIDS virus isolate in 1982 and 1983 had included the detection of HTLV-3 proteins, either with the rabbit antiserum or monoclonal antibodies — an impressive achievement, since Sarngadharan hadn't produced the first rabbit antibody until February 1984 and Sasha Arya hadn't made the first monoclonal antibodies until October of that year.[17]

The paper was a political exercise, a pollution of the scientific literature intended to help lay the groundwork for a defense against the French.[c] The ORI wasn't about to open a new misconduct investigation of Gallo without a signed confession. "I'm not going down that road again," Lyle Bivens said, "with anything less than an eight-gauge shotgun." But Sam Broder had the authority to pursue possible misconduct by one of his researchers, and he directed Gallo's boss, Dick Adamson, to bring closure to the questions raised by Dingell's staff.[18] When Gallo couldn't document any isolations of HIV from 1982 or 1983 that met the description in the *PNAS* paper — or any isolations at all prior to the arrival of LAV from Paris — Hadley wasn't surprised.[19] "More of the same old stuff," she said.

During one of the Dingell staff's Friday afternoon visits to the NCI, Broder announced that he had made a decision. It was time for Gallo to leave the NIH. "Sam said, 'Believe me, Bob is going to leave here one way or another,'" Hadley said. "Then he said, 'I'm trying to tell Bob it's time to retire. And if he doesn't, other things are going to happen. As far as I'm concerned, the books can be closed if Bob leaves. But the implications of his leaving will be clear: Bob has beat a rap. There won't be any ticker tape parades.'"

Broder had arranged for Gallo to be approached by an emissary and told that the time had come to go, or else. When Suzanne Hadley asked what else, Broder replied that if Gallo refused to retire he intended to order an NCI investigation of the apparent misrepresentations in the *PNAS* and other papers.

"Sam said, 'I told Bob to his face, "You can't only own the good stuff,"'" Hadley said. "'He said, "The mere fact that 3B equals LAV, in and of itself, requires an apology. Send me the documents that show me where you ever apologized." He said, 'I told Bob, "You've degraded the institute, you've degraded the public and you've degraded reporters by lying to them." I told him, "We owe things to the people of another time. They need to know what things were really like during this era of AIDS research." One of Bob's biggest sins is his overdriven compulsion to claim all the credit and to trace it all to his great intellect.'"

"'And,' said Sam, 'That is not the way it was. He was confused out of his mind. Bob was so thoroughly wrong. The AIDS virus had to fit the retroviruses as he knew them, and he was wrong. He needed to listen to his data, and he did not want to do that.' He said, 'Bob writes all these historical things that have no relationship to the way it really was. I told Bob, "I have not forgiven you for this. People are dying of real diseases, and this is not a game."' He said, 'Frankly, Suzanne, it was a Nobel Prize run. You guys don't talk about that, but I was there, and I know. And frankly, he almost got it. And if he had gotten it, he would have been truly invincible.' It was a very poignant conversation."

On a Sunday afternoon in mid-June of 1993 Gallo called Hadley from Charleston, home of the Medical University of South Carolina, where Peter Fischinger had been hired as vice president for research in hopes he could improve the school's NIH funding. At first Hadley didn't recognize Gallo's voice, which sounded lower in tenor, like a recording played at half-speed.

"He said 'Sam read me the riot act yesterday,'" Hadley recalled. "The words he used were 'brutal' and 'dastardly.' Sam told Bob he'd done a deal with the subcommittee — if Bob left quietly, nothing more would happen." At that moment the hotel operator had interrupted the conversation with the message that someone was waiting for Gallo in the lobby. "He said, 'I'm in Charleston,'" Hadley said, "'so you know who's downstairs.'"

It sounded to Hadley as though Gallo was resigned to leaving. "He wants to meet with me in person," Hadley said, "to find out why this is happening to him. He said, 'We can be adults and talk to each other. You don't need to talk to the director — there are rumors all over town about me being in trouble, I'm being bombarded with calls about my status.' He said, 'If you think I've made so many mistakes that I've hurt the whole system, I can make a different pathway and I don't fear it. I'm willing to make a transition. I don't want NCI or you or anyone else to get hurt. But I'll fight like an animal if I'm not told what it's about.'"

"MUSC courting Gallo, AIDS virus discoverer," the *Charleston Post & Courier* reported two days later, quoting Gallo as saying he was "listening" to offers from the university, and had "cut the umbilical cord with the National Institutes of Health," which under Harold Varmus was "not quite what it used to be." The university's president,

James Edwards, who had served as secretary of energy in the Reagan administration, hoped Gallo would be "working in our lab when he gets the Nobel laureate [*sic*]." Although the university was cutting back its staff for lack of funds, Edwards, evidently under the impression that Gallo was receiving the proceeds from the blood-test patent, didn't think money would be an obstacle. "Gallo's HIV test patent alone brings in millions," the newspaper said, "and his work would quickly pay its own way."[20]

The HHS inspector general had put what HHS investigators had learned about the Gallo case into a thirty-five-page "Investigative Memorandum," a record of a twenty-six-month inquiry undertaken "to determine if any statements made by Dr. Gallo in his patent application of April 1984 and his November 1986 declaration, filed in connection with the interference proceeding, were false."[21]

The IG's memorandum included several items that had never been made public, among them Gallo's admissions that he lied by insisting that it had been "physically impossible" to grow LAV, and that he now remembered from the tripartite meeting in Paris that the Gallo and Pasteur ELISAs were "quite comparable."

The inspector general doubted that "the 'pool' experiment, as described by Gallo/Popovic, had really been done," and noted that "there is no evidence there ever was a 3B isolate independent of LAV." But the most startling revelation was the acknowledgment by the examiner who issued the Gallo blood-test patent that she wouldn't have done so if she had known the Pasteur had already applied.[d]

News of the inspector general's findings broke on a Sunday in June 1994.[22] In France, the Tuesday papers were quoting Maxime Schwartz's pronouncement that a "turning point" had been reached in the Pasteur's nine-year struggle with the Americans.[23] Joe Onek dismissed the report as "filled with an extraordinary number of errors reflecting deliberate factual distortions, scientific illiteracy, and obvious bias"— evidenced, in Onek's opinion, by the IG's failure to mention that LAV_{Lai} had also contaminated Robin Weiss's CBL-1 culture, the virus that was being used by Burroughs-Wellcome to make the British AIDS test.[24]

When Suzanne Hadley saw Onek's statement, she recalled the passing reference in the appeals board's *Popovic* decision to LAV_{Lai}

having contaminated a virus culture in England. "I knew it," Hadley said. "The board got that straight from Gallo and Onek."

Having obtained an audience with Harold Varmus, Maxime Schwartz was about to catch the Concorde when the NIH called to put the meeting on hold, explaining that Varmus wanted to write Schwartz another letter. "I asked them why NIH was backing out," Rob Odle recalled. "They said, 'We think you'll like the second letter better than the meeting.'" Odle hoped so, because if it was anything like the first letter "I'm going straight to NIH and shove it down their throats."

The first letter had been written by the HHS lawyers, and Varmus felt badly when he realized how it had been received in Paris. Since then the inspector general's report had leaked, and Varmus now told Schwartz that, "were I to be persuaded that a change in our current arrangement for distribution of royalties is warranted, I would surely take steps to see that a change is made."[25]

As for the Pasteur's other demand, Varmus recalled that "when we last spoke, you reiterated your wish for an acknowledgment from me appropriate to the current state of knowledge: that the French virus was used by National Institutes of Health scientists in developing the American test kit. I am entirely open to taking steps that appropriately accomplish that goal, which you and I share."

"I didn't really know what to think," Schwartz said. "Obviously there was a doorway slightly open, but just for the official recognition and not much more." But *Nature* quoted a "senior NIH official" confirming that Harold Varmus had "shifted his position markedly" on the question of reparations to the French.[26] According to *Science,* the dispute with the Pasteur was now heading "for a showdown," thanks to an inspector general's report that "reads like a brief for the prosecution in a scientific fraud case."[27]

The annual meeting of the French and American AIDS Foundation was a few days away, and as it had done two years before, the Pasteur intended to introduce a new resolution altering the division of royalties in favor of the French. This time, however, it seemed possible that both sides would vote in favor. Pasteur's most recent demand was for 75 percent of future royalties. When Harriet Rabb called Mike Epstein and Rob Odle with the government's counteroffer, Odle termed it an insult: $200,000 a year, or $1.6 million over the remaining eight years of the patent, a tiny fraction of the $16 million Pasteur was seeking. Rabb's only sweetener would be a public acknowledgment by HHS that HTLV-3B was LAV.

Odle suspected that HHS was "going to screw us on the money and try to make it up to us in the statement." But Rabb wanted Harold Varmus to read the proposed resolution before giving it to Odle, and Varmus had gone off with his family on a bicycle tour of France. "Harriet tells us he's not in his hotel room," Odle said. "It's after midnight in France. I think she's playing games." When the statement finally showed up on Odle's fax, he took back his prediction of a few hours before. "They're going to screw us on both the money *and* the statement," he said.

"The Board of the French & American AIDS Foundation," the resolution read, "takes notice that Roche Molecular Systems concluded in a study published in 1991 that the virus used by the National Institutes of Health in developing its HIV test kit was actually a virus provided by the Institut Pasteur. The Board therefore concludes and RESOLVES that formal acknowledgment be and hereby is made that a virus provided by Institut Pasteur was used by National Institutes of Health scientists who invented the American HIV test kit in 1984."

When Bruce Chafin saw the statement he reached for the phone. The HHS language was impossible, Chafin told Rabb. It didn't begin to acknowledge the breadth of what had happened. Rabb reminded Chafin that, three days before, she had sat in the subcommittee's office while Dingell's staff told her the chairman would be happy as long as the French were happy. If the French were willing to buy the statement, didn't that fulfill Rabb's part of the deal? If the subcommittee now was pushing HHS to make a more forthcoming statement, it was changing signals in midplay.

"Harriet said, 'I knew this was going to happen,'" Chafin recalled. "She said, 'I knew we should have waited for your report. We might as well cancel the Monday meeting.' I told her, 'You didn't hear what we were saying. We want you to do your own deal with the French. We're not going to tell you how much money to give them or what your statement should say. That's not our function. We're an oversight committee. But at the end of the day, when we issue our report, we're going to pass our judgment on how you've handled this matter. And our standards for what you'll have to admit having done are going to be a lot higher than those of the French.'"

It was lunchtime on Saturday in Paris when Odle and Epstein reached Maxime Schwartz, who told them he was ready to sue. Harriet Rabb didn't have anything to add to the offer on the table, except that Harold Varmus hoped to continue counting Schwartz among his colleagues. Thinking Rabb had given him "something to work with," Odle suggested that since both Schwartz and Varmus were in France, perhaps they should have a conversation one-on-one.

Having tracked down Varmus at his hotel in Nice, Schwartz explained that Pasteur's bottom-line position was a 60–40 split of all future royalties, which worked out to an extra $1 million a year over the eight remaining years of the patent. Varmus replied that HHS's position, that each side was entitled to an equal share of the royalties, wasn't likely to change. "But it was a friendly talk," Schwartz said, "and it was clear that we would have a new discussion when we get back to the States. I didn't believe that nothing would happen. It was my impression that we would get some kind of agreement. But I still did not know whether on Monday morning we would have to announce that we are going to court."

As a member of the foundation's board, Gallo would be entitled to vote on the royalty question at the Monday board meeting. But when Gallo called Hadley over the weekend, he seemed less concerned about the reallocation of royalties than the statement being negotiated between HHS and the Pasteur.

"He was really bouncing all over the place," Hadley recalled. "He said, 'How can we go into this meeting with these people who have blood on their hands?' He said, 'Monday they'll probably feel good. I'll take more hits — maybe they'll get more money.' He's been in France. He said he had heard about Peter Stockton yelling at the NIH director that Gallo had harassed Barré-Sinoussi. He said she's a friend of his, and she's emotionally unstable, that she's been given a professorship and then it was taken away. I said, 'That's simply not true.'

"He said, 'It's not important, none of this is important ethically. Maybe we fudged a bit, but there was no cheating. It doesn't matter what I told a reporter. It's true I didn't look at Mika's books.' He said, 'You want to make a Saint Francis out of me, you want to hold me to a higher standard. I'm not three standard deviations above anybody else. I never deliberately deceived anyone in my entire life.'"

On Sunday afternoon, June 10, Maxime Schwartz and Harold Varmus landed at Dulles International Airport twenty minutes apart.

Despite attempts by Odle and Epstein to arrange a small dinner, Varmus went straight to his house, where he was joined by Harriet Rabb, Rabb's deputy, Beverly Dennis, and Phil Lee, an old colleague of Don Francis from the University of California who had replaced Jim Mason as the assistant HHS secretary.

Schwartz had been asked to call Varmus when he reached his hotel in Bethesda, and he placed the call with Raymond Dedonder, Alain Gallochat, and Mike Epstein looking on. But the Varmus camp had nothing yet to report. Over glasses of ice water — all the Varmuses had to offer their guests after two weeks in Europe — Beverly Dennis suggested increasing the Pasteur's future royalties to a point where each side would receive the same amount of money over the seventeen-year lifetime of the patent. That way, Varmus could present the reallocation of royalties as the rectification of a historical imbalance, rather than reparations for past sins.

It was all about appearances anyway, since the money was no longer enough to matter to either side. When Varmus returned Schwartz's call, he reported that HHS was willing to agree that the Pasteur would begin receiving two-thirds of what was left of the royalty pool after each side retained an initial 20 percent — a reallocation that should provide the French with about $6 million over the next eight years.

Schwartz sounded receptive, but he wanted the government's statement to include some linkage, to make the point clearly that the royalties were being reallocated *because* Gallo used the French virus. Varmus was equally adamant that there be no linkage, that the money and the acknowledgment be treated separately, lest the government appear to be admitting it had done something wrong. It was the HHS public affairs officer, Victor Zonana, who came up with the solution. Don't link them, Zonana said, but don't unlink them either. Just leave the question open, since everybody will make the connection anyway.

After midnight, Harriet Rabb and Mike Epstein talked for the last time. "Harriet said, 'Why don't we just leave it ambiguous?'" Epstein recalled. "'Let each side characterize it the way they want?'" With the board meeting less than ten hours away, the Pasteur's only choice was to accept Rabb's terms or take the government back to court. "I'll convince the client," Epstein told Rabb.

Monday morning, July 11, 1994, broke hot and clear in Bethesda. As they had two years before, the members of the board of the French and American AIDS Foundation trudged up the rolling NIH greensward to Stone House. Bernadine Healy, who had presided at the last such meeting, was far away in Cleveland, hosting TV health-care infomercials following a resounding defeat in her quest for the Republican senatorial nomination from Ohio.[28]

Schwartz, Raymond Dedonder, and Epstein, sitting in for Ira Mill-stein, voted in favor of the resolution. So did Montagnier, who arrived late. "My secretary put 9:30," Montagnier explained, "but the meeting was 8:30." The four American board members, Harold Varmus, Phil Lee, a Public Health Service lawyer named Dick Riseberg, and Gallo, made it unanimous — Gallo voting "aye" under orders from Varmus, then moving to include his own statement in the record: "I do not believe," it began, "that there is any truthful, new, substantive infor-mation since the 1987 agreement which bears upon the history of our respective scientific contributions."[e]

A few of the reporters who had covered Margaret Heckler's news conference a decade before were in the overflow crowd that gathered at Stone House for the postmeeting news conference. Gallo, appear-ing for an instant in the hallway, vanished just as Varmus began to speak, leaving a glowering Joe Onek behind.

"This is a pleasant occasion for us," said Varmus, in shirtsleeves but wearing an unaccustomed necktie. "I'm pleased to announce that as part of the meeting of the French and American AIDS Foundation, an agreement was reached today to put an end to the Institute Pas-teur's request for additional patent royalties from the sale of HIV test kits."

Varmus turned the microphone over to Schwartz, who declared how gratified *he* was "by what happened this morning. I am pleased, first, because there is today an official acknowledgment by the U.S. government, the secretary of health, that the virus which was used to develop the American AIDS test kit was in fact a virus which had been isolated at the Institut Pasteur and sent to the United States. This demonstrates and acknowledges the fact that all test kits which have been sold in the world have in fact been using a virus which had been isolated at the Institut Pasteur."

Schwartz had the grace not to mention that the acknowledgment had come after many years of denials by the NIH and HHS that had cost the French millions of francs to overturn. But he was also pleased, Schwartz said, "because a decision has been taken to change the distribution of royalties in a way that is much more fair than it was before. For the past seven years or so, the distribution was such that the NIH or HHS were receiving more royalties than we were. So now, for the second half-life of the patents, the Pasteur Institute will receive more royalties than the Department of Health and Human Services here."

"You said you hoped this puts things behind us," a reporter told Varmus. "Do you think that this is the end of this? That Congress is going to back off, Dingell's going to back off, everybody's going to back off and say, 'Now let's move ahead'? Or do we still have more episodes to come?"

"Well," Varmus replied, "I don't pretend to speak for all. But I'm pleased to receive a letter from Maxime saying that as far as they're concerned this is the end of deliberations over the patent component.[f] The problem of HIV and AIDS is a very big problem, and there are many components to it. If you're referring to disputes between the Pasteur and the NIH, my hope is that with the camaraderie that exists between the two of us, and today's proceedings, and the feeling of good fellowship that exists at the moment, we can say with some confidence that this will be the end."

Phillip Hilts of the *New York Times* wondered whether the inspector general's report had "any influence on this decision or not?"

"Very little," Varmus replied, but he was smiling.

Another reporter wanted to know the significance of HHS's acknowledgment that scientists at the NIH used a virus provided to them by Institut Pasteur to invent the American HIV test kit.[29]

"From my perspective," Varmus said, "it's simply placing it onto the record of this organization that we acknowledge the results of that test and the publication that ensued."

"From *our* perspective," Schwartz interrupted, "it's a major step. Because all there was so far was just a letter which had been sent in a scientific journal which is not for the general public. There was never so far an official acknowledgment by authorities in this country that the virus was coming from the Pasteur. So for us it is a very important point."

"Is the acknowledgment really more important than the money?" someone asked.

"I would say yes," Schwartz replied. "It's important that truth is known."

Another reporter wanted to know whether it was possible to put a few questions to Gallo and Montagnier.

Varmus looked around. Montagnier was standing by the door, but Varmus couldn't see Gallo anywhere.

"Dr. Gallo is no longer here," Varmus said.

EPILOGUE

"Rather Does the Truth Ennoble All"

Like the settlement of 1987, the settlement of 1994 was front-page news in the United States and abroad. This time, however, the story was being cast as a clear victory for the French.[1]

"U.S., France settle AIDS virus dispute," reported the *Chicago Tribune*, which had set the day's events in motion five years before. "Key patent on AIDS to favor the French," announced the *New York Times*. "U.S. admits French role in HIV test kit," the *Los Angeles Times* declared. "US climbs down in feud with French over Aids research," said the *Financial Times*. And, from *Le Monde*, "*Les États-Unis reconnaissent que le virus du sida a été découvert à l'Institut Pasteur de Paris*" (The United States recognizes that the AIDS virus was discovered at the Pasteur Institute of Paris).

"They broadcast it for a full day on the BBC," Abraham Karpas said, "that the U.S. has acknowledged it was the same virus. Pity they had to wait for nine years. They could have heard it from me in 1985."

Over a mid-August lunch in a nearly deserted Paris brasserie, Maxime Schwartz insisted that he had been emotionally prepared to take the United States government back to court. In deciding at the last moment to accept the American offer, Schwartz had assured Harold Varmus that the Institut Pasteur considered the matter closed. "The story is over," Schwartz said, then he paused for a moment. "Except there is the Dingell committee."

Françoise Barré's declaration about her disputed conversation with Mika Popovic had never been made public. Neither had the

Secret Service examination of Popovic's and Betsy Read's lab notes. But all those and more were in the hands of John Dingell's staff in November of 1994, when the Democratic Party lost control of the House of Representatives for the first time in forty years.

Dingell was reelected in his safe Detroit district, but he was no longer chairman of the Committee on Energy and Commerce. "After fourteen years of unchecked expansion," said the *New York Times,* "the empire of Representative John David Dingell Jr. is being dismantled. Like a plump Thanksgiving turkey, Mr. Dingell's House Energy and Commerce Committee is being readied to be carved up and dished out. Gleeful Republicans have begun to disassemble its muscular investigative unit and pass around its meaty legislative authority."[2]

Al Gilman, the most outspoken member of the National Academy panel that had accused Robert Gallo of "intellectual recklessness" and "essentially immoral" behavior, had just won the Nobel Prize. But with the Dingell investigation having come to an abrupt halt, Gallo had reason to rejoice. "Congressman Dingell is out of his chairmanship and all problems are over," Gallo wrote Francis Ford Coppola, whose acquaintance with Gallo had inspired a screenplay, *The Cure* by Diane Johnston, about the Gallo-Pasteur dispute. "The true story," Gallo assured Coppola, "is so much stranger and wilder than any fiction."[3]

For months the whole story, the 267-page "Institutional response to the HIV blood test patent dispute and related matters," had been emerging from Suzanne Hadley's word-processor.[4] Like a police detective laying out pieces of evidence on a table, Hadley had assembled what looked to her like an airtight case that Gallo must have known HTLV-3B was LAV long before he acknowledged it. But in assigning culpability the Dingell Report spared no one, starting with the Department of Health and Human Services.

"HHS did its best to cover up the wrong-doing," the report said. "Meanwhile, the failure of the entire scientific establishment to take any meaningful action left the disposition of scientific truth to bureaucrats and lawyers, with neither the expertise nor the will essential to the task. Because of the continuing HHS cover-up, it was not until the Subcommittee investigation that the true facts were known, and the breadth and depth of the cover-up was revealed."

In case anyone wondered why a congressional subcommittee had spent nearly five years sorting out the discovery of the AIDS virus, the report explained that "the very endurance of these issues shows that they are important."

"Without the investigations," it said, "without an authoritative accounting of the facts, the falsehoods would have remained as the definitive record. The people and the scientific community deserved to know the truth. One of the most remarkable and regrettable aspects of the institutional response to the defense of *Gallo et al.* is how readily public service and science apparently were subverted into defending the indefensible."

A number of prominent scientists, including Harvard's John Edsall, urged Dingell to make the document public in the interregnum between the election and the swearing-in of the new Congress.[5] But there hadn't been time for the chairman or the other subcommittee members to read the report, much less vote on whether to release it, before Dingell was replaced as chairman by Virginia Republican named Thomas Bliley.[6]

With Dingell dethroned, the report was turned over to the subcommittee's new Republican staff and locked away in some congressional archive, never to be released under the imprimatur of the United States Congress. But Gallo predicted that the report would soon be leaked.[7]

"US accused of 'cover up' in defence of Gallo claims," declared *Nature,* having obtained a bootleg copy of what Joe Onek termed "a classic example of 'lame duck lunacy'"[8] and Bernadine Healy dismissed as John Dingell's "final spasm." But *The Lancet,* which had actually read the report, concluded that "the carefully documented piece of work is difficult to ignore."

After a brief stint as dean of the medical school at Ohio State University, Bernadine Healy found her way back to Washington, this time as head of a troubled American Red Cross, operating under a court-ordered consent decree with the Food and Drug Administration and struggling with fiscal deficits traceable to its blood-banking business in the age of AIDS.[9] "This is exactly the kind of person the Red Cross needs as its president," said the chairman of its board of governors in announcing Healy's appointment.[10]

Within hours of the September 11, 2001, hijackings that killed thousands in the World Trade Center and the Pentagon, Bernadine Healy was on TV, with hourly appeals to Americans to donate their blood and money to the Red Cross "in this time of unprecedented need." Healy soon found herself forced out of her $450,000-a-year job by the ARC board of governors — unhappy, according to the *Washington Post,* with her surprise decision to set up the fund-raising effort, which garnered some $700 million in pledges and so much unneeded blood that some had to be thrown out. It was typical, said the *Post,* of Healy's "assertive, go-it-alone leadership, including a tendency to act on important matters without first seeking board approval." Other relief organizations were reportedly angered by the Red Cross's refusal to coordinate its post–September 11 efforts with theirs, and victims' families were shocked to learn that the Red Cross was holding back $200 million of the money donated for their benefit for "future disasters."

Abbott Laboratories, still selling its HIV blood test to the Red Cross, was hit with a $100 million fine — the largest ever imposed by the FDA — as punishment for what the agency said were repeated failures by Abbott to bring its manufacturing of hundreds of different diagnostic kits, including the AIDS blood test, into line with federal regulations. Inventories of scores of Abbott kits were ordered destroyed by the FDA, which feared they might produce false positive or false negative diagnoses.[11]

After nearly three decades of terrorizing Pentagon colonels, senior civil servants, and captains of industry in the name of better government, Peter Stockton retired to run a bed-and-breakfast and grow flowers in the Virginia countryside. Suzanne Hadley remained on the NIH payroll, but she never again set foot on the NIH campus, having been granted a permanent reassignment to George Washington University as a visiting associate professor of psychiatry, where she co-directed a program on medical ethics.

Mikulas Popovic, claiming the misconduct investigations had cost him four years of salaried employment and legal fees of $350,000, sued Hadley and the Office of Research Integrity for $5 million.[12] According to Popovic, by failing to conduct the investigation "in a reasonable, fair, thorough, and prompt manner," the OSI had violated his civil rights, invaded his privacy, and inflicted "severe emotional stress" on himself and his family. After sixteen months of wrangling between Popovic's lawyers and the government, the presiding federal judge dismissed Popovic's complaint.

"In the white hot glare of the international controversy surrounding discovery of the AIDS virus," the judge said, "the record is clear that NIH made an overall reasonable attempt to look into serious allegations of scientific misconduct. However emotionally distressing and expensive the investigation may have been for Popovic, nothing occurred in the proceedings that exposes the Defendants to civil liability after the fact."[13]

Among the appointees to a new government commission created to propose changes in the federal government's definition of scientific misconduct was a profoundly disillusioned Priscilla Schaffer. After eighteen months of hearings and debate, the commission recommended replacing the existing definition — "fabrication, falsification, plagiarism, or other practices that seriously deviate from those that are commonly accepted within the scientific community"— with a broader and more realistic definition of "significant misbehavior that improperly appropriates the intellectual property or contributions of others, that intentionally impedes the progress of research, or that risks corrupting the scientific record or compromising the integrity of scientific practices."[14] Five years later the proposed definition still hadn't been adopted, and it appeared certain to be watered down.

The Office of Research Integrity, shaken by the appeals board's reversal of Thereza Imanishi-Kari's misconduct finding in the Baltimore case,[15] continued to find misconduct in about a third of the cases it opened, but fewer cases were being opened every year.[a] Lyle Bivens, who had called the Baltimore case "as strong as any we've had in the office," retired from the federal government.

Imanishi-Kari's acquittal represented another victory for Joe Onek. But with the number of misconduct cases on the decline, Onek abandoned private practice for a job in the Justice Department. Under Bivens's successor, Chris Pascal, the ORI's mission was "refocused" to include "affirmative steps" to prevent fraud before it happened, by educating government and university scientists on "the responsible conduct of research."[16]

Following his retirement from the Centers for Disease Control, Don Francis joined the San Francisco biotech company Genentech, which was developing what Francis considered a promising candidate vaccine for AIDS. When the NIH, dubious about the vaccine's merits, decided against funding the large trial necessary to show whether the vaccine actually worked, Francis convinced Genentech to spin off the project into a new company, VaxGen, with Francis as CEO and Bob

Nowinski as chairman. After raising $20 million from private sources, including Hollywood luminaries who remembered Francis from *And the Band Played On,* VaxGen began testing the vaccine in thousands of HIV-negative homosexuals and drug users in the United States and Thailand.[17]

Harold Varmus headed off to New York City and the presidency of the Memorial Sloan-Kettering Cancer Center. Before departing Bethesda, Varmus had given journal editors heart attacks[18] by proposing the creation of an NIH-sponsored Internet site where any researcher in the world could post his latest data,[19] a plan that would effectively end the journals' stranglehold on the biomedical literature. Had such a thing existed in 1983, the world would have known about LAV much sooner than it did. The lessons of the Gallo case hadn't been lost on Varmus, who also imposed new regulations governing the sharing of NIH discoveries with other laboratories, discouraging patents on those discoveries, banning collaboration agreements that imposed "excessive" editorial control on their recipients, and providing an exemption for research materials whose primary usefulness was to further scientific discovery — materials like HTLV-3B and H-9.[20]

John Maddox, knighted by the queen, retired after more than twenty years as the world's most important scientist.[21] With unaccustomed leisure, Sir John had written a book on scientific discovery that took an unexpected swipe at Gallo.[22]

"The hunt for HIV and for remedies against infection," Maddox observed, "brought out the worst in the research community's innate competitiveness — not so much for riches as for fame." According to Maddox, Gallo "first sought to diminish the discovery of the virus by Luc Montagnier, a professor at the Pasteur Institute in Paris, and then to give his own comparable work the ring of authenticity. . . . This corrosive incident has reflected badly not only on those concerned, but on the research community as a whole."

By publishing Gallo's bogus claim to the first isolation of HIV, Maddox had done more than his share to lend Gallo's work the ring of authenticity. But Simon Wain-Hobson, now a full professor at the Pasteur, had sensed the pro-Gallo winds at *Nature* beginning to shift before Maddox's retirement. Wain-Hobson recalled a dinner with Maddox in Paris "over a very nice bottle" a few days after HHS had agreed to the French demand for future royalties. When the talk turned to Gallo, Maddox had "confessed that Gallo had initially charmed the pants off him, but that he got wise around 1986. When I pointed out that it had been hard to see this in the news pages of *Nature,* he suggested that *Nature* would have to 'stick the knife in Bob' a bit more."

When *Science* surveyed France's "hottest AIDS researchers," Wain-Hobson made the short list of seven.[23] Not included was Jean-Claude Chermann, who had spent much of his exile in Marseille testing a peptide, *THF Gamma 2,* that Chermann hoped would prove to be a treatment for AIDS. When it didn't work, the French biomedical research agency, INSERM, decided to close his lab, and Chermann took a job with a pharmaceutical company.

Also missing from the list was Luc Montagnier, now dividing his time between his Pasteur laboratory and New York City, where he had accepted an endowed professorship at Queens College and a promise of $30 million to found his own AIDS research institute.[24] "New York is the center of the disease," Montagnier said in explaining his decision.[25] But the college had been able to raise less than $5 million, and the center never opened. "You cannot just raise money on a name," Montagnier admitted. "My priority now is to get some research going and show we can do the work."[26]

With Gallo gone from NIH, Abraham Karpas had more time to devote to science, and he had come up with a genuine breakthrough — the first human myeloma cell line, Karpas 707H, capable of producing the monoclonal antibodies that were becoming the new vogue in cancer treatment.[27] Cesar Milstein, who shared the Nobel Prize for having worked out how to produce monoclonal antibodies in mice a quarter-century before, proclaimed that "Dr. Karpas has solved a puzzle which has bedeviled laboratories across the world for over twenty years."

Despite Karpas's best efforts, Robin Weiss, now heading an institute at University College, London, was finally elected to the Royal Society. Reviewing Montagnier's memoirs[28] for *Nature,* Weiss observed that "For a victorious general renowned throughout the world," Montagnier remained surprisingly bitter, portraying himself "as a prescient though misunderstood scientist who, almost alone, saw the danger of the AIDS agent contaminating the blood supply but was ignored." The memoir Weiss wanted to read, but doubted would ever be written, was "that of Françoise Barré-Sinoussi, the Rosalind Franklin of HIV."[29]

Sam Broder resigned the directorship of the National Cancer Institute, a casualty of "personality differences" with Harold Varmus and withering criticism of the NCI's bumbling response to the

Chicago Tribune's disclosure of the worst instance of fraud by an NCI-funded researcher in the history of breast cancer research.[30] Hillary Clinton was said to be foremost among those who thought it was time for Broder to go. When Broder telephoned Harold Varmus to say he was leaving the NCI, Varmus was too busy to take the call. Broder left a one-word message with Varmus's secretary: "Adios."

With the nearly simultaneous departures of Dick Adamson and Bruce Chabner, the last of the NCI's old guard, the way was cleared for a revamping of the National Cancer Institute, whose basic structure and focus had scarcely changed since the early days of the War on Cancer. The surprise choice as Broder's successor was Richard Klausner, one of Bernadine Healy's erstwhile Wise Men and the first non–cancer researcher in history to lead the NCI. Three years into his tenure, Klausner, who had shifted more resources toward cancer prevention while investing heavily in potentially revolutionary genetic approaches to cancer treatment, was being acclaimed by many as the best director in the institute's history.

Broder had warned Gallo that the Laboratory of Tumor Cell Biology was soon to become extinct, and on the day of Broder's departure Gallo requested permission to retire from the Commissioned Corps of the U.S. Public Health Service. "I should have done it seven years ago," Gallo said. "If I'd made the move at that time, I think a lot of the problems I went through wouldn't have happened. They certainly wouldn't have happened without a lot of counterpunching."[31] Mal Martin, just elected to the National Academy, agreed with Gallo for once. "If he'd done it years ago," Martin said, "he'd have been left with a little bit more honor, instead of leaving as a disgraced person."

Now that Gallo was soon to be without a job, the only expressions of interest were from a handful of third-rate institutions: Gallo's alma mater, the Jefferson Medical College, Virginia Commonwealth University, and Peter Fischinger's Medical University of South Carolina. Gallo appeared headed for Virginia when the governor of Maryland, Parris Glendening, whose brother had died of AIDS, launched a personal "full-court press" to bring Gallo to the University of Maryland in Baltimore.[32] Despite the hourlong commute, Gallo liked the idea of working in "a very important city in the history of American medicine." But like Montagnier and Robin Weiss, he wanted his own institute. "If place 'A' comes up with three times the amount of money as place 'B,'" Gallo said, "there's no way I can go to place 'B.'"

The state of Maryland had no money in its budget to finance AIDS research. But Glendening put together a $9 million package from a "Sunny Day" fund intended to assist companies in relocating to Maryland.[33] Another $3 million in economic development money earmarked for inner-city Baltimore carried the day. The governor and the mayor of Baltimore explained that Gallo's new Institute of Human Virology,[b] a renovated department store warehouse in downtown Baltimore, was really an investment in the city's future. Not only would the Gallo institute create jobs, it would generate income from the sale of the biotechnology products that were certain to be invented there.

It was also Glendening's hope that the IHV would "catapult" the University of Maryland, which had languished for decades in the shadow of Johns Hopkins, to "a worldwide leadership position" in the biotechnology industry. Not everyone shared Glendening's vision, including several prominent members of the Baltimore AIDS community. "The money could have been better spent to help AIDS assistance workers do their jobs," said Lynda Dee, a lawyer and director of AIDS Action Baltimore. "The mayor hasn't spent a dime on HIV throughout his administration. It's almost a smack in the face for him to cough up $3 million. I'm still waiting for Dr. Gallo to do something for AIDS. I've seen a lot of self-promotion and never any results."[34]

Gallo's salary would be $300,000 a year, higher than all but two members of the university's medical faculty, not counting his annual $100,000 in patent royalties. Suzanne Hadley was astounded when she learned that Gallo had invited Mika Popovic to join his institute as a full professor of medicine. "What does Mika know that's so important to Bob?" Hadley wondered. "That he could leverage it into a job after everything that's gone on?"

With the NCI's approval, as Gallo departed Bethesda he took with him a gift from the taxpayers: $50,000 worth of scientific equipment and computers and the furniture from his NCI office, including "one executive style desk, one leather chair, one credenza, one matching (rosewood) file cabinet, one book case, one conference table with eight chairs, five wooden display cases, one metal display case, one three-piece sectional sofa and one side table."[35]

Leaving NIH, Gallo complained that "years of my life and of my work have been lost. I don't know what, scientifically, we would have done if we didn't lose those years. And essentially we lost them."[36] But Gallo hadn't returned any tax dollars from his laboratory's budget,[c] and even while the investigations were at their peak Gallo had continued to lead the world's AIDS researchers in the sheer number of articles published, nearly two hundred in four years, fifty more than his closest competitor.[37]

But every road down which Gallo had searched for an AIDS cure had been a dead end. Gallo had nominated HHV-6 as a potential cofactor in AIDS,[38] as well several blood cell cancers.[39] HHV-6, which didn't have anything to do with AIDS or cancer, had turned out to be a ubiquitous virus that infected nearly everyone;[40] the only medical condition with which it appeared to be associated was a childhood rash called roseola.[41] The unidentified compound Gallo had touted "that wipes out the Kaposi's sarcoma in a way I have never seen before" turned out to be an old drug, SP-PG, a relative of another failed AIDS treatment, dextran sulfate. When SP-PG was tested in patients with Kaposi's sarcoma, it didn't have any therapeutic value at all.[42]

During the Popovic appeal hearing, the NCI had issued a six-page news release trumpeting Gallo's work on several other potential AIDS treatments, existing drugs like hydroxyurea and new ones with exotic names like GEM-91 and SLWDQ.[43] After a *New York Times* story about Gallo's research with hydroxyurea, AIDS patients had begun clamoring for the compound.[44] But when Gallo submitted a paper to *Nature* reporting that hydroxyurea could prevent HIV from reproducing in a test tube, it hadn't been published. Another hydroxyurea paper, sent to *The Lancet,* had ended up in Dani Bolognesi's *AIDS Research and Human Retroviruses.*

Like SP-PG, hydroxyurea had nothing to offer AIDS patients.[45] Neither did GEM-91, a short strand of HIV DNA, whose testing in AIDS patients Gallo had heralded as "a new and important chapter of clinical research and therapy for AIDS." On the heels of GEM-91 had come another apparent breakthrough, SLWDQ, a discovery by Daniel Zagury's son, Jean-François, working as a postdoc in Gallo's lab.

Gallo declared that SLWDQ, a short string of amino acids, "explains the pathogenesis of HIV infection." In submitting the manuscript to *Nature,* he had predicted that it would be "among the most important in AIDS research since 1984." When the SLWDQ paper was rejected, Gallo submitted it himself to *PNAS,* where it eventually appeared in print — only to be quickly forgotten.

According to the *Baltimore Sun,* as part of his deal with the state of

Maryland Gallo was "expected to attract private investors who would establish a private company that would market products spawned in laboratories run by Dr. Gallo and colleagues."[46] A week before the Maryland legislature was due to vote on his institute's budget, Gallo announced his discovery of "the long sought-after suppressor factors which block HIV infection."[47] Without mentioning that the existence of the suppressor factors had first been proposed years before by Jay Levy, Gallo remarked that many labs had been "intensively working for years in an effort to find the chemical nature of these factors and to purify them."[48]

Levy had published a number of papers on something he called CAF, for cellular antiviral factor. But he hadn't managed to isolate CAF. Now, after "Levy's eleven years of talk," Gallo claimed to have found the suppression factor — or, rather, factors: a triad of biochemicals, known as chemokines, which direct white blood cells to infected areas of the body. These particular chemokines, Gallo said, blocked the replication of the AIDS virus. Levy dismissed Gallo's claim out of hand. In searching for CAF, Levy said, he had already tested, and rejected, the very chemokines Gallo now claimed to have discovered.

If the subtleties of HIV regulators were lost on the Maryland legislature, the headlines generated by Gallo's announcement were not.[d] According *Business Week,* Gallo had opened "a whole new avenue for thinking about how to control HIV."[49] *Newsweek* thought that "rarely in fifteen years of AIDS research have lab findings held such promise."[50] *Science,* where Gallo's chemokine paper had appeared, voted it the "Breakthrough of the Year," and predicted that chemokines "may one day blossom into new treatments or even vaccines." Attempting to set the record straight, Harold Varmus declared in a letter to *Science* that it was not Gallo, but an NCI scientist named Ed Berger, who explained how chemokines suppressed HIV and had made the "pivotal finding."[51]

His well-timed discovery in hand, Gallo appeared in person to convince the Maryland legislature that he was worth an eight-figure investment of the taxpayers' money. "Our group is doing more with one hand tied behind our back than any other group in the world," Gallo told the legislators. As for who had discovered the AIDS virus, "it is nonsense to talk about relative credit. Historians will decide that."[52]

It emerged at the hearing that the real cost of the Gallo institute to the taxpayers would be not $12 million, but $20 million. Even so, state finance analysts predicted that by 1999 the IHV would be "largely self-supporting." The AIDS blood test had earned some $40 million in royalties, and Gallo had "expressed confidence that the institute will generate research findings not unlike his previous efforts."[53]

Dazzled by the prospect of patent royalties and biotech spin-offs, the legislators approved the appropriation, though with the stipulation that, "given the seriousness of the ethical concerns raised" about Gallo's previous research, the University of Maryland should "be sensitive to those issues and take actions it deems appropriate to assure the public that its reputation for high scientific standards will be maintained."[54] The two legislators who chaired the committees that had passed on Gallo's appropriation were promptly installed on the board of advisers of the institute they had just funded, joining Jim Wyngaarden, Bernadine Healy, Barbara Culliton, and Robert K. Gray, who had become Gallo's chief fund-raiser after resigning as chairman of Hill & Knowlton.[e]

The following month, when *Time* magazine picked its Man of the Year for AIDS, the choice was David Ho of the Aaron Diamond AIDS Research Center in New York City, credited with delivering the first good news about AIDS in more than a decade: a new class of drugs, called protease inhibitors, that eliminated HIV from the circulation by disabling the enzyme that plays a crucial role in the manufacture of new virus copies.[55] "After fifteen years of horror, denial and despair," said *Time,* "science may finally be turning the tide on AIDS." Gallo, "famous for his temper and his contempt for authority," was among the also-rans.[56]

Three years after its creation, the Institute of Human Virology had ninety employees, far short of the 350 jobs Gallo had pledged to create.[57] Nor had it become self-supporting. Gallo had formed a succession of paper companies, with names like Human Virology, Inc., Virex, Omega Biotherapies, and GBR Scientific, but they had lain fallow, with no discoveries to sell. Despite Bob Gray's efforts to tap major AIDS contributors in Los Angeles and New York, private donors had anted up barely half a million dollars. Thanks to funding extensions by the legislature, nearly half the institute's money was still coming from the state of Maryland. "In light of what we were told at the outset," one state senator said, "I think that we've been more than generous on this project."[58]

Like Montagnier, Gallo had fallen into eclipse, rarely quoted in the newspapers or seen on television. Their surprise appearance together, in Boston in 1998, to accept a joint award from a private foundation, prompted the *Boston Globe* to suggest that the occasion "might clear the way for Gallo and Montagnier to share ultimately in a Nobel Prize."[59]

The Nobel buzz became audible when Gallo was accorded the Paul Ehrlich Prize, Germany's top scientific honor, conferred by the first German researcher to receive HTLV-3B and H-9. The buzz intensified when the Ehrlich Prize was followed by an essential precursor for any Nobel candidate, an honorary doctorate from the Karolinska Institute in Stockholm,[60] now directed by Gallo's Swedish friend, Hans Wigzell.

But the buzz was all for nothing, and the Nobel for medicine had gone to three other Americans. As the millennium arrived, Gallo was publishing mostly by communicating his own papers to *PNAS*, or in his own institute's new bimonthly, the *Journal of Human Virology*, of which Gallo was founder and consulting editor.[61] Gallo hadn't published a research article in *Science* for more than four years,[62] and nothing in *Nature* since a 1995 report that a protein found in the urine of pregnant women appeared to cure Kaposi's sarcoma in mice.[63]

The protein, called hCG, had been introduced by Gallo with predictable hype, as possibly "the first effective treatment for Kaposi's sarcoma in AIDS patients."[64] According to *Newsweek*, it was "an open secret in the AIDS research community that Gallo's lab is in hot pursuit" of hCG's effects on the AIDS virus itself. "If Gallo's next study of hCG and AIDS is as stunning as the buzz among researchers suggests," *Newsweek* said, "then Kaposi's will loom even larger in AIDS history."[65]

Other groups reported being unable to reproduce important parts of Gallo's chemokine work,[66] and when AIDS clinicians rushed to try hCG in their patients, it hadn't worked at all.[67] Four years after announcing the discovery of hCG, Gallo conceded he had been wrong. The active ingredient in his preparation wasn't hCG after all. It was something he couldn't identify.[68]

During its first five years of life, the Institute for Human Virology hadn't come up with any marketable discoveries. "We haven't seen any payback yet. And we're getting a little testy," said one of the Maryland legislators who had voted to fund Gallo's institute for a three-year period that was about to become six. Gallo, who didn't remember any three-year limit on his public funding, dismissed such criticisms as "ridiculous." His institute, Gallo said, provided "international visibility to the city and the state."[69]

To make up the shortfall from the impending loss of state money Gallo turned to "sponsored research," a euphemism for deals with pharmaceutical companies — including one contract, according to CBS News, to develop a blood test for the malady of the moment, mad cow disease. In case some viewers hadn't recognized Gallo's name, CBS identified him as "the same man who discovered HIV."[70]

Gallo launched an urgent search for the mystery molecule he now called hCG Associated Factor, or HAF, but it hardly mattered.[f] A new generation of molecular biologists, many of them working for companies like Genentech, ImClone, and Sugen, was using computers to design monoclonal antibodies and other exotic proteins that were recording dramatic rates of remission in Kaposi's sufferers and other cancer patients.[71]

Molecular medicine was moving forward at lightning speed — "the beginning of the end" for cancer, said David Golde, who had replaced Vince DeVita as physician-in-chief at Sloan Kettering after DeVita moved to the Yale Cancer Center. The classical laboratory scientists, with their pipettes and flasks, were being left behind. "The older generation in AIDS research," observed John Moore, "their place in the sun is going, or gone in some cases, and they hanker for their youth. Tough luck."[72]

Some intractable cancers already were being cured by the new molecular drugs — one, called STI571, had racked up a near-100 percent cure rate for chronic myelogenous leukemia.[73] But there were no comparable advances in AIDS. Although the AIDS death rate had slowed following the introduction of protease inhibitors, epidemiologists noted that the fall coincided with a sharp drop-off, ten years before, in the rate of new HIV infections — ten years being the average latency for AIDS. The protease inhibitors, for which there had been so much hope, did reduce, or even eliminate, detectable HIV in the blood of many patients. But they didn't eradicate HIV entirely, and when patients stopped taking the drugs the virus came back.

By the century's turn eighteen million people worldwide had perished from AIDS. But not much more was known about the disease, or the virus that caused it, than a decade before. Why HIV gave rise to Kaposi's sarcoma, or infections with relatively rare microbes like

Pneumocystis carinii — but not other fatal cancers or diseases — still wasn't understood. Neither was the precise mechanism by which HIV killed T-4 cells, or even the complete functions of all of the virus's nine genes. Twenty years after Mike Gottlieb reported the first cases of AIDS, the most important advances in AIDS research remained the discovery of the virus and the invention of the blood antibody test.[74]

Gallo still credited himself with "the independent discovery" of the AIDS virus,[75] but his place in history varied according to the source. To the *Irish Times,* he was "the doctor who first identified the AIDS virus and developed a test for it."[76] *Forbes* thought Gallo was "the man who codiscovered the HIV virus."[77] In the *Washington Post,* Gallo was remembered as the researcher who "published key papers linking the retrovirus now known as HIV to the disease."[78] The best accolade *Science* could muster was "credited with speeding the development of the HIV blood test."[79]

Not long after settling himself in Baltimore, Gallo had given a talk titled "Is There Life after NIH?" He remembered a time, Gallo said, when "all of us were awestruck by NIH, so privileged to be working there. There were already two or three Nobel prize-winners there. Another was about to occur. This was a period of enormous opportunity. I became a lab chief at twenty-seven. This would be impossible today. This was a great time to be young, and a great time to be at NIH. I used to wear loafers, because I couldn't wait to tie my shoes and get to work."

Somehow it all had gone wrong. The National Cancer Institute had experienced what Gallo saw as "loss of innocence," marked by "increased competition, a decreased interest in Congress, patents, lawyers, increased things related to money, increased media attention, over-ambitious, righteous, not well-informed, zealots on a congressman's staff. When I came there was no such thing as how you kept your notebook. In fact, nobody ever even asked me if I kept a notebook. Later, you could get investigated for not having the right notebook. I have two Laskers, I got every cancer prize. I got everything short of the Nobel prize — and the patent."

Robert Gallo played the game of Big Science better than it had ever been played before. He had published, by his own count, over a thousand scientific papers, including the ones he had actually written. His *curriculum vitae* listed eight single-spaced pages of prizes, honors, and awards. He had become the most famous AIDS researcher in the world, treated like scientific royalty on three continents.

But for the tens of millions of dollars that flowed into Gallo's lab the taxpayers had gotten precious little beyond HTLV-1 and T-Cell Growth Factor. They had also gotten a French virus renamed HTLV-3B; a T-cell line renamed H-9; HL-23; HTLV-1B; HBLV; a nonexistent Nigerian AIDS virus; the New Jersey Pair; and a surfeit of preposterous notions: the "reverse contamination" in Paris, Frédéric Brugière's acquisition of HIV in New York, Mika Popovic's inability to grow LAV, and many others. The many misstatements in Gallo's four landmark 1984 articles in *Science* have yet to be corrected.[g]

Being wrong in science is hardly a sin. Scientists are wrong every day, and in a curious way mistakes are what pushes science forward. What set Robert Gallo apart was his profound disinclination to acknowledge his mistakes, preferring instead to ignore them, insist they hadn't occurred, blame someone else, or propagate outlandish explanations and outright fictions that only confused science further and slowed its forward march.

Not that Gallo didn't wish things had turned out differently. He wished, for example, that he had invited the French to Margaret Heckler's news conference,[75] that Popovic's *Science* paper had identified LAV and HTLV-3 as two names for the same virus, and that he had never signed the sworn declaration. "I'm not proud of that," he admitted.[76] But in the end, the most compelling question was one only Gallo could answer: Had he somehow convinced himself that all the lies were true? Or had he known better all along?

Shortly after settling in Baltimore, Gallo had come across a quote that he liked from a ninth-century Arab philosopher. With no apparent sense of irony, he announced that he planned to inscribe it over the door of his new institute.[77]

"We ought not to be ashamed," it went, "of appreciating the truth and of acquiring it wherever it comes from, even if it comes from races distant and nations different from us. For the seeker of truth nothing takes precedence over the truth, and there is no disparagement of the truth, nor belittling either of him who speaks it or him who conveys it. No one is diminished by the truth; rather does the truth ennoble all."

NOTES

Superscript letters in the text indicate informational notes, which follow. The superscript numerals appearing in the text indicate citational notes, which are available online at www.sciencefictions.net.

Readers should take care not to confuse references to the OSI (the now-defunct NIH Office of Scientific Integrity) with references to the SOI (the Subcommittee on Oversight and Investigations of the United States House of Representatives).

Prologue. "*This* Is What We're Going to Work On"

[a.]Writing in the July 1990 *Journal of NIH Research*, Baltimore said he hadn't known of Temin's talk at the time of the call.

[b.]To settle arguments over priority, *Nature* and some other journals include the dates of receipt and acceptance for the papers they publish. Temin's manuscript was marked by *Nature* as received on June 15, Baltimore's on June 2.

Chapter 1. "Too Lucky to Be True"

[a.]At the time of the conference the term used for the disease was Acquired Immune Disorder.

[b.]"It's quite likely we were detecting an alternative enzyme that probably wasn't reverse transcriptase," recalled Robert Gallagher, one of Gallo's co-authors. "We didn't know enough to be really sure." Gallo's other co-author, Sue Yang, later agreed that she could "not rule out [the] possibility" that the experiment had detected a DNA polymerase.

c. Articles submitted to *PNAS* now undergo peer review, although reviewers are frequently selected by the communicator, not the journal.

d. Poiesz, B., *et al.* "Detection and isolation of type C retrovirus particles from fresh and cultured lymphocytes of a patient with cutaneous T-cell lymphoma." *PNAS* 77:7415–7419. December 1980. Communicated by Henry S. Kaplan, August 4, 1980. Robin Weiss thought a more appropriate title for Poiesz's paper might have been "Detection and characterization of type C virus particles . . . ," omitting the term "isolation" (R. Weiss to the author, October 14, 1996). Asked whether he had actually *isolated* HTLV at the time the article appeared, Poiesz said he had: "We purified the virus particles and their individual proteins and nucleic acids and characterized them as clearly retroviral in nature. We could even take pictures of the particles adjacent to cells or by themselves after we had purified them." Asked why the paper contained no mention of Elizabeth van der Loo or adult T-cell leukemia, Poiesz noted that "several of our early papers . . . had already been written by the time we knew of the van der Loo and ATL papers." Van der Loo was finally acknowledged in a subsequent article, after several of Gallo's colleagues brought her paper to the attention of NCI officials. (Poiesz, B., *et al.* "Isolation of a new type C retrovirus (HTLV) in primary uncultured cells of a patient with Sezary T-cell leukaemia." *Nature* 294:268, November 19, 1981.)

e. Nearly twenty years later, patients with mycosis fungoides, Sezary syndrome and other cutaneous T-cell lymphomas were still negative for HTLV-1. Kikuchi, A., *et al.* "Absence of human T-cell lymphotropic virus Type I in cutaneous T-cell lymphoma. *N. Engl. J. Med.* 336:296–297, January 23, 1997.

f. It was not a view shared by all of Gallo's colleagues, including Adi Gazdar, who had established HUT-78 without T-Cell Growth Factor, or Gallo's old boss, Ted Breitman. "Most of these cells don't need it," Breitman said. "If you have a good, productive, permanent T cell line, why pay someone to come in every three days and add T-Cell Growth Factor?"

g. Just how many of the patients tested by Guroff were HTLV-positive has never been made clear. In his 1991 memoir "Virus Hunting," Gallo asserts that "[b]y late 1980/early 1981," the time of Lake Biwa, "we found that eight out of eight Japanese cases of [ATL] had serum antibodies against HTLV." Gallo's NCI associate, William Blattner, maintained in a 1993 letter to the journal *Leukemia Research* that all the ATL sera tested by Gallo were positive for HTLV-1, and that "[t]his finding had been reported in the presence of Dr. Hinuma some weeks earlier at a workshop in Kyoto. . . ." Guy de Thé recalled that Guroff did not disclose in her Lake Biwa talk how many of the blood samples were positive. A report on the Kyoto meeting, published by Gallo, de Thé, and Ito in *Cancer Research* (41:4738–4739, November 1981), states only that HTLV-1 antibodies were found "in sera of *some* patients with these diseases, including sera from *some* Japanese patients with adult lymphoid cancers [emphasis added]." When Guroff published her blood test data nearly a year after Lake Biwa (*Science* 215:975, February 19, 1982), she reported that six of seven ATL patients had been positive for HTLV antibodies, while some eighty healthy individuals were negative. In a 1995 article in *Nature* (Wong-Staal, F., and Gallo, R.C. "Human T-lymphotropic retroviruses." *Nature* 317:395, October 3, 1985) Gallo claimed that the same data published by Guroff in *Science* in February 1982 had been presented at the Lake Biwa conference in March 1981.

[h.] Miyoshi, I., *et al.* "Type C virus particles in a cord T-cell line derived by co-cultivating normal human cord leukocytes and human leukaemic T cells." *Nature* 294:770, December 24/31, 1981 (received by *Nature* on July 13, 1981, four months after the Lake Biwa meeting). Hinuma, Y., *et al.* "Adult T-cell leukemia; antigen in an ATL cell line and detection of antibodies to the antigen in human sera." *PNAS* 78:10, 6476, October 1981 (communicated by Werner Henle, June 26, 1981). Although the title of Hinuma's paper refers to an "antigen" rather than a virus, the paper contains electron micrographs of a type-C retrovirus which Hinuma concluded was "the most probable candidate" for what the Japanese were then calling "Adult T-cell Antigen." Hinuma's paper states that "[t]he present results suggest, but do not prove, a causal relationship between a type C virus and ATL."

[i.] When Ed Scolnick, who had left George Todaro's lab to join Merck, tried to wangle a sample of HTLV from Dani Bolognesi, Gallo warned Bolognesi that "I in no way would want any materials sent to [Scolnick] on HTLV. You explain to me, or at least have him explain to you, what is the reason for his interest? I am sure it is not to foster our careers or to help solve any of the problems that we are interested in . . . he certainly has shown evidence that he is not someone to trust and that he is not a friend" (R. Gallo to D. Bolognesi, July 25, 1983).

[j.] Charlie Robinson's diagnosis also was revised, posthumously, from mycosis fungoides to adult T-cell leukemia, a change with which Adi Gazdar disagreed. "It's not really adult T-cell leukemia," Gazdar said later. "It's HTLV-associated disease. It's different." But the new diagnosis allowed Gallo to change the "L" in HTLV to "leukemia." In retrospect, Robinson probably hadn't had mycosis fungoides. "These patients came from the navy, from what was then the VA oncology branch," recalled an NCI epidemiologist, Doug Blayney, "and they had an interest in carving out mycosis fungoides as their thing. They couldn't be seen as doing lymphoma work, because that was the province of the medicine branch. So they got this guy C.R., who did not behave like the normal mycosis fungoides, but they called him that anyway."

[k.] $HTLV_{CR}$, the Robinson virus, was isolated not from fresh leukemic T-cells but from cells Adi Gazdar had transformed into the HUT-102 cell line. In the interim, any number of animal retroviruses could have contaminated and grown in HUT-102. Although Poiesz and Ruscetti had gone to great lengths to make sure that hadn't happened, Karpas pointed out that the way to *prove* that Robinson was infected with

HTLV$_{CR}$ was to see whether the T-cells circulating in Robinson's blood contained HTLV$_{CR}$ DNA. According to Bernie Poiesz, that experiment had never been done because, shortly before his death, Robinson had undergone a dramatic remission that depleted his stock of leukemic T-cells. By contrast, another patient, M.B., from whom Poiesz had isolated HTLV$_{MB}$, had never gone into remission and had plenty of leukemic T-cells. Using a technique called cross-hybridization, Poiesz had done the only experiments possible: comparisons of HTLV$_{CR}$ with HUT-102; with CTCL-2, the cell line that had yielded HTLV$_{MB}$; with M.B.'s fresh leukemic cells; and with normal human tissue. Karpas thought it suspicious that, at the genetic level, HTLV$_{CR}$ and HUT-102 were only 45 percent alike, and even more suspicious that HTLV$_{CR}$ and CTCL-2 were only 21 percent alike — considering that HTLV$_{CR}$ and HTLV$_{MB}$ were supposedly the same virus. Odder still, the similarity between HTLV$_{CR}$ and the DNA from M.B.'s fresh leukemic cells was only 17 percent — not much more than with normal human DNA. The explanation later offered by Gallo was that "some non-related nucleic acid sequences exist in the HTLV isolates." How this could have been determined is unclear, since HTLV$_{MB}$ was never characterized. But all the HTLV isolates whose genomes *have* been decoded are virtually identical, and questions remain about whether patient M.B. was indeed infected with HTLV.

[l.]Poiesz, B.J., *et al.* "Isolation of a new type C retrovirus (HTLV) in primary uncultured cells of a patient with Sezary T-cell leukemia." *Nature* 294:268, November 19, 1981. According to Poiesz, the blood sample from the child — actually a teenager — with T-Cell Adult Lymphocytic Leukemia "was not an NIH sample but came from off-campus and had been stored frozen at the Laboratory of Tumor Cell Biology some time before I discovered HTLV. I did not isolate HTLV from this sample nor was there any plasma available to test for antibodies to HTLV. The clinical information on this sample was scanty. It simply stated that he was a sixteen year old male with T-cell ALL. In retrospect I suspect he had ATL. We were unable to obtain any more samples from this patient nor further clinical data. The hybridization data on his leukemic cells, while seemingly accurate, was all that we had." Poiesz thought the data had been included in two later articles, one by Gallo and another by a Gallo assistant, Marvin Reitz. However, the Gallo article reports only that "HTLV nucleotide sequences were found in the DNA of uncultured leukemic cells of a 16 yr old young man with T-cell ALL," without elaboration. The second article (Reitz, M.S., *et al.* "Characterization by nucleic acid hybridization of HTLV, a novel retrovirus from human neoplastic T-lymphocytes," *Haematology and Blood Transfusion,* 1981) contains no supporting data and does not identify the virus in question as having come from a child — surprising, given the importance of such a rare event.

[m.]Sanger received his first Nobel Prize in 1958, for the amino acid sequence of the protein insulin, and his second, in 1980, for his method of sequencing DNA. In the interim, an American, Robert Holley, using Sanger's sequencing technique, published the first partial genetic sequence of RNA, followed closely by Sanger himself. Holley's Nobel Prize is sometimes referred to as "Fred Sanger's third Nobel"— but never by Sanger himself.

[n] Crewdson, J. "The Great AIDS Quest." *Chicago Tribune,* November 19, 1989. When the ATLV sequence was published in the summer of 1983, it was evident that ATLV did indeed bear a remarkable resemblance to the cancer-causing animal viruses. The first gene, called *gag,* for *group-specific antigen,* contained the genetic code for assembling the proteins that formed the virus's core. The second gene, *pol,* the viral *polymerase,* held the code for the virus's reverse transcriptase. The third gene, *env,* was the genetic blueprint for the viral *envelope,* the balloon-like structure of fat and protein that enveloped the viral core. So far, nothing new. But lying downstream of *env* the Japanese found something they couldn't explain. It seemed that ATLV had a mystery gene. The mystery gene wasn't an oncogene, like the cancer-causing genes found in the Rous sarcoma virus and some other animal cancer viruses. The Japanese had no idea what the gene did, but the fact that it existed probably meant it did something. Until they could say what, they called it the X gene.

[o] Gallo, R. C., and Reitz, M. S., Jr. "Human retroviruses and adult T-cell leukemia-lymphoma." *J. NCI,* 69:6, pp. 1209–1212, December 1982. One Gallo article maintained that it had been Gallo, not the Japanese, who first identified Kyushu as the area of Japan where HTLV was endemic (Shaw, G. M., *et al.* "Human T-cell leukemia virus: Its discovery and role in leukemogenesis and immunosuppression." Year Book Medical Publishers, 1984). According to Gallo, Hinuma had reported at Lake Biwa only that "some ATL patients had antibodies reactive with some ATL cell surface antigens" (Gallo, R. C. "The family of human lymphotropic retroviruses called HTLV: HTLV in adult T-cell leukemia (ATL), HTLV-2 in hairy cell leukemias, and HTLV-3 in AIDS." In M. Miwa *et al.,* eds. *Retroviruses in Human Lymphoma/Leukemia.* Tokyo: Japan Sci. Soc. Press, 1985). In fact, *all* the patients presented by Hinuma at Lake Biwa were antibody-positive, in contrast to *some* of the patients presented by Marjorie Guroff.

[p] The citations for these statements are to Marjorie Guroff's *Science* article and another article by V. S. Kalyanaraman (*PNAS* 79:1653–1657, 1982]. However, neither contains any data reflecting the detection of HTLV antibodies in healthy Japanese. Instead, both state that "[a]ll of 79 sera from normal Japanese, including 39 collected from the endemic ATL area of southwest Japan, were negative for antibodies to HTLV p24."

[q] Working at the University of California medical school in San Francisco, Bishop and Varmus had focused on a strain of RSV that contained a gene, *src,* in which the presence or absence of a tiny mutation appeared to determine whether the infected chicken got cancer. According to the existing hypothesis, cancer-causing oncogenes had been deposited in the human genome by retroviruses long ago and been passed from generation to generation. Bishop and Varmus established that oncogenes like *src* weren't retroviral genes after all, but normal cellular genes that had mutated in a way that enabled them to trigger the proliferation of a previously healthy cell. The observation that *src* existed in humans *and* chickens, and probably every other species, meant the virus-hunters had it backward: the *src* oncogene had been

acquired by some strains of Rous sarcoma virus from their chicken hosts, then carried by those viruses through the eons, only to be discovered by twentieth-century virologists who mistakenly assumed that the onco-retroviruses must have *delivered* cancer-causing oncogenes. Oncogenes might well cause cancer in humans — that remained to be shown — but they were *human* genes. "The first time I read this thesis, I thought I had misunderstood it," said Gosta Garthon of Sweden's Karolinska Institute. "Imagine: the likely cause of cancer comes from us, and all that the outside factors have to do is to push the right button."

Chapter 2. "These Guys Have Found Something Important"

[a.]Crewdson, J. "The Great AIDS Quest." *Chicago Tribune,* November 19, 1989. In his memoir, *Virus Hunting,* Gallo recalls having first heard about AIDS during a talk at NIH in late 1981 by James Curran of the Centers for Disease Control, who recalls having given such a talk.

[b.]Kalyanaraman, V. S., *et al.* "A new subtype of human T-cell leukemia virus (HTLV-2) associated with a T-cell variant of hairy cell leukemia." *Science* 218:571, November 5, 1982. Although HTLV-2 was isolated in Gallo's lab, the cell line from which it had come was established by a UCLA researcher, David Golde, from the spleen of a Seattle seafood salesman with an extraordinarily rare cancer called hairy cell T-cell leukemia (the salesman, John Moore, code-named "Mo," later sued UCLA, unsuccessfully, for appropriating his body for commercial purposes). At the genetic level, the HTLV isolated from Moore differed dramatically from the viruses found in Charlie Robinson and the Japanese patients — so much that Gallo now proposed calling the original virus HTLV-1 and the "Mo" virus HTLV-2. The NCI epidemiologists cautioned that no causal link between HTLV and hairy-cell T-cell leukemia could be forged on the basis of a single virus isolation. It was entirely possible, they said, that Moore had become infected with the virus *after* contracting leukemia. Beyond that, Moore was only the fourth case of hairy-cell T-cell leukemia ever recorded — an extraordinarily low incidence for any transmissible disease.

[c.]Hoping to show that people somewhere besides Japan were infected with the new virus, the NCI had begun screening blood samples from Europe, the Caribbean, and Africa for antibodies to HTLV. But only a few pockets of HTLV infection had been uncovered in Jamaica and Haiti.

[d.]Morens, D. M. *JAMA* 269:9, p. 1115, March 3, 1993. According to Morens, Don Francis first outlined his HTLV hypothesis in October of 1981, "at the end of a long phone conversation concerning other matters. . . ." (letter to the author from D. Morens, March 13, 1993). That version of events is contradicted by a May 27, 1993, letter to Gallo in which Harvard's Max Essex recalls that Francis, who earned his doctorate in Essex's lab, telephoned him in the summer of 1982 "to discuss the AIDS epidemic with me, and to emphasize his feeling that it was an infectious disease. I assured him I agreed with the infectious hypothesis and we discussed the types of infectious agents that might be considered. He suggested viruses such as hepatitis B, cytomegalovirus, and Herpes simplex. I told him that the 'new class of human retroviruses' should also be considered. He replied that he and his colleagues at CDC were not aware of these viruses and I told him about them. . . ." Francis disputes Essex's recollections, noting that "some months before" his call to Essex he had asked for, and received, HTLV-1 reagents from Gallo's lab for use in testing blood samples from Haitian refugees with AIDS.

e·Barré's lab notes for January 26, 1983, show reverse transcriptase levels for Flask 2 of 7400/1700 counts per minute of radiation, and of 5600/1600 cpm for Flask 3. On January 29 the levels increased to 22,000/4,000 cpm and 24,000/4600 cpm, respectively.

f·According to Ersell Richardson's log, the patients who followed E.P. — A.C.R., J.L.W., C.M., and D.B. — were all negative for antibodies to HTLV proteins.

g·Crewdson, J. "The Great AIDS Quest." *Chicago Tribune,* November 19, 1989. Claude Chardon's widow assured his doctors that her husband was not a homosexual. In his book *A Strange Virus of Unknown Origin* (New York: Ballantine, 1985) Leibowitch describes "Monsieur C" as "a French geologist of about 40 years of age" who had left his wife and family in Paris to live "in the company of a young Haitian woman"— who ultimately ended their relationship by casting a "wicked spell" upon him.

h·Memorandum dated February 9, 1983. "AIDS Serum & Cells." Dr. Jacque [*sic*] Leibowitch/Paris, France.

i·"Human T-cell leukaemia virus related antigens were shown to be expressed on this patient's blood cells, by R. Gallo and his group at the National Institutes of Health. Details will be published later."

j·Although one of the patients was Claude Chardon, Gallo's addendum mistakenly describes both patients as female. His use of the term "isolates" is also inaccurate, since no virus was ever isolated from M.A.

k·Gallo's March 15, 1983, letter predates by nearly two months Fischinger's directive that Gallo sever his ties with Cambridge BioScience, and there is some question about when — or even whether — the letter was actually received by the company.

l·Gallo's chief molecular biologist, Flossie Wong-Staal, sent Montagnier the HTLV DNA probe on March 23, 1983.

m·Within a few weeks the French had determined that this was, indeed, the case. Montagnier, L., *et al.* "Isolation of a new retrovirus from a patient at risk of AIDS." Presented June 18, 1983. *Proceedings of the First German Round-Table Discussion on AIDS and its Implication in Hemophiliacs,* June 18, 1983. Stuttgart: *Schattauer Verlag. Ann. Virol,* March 1984.

[n]The Pasteur's micrograph of LAV evoked differing interpretations. Robert F. Zeigel, an electron microscopist at the Roswell Park Memorial Cancer Institute in Buffalo, wrote *Science* that he would "stake my interpretive reputation" on his conclusion that the virus in the picture was *not* HTLV, but an Arena-virus (R. Zeigel to *Science,* May 16, 1983). *Science* didn't publish Zeigel's letter but instead sent it to Gallo, who replied that while some of the particles in the photograph "may very well be Arena viruses," the patient from whom the virus came "assuredly had antibodies to HTLV-like virus or to an HTLV related virus" (R. Gallo to R. Zeigel, July 26, 1983).

[o]R. Gallo to R. Kulstad, April 19, 1983. On April 20, Kulstad wrote Montagnier that "I understand Dr. Gallo has already discussed some changes in the paper with you. I am making some minor editorial changes and will seek Dr. Gallo's advice if I have any questions and cannot reach you. I am hoping to send it to the printer tonight, and will send you a copy of the galley proofs immediately." Although Montagnier subsequently received proofs of the article and the abstract, he let the paper go forward without protest. In a March 26, 1991, letter to the NIH's Office of Scientific Integrity, Montagnier explained that he felt "I had no other choice for having our manuscript accepted for publication than to accept the modifications introduced by Dr. Gallo, who was the referee of this work."

[p]"The AIDS mystery: New clues." *Newsweek,* May 25, 1983. Only Max Essex's paper contained any serological data. No blood antibody testing was performed or reported by Gallo or Pasteur.

[q]V. DeVita to NCI staff, April 14, 1983. Despite his complaints, Gallo took advantage of his new responsibilities to appeal for more space and personnel: five new technicians, six new postdocs, another full-time secretary, and "1-1/2 clerk typists." Gallo also wanted the space in NIH Building 37 occupied by the NCI's travel and computer staffs, assuring his division chief, Bruce Chabner, that "I believe this addition will satisfy [me] forever more. Please realize this is not a new request. I have always felt these were our needs, and with the pressing added work on AIDS it is mandatory." Then-associate NCI director Peter Fischinger later informed DeVita that Gallo's request for the remaining space on the sixth floor was moot, because it had "already been *defacto* exappropriated [*sic*]. . . ."

[r]The idea that significant numbers of Haitians were succumbing to AIDS was based not on epidemiological studies in Haiti, but on the early appearance of AIDS cases among Haitian refugees in Miami.

[s]The day after Gruest's arrival Gallo implored Montagnier "We desparately [*sic*] need more DNA. The data is critical for you, us and the field, so please do everything possible to get a good amount of DNA to us as soon as possible. There was only 30 [micrograms], enough just of [*sic*] a few blots. Many questions will go unanswered. There is at this point no higher priority" (letter from Gallo to Montagnier, April 19, 1983). Despite Gallo's letter, his lab records show that 1,600 micrograms of LAV

DNA, not thirty micrograms, was delivered by Gruest on April 18, 1983. Experiments comparing LAV and HTLV, designated A31 and A32, were begun on April 19 and finished a week before the *Science* articles appeared. According to an August 6, 1990, letter to Gallo from Beatrice Hahn, who performed the experiments, they showed that the French virus had nothing in common genetically with HTLV-1 or HTLV-2.

[t.]In an April 27, 1983, memo to Gallo, Marvin Reitz suggested that only ten more AIDS patients be tested for HTLV. "If we fail to find it in 10 cases," Reitz said, "we probably should look no further with HTLV probes."

Chapter 3. "We Were Wrong, and Barré-Sinoussi Was Right"

[a.]In a December 12, 1994, letter to the author, Edlinger recalled a conversation with Montagnier in the Pasteur cafeteria, in the late spring of 1983, in which "I mentioned to Montagnier that the Equine Infectious Anemia Virus has apparently a very similar pathology . . . to LAV."

[b.]After returning to Paris, Montagnier reminded Gallo that "the more common meaning of HTLV is Human T Leukemia Virus," and that "there is not a single data suggesting that our virus, which we call now Lymphadenopathy Associated Virus (LAV), is involved in human leukemia. I should be grateful to you if this could be brought to the knowledge of the other members of the group" (L. Montagnier to R. Gallo, September 2, 1983).

[c.]In January 1983 the CDC supplied Gallo's lab with blood and cells from nine AIDS patients and blood from fifty Haitian refugees. Only nine of the fifty-nine samples had antibodies to HTLV (J. Curran notes, February 14, 1983).

[d.]What Mullins thought might be a new human retrovirus turned out to be a Syrian hamster virus that somehow contaminated the CDC's viral cultures.

[e.]In a March 23, 1992, letter to the author, Robin Weiss acknowledged that the more generous of the two referees "could be me," and wondered whether the harsher reviewer had been Howard Temin. However, some stylistic features of the harsher review, such as the use of "no-one" rather than "no one," bear a closer resemblance to grammatical usage in Britain than Wisconsin.

[f.]The only cloud on Gallo's horizon was the sudden evaporation of a potentially important breakthrough on HTLV from one of Gallo's postdocs, Beatrice Hahn, who had reported in *Nature* that when HTLV inserted itself into the DNA of a cell, it often did so in exactly the same place (Hahn, B., *et al.* "Common site of integration of HTLV in cells of three patients with mature T-cell leukaemia-lymphoma." *Nature* 303:253, May 19, 1983). Given the number of possible insertion points, Hahn's observation seemed significant; the point chosen might determine whether HTLV caused cancer or something else. Too late, it was discovered to be the product of a laboratory contamination, and Gallo's retraction appeared in *Nature* just as the Cold Spring Harbor meeting opened (Hahn, B., and Gallo, R. C. *Nature,* 305:340, September 22, 1983). "After the retraction," Hahn said, "I was so disturbed that I worked another three months to find out what happened. There were bottles that were used by the entire laboratory to spin down DNA. These bottles were washed by the dishwashers but not autoclaved. What happened was that people were using the bottles for phage and plasmid preparations as well as for genomic DNA preps, and they were not given back to the room they came out of. The dishwashers washed them, put them back on the tray and they were redistributed, but not in the same way." The embarrassment for Gallo was softened by the publication, also in *Nature,* of new data to which Gallo had been alluding for months, and which might yet solve the mystery of how HTLV could cause leukemia in some patients and AIDS in others (Clarke, M. F., *et al.* "Homology of human T-cell leukaemia virus envelope gene with Class I HLA gene." *Nature* 305:60, September 1, 1983. Submitted May 5, 1983, accepted June 7, 1983). Ironically, that article, which described a protein, known as an HLA antigen, found on the surface of HTLV-infected T-cells, would later be retracted as well. According to the article, there were enough genetic similarities between the HLA protein and the HTLV envelope protein that the appearance of the HLA protein might be related to the cell's infection by HTLV — an idea not unlike that behind Max Essex's HTLV-MA. Because the HLA protein wasn't an ordinary cell-surface protein, its presence might impair the infected T-cell's ability to regulate the immune system, thereby providing "a possible mechanism for the induction by a retrovirus of leukaemia or other immune disorders." The "other immune disorders" weren't specified, but the only immune disorder with which anyone had associated HTLV was AIDS. It was Gallo's longtime assistant, Marvin Reitz, who had hybridized the HTLV envelope gene with the gene containing the code for the HLA protein and found what appeared to be a significant match. Unfortunately for Reitz, a week after the paper was accepted by *Nature* the Japanese published the full genetic sequence of HTLV. The Japanese sequence didn't contain the similarities Reitz thought had existed, and he had asked *Nature*'s permission to add a note to that effect at the end of his manuscript. According to Reitz, *Nature* refused, leaving its readers to learn of the problem six months later in a letter from two Cambridge researchers (Jennings, P. A., and Even, J. "No real homology of human T-cell leukaemia virus envelope with class I HLA." *Nature* 308:85, March 1, 1984). Reitz acknowledged that the paper's conclusion "eventually turned out not to be correct" (M. Reitz to the author, December 21, 1988). But the closest Gallo came to explaining how Reitz's finding might have raised "interesting possibilities in relation to immune suppression" was in his remarks to an NCI advisory board on September 30, 1983 — a full month *after* Reitz's *Nature* paper had been published and, by Reitz's own account, after it had become clear that the predicted homology didn't exist. According to the minutes of the meeting, Gallo "outlined several hypotheses related to HTLV and immunosuppression," including the possibility that HTLV infection caused "aberrations in HLA recognition signals. . . . Dr. Marvin Reitz of the LTCB recently discovered that the envelope of Type 1 HTLV shares some homology with the HLA Class One genes. . . . Dr. Gallo stated it may therefore be possible that the antigen is [*sic*] the envelope of

HTLV and shares a determinant with HLA genes." Although Gallo was chief of the lab where Reitz worked and had touted Reitz's results in meetings, and although the *Nature* article thanks him "for helpful discussions and a critical reading of the manuscript," Gallo later disclaimed any responsibility for its conclusions. "I'm not on the paper," Gallo said, "I was nowhere near close to the data. It's entirely Marv's work and independent."

[g.]Told that Francis, a decade later, did not remember cutting Montagnier off, Montagnier only smiled.

[h.]Two weeks earlier, Marjorie Guroff advised Montagnier she was sending him twenty coded blood samples positive for HTLV antibodies, which Gallo wanted the French to test with their LAV ELISA. A September 2, 1983, letter from Guroff to Montagnier states that the samples were "enclosed." But neither Montagnier nor Barré recalls receiving any blood samples from Gallo's lab. Nor does Guroff remember ever having received the results of any such tests from Pasteur (M. Guroff to the author, September 24, 1992).

[i.]A month before, Gallo had claimed to have "approximately twelve isolates of different types of HTLV from AIDS cases. Most of them fall into what I call HTLV class I" (R. Gallo to S. Sprecher, August 4, 1983). Six weeks later, Gallo would put the number of AIDS patients from whom he had isolated HTLV-1 at eleven (R. Gallo to R. Pearce, September 20, 1983). However, there is nothing in Gallo's laboratory records reflecting any isolations of HTLV from AIDS patients except E.P. and Claude Chardon. Gallo may have been referring to *detections* of HTLV proteins, but these do not constitute isolations, and according to Ersell Richardson's log there were fewer than a dozen such detections.

[j.]The last Chardon culture, maintained by Ersell Richardson, was declared dead on August 10, 1983. In a June 3, 1994, memo to S. Broder, Gallo stated that Popovic had also given up working with cells from an HTLV-2-infected AIDS patient, J.P.

[k.]Popovic's lab notes for September 10, 1983, show that the two cord-blood-cell cultures were designated C306/LAV and C310/LAV.

[l.]Betsy Read's lab notes show C310/LAV as RT positive on September 20, 1983.

[m.]The three patients doubly infected with both HTLV-1 and LAV were E.P., M.J., and J.K. Besides Brugière, cells from AIDS patients Ch.C., E.T., and S.N. reacted *only* with LAV (LTCB response to OSI question 1b, and submission to OSI on "The Use of LAV in LTCB," May 15, 1990).

[n.]The French patent application didn't describe the ELISA as a test for antibodies to the AIDS virus, since there wasn't conclusive proof that LAV was the cause of AIDS. If LAV were ultimately shown to cause AIDS, the ELISA would be an AIDS virus antibody test. If LAV didn't cause AIDS, it would simply be a LAV antibody test, for whatever that was worth.

o.According to Montagnier's lab notes, the sixth isolate, from patient deLongre, was made on October 1, 1983.

p.M. Popovic to OSI, June 26, 1990. The virus was shipped from Paris on September 21, 1983, by overnight air-express, arriving in Bethesda on September 22. The non-commercialization agreement was signed and dated by Popovic on September 23, 1983.

q.HUT-78, HOS, and SRA, were moderately RT positive, and Ti7.4 was strongly RT positive. B. Read lab notes, October 27, 1983; M. Popovic lab notes, November 9, 1983.

r.Schupbach, J., *et al.* "Antigens on HTLV-infected cells recognized by leukemia and AIDS sera are related to HTLV viral glycoprotein." *Science* 224:607, May 11, 1984. At the time the Schupbach paper was submitted in December 1983, the idea that the Essex protein, p65, originated from an infection with HTLV-1 provided convenient support for Gallo's hypothesis that HTLV-1 or a closely related virus caused AIDS.

s.The Biotech Research Laboratories ELISA that Guroff used employed the whole HTLV virus as a target for viral antibodies, and required the use of a detergent that dissolved the viral envelope, exposing the DNA core. Such a test, the paper said, would naturally be more inclined to detect antibodies to core proteins than to envelope proteins.

t.In an April 6, 1990, letter to Gallo, Hahn states: "It became apparent that the mislabeling had occurred in Mika's lab."

u.According to Hahn, the paper was rejected by *Science* before it could be withdrawn. When HTLV-1B was finally reported in the *International Journal of Cancer,* it was correctly described as having come from "an African patient with adult T-cell leukemia-lymphoma." Jacques Leibowitch, who had gone to great lengths to provide Gallo with the blood sample from Elomata, complained that "I was not even acknowledged in the paper. It's not fair. It was the first-ever isolate they had from Zaire. It was many hours of work on the Elomata case to bring the cells eventually to them. I wrote to them, and I got a letter from Gallo. He said, 'It's not my fault.'"

v.January 15: LAV/*Bru;* May 30: LAV/*Loi;* June 9: LAV/*Lai;* June 26: LAV/*Pri;* September 3: LAV/*Eli;* October 1: LAV/*Del;* October 13: LAV/*Lap,* LAV/*Par;* October 14: LAV/*Hec,* LAV/*Van;* November 22: LAV/*Rem;* December 14: LAV/*Rab.*

w.When Beatrice Hahn tested the LAV DNA delivered by Montagnier to Gallo's house in July 1983, she got the same results as she had with the DNA delivered by Jacqueline Gruest just before Easter: genetically, LAV and HTLV were quite different viruses. In a September 23, 1992, interview with the staff of the House Subcommittee on Investigations, Hahn recalled that "we probed with HTLV-1 and HTLV-2," and that both probes were "negative." Hahn's account is confirmed by Flossie Wong-Staal's memo to Gallo of October 1, 1992.

Chapter 4. "This Looks Like It Could Be the Cause"

[a.]A tape recording of the Park City proceedings was kindly provided to the author by F. Brun-Vézinet.

[b.]Elomata was presented to Gallo by Jacques Leibowitch as "a typical case of HTLV-related lymphoma from Zaire," not an AIDS patient.

[c.]Neither Brun nor Rouzioux retained a copy of the letter that accompanied the manuscript, but Rouzioux recalled editing the final version of the paper a few days after the birth of her baby on December 14, 1983.

[d.]Chermann, J. C., *et al. UCLA Symposia on Molecular and Cellular Biology* (New Series 16), M. S. Gottlieb and J. E. Groopman, eds. (Liss: New York, 1984). Brun hadn't been invited to speak at Park City, but she and Christine Rouzioux submitted an abstract reporting that, using a radioimmuno precipitation assay (RIPA), 40 percent of AIDS patients and 88 percent of pre-AIDS patients had antibodies to the core protein of LAV.

[e.]B. Read to OSI, June 7, 1990. NIH Lock Record for Building 37, Rooms 6B03-A and 6B03-B, shows that locks were installed on February 14, 1984, the same day Chermann presented his seminar.

[f.]Montagnier created the line, which he named FR-8, on Nov. 17, 1983, by transforming normal B-cells into leukemic B-cells via exposure to the Epstein-Barr virus.

[g.]Lab notes kept by Montagnier's assistant, Sophie Chamaret, show the date of the call as February 27, 1984.

[h.]According to M. G. Sarngadharan, MOV was short for Mo Varient — Mo being the code name for John Moore, the Seattle seafood salesman whose T-cells had yielded the first isolate of HTLV-2. In testing the Popovic virus, Sarngadharan claimed to have noticed "a low but identifiable reaction" with HTLV-2, which had been growing in Popovic's lab "for a long time prior to and during this period. We entertained the thought that he might have some minor contamination with MO virus. But we were confident that if there was a MO virus component in the new virus culture it had to be a very minor one. . . . Mika pointed out that there was another virus-positive culture coming up, but it was a little bit behind the MOV culture. As soon as that culture was ready we would start using that one," evidently a reference to the "pool" virus HTLV-3B (M. Sarngadharan to OSI, January 29, 1991).

[i.]M. Sarngadharan lab notes, January 20, 1984. The previous summer, Zaki Salahuddin's partner, Phil Markham, had flown to Yale to pick up the cells from the mother and child. Both were positive for reverse transcriptase (S. Z. Salahuddin lab notes, July 11, 1983). But Salahuddin, who had been looking for an HTLV-like virus, hadn't been able to isolate any virus from either culture. Now the ELISA had confirmed that the mother and child had blood-borne antibodies to Popovic's new virus.

j.According to an April 6, 1990, letter to Gallo from Beatrice Hahn, the cloning of HTLV-3 did not begin until May 2, 1984. The cloning experiments begun on March 7 involved a virus designated as "LAV." Those clones, however, contained DNA "related to HTLV-1 and HTLV-2 and not the AIDS retrovirus."

k.Popovic erroneously assumed his technician, Betsy Read, had co-cultured R.F. with the H-4 cell line. Read maintained to the Office of Scientific Integrity that she had used uncloned HUT-78. (R. Gallo, "Introductory Remarks" to OSI, July 18, 1990).

l.Following the demise of the original S.N. culture on February 27, 1984, Betsy Read co-cultured primary S.N. cells with the H-4 cell line. That culture briefly showed low-level virus production before being discontinued in May (LTCB "S.N. History," April 26, 1990).

m.Speaking at Park City, Gallo defined a viral isolation as "when we've characterized what we have in detail and when we've been able to successfully transmit it, to be able to hand it out to somebody." According to the article, however, "Evidence for the presence of HTLV-3 included: (i) viral reverse transcriptase (RT) activity in super-natant fluids; (ii) transmission of virus by coculturing T cells with irradiated donor cells or with cell-free fluids; (3) observation of virus by electron microscopy; *and* (iv) the expression of viral antigens in indirect immune fluorescence assays using serum from a patient positive for antibodies to HTLV-3 as described, *or* antisera prepared against purified, whole disrupted HTLV-3 [emphasis added]." The legend for the table summarizing the forty-eight "isolations" states that samples exhibiting *any two* of these markers were considered positive for HTLV-3 — criteria that would not exclude HTLV-1 or HTLV-2, or some yet-undiscovered retrovirus.

n.Editing an earlier draft of the manuscript, Gallo inserted a note that LAV "grows in H-4 and produces similar cytopathic effects" as HTLV-3 — a fuller disclosure of Popovic's work with LAV than Popovic himself had made. By the final draft Gallo had substituted the assertion that LAV "has not yet been transmitted to a permanently growing cell line."

o.No independent record of Gallo's talk exists, because Gallo insisted that the press not be allowed into the auditorium, explaining that he "was afraid in the United States of what would happen" if his remarks reached Washington (R. Gallo to OSI, April 11, 1990).

p."I sat where I am," Gallo told the Office of Scientific Integrity on July 27, 1990, "and they were working on a corner of a circled table but I didn't know why Don Francis was there. He said, 'Oh, you know, the results were quite comparable in the blind comparative test.' I was saying, 'I am going to get right sucked into this. They are going to' — I said, 'Look, I am not publishing CDC data sera. We have our own publications planned.' . . . I was getting worried that they were going to — this is what was happening. . . . I saw that data from six feet away for two milliseconds. I saw no real numbers. I never got them to analyze and they were never published." Years later, Gallo left a message on Don Francis's answering machine acknowledging that he had been "well-aware of the serology data that you gave for me to look over on one occasion during the visit to Pasteur" (D. Francis telephone notes, March 25, 1992).

Chapter 5. "Our Eminent Dr. Robert Gallo"

[a.]L. Arthur to R. Ting, May 13, 1988. The technician at Biotech Research Laboratories who prepared the virus for shipment to Frederick noted on her calendar for April 9, 1984, that she sent "1 roller bottle HTLV3B to Dr. R. Gilden at Frederick Cancer Center. (L. Fang to SOI, May 7, 1993). The term "HTLV-3B" raises the obvious question: What happened to HTLV-3A? Fang later told the SOI that the company's scientific director, Bob Ting, had presented her a few days before with eight flasks of the Gallo AIDS virus, which Ting had prepared himself. Four of the flasks were labeled HTLV-3A, and the other four HTLV-3B. In a letter to Gallo dated June 13, 1984, Ting stated that the designation HTLV-3B had been given to him by somebody in Gallo's lab. According to Ting, HTLV-3A was the name he himself had given to MOV (R. Ting to R. Gallo, June 13, 1994).

[b.]M. Popovic to OSI, June 26 and December 1, 1990. In his June 13, 1990, interview with OSI, M. G. Sarngadharan confirmed that "R.F. was, I think behind. I don't think R.F. was available then."

[c.]A copy of the interview tape was kindly provided to the author by M. Redfern.

[d.]Draft announcement by Edward N. Brandt, Jr., for release Wednesday, April 18, 1984. Brandt's statement credited "Dr. Robert C. Gallo, Jr. [*sic*], chief of the NCI Laboratory of Tumor Cell Biology, who directed the research," with having "isolated the new group of viruses," which Brandt described as "variants of a family of viruses known as human T-cell leukemia/lymphoma virus (HTLV), of which HTLV-I and II are members." Although their only contribution had been to supply Gallo with some AIDS patients' blood samples, Brandt's announcement also credited scientists from Memorial Sloan-Kettering, Duke, and the University of North Carolina with having isolated HTLV-3. Despite Brandt's memo to Margaret Heckler of two months before about "the apparent importance" of LAV, nowhere did Brandt's statement mention the Institut Pasteur.

[e.]Gonda's lab notes for February 15, 1984, show a virus-positive micrograph of the virus from patient J.S. According to Salahuddin's lab notes, the J.S. virus was isolated on January 17, 1984.

[f.]An article in the April 18, 1987, edition of the Dutch newspaper *Volkskrant* paraphrases Gallo as saying that "this news leaked because of a freelance journalist who also was working for *New Scientist*. During an interview that journalist had stolen a few documents when Gallo was out of his room for a while." Another respected Dutch paper, the *Financiel Dagblad,* quoted Gallo the same day as saying that "Just before publication a British freelance journalist had come to see me about oncogenes. I told him also about the AIDS virus but also said to him that this should be confidential until June 1984. After the interview when I left my room for lunch he took private documents from my desk and sold them later on to *New Scientist*." In *Virus Hunting,* Gallo gives yet another version, stating that he told Redfern "he could take materials from our office library," but that Redfern instead had taken "copies of the papers that were in press for *Science*." According to Sarngadharan, the real source of the leak had been a scientist who provided Zaki Salahuddin with some blood samples and who was named as a co-author on one of the *Science* articles (M. G. Sarngadharan to OSI, January 29, 1991).

[g.]Weiss didn't recall exactly what he said to Gallo in Wyngaarden's hearing, but he agreed that "clearly I made some impression on him, perhaps more so than I had intended" (R. Weiss to the author, November 1, 1993). Wyngaarden's chief recollection of the occasion was Weiss asking Gallo how he could "dismiss the French work" (J. Wyngaarden to the Office of Scientific Integrity, September 27, 1993).

[h.]Weiss achieved the successful transmission of LAV to the CEM cell line on February 29, 1984, four days after Popovic infected H-9 with HTLV-3B.

[i.]R. Weiss to L. Montagnier, April 12, 1984, and L. Montagnier to A. Karpas, Aug. 11, 1992. In a May 18, 1987, letter to Robin Weiss, Montagnier wrote that "The RT was low (around 10,000 cpm) but within two weeks of culture in our lab, the titer went up to 2,000,000 cpm."

[j.]**May 20, 1983:** Isolation of new human retrovirus from patient BRU (*Science* 220:868). **June 18, 1983:** Antibodies to LAV/*Bru* in 63 percent of patients with pre-AIDS. LAV is described as morphologically and biologically different from HTLV, and tropic for human T-4 cells (L. Montagnier, First German Round-Table on AIDS, Frankfurt; F.K. Schattauer Verlag, 1984). **June 25, 1983:** Partial characterization of LAV core protein p25 and reverse transcriptase; virus infects only T-4 lymphocytes. (J. C. Chermann, *et al.,* First European Conference on AIDS, Naples, Italy; *Antibiot. Chemother.,* 32:48–52. Basel: Karger, 1984). **September 15, 1983:** Further characterization of LAV, isolation of three new viruses from a Haitian, a French hemophiliac, and a French homosexual with Kaposi's sarcoma, and homology with a member of the animal lentivirus family. LAV antibodies found in 63 percent of patients with pre-AIDS, 20 percent of AIDS patients and 17.5 percent of healthy homosexuals, but only 1.9 percent of controls (L. Montagnier, Presented at Cold Spring Harbor Laboratory September 15, 1983. In Gallo, R. C., *et al. Human T-cell Leukemia Viruses.*

New York: Cold Spring Harbor Press, 1984. **November 13, 1983:** Total of seven LAV samples from a Haitian, a British Caucasian living in Trinidad, a hemophiliac, a Zairian, two homosexuals, and a Caucasian living in Africa. LAV antibodies in 37.5 percent of AIDS patients and 74.5 percent of pre-AIDS patients, but less than 1 percent of healthy controls (F. Barré-Sinoussi, "A new human retrovirus associated with acquired immunodeficiency syndrome (AIDS) or AIDS-related symptoms." In Aoki, T., *et al.* (eds). *Manipulation of Host Defence Mechanisms.* Tokyo: Excerpta Medica, 1983). **November 15, 1983:** LAV infects and kills T-4 cells. (D. Klatzmann, "Immune status of AIDS patients in France: Relationship with lymphadenopathy associated virus tropism." *Ann. N.Y. Acad. Sci.* 437, 1984). **December 1983:** Antibodies to LAV in 74 percent of pre-AIDS patients and 40 percent of AIDS patients (L. Montagnier, *et al.,* Actualities Hematologiques, 1984). **February 28, 1984:** Total of 10 LAV isolates from patients with AIDS or pre-AIDS. LAV is not a type C retrovirus, has an Mg^{2+} preferring RT and a core protein of 25,000 weight. (J. C. Chermann, *et al. Bull. Acad. Nat. Med.*). **March 4, 1984:** LAV has structural and antigenic relatedness to equine infectious anemia virus but shows no relationship to HTLV-1. (L. Montagnier, *et al. Ann. Virol.* 135E:119). **March 27, 1984:** Biochemical characterization of RNA dependent DNA polymerase (reverse transcriptase) produced by LAV. (F. Rey, *et al., Biochemical and Biophysical Research Communications,* May 31, 1984). **April 7, 1984:** Isolation of LAV from two siblings with hemophilia B, one ill with AIDS, the other not. First report of a healthy-carrier state in AIDS. Article contains first published description of Pasteur LAV ELISA (E. Vilmer, *et al., Lancet* i:753–757).

[k.]The application's single allusion to LAV is an oblique sentence copied from Sarngadharan's *Science* article: "Isolation of another retrovirus was reported from a homosexual patient with chronic generalized lymphadenopathy, a syndrome that often precedes AIDS and therefore [is] referred to as 'pre-AIDS.'" However, the Material Information Disclosure supporting the Gallo application, filed on June 26, 1984, cited only articles from Gallo's laboratory as prior art, failing to mention any of the Pasteur's dozen or so publications or public presentations, including Cold Spring Harbor and Park City. When Gallo, Popovic, and Sarngadharan filed their declaration of inventorship with the Patent Office on July 27, 1984, they affirmed that "no blood test for AIDS was ever *known* or used in the United States before our invention thereof or patented or described in any printed publication in any country before our invention thereof . . . [emphasis added]."

[l.]Although Martin received LAV on April 12, 1983, his signed receipt is dated April 13.

[m.]C. Haddow to SOI, June 22, 1992; R. Gallo to OSI, July 27 and August 4, 1990; V. DeVita to the author, December 6, 1994. Gallo remembered having assisted Margaret Heckler with her statement, but not demanding that the French be given no credit. Neither did Vince DeVita. "If Dr. Gallo asked that any reference to the French contribution be deleted, he did so without my knowledge," DeVita said. "There was a meeting with the secretary, but that was separate from the meeting with Mr. Haddow, Dr. Gallo, Dr. Fischinger, and myself. No mention was made of any reference to the French contribution at that time. Perhaps this happened at another meeting, and if so I was not present." Haddow's recollection is that Gallo's demand came during a telephone conversation rather than in a meeting.

[n.]Heckler did not reply to a January 18, 1997, letter from the author asking why she omitted the paragraph from her remarks.

Chapter 6. "We Assumed That Was *Your* Job"

[a.]L. Montagnier to R. Gallo, July 8, 1984. Gallo later denied having made such a claim. "I said you had cell lines from us," Gallo wrote Barré a month after the news conference, "and that you were at one time in our lab to learn about some cell cultures. I did not say for T-cells. I think this is a minor point. I was responding to the dirt flung from Paris that the French had sent me so much and we hadn't sent them anything. You must have seen the many, many articles to this effect, so if I were you I wouldn't feel very sensitive. Clearly our work has given you all rather dramatic credit and visibility" (R. Gallo to F. Barré-Sinoussi, June 27, 1984).

[b.]Gallo, R. C., *et al.* "The Family of Human Retroviruses Called Human T-Cell Leukemia/Lymphoma Virus (HTLV): Their Role in Lymphoid Malignancies and Their Association with Lymphosuppressive Disorders (AIDS)." Gallo, R. C. "Human T-cell leukemia lymphoma virus." Presented at Cold Spring Harbor Laboratory, N.Y., September 15, 1983. In Gallo, R. C., and Essex, M., eds. *Human T-cell Leukemia/Lymphoma Viruses.* New York: Cold Spring Harbor Press, 1984. Although it was clear from the citations it contained to Gallo's May 1984 *Science* papers that the updated paper couldn't have been presented in September 1983, the preface to the volume states that all presentations were made to the HTLV meeting held at Cold Spring Harbor in September 1983. "I wouldn't do it," Robin Weiss said later. "I don't like the idea of Gallo talking at Cold Spring Harbor without even knowing about HTLV-3, and slipping in a paper five months later." What offended Weiss most was Gallo's failure to include a citation for Montagnier's talk, "the most important paper in this volume in terms of AIDS."

[c.]Markham., P. D., *et al.* "Correlation between exposure to human T-cell leukemia-lymphoma virus-3 and the development of AIDS." In Selikoff, I. J., *et al.,* eds. *Acquired Immune Deficiency Syndrome. Ann. N.Y. Acad. Sci.* 437, 1984. The Markham article refers to another article, by Suresh K. Arya of Gallo's lab, that appeared in *Science* in August 1984, as "submitted for publication." According to *Science,* Arya *et al.* was received May 1, 1984. Thus, the Markham article must have been updated some time after that date.

[d.]A footnote indicated that the Gallo-Markham paper "was not presented at the conference" — although not that the data it contained hadn't been obtained until months after the conference.

e·Robin Weiss observed that Jay Levy in San Francisco was growing ARV-2 in the HUT-78 cell line, and that the CDC in Atlanta was growing LAV, and that even if Gallo's lab had never worked on AIDS, companies interested in making an AIDS test could have sought a license from another laboratory "or done a deal with Institut Pasteur for the U.S. market. I have a feeling that the screening of blood might not have been delayed by a single day without Gallo" (R. Weiss to the author, January 15, 1993).

f·Arthur's notebooks show that the viability of the AIDS virus culture declined from 34 to 31 percent on April 20, 1984.

g·In a July 15, 1981, deposition in the case of *Hoffman-LaRoche, Inc., v. David W. Golde, et al.*, Gallo confirmed that NIH's policy was to make cell lines available "to everybody on publication who asks who's a qualified investigator, whether they work in any place, any affiliation, race, color, or creed, and so on. The lines are available on publication."

h·Many of those who signed the agreement never included Gallo as an author on their subsequent papers, but many others did.

i·P. Fischinger to J. Wyngaarden, June 27, 1984. Fischinger and Lowell Harmison backed down on the secrecy clause, which Ed Brandt hadn't known about and wouldn't have agreed to (E. Brandt, to SOI, February 24, 1993). Their retreat came after Elkan Blout, dean for academic affairs at the Harvard School of Public Health, protested that the clause placed "unacceptable restrictions on research, is inconsistent with long-standing policies of this and many other major research institutions and threatens to inhibit vital research activity on a major threat to public health" (E. Blout to P. Fischinger, October 10, 1985). In an October 23, 1985, reply, Fischinger assured Blout "that in the University or any other non-profit research environment, secrecy agreements or any attempt from [*sic*] public disclosure be disregarded."

j·In chronological order: Daniel Zagury; Dani Bolognesi and Bolognesi's Duke University colleague Bart Haynes; Mark Wainberg, a young Canadian researcher who had worked in Gallo's lab; Robin Weiss; the New York Blood Center's Fred Prince (3B only); the CDC's Fred Murphy (3B only); John Sever of NIH (3B only); Gallo's Italian colleague Paolo Rossi; Luc Montagnier; Louis Gazzolo, a French researcher who had worked in Gallo's lab; Antti Vaheri; Martin Hirsch and Bill Haseltine from Harvard; Gallo's cancer-virus colleague Wade Parks, then at the University of Miami; Jean-Claude Chermann; Rubin Sher; Reinhard Kurth; Paul Jolicoeur; George Miller; Fred Jensen of the Cytotech Corporation (3B only); Ian Gust; Fausto Titti; Max Essex; Carel Mulder (3B only); John Sullivan (3B only); M. A. Koch; Friedrich Deinhardt; Gunnel Biberfeld of the Karolinska Institute in Stockholm; Tony Chu (3B only); Gerhard Hunsmann; Gerry Robey at the NCI's Frederick center (3B only); Olivia Prebble (3B only); Jim Curran of the CDC (3B only); Leon Epstein (3B only); Sam Broder (3B only); Francis Barin; Don Burke of San Francisco General Hospital (3B only); Hubert Schoemaker (3B only); Paul Bunn, Adi Gazdar's boss; Kai Krohn; Murray Gardner; Steve Sherwin (3B only); Fredrich Dorner; Arye Rubinstein (3B only);

Joseph Pagano (3B only); Arwin Diwan (3B only); Jerry Groopman; Emin Kansu; Ferenc Toth; Jaap Goudsmit; Otto Thraenhart; Jeff Laurence (3B only); Franz Heinz; John Fahey; Richard Emmons (3B only); Robert Downing; Jun Minowada; Arsene Burny; Volker terMeulen; Peter Wernet; Jim Hoxie; and Phil Hartig.

[k.]On April 13, 1984, ten days before the Heckler news conference, Zagury signed a receipt stating that "I received from Dr. Robert C. Gallo (LTCB, NCI, NIH) HT cells (clone 4) and HT cells infected with HTLV3 from AIDS patients as well as antibody anti HTLV3 virus only for research purposes. This material will not be used for any other reasons."

[l.]F. Wong-Staal to G. Franchini (undated). When a similar request arrived from Jim Mullins, Ann Sliski advised Gallo that "Flossie may want to write in some further restrictions as she did with Haseltine" (handwritten note appended to letter from J. Mullins to R. Gallo, June 4, 1984).

[m.]Weiss's noncollaboration clause proved helpful on at least one occasion. A month before the Heckler news conference, Marguerite Pereira of the Public Health Laboratory Service in London wrote to thank Gallo for having sent HTLV-1 reagents to aid her in tracking the U.K.'s incipient AIDS epidemic (M. Pereira to R. Gallo, March 15, 1984). Gallo waited until the day of the news conference to let Pereira know that he had sent her the wrong virus, and that the actual cause of AIDS was "a new variant" called HTLV-3. Even though Daniel Zagury in Paris had had the virus for over a week, Gallo told Pereira he wasn't able to send the British Public Health Service any HTLV-3 because "we have to have papers published and other assurances" (R. Gallo to M. Pereira, April 23, 1984). When no HTLV-3 was forthcoming from Bethesda, Pereira simply borrowed some from Robin Weiss (M. Pereira to H. Streicher, February 20, 1985).

[n.]J. Levy to R. Gallo, May 4, 1984. The letter bears a handwritten notation by someone in Gallo's lab: "Save for staff meeting to decide what to do." Gallo told another researcher, James McDougall of the Fred Hutchinson Cancer Research Center in Seattle, that "we are still in the middle of characterizing some clones. It will be a while before we can distribute them." Gallo added a handwritten note: "Jim, write to me again in about 6 weeks." When McDougall asked again six weeks later, Gallo scribbled "No" across the top of his letter.

[o.]M. Sarngadharan to OSI, June 13, 1990. Montagnier named the core protein of LAV p25, to reflect its molecular weight of almost exactly 25,000 daltons. Gallo incorrectly labeled the same protein p24, to artificially enhance the similarities between HTLV-3B and HTLV-1 and HTLV-2, whose core proteins weigh closer to 24,000 daltons.

[p.]"We could not detect gp41," Montagnier said later. "Sarang used a Western Blot and he could detect gp41. I could detect a p42, but it was cellular. We missed the gp41 at that time. That's Gallo's contribution. We didn't use the Western blot. We used only immune precipitation, and if you label the virus you don't label this protein." In less than three weeks Sarngadharan had resolved the temporary discrepancy by putting both HTLV-3B and LAV through a Western Blot. In the middle of the LAV blot was gp41, the protein Montagnier had missed (M. Sarngadharan laboratory notes, June 15, 1984; M. Sarngadharan to OSI, June 13, 1990).

q·D. Francis telephone notes, May 21, 1984. "Competition — Sarang — infected cells: competition by Françoise — p25 [the viral core protein] same. French side of comparison done."

r·*Wall Street Journal,* July 5, 1984. Three weeks after Nowinski's announcement, Gallo and Popovic applied for an American patent on the CEM cell line as a method of producing the AIDS virus (U.S. Patent Application 602,946, July 29, 1984). However, Betsy Read's lab notes show that she first infected CEM with the AIDS virus on May 28, 1984, a few days after Sarngadharan's return from Paris — where, according to Robin Weiss, Sarngadharan encountered Weiss's assistant, Rachanee Cheingsong-Popov, delivering the LAV-producing CEM line infected by Weiss three months before.

s·Brun-Vézinet, F., *et al.* "Detection of IgG antibodies to lymphadenopathy-associated virus in patients with AIDS or lymphadenopathy syndrome." *Lancet* (8389): 1253, June 9, 1984. Ian Munro, editor of *The Lancet* at the time the paper was published, said he could not recall why the manuscript was held up, although he was certain it had not been negatively reviewed by Dr. Gallo "or any of his close (or even remote) colleagues" (I. Munro to the author, August 2, 1993). As for whether Gallo's March 5, 1984, letter to Munro, touting the discovery of HTLV-3 and denigrating the Pasteur's discovery of LAV, had played a role in delaying publication of the Pasteur paper, Munro replied that "I cannot refrain from refuting in the strongest terms the apparent implication that the *Lancet* was a party to some scheme to delay publication of the French paper." Munro's successor, Robin Fox, agreed that any suggestion the journal might intentionally have delayed publication on the basis of Gallo's letter is "far from *The Lancet*'s way of working — then and now. . . ." (R. Fox to the author, August 24, 1993).

t·Judging from his published data, Levy's first isolate of ARV was accomplished prior to November 15, 1983 — the day the cells that produced four of the five isolates identified in Popovic's *Science* article — R.F., B.K., L.S., and W.T. — were first unfrozen and placed in culture. The fifth *Science* isolate, from the patient S.N., was first cultured in cord blood cells on November 16 (C359/SN; B. Read lab notes. R. Gallo to OSI, December 10, 1990). Levy delayed announcing his discovery until he could complete an experiment that hadn't been attempted by either Gallo or the French. "Hemophiliacs had gotten AIDS," Levy said. "The only thing I couldn't explain was how could a retrovirus get into Factor VIII. So I decided before we published we better put a retrovirus through Factor VIII treatment and show that it does, or does not, survive. If it doesn't survive then this is not the cause." Levy had gotten in touch with Cutter Laboratories, a principal manufacturer of Factor VIII, across the

San Francisco Bay in Berkeley. "We set up an experiment in which we used a mouse retrovirus, because it was easy to measure," Levy said. "That took three months, and in March we saw that the mouse retrovirus survived. We realized that a human retrovirus could do it as well, and we set out to find out how do we get rid of it. And we did a heating experiment, which shows that you have to heat it for three days in order to kill it. We put that together and we sent it off to *Lancet*. And then we put together the paper on the isolation for *Science*."

Chapter 7. "Only Because There Are So Many"

a. "I enclose a complete 1981 list of the Academy including sectional breakdowns," Gallo wrote Fischinger on July 30, 1982. "As we discussed the section most appropriate for me would have been #41 (Medical Genetics, Hematology, and Oncology). Hillary [Koprowski] has, however, nominated me for section 22, Cellular and Developmental Biology. This is likely to be more difficult. I have circled what I feel sure are friends in 41, and those who I hope are at least useful in 22 — just in case you have any chances. Takis Papas has contacts to Dr. Kafatos. He is very good and respected. He is at Harvard. Takis feels he could and would really help. However, he is in Greece until early September. There is a 'straw' vote mid-late August. If I make it in section 22 that is the time for the contacts to key people in this section via Kafatos and Hillary or anyone else."

b. "Four win awards for cancer work." *New York Times,* June 21, 1984. "Dr. Gallo, a physician, was cited for discoveries that have 'profoundly influenced modern cancer research' by showing that a virus called HTLV-1 is a cause of leukemia in humans . . . [h]is team has recently discovered two related viruses, HTLV-2 and -3. The latter is strongly suspected of causing acquired immune deficiency syndrome, known as AIDS."

c. According to Gallo's lab records, the four other *Science* cultures, B.K., L.S., S.N., and WT, were discontinued either shortly before, or shortly after, the *Science* paper was published. Betsy Read's lab notes show that while 80 percent of the cells in the H-4/R.F. culture were producing virus on March 1, 1984, by April 11 the number had fallen to less than 20 percent. That none of the five original isolates had been distributed to other laboratories bothered Robin Weiss. "One should be able to continuously propagate them," Weiss said. "If one couldn't, I'd say, 'Well, hold on a minute, they ought to be hardy enough to send to other labs.'"

d. B. Read lab notes, June 28, 1984. The R.F. culture reported in *Science* was in the less-productive H-4 cell line.

e. B. Hahn to R. Gallo, April 6, 1990. The viruses were J.K., J.R., L.S., M.R., L.W., and mROD.

f. In her April 6, 1990, letter to Gallo, Beatrice Hahn states that R.F. was "identified as an independent and genetically distinct isolate" on June 5, 1984.

ᵍ·According to an October 25, 1984, memo from Gallo to Vince DeVita, the call to Montagnier occurred on August 23 of that year. In a June 18, 1991, letter to the OSI, Montagnier remembered it as having taken place sometime in July. Gallo's memoir *Virus Hunting* dates the call in June — impossible, since the LAV B-cell culture with which HTLV-3B was compared didn't arrive in Bethesda until mid-July. In an April 11, 1990, interview with the OSI, Gallo said the conversation took place in October. Because of its proximity to the time of the call, Gallo's memo to DeVita is probably most accurate. A New Jersey scientist, Stanley Weiss, recalled an appointment with Gallo on the afternoon Gallo got the news about the genetic divergence of R.F. In a November 5, 1990, letter to the OSI, Weiss recalled that "Dr. Gallo was delayed" for their meeting, and that "George Shaw was waiting as well. He was scheduled to meet with Dr. Gallo first. While we both were waiting, Dr. Shaw talked to me a bit concerning some data he was about to present to Dr. Gallo for the first time. This was the result of the molecular analyses he and Dr. Hahn were doing on HTLV-3B and LAV. They appeared to be the same. At the end of Dr. Shaw's meeting with Dr. Gallo they both came into the hallway and involved a few of us who were around in a brief discussion." In a December 8, 1992, letter to the Subcommittee on Oversight and Investigations, Weiss said he particularly remembered "the emotional reaction that I observed from one of the pre-eminent scientists in the world. I had never heard him speak frankly. I think he may have cursed at the time. That made an impression on me." Following the discussion in the hallway, Weiss said, Gallo "retired to his office to solicit advice from other colleagues around the country. I believe he eventually called Dr. Montagnier later that evening to relate that it looked like the French had contaminated their LAV with material from LTCB." In a September 23, 1992, interview with the SOI, Shaw said he had no recollection of having met with Gallo on a single occasion to present data on the genetic dissimilarity between R.F. and 3B, and that the genetic divergence between R.F. and the other AIDS viruses in Gallo's lab had been the subject of many less dramatic conversations among himself, Wong-Staal, and Gallo. The recognition that LAV and HTLV-3B were too much alike to be independent isolates from different patients, Shaw said, had been a gradual one, rather than a sudden flash of insight that would have occasioned the moment recalled by Weiss. Ten days after Weiss's letter to the SOI, Gallo wrote to Weiss's department chairman at the New Jersey University of Medicine and Dentistry, "enthusiastically" recommending Weiss for promotion to associate professor with tenure.

ʰ·Gallo to OSI, April 4, 1990. Gallo's October 25, 1984, memo to Vince DeVita states that "the cell line we received from them probably contains our virus. They had our producer cell line for months before we received theirs."

ⁱ·According to Montagnier's lab notes, the BJAB B-cell line, obtained from George Klein, was infected on April 27, 1984, with LAV from its predecessor, the FR-8 B-cell line created by Montagnier the previous November.

ʲ·When epidemiologists pointed out that if the AIDS virus could be transmitted through saliva, millions of Americans would have AIDS, Salahuddin and Groopman countered with the case of a sixty-one-year-old woman who they claimed had contracted the virus merely by kissing her husband (Salahuddin, S. Z., *et al.* "HTLV-III in symptom-free seronegative persons." *The Lancet* ii:1418, December 22/29, 1984). When the CDC tried to follow up the "case of kissing AIDS," repeated efforts to isolate the virus from the woman were unavailing (Curran, J. W., *et al.* "Epidemiology of HIV infection and AIDS in the United States." *Science* 239:610, February 5, 1988). Groopman told the *New York Times* he planned to send a retraction to *The Lancet* ("A flaw in the research process: Uncorrected errors in journals," *New York Times,* May 31, 1988). When no correction was forthcoming, Groopman explained that Gallo had advised waiting until the woman's T-cells could be analyzed with DNA probes to make certain they contained no AIDS virus. By then the woman couldn't be located, and the analysis was never performed. It was left to Groopman's Harvard colleague, David Ho, to report that the AIDS virus was rarely found in saliva, and that "casual transmission of HTLV-3 does not occur, even among household members exposed to the saliva of infected persons" (Ho, D. D., *et al.* "Infrequency of isolation of HTLV-3 virus from saliva in AIDS." *N. Engl. J. Med.,* 1606, December 19, 1985). In a November 27, 1996, letter to the author, Groopman acknowledged that "there is no compelling data to suggest salivary transmission of HIV," and that the isolation of HIV from saliva "is probably a laboratory finding which is not recapitulated epidemiologically." Not until 1997 did the CDC report the first apparent case of HIV transmission through kissing, in a heterosexual couple with severe gum disease.

k. Simon Wain-Hobson confirmed that "Montagnier talked to them and said, 'Get that out, it's not correct.' He was in contact with the CDC, saying, 'My people can't reproduce this, I don't want that in the paper.' He tried a number of times, to no avail."

l. R. Gallo to J. McDougall, May 19, 1984. According to the fine print in Gallo's paper, the conditions under which the experiments were conducted created an environment in which two pieces of DNA with very little in common would still be likely to display some apparent biochemical attraction. Years later, Gallo admitted that "there were conditions of hybridization that were too loose. There's only a few percent homology. You know, you can get into things because this is what you think and because this is what you believe. What I'm trying to say is, if you knew too much it prejudiced one" (R. Gallo telephone interview with the author, September 26, 1988).

m. Not only did Wong-Staal's unpublished manuscript belie Gallo's insistence that the French "didn't have enough material to send us" to make any comparisons with HTLV-3B, it undercut Gallo's claim that 3B had contaminated Montagnier's LAV cultures following Sarngadharan's visit to Paris. One of the restriction enzymes used in the experiments, *SST-1,* cleaved the DNA of one HTLV-3B clone, HXB2, and one Ti7.4/LAV clone, J-81, at precisely the same point, about 5,500 nucleotides downstream from the 5-prime terminus. Another enzyme, *Bgl* II, produced a similarly unique dual fingerprint. Gallo told the OSI the comparisons had been done by Beatrice Hahn in the late summer of 1984, and Hahn's notebook showed that she indeed compared HTLV-3B with LAV in late August and early September of that year (experiments B_6 and E_6, completed on September 2, 1984). But when Hahn was shown a copy of Wong-Staal's manuscript during a September 24, 1992, interview with the Subcommittee on Oversight and Investigations, she replied that "I don't think I have ever seen this," and "I don't recall having ever analyzed Ti7.4/LAV." In his memoir, *Virus Hunting,* Gallo states that it was Wong-Staal who "compared the genetic material of LAV with our isolates."

[n.]Bryant recalled Lee Ratner telling him that his manuscript had been discussed at a Gallo staff meeting.

[o.]M. Gardner to SOI, February 1, 1993. In a December 20, 1988, letter to Gallo, written at Gallo's request, Gardner stated that "In no way was I prevented from publishing our data on these virus comparisons. I agreed of my own free will and still believe strongly it was the right decision. . . . [M]y research program has not been delayed or influenced in any way by this course of events."

[p.]According to Beatrice Hahn's April 6, 1990, letter to Gallo, preparation for the cloning experiment which produced the first full-length clone of HTLV-3B, named BH10 ("BH" for "Beatrice Hahn"), began on May 29, 1984. Prior to the cloning of BH10, Hahn and George Shaw derived a partial HTLV-3B clone, designated BH5. The first reference in Shaw's notes to BH5 is dated June 8, 1984 — more than two months after the Pasteur's first partial clone of LAV. In explaining the lack of dates on several of her subsequent notebook pages, Hahn told the SOI that "I have a mental block when it comes to dates." However, the government's application for a patent on BH10 was filed August 22, 1984, suggesting that the clone was completed on or shortly before that date. Wain-Hobson's notes show that the first full-length clone of LAV, J-19, was obtained on August 16, 1984.

[q.]The first two genes, which contain the genetic code for the core proteins and the virus's reverse transcriptase, were roughly in the same spot, although in LAV the ends of the genes overlapped. But LAV had a third gene, which Wain-Hobson named Q, that was missing altogether from HTLV-1. The fourth gene contained the DNA code for the proteins that formed the protective viral envelope.

[r.]John Maddox promised to "dig that paper out" of *Nature*'s archives and provide "a yes or no answer" to the question of whether it had been changed between submission and publication. Despite repeated reminders to Maddox of his promise, no answer has ever been forthcoming.

[s.]The first three genes of HTLV-3B were the same as LAV. The fifth gene, which Wain-Hobson had named F, was more problematic. The Gallo group had sequenced two clones of HTLV-3B. The first didn't appear to have the fifth gene, but the second did. Or did it? Because HTLV-1 didn't have five genes, the prevailing opinion in Gallo's lab was that the AIDS virus didn't either, and that what looked like a fifth gene was an artifact. "Nobody was believing that it was a functional gene," said Nancy

Chang, one of the Gallo sequencers. The most glaring difference, however, was in the fourth gene, the envelope gene. According to Gallo, the envelope gene in HTLV-3 was the same length as its counterpart in HTLV-1, which made it only half as long as the one in LAV. The extra space in Gallo's gene map was occupied by a region named *lor*, for *long open reading frame*, that might or might not contain the genetic code for a protein — hence the ambiguous name. Bill Haseltine suggested that the fourth gene of HTLV-3B must be a fusion of *env* and *lor* — Haseltine gave it the name *env-lor* — that contained the DNA code for *two* proteins: the envelope protein, and a second protein analogous to a mystery protein produced by the HTLV-1 called *pX*. But Haseltine had been wrong — there was no *"env-lor."*

t. The fourth gene in ARV was a very long envelope gene and nothing else, and ARV also had the *F* gene.

u. Wain-Hobson recalled that Sam Broder hadn't asked for a copy of his symposium paper until six weeks after the seminar, just before the Pasteur's LAV sequence was about to come out in *Cell*. By then, Wain-Hobson said, there hadn't seemed any point in submitting the paper to the NCI.

v. According to Gallo, the footnote "was not added by Dr. Wong-Staal, and she has never claimed priority for the content of one symposium paper based on the time or presentation." Wong-Staal told the OSI that in March and April of 1985 — three months after the December NIH symposium — "we and independently Haseltine's group were able to functionally map the transactivator gene precisely. The paper describing this work was submitted to *Science* in May and published in July. Obviously, knowing the precise location of this gene, it would have been silly and wrong to still refer to *env-lor* in the *Cancer Research* paper that was published two months later." But Wong-Staal couldn't explain why her published paper claimed the gene map had been presented at the symposium.

w. Chermann, J. C., *et al.* "Comparative immunological properties of LAV and HTLV-3." Unpublished manuscript. L. Montagnier to R. Gallo, January 2, 1985. Although the protein comparison paper was written at Pasteur and was to have been one of three joint publications with Gallo's lab, Gallo evidently intended to take primary credit for those experiments. When he noted, in a *Science* article (226:1165) published in December 1984, that 3B and LAV were "immunologically indistinguishable," the footnote referred not to Chermann's paper but to a paper by "M. G. Sarngadharan *et al.*, in preparation."

Chapter 8. "Let Them Bark in the Wind"

a. Popovic's lab notes show that the pool from which he claimed to have isolated HTLV-3B was created on November 15, 1983, from samples received by Gallo's laboratory during the preceding four months. None of the ten pool patients was from New York City. Four were from Long Island, the rest from Washington, D.C., and North Carolina, and the majority weren't gay men.

b.B. Read lab notes, June 28, 1984. To Popovic's consternation, by the time the *Science* papers were published in May of 1984 Matt Gonda hadn't been able to photograph any virus in R.F.'s cells (Visiting Associate, LTCB, DTP, DCT, NCI, to Chief, Laboratory of Tumor Cell Biology, DPT, DCT, NCI. November 28, 1984). Struggling over the summer of 1984 to get HTLV-3$_{RF}$ "out the door" of Gallo's lab, Popovic asked Gonda to try one more time to find the AIDS virus in the original R.F. cells. "Mika was extremely aggravated," Gonda recalled, "and wanted us to go back until we found virus." In October 1984, after re-examining the original R.F. sample from early in the year, Gonda finally found a solitary particle of HTLV-3 — the equivalent of one virus per six thousand cells, an indication that the R.F. culture hadn't been very productive (M. Gonda to M. Popovic, October 17, 1984; M. Gonda to OSI, August 13, 1990).

c.According to a summary of Francis's March 11, 1992, interview with the General Accounting Office, "Dr. Gallo telephoned Dr. Francis to express in a caustic manner his displeasure that he had hired 'Kaly' away from him. During the conversation Dr. Gallo made direct references to Dr. Francis that he would prevent him from publishing in the future or perform any work in the area of retrovirology."

d.In a letter to the author dated June 14, 1991, Kalyanaraman's attorney stated that "Dr. Kalyanaraman did not make the statements referred to" by Omar Sattaur.

e.Abbott Laboratories, Inc. Product License Application for the Manufacture of Human T-Lymphotropic Virus, Type III, December 19, 1984. Of 7,758 blood samples from "normal healthy donors," forty-two tested positive. Of these, seventeen were true positives and twenty-five false positives.

f.FDA AIDS workshop, December 26, 1984. "Initial studies indicate that all tests successfully identify HTLV III reactive samples but confirmatory testing will be required since a significant proportion of donor samples yield false positive results."

g.Electronucleonics received its license on Thursday, March 7, 1985.

h.Philadelphia got 8,000 tests, followed by Boston (7,300), Los Angeles (7,000), Detroit (6,000), Cleveland (5,000), Washington, D.C. (4,500), and Atlanta (4,000).

i.At the time Gallo spoke, between 200,000 and 300,000 Americans were believed to be infected with the AIDS virus. Subsequent epidemiological studies have shown that, even at the epidemic's peak, there were never more than 750,000 at any one time, and probably substantially fewer.

j.By the end of 1999, according to the U.K. Public Health Laboratory, 32,200 British had been diagnosed as infected with the AIDS virus, and 15,500 of those had subsequently developed AIDS, 12,800 of whom had died.

k.Montagnier credited Robin Weiss for "the beginning of our knowledge that the virus could grow in CEM." According to Montagnier, however, the LAV-infected CEM line Weiss delivered to Pasteur in the spring of 1984 contained mycoplasma. Rather than go through the laborious process of removing the bacteria, Montagnier had obtained a mycoplasma-free sample of CEM from the American Type Culture Collection and given it to Klatzmann to clone.

[l.]The patent office case file shows the Pasteur application, "Antigens, Means and Method for the Diagnosis of Lymphadenopathy and Acquired Immune Deficiency Syndrome," was filed on December 5, 1983, but not "docketed" until December 27, 1984. The examiner's interference search was performed on November 15, 1984.

[m.]D. Bassett to S. Nunn, July 26, 1985; B. Chabner to A. D'Amato, August 8, 1985; P. Fischinger to C. Dodd, July 22, 1985. To Senator Christopher Dodd of Connecticut, Peter Fischinger replied that HTLV-3 was "very similar to but clearly different from the LAV isolate. Accordingly, Dr. Gallo did not 'steal' the virus from France. In fact, he had many of his own isolates, each of which could have been used for the development of diagnostic tests."

[n.]The "Chermann history" provided by Gallo to the OSI was dated July 1985. However, in a September 8, 1986, note to James Wyngaarden, Gallo gives March 8, 1986, as the date Chermann signed the document "in the presence of Professor Daniel Zagury and Dr. Escoffier-Lambiotte." In a letter to the author dated August 4, 1995, Escoffier-Lambiotte stated that "Of course, I was *not present* at Zagury's home" when the history was written. NIH travel order 636356 shows that Gallo was supposed to have been attending an AIDS symposium at the University of Genoa on March 8.

Chapter 9. "I Don't Want to Go to Jail"

[a.]Transcript of telephone conversation between B. Hampar and J. Roberts, August 7, 1985, as provided by Roberts to the SOI. Although Hampar was unaware at the time that Roberts was recording their conversation, he agreed to the use of the transcribed conversation in this book.

[b.]M. Popovic to OSI, December 21, 1990, p. 29. According to Betsy Read's notes, on September 20, 1983, reverse transcriptase was detected in fresh lymphocytes infected with the July LAV sample, the cells in which Matt Gonda first photographed the AIDS virus. The September LAV grew continuously from October 24, 1983 — not in "fresh T-cells" but in two continuous T-cell lines, HUT-78 and Ti7.4.

[c.]In a July 16, 1992, interview with the General Accounting Office, Fischinger acknowledged having known about the CDC blood-test results with the French ELISA in the spring of 1984, and having concluded at that time that LAV was the cause of AIDS.

[d.]Fischinger's report conceded the French apparently had some kind of test, but one designed to pick up antibodies primarily to the core protein of the AIDS virus, p24. "We now know that many AIDS patients do not have detectable anti-p24 antibodies,"

Fischinger told Harmison, "while all have antibodies to the envelope gp41 component" — which happened to be the primary "target antigen" of the Gallo test. But when Harmison asked Sarngadharan how many proteins in Western Blot should be positive before concluding that a person was infected with the AIDS virus, Sarngadharan replied that either p24 or gp41 alone would be enough.

e.The "December 1982" isolates surfaced when the search for Mika Popovic's lab notes turned up a musty piece of paper showing that the cultured cells from two AIDS patients, H.R. and C.M., had scored as "plus-minus" for reverse transcriptase and negative for the presence of HTLV-1 on December 26, 1982. Since the only AIDS patients of interest to Gallo's lab were those infected with HTLV-1, no attempt had been made to culture a virus from those patients (LTCB response to OSI question 4a). So insignificant were the two samples that Ersell Richardson's logbook records C.M. as "negative" for RT and contains no mention of H.R.

f.Fischinger referred to a recent article in *Science* (Wong-Staal, F., *et al.* "Genomic diversity of human T-lymphotropic virus type 3 (HTLV-3)." *Science* 229:759, August 23, 1985) reporting that an AIDS virus had been isolated from a New Jersey homosexual, S.L., that was a virtual twin of $HTLV3_{MN}$ — a difference of 1 restriction site in 23. The fact that M.N. was an infant excluded any sexual contact. But M.N. had been born in New Jersey, and Gallo concluded, erroneously, that the baby's mother, an intravenous drug user, had picked up and passed on to her child the same virus that infected S.L.

g."This is considered to be very critical," Fischinger wrote Gallo. "We understand that pools of several patients' samples were used and on more than one occasion. What is needed is: what samples were used and at what times, how much of each, the patients' initials and the clinical source of each, when the first positive tests occurred, and the sequence of that documentation. We need an oral description as well as copied pages from relevant notebooks."

h.Wong-Staal, F., and Gallo, R. C. "Human T-lymphotropic retroviruses," *Nature* 317:395, October 3, 1985. Six weeks later, in a less-than-mainstream journal where it was not likely to be seen by many people, Lee Ratner acknowledged that the AIDS virus had "a distinct genetic structure" from HTLV-1 and HTLV-2, and "shares only very distant nucleic acid similarities with them" (Ratner, L., *et al.* "Polymorphism of the 3' open reading frame of the virus associated with the acquired immune deficiency syndrome, human T-lymphotropic virus type III." *Nucleic Acids Research* 13:8219, November 25, 1985).

i.M. Popovic to R. Gallo, September 6, 1985. According to Popovic's February 13, 1992, submission to OSI, the draft of Popovic's memo is in Gallo's handwriting.

j.The Pasteur serology reported at Park City was performed in November and December of 1983. According to the CDC's "Calendar of Events June 1983–June 1984," Kalyanaraman and another CDC scientist, Jane Getchell, did not arrive in

Paris until April 22, 1984 — not to assist the French, but to "consult with Dr. Chermann, to learn serological techniques and perform serology on AIDS-related sera [and] to obtain information on virus growth and isolation techniques. . . ."

[k.]There are only about ninety nucleotide differences between 3B and LAV, not 150, and those ninety differences would have been more or less evenly divided between the two virus cultures, with forty-five occurring in Paris and the other forty-five in Bethesda. Before HTLV-3B was cloned by Beatrice Hahn it had been growing in Gallo's lab for more than six months, not six weeks. Fewer than fifty nucleotide changes over six months is well within the mutational realm of a retrovirus comprised of more than nine thousand nucleotides and which changes its overall genetic makeup by 5 percent a year.

[l.]Popovic evidently referred to the restriction analyses showing the genetic identity of LAV and HTLV-3B contained in the unpublished paper by Flossie Wong-Staal.

Chapter 10. "French Virus in the Picture"

[a.]E. Esber to D. Awberry, February 19, 1986. Abbott's application for an FDA license was filed on December 24, 1984, and granted March 2, 1985. Genetic Systems's application was filed on May 16, 1985, and granted on February 19, 1986.

[b.]Genetic Systems news release, February 19, 1986. A few months earlier, Genetic Systems had been purchased for $300 million by Bristol-Myers, which retained Bob Nowinski and George Todaro as the company's chief executive officer and scientific director.

[c.]First to successfully infect CEM with the AIDS virus was Robin Weiss, on February 29, 1984. The first mention of CEM in Gallo's lab notes is dated May 28, 1984, a month after Weiss had told Gallo of his success with CEM in Cremona.

[d.]According to Montagnier's notebook, the cells, code-named *Mir,* sent by a Portuguese microbiologist, Odette Santos-Ferreira, arrived in his laboratory on September 16, 1985.

[e.]In the current nomenclature, HTLV-3B and LAV_{Bru} are designated $HIV-1_{Lai}$. ARV-2 is $HIV-1_{SF2}$. $HTLV-3_{RF}$ is $HIV-1_{RF}$. For consistency, the original designations will be retained throughout this book.

[f.]Besides Robin Weiss, the other signatories were John Coffin, Ashley Haase, Jay Levy, Luc Montagnier, Steven Oroszlan, Natalie Teich, Howard Temin, Kumao Toyoshima, Harold Varmus, and Peter Vogt.

[g.]The correction states that "In the several months preceding preparation of the composite in question, electron micrographs of cultures infected with our HTLV-3 isolates were available from specimens obtained from known ARC and AIDS patients. One appeared in Gallo *et al.;* others were used in Popovic *et al.* and Shaw *et al."* In fact, Gallo had only one micrograph of an AIDS virus other than LAV, the picture in Gallo *et al.* of Zaki Salahuddin's J.S. As Gallo later acknowledged, the micrographs in Popovic *et al.* and Shaw *et al.* were also pictures of LAV.

h·Gallo wrote Bernard on February 10, 1986, that "What [Montagnier] sent us was an extremely small amount of virus particles present in media from a temporarily infected dying T-cell. What we did is what we were supposed to do. We temporarily transmitted the virus to human fresh blood T-cells (which soon die) to confirm it was a virus. We also determined that the particles had some reverse transcriptase-like activity and, therefore, confirmed that it was probably a retrovirus. (However, the amount was so small we could not characterize the enzyme.) . . . We did nothing more with this virus which they stated could not be grown in a permanent cell line, which is, of course, exactly what we succeeded in doing with several of our isolates of HTLV-III."

i·That didn't square with Gallo's bombastic telephone call to Matt Gonda over Gonda's identification of LAV as a lentivirus; or with Montagnier's recollection of the Palais des Congrès meeting where Gallo told Montagnier "that he had seen under the electron microscope the virus I gave to him"; or with the Tokyo taxi ride in which Gallo told Françoise Barré he had pictures of a T-cell-killing virus that looked "just like LAV."

j·Crewdson, J. "The Great AIDS Quest." *Chicago Tribune,* November 19, 1989. According to Hampar's later recollection to the OSI, it was a few days *before* Gonda's meeting with Swire that Gonda discovered the *Science* pictures were LAV. That revelation, Hampar said, had been prompted by a request from someone in Gallo's lab "to recheck the origin of the photos used to make the composite." If Hampar's recollection is correct, someone in Gallo's lab discovered the mislabeling on his or her own. Another indication that Gallo's lab knew of the mislabeling before Gonda heard about it from the Pasteur lawyers was Gonda's recollection to OSI of a "frantic" call from Mika Popovic prior to Gonda's meeting with Jim Swire. "He was mad at me for something," Gonda said. "I had absolutely no idea what. He says, you know, 'I want you to get some photographs for me,' or 'I want to know who you gave these photographs to.' Mika doesn't make a lot of sense when you try to talk to him. When he is mad, it is even worse." It was at that point, Gonda said — not after his meeting with Swire — that "I notified government officials, we have got a problem. These are LAV." However, in a subsequent letter to the OSI, Gonda dated the call from Popovic as March 14, 1986 — more than a month *after* his meeting with Jim Swire. That date seems implausible, since Gallo and his assistants learned of Gonda's meeting with Swire shortly after it occurred. Gallo further confused matters by telling the *New York Times* that the mislabeling of the LAV micrographs had been discovered in his own lab, during "a thorough review of documents after the recent pretrial questioning of Dr. Gonda by the Pasteur Institute's attorneys." However, the fact that George Todaro learned of the mislabeling in December of 1985 suggests that it was known within NCI at least two months before Gonda's meeting with Swire, and it seems likely that Gallo or someone in his lab would have been informed at that time. Nevertheless, the micrograph mix-up might never have become public had Todaro not been tipped off.

[k.]Gonda recalled having chosen the pictures the day before beginning a vacation to England. In a September 21, 1990, letter to OSI, Gonda said he departed for London on April 19, 1984, the day the Gallo manuscripts were accepted for publication by *Science.* That chronology would date the selection of the pictures as April 18. However, Gallo's talks in Zurich on April 5, and at the Pasteur on April 6, were both illustrated with a picture of "HTLV-3" (R. Gallo to OSI, December 2, 1990). No copy of the picture shown at the Pasteur is known to exist, but one of the slides Gallo presented in Zurich the previous day is the same collage of HTLV-1, HTLV-2, and HTLV-3 (actually LAV) that appeared in *Science.* The only apparent explanation is that the picture of LAV was selected by Gonda prior to Gallo's departure for Zurich on Sunday, April 1 — nearly three weeks before the April 18 date given by Gonda. The April 1 date coincides with the purported reason for creating the collage — to counter objections at *Science* about the insubstantiality of Jorge Schupbach's paper, which was submitted to *Science* on Friday, March 30. If the LAV micrographs were selected following the Schupbach paper's receipt at *Science* and prior to Gallo's departure on April 1, the most likely date would then be Saturday, March 31.

[l.]Popovic's *Science* article included a micrograph of an AIDS virus identified only as "clone H4/HTLV-3," which Gallo later admitted was also HTLV-3B, i.e., LAV (R. Gallo, "Introductory Remarks" to OSI, July 18, 1990).

[m.]In an August 10, 1995, letter to Peter-Hans Hofschneider, Gallo declared that an "error was obviously made by our collaborating microscopist, Matt Gonda, working in Frederick, Maryland, forty miles away from me."

[n.]Gonda told the OSI on August 13, 1990, that when he was shown the micrograph "I said that is not HTLV-3." Gallo acknowledged to OSI (May 25, 1990) that Gonda "did not feel confident" that the virus depicted was HIV, and that because Gonda was a co-author of the *Science* correction Gallo "had no other choice" but to withdraw the EM.

[o.]Patient Sample	Test or assay	*Nature* letter	LTCB notebooks
G. W.	Reverse transcriptase	Positive	+\−
G. W.	HTLV-1 p24	Negative	Not Done
B.U.	Reverse transcriptase	Positive	+\−
M.A.	Reverse transcriptase	Positive	+\−
M.A.	HTLV-1 p19	Negative	Positive

M.A.	HTLV-1 p24	Negative	Not Done
C.C.	HTLV-1 p19	+\−	Positive
C.C.	HTLV-1 p24	+\−	Positive
R.F.	Electron microscopy	Positive, Oct. 18, 1983	Positive, Oct. 17, 1984
S.N.	Electron microscopy	Not Done	Negative (Gonda to Popovic, Feb. 22, 1984).

p. Ersell Richardson's lab notes show that G.W. was negative for reverse transcriptase on December 15, 1982, positive on February 17, 1983, and negative thereafter.

q. Gallo, R. C., *et al.* "Isolation of human T-cell leukemia virus in acquired immune deficiency syndrome (AIDS)." *Science* 220:865, May 20, 1983. Although neither of the French AIDS patients is named in the article, only M.A. and Claude Chardon were positive for HTLV-1. Ersell Richardson's cell sample log records M.A. (3735) as positive for HTLV-1 *p19* antibody at day 29.

r. In his May 16, 1990, interview with the OSI, Gallo stated that "experiments to separate the HIV-1 component of C.C. from HTLV-1" were carried out on April 2, 1986 — two weeks before the letter describing Claude Chardon as an AIDS virus isolate was mailed to *Nature*.

s. The electron micrographs published in the Pasteur's May 20, 1983, *Science* article were made on March 29 and April 5 of that year.

t. J. Lemp to R. Gallo, December 11, 1985. The letter states that "Your Accession No. W3731 was received on May 9, 1983, from Ms. E. Richardson in your LTCB. Dr. Kramarsky prepared blocks from the infected cell pellet, and the EM photomicrographs #7083-4 and #7084-4 were actually finished on May 26, 1983, from the virus-infected cells received from NCI on May 9, 1983."

u. In his August 19, 1985, memo to Peter Fischinger, Gallo states that "Numerous isolates from AIDS patients' material were obtained in our laboratory prior to receiving any LAV and prior to receiving viable LAV. . . . These isolates showed R.T. activity, were co-cultured, and were negative for p24 and p19 of HTLV-1. We felt EM would not be more informative at this stage." While the *Nature* letter was being prepared, however, Mika Popovic asked the electron microscopist at Electronucleonics, Bernhard Kramarsky, to reassess a picture Kramarsky had taken of cells from the patient L.S. on February 29, 1984. On March 25, 1986, Kramarsky wrote Popovic that the virus particle in the picture "is considerably smaller than the usual HTLV-3 virion. But when an irregularly shaped particle is sectioned at a certain angle this profile may result. The dense core is about right for HTLV-III. On this basis I conclude that if confirmed by reverse transcriptase and immunofluorescence data the culture should be considered positive for HTLV-3." No picture of HTLV3$_{LS}$ has ever appeared in print.

^{v.}A May 26, 1983, report from Electronucleonics to the Laboratory of Tumor Cell Biology states that plates 7081-7086, made from virus extracted from C-103 + W3731 (Chardon co-culture with C103 cord blood cell line) and W-3731 contain "C-type particles." HTLV-1 and HTLV-2 are type-C retroviruses — but not the AIDS virus, which has some features of a D-type retrovirus but belongs to the lentivirus subgroup of retroviruses.

^{w.}An Electronucleonics technician wrote Gallo in December 1985 that "Relative to my discussion with you and Dr. Striker [*sic*] about early HTLV cultures which we received from your laboratory for cultivation and EM, Dr. Kramarsky has found two thin, cell pellet sections (attached) which have aberrant morphology, neither HTLV-1 nor HTLV-2." Electronucleonics produced a second version of the letter, dated the same day but with a different first paragraph, in which the new particles were described as "morphologically-distinct HTLV-3 virus."

Chapter 11. "Bingo. We Win"

^{a.}When Weiss asked Karpas for samples of the "Karpas T-cell line" and the AIDS virus, C-LAV, Karpas claimed to have isolated in December of 1983, Karpas pretended not to be reassured by Weiss's promise that neither the virus nor the cell line would leave Weiss's laboratory. "I regret very much having to say that I do not feel able at present to place my trust and confidence in your assurances," Karpas wrote Weiss. "Might not my cell line end up with a new name and a rediscovery?" Weiss replied that he was "dismayed that you express doubt as to my academic propriety and integrity, which remarks I must ask you to withdraw. . . . I am returning your letter with this one, and I invite you, upon reflection, to destroy both of them. I have kept copies of this correspondence, but will be happy to destroy these on hearing within the next two weeks that you have done the same to the originals." Karpas responded by thanking Weiss for his letter, "which in fact I will not destroy. I may even frame it next to mine. Unfortunately I remain tormented by doubts and therefore am unable to withdraw any of my remarks about your academic propriety and integrity. I am also reminded of your writing in *Nature* about the French '. . . skimpy data . . .' — an odd way of thanking Dr. Montagnier for providing you with the French AIDS virus isolate."

^{b.}According to Sarngadharan's May 1984 article in *Science,* the original Gallo ELISA detected HTLV-3 antibodies in 88 percent of AIDS patients tested, a 12 percent false-negative rate. There is no indication in the article that the sera tested were coded, which would represent a major protocol violation. With coded sera sent by other laboratories, however, the Gallo ELISA did much worse. When Sarngadharan tested blind samples from Sloan-Kettering, 52 percent of AIDS patients were negative (Safai, B., *et al.* "Seroepidemiological studies of human T-lymphotropic retrovirus Type III in acquired immunodeficiency syndrome." *Lancet* 1438. June 30, 1984), and only 60 percent of the coded AIDS sera provided by David Ho at the Massachusetts General Hospital (D. Ho to M. Sarngadharan, May 25, 1984). In both

cases, Gallo's score was about the same as his original tally with the CDC blood samples before it was enhanced by Jim Curran.

c. In a May 20, 1986, letter to Abbott's Sally Hojvat, Nancy Dock of the Red Cross blood center in Syracuse wrote that "[w]e are extremely concerned about the Abbott modified EIA which detects this sample as reactive only 2 of 3 times tested, and about certain lot numbers of the current Abbott assay which do not detect it as reactive at all . . . the donor of this sample has been documented to be an HTLV III/LAV seroconverter and is viral culture positive by RT assay. Information regarding this sample was brought to the attention of Mr. Bill Stall at Abbott by Dr. Harold Lamberson on April 28, 1986, and they have discussed the problem at length." Tabulation of the Syracuse data shows that the modified Abbott ELISA missed HIV antibodies in two AIDS patients. See also M. Klamrznski telephone notes (conversation with S. Risso), May 15, 1986.

d. FDA Conversation Records, S. Risso and M. Klamrznski, May 15, 1986; S. Risso and M. J. Sidote, May 16, 1986. Of her conversation with Abbott's Sidote, the FDA's Sharon Risso wrote "that at least one site [Red Cross Syracuse] indicated to FDA that they had data from a study requested by Abbott, but that Abbott had not asked that the data be reported to them. I asked her to contact all sites in order to provide assurances to FDA that all data requested had been received and for her to submit any additional data to FDA. She assured me that Abbott had not censored any data and had provided all data available to them. She said they had contacted Syracuse based on my call yesterday and that Syracuse had indicated that all data had been received to Abbott except raw data listings which they would provide." In a May 27, 1986, letter to the FDA, Abbott acknowledged that the problem with Syracuse sample 313 had been discussed by the Syracuse center director, Dr. Harold Lamberson, and Abbott's William Stall on April 29, 1986 — but that Lamberson's call had been recorded by Stall "as a current product quality issue," not a false-negative report.

e. According to the *Philadelphia Inquirer,* by 1988 fifty-nine cents of every dollar spent by the Red Cross went to operate its blood program, while less than ten cents went to disaster relief. The best account of the American Red Cross's blood business is contained in the Pulitzer Prize–winning *Inquirer* series by Gilbert M. Gaul, which appeared in that newspaper September 24–28, 1989.

f. Defendant's Reply to Plaintiff's Opposition to Defendant's Motion to Stay Discovery. *Institut Pasteur v. The United States,* 730-85C. United States Court of Claims, May 19, 1986. Although the government informed the court that the genetic difference was 1.8 percent, or about 165 nucleotides out of 9,213, the actual difference is only 86 nucleotides, or less than 1 percent (Weiss, R. A., *et al. RNA Tumor Viruses,* 1107–1123. New York: Cold Spring Harbor Laboratory, 1985). Gallo later acknowledged that the real difference was less than 100 nucleotides.

g. Reply Affidavit of James B. Swire in Further Support of Motion to Compel. *Institut Pasteur v. The United States.* United States Claims Court, 730-85C, May 8, 1986. In an April 1, 1986, letter to acting assistant HHS secretary Anthony McCann, Swire maintained that "Although the Department claimed to have identified approximately 16,000 pages of responsive documents, it has thus far managed to provide only 4,600 pages of material. Further, of these 4,600 pages, only 1,600 or so are at all responsive to the narrowed request."

[h.]R. Gallo to V. DeVita, August 4, 1983. A May 12, 1986, letter to Swire from the HHS FOIA officer, Russell Roberts, lists 26 documents being withheld under the various exemptions in the FOIA law, including Gallo's August 19, 1985, memo to Fischinger, an August 21, 1985, memo from Gallo to Fischinger, and an August 7, 1985, memo from Fischinger to Gallo concerning the HHS meeting with Dedonder. At least one of the withheld documents, a two-page memo from Gallo to Fischinger dated August 29, 1985, has never been located. Other key documents, withheld in whole or in part on the ground that they contained "a predecisional exchange of opinions and ideas," included an August 27, 1985, memo from Fischinger to Harmison summarizing his investigation of Gallo's research; a September 10, 1985, memo from Fischinger to Gallo containing Mal Martin's questions; Gallo's September 18 reply, and his November 26, 1985, memo to Harmison.

[i.]Betsy Read's lab notes for October 6, 1983, consist of two pages, "A" and "B." The Eureka! experiment is recorded on the "A" page. Swire got only the "B" page, which showed that the virus in the July LAV sample wasn't HTLV-1 — which the French already knew. Another withheld page, dated October 27, 1983, showed Popovic's original LAV cultures producing reverse transcriptase. Also withheld was the page from Prem Sarin's notebook showing "HUT-78/LAV" and "Ti7.4/LAV" as RT positive at the end of October 1983, and a January 4, 1984, page in Popovic's handwriting headed "Rescue of LAV."

[j.]One of Popovic's pages, dated November 10, indicated that HUT-78 and Ti7.4 were still viable. The next day, both cultures, now identified as "HUT 78/v" and "Ti7.4/v," were still producing virus. Five days after that, material from "HUT 78/inf" and "Ti7.4/inf" had been sent to Sarngadharan. Six days later, on November 21, HUT-78/v and Ti7.4/v were still "O.K."

[k.]*October 21, 1983:* **LAV** *transmission to* **HUT-78, Ti7.4,** *CL-7, SR-2 and HOS* [*Read*]

October 24: *Additional LAV transmissions to* **HUT-78, Ti7.4,** *CL-7, SR-2 and HOS* [*Read*]

November 7: **HUT-78** *and* **Ti7.4** *cell increase slow. Giemsa: giant cells multinucleated more in HUT-78 RT — Sarang* [*Popovic*]

November 10: *HOS-does not grow-discarded.* **Ti7.4** *O.K. viability 70%* **HUT 78** *O.K. viability 65%* [*Popovic*]

November 11:   **HUT 78/v** *cell number* 6 × 10^5/ml **Ti7.4/v** *cell number* 4.3 × 10^5/ml [Popovic]

November 15:   1) Att: M. White [Gonda's assistant, Marty White] EM Studies 11/15/83 (Popovic) **HUT 78/LAV Ti7.4/LAV** (Popovic) 2) Culture fl. To Sarang for RT. **HUT 78/inf** +++ **Ti7.4/inf** +++ [Popovic]

November 21:   **HUT-78/v** *and* **Ti7.4/v** *O.K.* [Popovic]

November 22:   **HUT 78/v** *and* **Ti 7.4./v** = **MOV** [Popovic]

November 29:   Infection sup **HUT-78/MOV** usual procedure → Htu4 [Popovic]

December 5:   **HT/MOV** for concentration. Conc. **MOV** – Sarang [Popovic]

December 14:   1) **HUT 78/LAV** and **Ti7.4/LAV** are positive for lentivirus particles [Gonda]

December 28:   Conc. of culture fluids from **HT/MOV** . . . Sarang RT [Popovic]

January 2, 1984: Conc. virus **HT/MOV** Sarang RT. Cells for Schupbach [Popovic]

January 29:   **Mo variant** for RT Sarang [Popovic]

March 6:   RT Assay Tube 49; Sample #1 **Movariant** Counts 6731 [Popovic]

March 20:   RT . . . **Mo Variant**! + [Read]

April 13:   Extraction of high m.w. DNA from **MOV** [Shaw]

l.Except for the original Popovic–Betsy Read protocol, the only documents referring to the LAV-infected cultures as "LAV" were found in Matt Gonda's files: a November 15 note from Popovic to Gonda transmitting HUT-78/LAV and Ti7.4/LAV for electron microscopy, and Gonda's December 14 reply that HUT-78/LAV and Ti7.4/LAV were producing lentivirus. In his own notebook on November 15, Popovic first called the cultures HUT-78/v and Ti7.4/v, for "virus," and then HUT-78/inf and Ti7.4/inf, for "infected" (LTCB submission to OSI on MOV, May 10, 1990).

m.According to Swire, the redacted version of the December 14, 1983, Gonda-to-Popovic letter, which someone had photocopied after crudely taping over Gonda's observation of lentivirus particles in the two LAV-infected cell lines, was produced with other documents provided under the Freedom of Information Act on February 22, 1986. Gallo later denied knowing anything about it.

[n.]*November 15, 1983:*   *Isolation of HTLV/AIDS HUT-78 (preferred) infected with sup. From W6233 W6592 F 6367. RT +/–. Cultured in flasks 25 RPMI 1640-20 [Popovic]*

November 22:   *HUT 78 infected again. F6367 W6233 W 6592? Few Cells Multinucl. [Popovic]*

December 5:   ***HT/3 pooled.** Few conc. cells. [Popovic]*

January 2, 1984:   *W7644 W 7645 W7647 W 7675 W 7650 W7780 W7777 **HT/V pool** = conc. 1 ml after polybrene treatment [Popovic]*

February 25:   *Sup conc. **HT/pool:** H3; H4; H6; H9; H17; H35; H38 infected in the same time [Popovic]*

[o.]When Matt Gonda sent Popovic his results for twelve single-patient cultures on January 18, 1984, all were EM-negative for virus. Twenty-two additional samples, sent at the end of January, were also negative. When single-patient cultures were tested by immunofluorescence in early February, the number of virus-producing cells rarely crept above 10 percent (B. Read lab notes, February 2, 1984. On this day, R.F. was 5 percent positive, WT 2 percent, Charles King 2 percent, Ivan Hunt 4 percent. Only HP/H and Dm82631 surpassed 35 percent). According to Read's lab notes, several new S.N. cultures were begun as late as February 15, 1984.

[p.]*(**4BT**) shipment **Mo(v)** 5ml × 2.4×10^{10} parti.*
***LAV (MOV)** from Biotech (#**4BT**): Virus prep. And cDNA synthesis.*
*(**5BT**) shipment **Mo(v)** 5m. × 3.2×10^{10} parti.*
***LAV (5BT) (MOV):** Virus prep. And cDNA synthesis.*
*"shipment **HTLV-3B (H9)** banded 1 ml from Electronucleonics which was 3.2×10^{11}/ml resuspended in 1 ml TNE."*

Chapter 12. "A Small Guy Who Stumbled"

[a.]A tape of the September 19, 1986, interview, kindly provided by Maddox to the author, contains a gap of several minutes during which the conversation is obliterated by music. Efforts to recover the missing conversation electronically were unavailing.

[b.]The first reference to LAV in the notes mentioned by Maddox is dated January 19, 1984; the last, April 2. The collaboration of which Gallo spoke was not proposed until the April 6, 1984, tripartite meeting at the Pasteur, and not initiated until Sarngadharan's May 15, 1984, visit to Paris.

c.Although Gallo has alluded to a "break-in" at his laboratory, he has never produced any evidence that his laboratory was broken into, much less by anyone affiliated with the Institut Pasteur.

d.Through George Todaro's contacts at Frederick, Swire had received hints that Berge Hampar had landed in some trouble and might consider cooperating with the Pasteur. The allegations against Hampar came from an employee of the NCI's Frederick Cancer Research Facility, where Hampar had just retired as general manager. According to the employee, a group of Frederick researchers had agreed to use the NCI's laboratories to manufacture monoclonal antibodies, the diagnostic "silver bullets" worth considerable money on the open market. NIH investigators couldn't find evidence that any laws had been broken, and the only outcome of the investigation had been a minor disciplinary action against Hampar for failing to inform the NIH that he owned stock in a biotech company. Hampar suspected the investigation amounted to retribution for his questioning of the government's veracity in the Gallo case, and his "refusal to 'fall in line' as a supporter of the NCI's position." On a Sunday morning at the end of July 1986, Hampar got a call from Swire, who had heard about "recent events" at Frederick. According to Hampar's subsequent memo to the record, Swire "sympathetically referred to what he described as my abrupt dismissal as manager of the facility and my transfer from the FCRF. I responded that my departure was not unexpected since I had announced my intention to retire some time ago and that my replacement had been on board since May. He indicated he was aware of my plans to retire and asked if I had a lawyer. I replied that I wasn't aware that I needed one. He said he was not implying that I did. Mr. Swire then said that he had learned that I had abruptly changed my position concerning Dr. Gallo's role in the AIDS matter, and that two individuals would say that at a dinner meeting with me in December 1984 I stated that I had convincing evidence that Dr. Gallo had relabeled *LAV* to read HTLV-3. . . . I answered emphatically that this was impossible since I was not aware of any such evidence. He persisted in his claim concerning the individuals and said something to the effect that there also were notebook pages. I replied that my knowledge concerning AIDS work was limited to Frederick and I had no knowledge of what occurred in Dr. Gallo's lab. . . . I said that there was no possibility that any alleged mix-up of viruses could occur at Frederick. He reminded me of his meeting with Dr. Gonda where he indicated that the published pictures were *LAV* and not HTLV-3, and that subsequent events proved him correct. I replied that any comments on that situation would have to come from the Government. . . . I made a comment to the effect that I didn't see how the events at Frederick were related to the AIDS issue. Mr. Swire made some comments concerning mutual benefit and said if I would help them, they would help me. (I took this to mean that if I helped the French in the AIDS matter, the allegations against me at Frederick would disappear. . . .) After hanging up . . . I immediately reported the incident to the Government." When the HHS lawyers learned about the phone call, they asked the Justice Department whether Swire had violated the Code of Professional Responsibility (S. Trebbe to T. White, August 4, 1986). When Justice concluded that Swire hadn't, the HHS attorneys asked if it was legal to set up an electronic intercept of Swire's future telephone conversations. Justice replied that it might technically be legal, but that it didn't want anything to do with eavesdropping on a lawyer who was opposing the government in court. If HHS wanted to tap a lawyer's telephone, it would have to do so on its own (T. Byrnes to R. Charrow, August 6, 1986). "Crim Division said that our OIG [the HHS Inspector General] should do the intercept on Frederick/Swire," an HHS lawyer wrote (unsigned HHS attorney's notes, August 5, 1986). "Hot potato high visibility case — have to be extremely careful." There is no indication of whether such a tap was ever installed or, if it was, what it produced.

e. The incident to which Gallo referred occurred a few days after the *Science* correction appeared in print, while Myron Weinberg, Jim Swire's scientific consultant, was enjoying a postmovie snack with his wife at a delicatessen not far from the NIH. While the Weinbergs waited for their food, their attention was captured by snatches of conversation from the next table, which Weinberg recalled as concerning "an Oriental technician" who was going to "take the fall for mixing up some photographs," and a "convoluted story that Matt was sick that day." Weinberg's wife, who had had the best view of the other table, later identified the speaker from photographs as an NCI–Frederick researcher named Tom Wood. As Wood subsequently described the experience in an affidavit, he and his wife were dining on April 17, 1986, after attending a wedding in Frederick, Maryland. "We arrived at the restaurant at approximately 10:30 PM," Wood wrote. "Earlier that evening, while attending [a] wedding reception, a major topic of conversation had been the recent news articles regarding the alleged involvement of [the Frederick Cancer Research Center] personnel in the AIDS virus discovery. I had not discussed any aspect of this situation with my wife prior to attending the reception, consequently over dinner she asked several questions regarding the virus, the individuals mentioned in the article and the general controversy that had arisen. During our conversation I became increasingly aware that the gentleman sitting at the table adjacent to ours appeared to be paying an inordinate amount of attention to our conversation. His behavior was such that we discontinued the conversation and finished our dinner. A few weeks later on a Friday about 4:30 PM, I received a call from a gentleman who identified himself as a private investigator working for Colonial Insurance Company. He asked if I had been in Rockville, Maryland, on the night of April 17, 1986. I said I had. He asked if I had dinner at a restaurant called New York, New York. I asked why he wanted to know. He stated that there had been an accident and someone thought that a doctor with a beard who worked for PRI might have seen something. Since I had not observed an accident, I so stated and our conversation essentially ended. I still wanted to know where he got my name. The following Wednesday I received a call from a Mr. Swire, who identified himself as an attorney for the Pasteur Institute. He said that I should know why he was calling. He informed me that he had witnesses who were willing to state that I had evidence of a cover-up regarding the AIDS virus discovery and if I did not admit what I knew he would see that I "go down with the rest of the crooks." I said I didn't know anything and that I also had no way of knowing if he was who he said he was. He gave me a phone number and said to call it, they would verify his authenticity. I stated that as an employee with PRI under government contract I could not discuss this issue without informing my supervisor. He said that he considered me a hostile witness and that he would put me on the stand and ask me these questions. If I didn't answer them then he would prove that I was withholding information and that I had perjured myself."

f·Less than three weeks earlier, Gallo met with HHS lawyers and outside patent counsel "to review drafts of motions and preliminary statements" in the case against the French (unsigned HHS attorney's notes, September 1, 1986). The June–July 1986 billing statement from Cushman, Darby & Cushman, patent specialists retained by HHS, reflects conferences and telephone conversations with "Drs. Gallo, Sliski and Striker [*sic*]" regarding "initial drafting of motions and consideration of preliminary statement." Many of the documents filed by the government in claims court also contain routing slips showing they were sent to Gallo for comment.

g·Montagnier recalls shaving his mustache around this time, but only because "I was tired of it."

h·By his own admission to OSI, Gallo, not Popovic, selected HTLV-3B over R.F.

i·The second AIDS patient to go into the Popovic pool was a Jamaican.

j·Gallo never deposited HTLV-3$_{RF}$ with the ATCC.

k·"Pasteur plans to pursue patent suit on virus." *Nature* 320:96, March 13, 1986.

l·In his April 17, 1990, statement to OSI, Gallo claimed to have ordered Popovic to discontinue his work with LAV in early January 1984, some three months after Popovic's first cultures of LAV. However, there is no evidence that such a discontinuation ever occurred, except for a January 13 notepage showing that one of Gallo's freezers contained "frozen samples" of HUT-78/LAV and Ti7.4/LAV, the LAV cultures created by Betsy Read the previous October. Gallo construes this note as indicating that Popovic abruptly placed *all* his active LAV cultures "in the freezer" on January 13. However, a February 22, 1984, letter from Matt Gonda to Popovic reports electron microscope examinations of "HTU/31 LAV," "H/9 + LAV," "HUT 78/LAV," and "HUT/LAV." Since cell samples from those cultures were received by Gonda on February 15, even if all of Popovic's LAV cultures were frozen on January 13, some of them must have been unthawed a few weeks later to reinfect HUT-78 and the new clones. Asked if she remembered unthawing LAV in February 1984, Betsy Read told the SOI staff that "I don't recall *any* of that." Gallo concedes "there is no notebook entry" showing the thawing or reinfections, but maintains that "Dr. Popovic has stated this repeatedly at the time and since." The fact that Gonda saw no virus in any of the samples designated as "LAV" may have been due to the fact that those cultures were newly infected. Whatever the reason, the government lawyers relied on the February 22 Gonda letter as "evidence" that the French virus was unable to grow in Gallo's lab. The SOI staff concluded that the reinfections with LAV were red herrings created after Park City, to support Gallo's later claims that LAV never grew in Bethesda. As the SOI noted, "Why would Dr. Popovic, in the middle of the 'rush to save the blood supply'. . . suddenly decide to perform a laborious experiment" by attempting to culture a virus he had already grown for more than three months, and then send those cultures to Gonda when he already had plenty of pictures of LAV?

[m.]S. Arya laboratory notes, January 19, 1983, *et seq.* The page dated January 19 is headed, "HTLV cloned DNAs x LAV (BN1) cDNA." Similar entries exist dated January 27, January 30, February 5, February 7, February 23 ("LAV provirus Human cells"), February 25 ("LAV/Htu [Bn-1] [Mika virus]"), February 29 ("LAV/Htu [Bn2]: Mika Cell Culture"), March 5 ("Probe cDNA LAV [Bn2]"), March 16, March 21 ("Hybridization c LAV cDNA"), March 29 ("LAV [Mo(v)] from Biotech [#4BT]"), April 2 ("LAV (PZ-2)").

[n.]A September 21, 1986, memo from Arya to Gallo fails to mention that the first appearance of LAV in Arya's notebook actually occurred on January 19. A number of Arya's other LAV entries are also missing, including those for restriction and hybridization experiments performed on January 27 and 30, February 5, 23, and 29, and March 5 and 21.

[o.]S. Arya lab notes, January 19, 1984. As Maddox, Newmark, and Palca could have deduced from Popovic's notes, the only other candidate AIDS virus was MOV, then growing in sufficient quantities that Popovic had been able to send liters of concentrated virus to Sarngadharan two weeks before.

[p.]M. Popovic lab notes. "Infection sup HUT 78/MOV →Htu4." November 29, 1983. Gallo to S. Broder, June 3, 1994. The evidence that MOV had been used to make the DNA probes used in Arya's experiments was deleted from documents provided by Gallo's lab to OSI but was uncovered by the House Subcommittee on Oversight and Investigations.

[q.]Sarngadharan, the third inventor listed on the blood-test patent, also qualified for annual $100,000 payments. But under Sarngadharan's arrangement with his employer, Litton Bionetics, all such royalties were owned by the company.

Chapter 13. "Just Show Us the Proof"
[a.]"Abbott can't make enough gp41 to coat beads with 13% enriched lysate," wrote one attendee at the July 29 meeting. "At best can enrich about 4%."

[b.]The principal difference between the two tests, declared Byrnes, was that the French ELISA was attuned to antibodies to p24, while the Gallo test was focused on gp41. What Byrnes didn't mention was that the Gallo test had been producing false-negatives precisely *because* it failed to pick up antibodies to p24 — the flaw Abbott was working frantically to resolve. Byrnes next argued that the two tests were different inventions because the virus used in Gallo's test was being grown in the H-9 cell line, the availability of a permanent cell line being "absolutely essential to produce the virus for use in any detection method if meaningful results are to be obtained." But the French were contesting the patent on the blood test, not the separate patent for H-9. Considering the false positives H-9 was causing, the Pasteur was happy to grow its virus in CEM and leave H-9 to the Americans. The two blood tests were also different, Byrnes maintained, because the viruses from which they were produced had been isolated from different patients — an assertion very much at issue. And, finally, they were different because at the time the Pasteur application was filed, the French ELISA could identify LAV antibodies in only 20 percent of patients with AIDS. "Montagnier may have disclosed some kind of 'test method,'" Byrnes told the patent office, "but it was certainly not a method of detecting AIDS antibodies." Without mentioning the CDC comparisons, Byrnes told the patent office that there hadn't been any evidence prior to the Heckler news conference "that Montagnier had determined the cause of AIDS or had an effective blood test" (Motions I, II and IV by *Gallo et al.* for Judgment under 37 C.F.R. 1.633(b). Interference No. 101,574. Filed October 13 and November 10, 1986).

c. Declarations of Professor Luc Montagnier and Dr. Jean-Claude Chermann. Interference No. 101,574. Filed October 9, 1986. Montagnier declared: "Dr. Donald Francis of the Centers for Disease Control in Atlanta was also in Paris at this time, and was in possession of the results of serological tests of a large number of specimens from patients with AIDS or related conditions which showed similar results when either LAV or HTLV-3 antigens were used. Based on these discussions in Paris, it was my understanding that as of April 6, 1984, Dr. Gallo was aware of substantial evidence of the similarity of LAV and HTLV-3 including the facts that they have the same appearance by electron microscopy; they are both lymphotropic and cytopathic for OKT-4 cells; isolates from American AIDS patients, when compared, were immunologically indistinguishable from LAV; and serologic tests of a large number of specimens from patients with AIDS or related conditions show similar results when either of the prototype viruses is used as antigen."

d. 35 United States Code 102(g) states: "In determining priority of invention there shall be considered not only the respective dates of conception and reduction to practice of the invention, but also the reasonable diligence of one who was first to conceive and last to reduce to practice, from a time prior to conception by the other."

e. In an October 1986 interview with the *New York Native* Gallo dredged up H.R. and C.M., declaring that "[t]he first time we detected [HIV], without an EM, in retrospect, is December '82. Prem Sarin's lab has the proof of that, which we'll be using in court. In February '82 we had three or four virus types — the first mass production of the virus by anybody in the world — which solved the problem of reagents, blood test, proof of etiology, and the ability to type forty-eight isolates" ("Disputed territory." *New York Native,* October 6, 1986).

f. Preliminary Statement of the Party *Gallo et al.* Interference No. 101,574. Filed November 14, 1986. The only basis for Gallo's statement remained the two scraps of paper on which someone had recorded barely minimal reverse transcriptase levels for H.R. and C.M. (both under 1,200 counts per minute, compared with 24,000 counts for LAV_{BRU}). When Simon Wain-Hobson saw the RT data, he laughed. "Unquestionably negative by any score," he said. "Not even suggestive."

g.In an August 4, 1983, letter to S. Sprecher, Gallo stated that he had "approximately twelve isolates of different types of HTLV from AIDS cases. Most of them fall into what I call HTLV class I." In a September 20, 1983, letter to R. Pearce, Gallo put the number of AIDS patients from whom he had isolated HTLV-1 at eleven. In a September 27, 1983, letter to P. Hofschneider, Gallo said he had "ten HTLV isolates from frank AIDS cases in approximately 40 attempts."

h.Withheld from the Pasteur were the July 21, 1983, letter from John Lemp of Electronucleonics to Popovic reporting that the Chardon culture was "not growing well," and the two versions of the December 11, 1985, letter from Lemp to Gallo stating that "the electron micrographs were finished on May 26, 1983."

i.R. Gallo to R. Robertson, May 8, 1986. Attached to this memo is the December 11, 1985, letter to Gallo from John Lemp stating that "EM photomicrographs #7083-4 and #7084-4 were actually finished on May 26, 1983, from the virus-infected cells received from NCI on May 9, 1983."

j.R. Riseberg to D. Grinstead, January 24, 1986. According to a December 12, 1987, memo from Howard Walderman of the HHS Office of General Counsel to his counterpart at CDC, "everything CDC had on Gallo/Pasteur dispute was given to Riseberg and Harmison in 1986."

k.Salk's peers recognized that the real triumph had been John Enders's solution to the problem of how to grow the polio virus in the laboratory, and that Salk had merely produced his vaccine by following Enders's recipe, then killing the virus with formaldehyde and inoculating the dead virus into children. As with the manufacture of any killed-virus vaccine, however, it was impossible to know whether every last virus particle in every batch was dead. The "Salk vaccinations" were suspended after only two weeks when five California children, all of whom had received vaccine manufactured by Berkeley's Cutter Laboratories, suddenly contracted polio. The Cutter vaccine was found to contain live polio virus; by June 1955, the Public Health Service had recorded 113 cases of polio, and five deaths, traceable to the vaccine. Salk blamed Cutter for laxity in manufacturing, but the fact that only sixty-nine of the sick children had received the Cutter product suggested that the danger of killed-virus vaccine was inherent; the remaining victims had received vaccines made by Wyeth, Lilly, Parke Davis, and other manufacturers. Public confidence in the Salk vaccine had been shaken, and many parents withdrew their children from the program. In the summer that followed, thousands of children got polio, including nearly four thousand in Boston. Within a few years a safer and scientifically more elegant vaccine, containing live poliovirus whose infectivity had been genetically disabled, was developed by Albert Sabin at the University of Cincinnati. Children much preferred swallowing Sabin's cherry-flavored pink sugar cube to the sting of Salk's hypodermic needle. The two men remained bitter enemies, and years later Sabin was still grumbling that Salk "didn't discover anything."

[i.]V. Schmitt to S. Sandler, March 19, 1987. According to Terry Bieker, Abbott also agreed to cut the price of its Hepatitis-B test by 36 percent, and to throw in a free data management system.

Chapter 14. "We Were Going to Get Killed"

[a.]To the entry on Cold Spring Harbor, Montagnier added the Pasteur's 1983 reports of LAV-like viruses in hemophiliacs and Haitians with AIDS as well as homosexuals, and the resemblance between LAV and the equine infectious anemia virus. Where Gallo attributed the invention of the reverse transcriptase assay to "R. Gallo, S. Spiegelman and others," Montagnier noted that the inventor of the RT test had been Sol Spiegelman. Montagnier also thought Miyoshi and Hinuma, not Gallo, deserved credit for establishing the link between HTLV-1 and adult T-cell leukemia. If Gallo insisted that the official history include his lab's discoveries of IL-2 and HTLV-1, which had nothing to do with AIDS, then Montagnier wished to include *his* discovery of the integration of infectious DNA (Montagnier, L., *et al. C. R. Acad. Sci. Paris* 274D 1977–1980 [1972]) and his pioneering use of interferon antibodies (Barré, F., *et al. Ann. Microbiol.* [Inst. Pasteur] 130B 349–362 [1979]). Montagnier also added a citation Gallo had forgotten, or wished to forget: the article in which Gallo and Ed Gelmann had reported detecting HTLV-1 in four AIDS patients, and which had appeared in the same issue of *Science* with the Pasteur's discovery of LAV.

[b.]*Institut Pasteur v. The United States.* Appeal No. 86-1541, United States Court of Appeals for the Federal Circuit. March 9, 1987. The Contract Disputes Act, the appeals court said, was intended to cover business arrangements in which people sold things to, or bought things from, the federal government (814 F.2d 624 at 628).

[c.]One reference mentioned a nonexistent Gallo isolate named "C.S." Another entry had Popovic's "W.T." isolate growing in the H-4 cell line rather than H-9.

[d.]HHS had set aside $350,000 to pay its outside patent counsel, Cushman, Darby and Cushman, and Burston-Marsteller, the public relations firm that handled publicity for the settlement. Nobody even tried to add up the cost of the months of man-hours devoted to the case by the Justice Department and the HHS General Counsel's office [unsigned HHS attorney's notes, June 5, 1986; memo from W. Forbush to Associate Director for Administration, NIH. April 13, 1987; R. Charrow to W. Pines, May 18, 1987; memo from J. Jarman to "Mr. Mansfield," June 16, 1987; R. Charrow to W. Pines, May 18, 1987].

[e.]According to the March 31, 1987, Joint Public Statement by HHS and Institut Pasteur, "The agreement resolves a difference between the two parties concerning the patent rights for the blood screening test for the HIV infection responsible for AIDS."

^{f.}The first mention of the New Jersey Pair occurred in a 1985 article by Flossie Wong-Staal (Wong-Staal, F., *et al.* "Genomic diversity of human T-lymphotropic virus Type III (HTLV-3)." *Science* 229:759, August 23, 1985). The following year, Marvin Reitz told the Park City AIDS symposium that the New Jersey Pair represented evidence that "viruses obtained from different individuals within a fixed time period and geographic area can have very similar DNA sequences" (Reitz, M., *et al.* "Variability of nucleotide sequence of different isolates of HTLV-3." UCLA Symposium on Viruses and Human Cancer, Park City, Utah, February 2–9, 1986). A few months later, Gallo assured John Maddox and Abraham Karpas that "We have now sequence data on two very independent isolates from 1984 New Jersey homosexuals in which there are only about 80 nucleotide differences" (R. Gallo to A. Karpas and J. Maddox, July 31, 1986).

^{g.}The conference program states that Gallo's abstract was "not available at the time of printing," and no abstract ever was provided. According to the National Cancer Institute, Gallo did not speak from a prepared text and no written record of his remarks exists.

^{h.}Daniel, M. D., *et al.* "Isolation of T-cell tropic HTLV-3-like retrovirus from macaques." *Science* 228:1201, June 7, 1985, received February 19, 1985, and accepted April 12, 1985. The idea that some monkeys might be carrying an HTLV-like virus wasn't new. The Japanese had published circumstantial evidence that so-called Old World primates from Asia were infected with such a virus (Miyoshi, I., *et al. Int. J. Cancer* 32:333 [1983]). All that remained was to identify the monkey equivalent of HTLV-3. In rather short order it was found, by Muthiah Daniel, a Harvard virologist with nearly a dozen monkey-virus discoveries to his credit, who isolated the new virus from four macaques — Mm251-79, Mm239-82, Mm220-82, and Mm142-83. Exercising the discoverer's prerogative, Daniel named his find the macaque immunodeficiency virus, or MIV. When Essex offered to help characterize the new virus, Daniel's boss, Ronald Desrosiers, agreed over Daniel's protests to send Essex a sample of MIV. Plans were laid to publish two papers back-to-back, one from Daniel on the discovery, the other from Essex on its biological characteristics (Kanki, P. J., *et al.* "Serologic identification and characterization of a macaque T-lymphotropic retrovirus closely related to HTLV-III." *Science* 228:1199, June 7, 1985). But when the papers appeared in *Science,* Daniel's new virus was no longer called MIV. Now it was named STLV, for simian T-lymphotropic virus. According to Daniel, Essex had prevailed on the *Science* editors to change the name without his knowledge. STLV didn't appear to have much in common with HTLV-1. It did, however, have "striking similarities" with HTLV-3 — so striking that Essex subsequently renamed Daniel's discovery again, to STLV-3MAC.

^{i.}Hirsch, V., *et al.* "The genome organization of STLV-3 is similar to that of the AIDS virus except for a truncated transmembrane protein." *Cell* 49(3):307–319, May 8, 1987. Of Essex's three isolates of HTLV-4, two were identical to STLV-3$_{AGM}$. The third isolate differed in one restriction site out of thirty-two. One of Muthiah Daniel's

isolates of STLV-3$_{MAC}$ was identical to *both* STLV-3$_{AGM}$ *and* HTLV-4. Two of the other STLV-3$_{MAC}$ isolates, identical to one another, differed from STLV-3$_{AGM}$ and HTLV-4 by two restriction sites out of twenty-three.

[j.]In an April 5, 1990, telephone conversation, Zagury confirmed that he had obtained Gomez's serum "from the hospital" and delivered it to Gallo.

[k.]Zagury's subsequent paper (Zagury, J. F., *et al.* "Sequence of NIH-Z," *PNAS* 85:5941–5945 [1988]) states that "We isolated HIV-2$_{NIH-Z}$ in 1986 from the peripheral blood of an immunodeficiency patient who originally lived in Guinea Bissau. A virus, isolated from the same patient and designated lymphadenopathy-AIDS virus (LAV)-2$_{FG}$, from the Guinea Bissau patient named Fernando Gomez, was described by Clavel *et al.* (11) and is likely highly similar." The reference is to the July 1986 *Science* article by Clavel *et al.* However, the only LAV-2 isolates described in that article are from the patients MIR and ROD, not from F.G.

[l.]"Too seldom," said *Nature* in an editorial, "do researchers in this field retract data found to be erroneous," but *Nature's* admiration proved premature. Writing the next year in the *Scientific American,* Essex admitted only to the "possibility" that *one* of his "early isolates" of HTLV-4 might have been taken from a cell culture contaminated with the monkey virus (Essex, M., and Kanki, P. J. "The origins of the AIDS virus." *Scientific American* 259:4, 64, October 1988).

[m.]Montagnier, L., *et al.* "Retrovirus capable of causing AIDS, antigens obtained from this retrovirus and corresponding antibodies and their application for diagnostic purposes." United States Patent 4,839,288, filed March 3, 1986, issued June 13, 1989. In a cross-licensing agreement, Pasteur licensed HIV-2 to Max Essex's company, Cambridge BioScience, while Harvard licensed Essex's claimed discovery of the HIV-1 gp120 protein to the Pasteur, which had filed a claim of its own for that discovery.

Chapter 15. "The Whole Thing Was Sordid"

[a.]Unfortunately for a book that had such a broad impact, Shilts's work contained a number of historical errors: Shilts credits Gallo, rather than Hinuma and Miyoshi, with having "shown that a retrovirus caused a leukemia common in Japan." He has Gallo having growing up in New Jersey rather than Connecticut. He confuses Françoise Barré with Françoise Brun, placing the former rather than the latter in the operating room while Frédéric Brugière's lymph node is being extracted. He locates the Institut Pasteur, which sits in the fifteenth arrondissement of Paris, in the Latin Quarter, which is the fifth arrondissement. He has Barré adding fresh lymphocytes to the *Bru* culture on January 18, 1983 — before the first RT peak — rather than the actual date of February 9, and he dates the RT peak as January 23 rather than January 29. He has Barré proclaiming to Montagnier and Chermann on that day that she had found a new human retrovirus, when several weeks of experiments remained to prove that discovery. Shilts describes Frédéric Brugière as a "flight steward" (Brugière was a couturier). Shilts credits Gallo, rather than Howard Temin and David Baltimore, with discovering reverse transcriptase. He misconstrues the discovery of T-cell Growth Factor as an outgrowth of Gallo's search for a way to grow lymphocytes in culture, when in fact Gallo was searching for a growth factor for myeloid cells. He credits Gallo with the discovery of HTLV-1 in 1978, whereas the first report of HTLV-1 was published in December 1980. Shilts dates the isolation of HTLV-2 to the spring of 1983 rather than November 1982. He has Jacqueline Gruest bringing "a lymph node" to Gallo, rather than the *Bru* virus DNA she actually carried. Shilts recounts Gallo's abuse of Max Essex at the CDC meeting in the summer of 1983; in fact, Gallo's target was Jim Mullins. Shilts describes NIH Building 37, the glass-and-steel high-rise where Gallo had his laboratory, as a "red brick" structure. He has Jerry Groopman, rather than Gallo, moderating the Park City panel at which Chermann spoke in February 1984, and has Gallo asking questions of Chermann that, according to the tape recording of that session, were not asked by Gallo or anyone else. Shilts claims that LAV first arrived in Atlanta on February 26, rather than the actual date of February 6. He states that Ed Brandt was informed of the discovery of HTLV-3 in February, rather than the actual date of March 30. Shilts claims Gallo submitted six papers to *Science* rather than the actual four. He credits Kalyanaraman, rather than Paul Feorino, with the isolation of the CDC's transfusion-pair viruses. Shilts claims Gallo called the French "whores for lecturing all the time" in a March 27, 1984, conversation with Don Francis; the actual date was June 12. Shilts claims, without attribution, that Martin Redfern persuaded Gallo's secretary to give him advance copies of the *Science* articles, whereas Redfern maintains that he received the articles from Gallo himself. Shilts says Gallo flew all night from Italy to arrive in Bethesda on the Monday morning of the Heckler news conference. There are no overnight flights from Europe to the United States, and Gallo had returned home at least by Saturday evening, April 19, when he called Mal Martin at home. Shilts says Gallo only learned on Sunday, April 22, that his presence would be required at the next day's news conference; in fact, Ed Brandt had informed Jim Wyngaarden and Gallo by telephone in Cremona the previous Wednesday. Gallo could not have been "stunned" on Monday morning "to hear that the previous day's *New York Times* carried a page-one story" in which Mason gave the credit to the Pasteur, since Gallo had called Mal Martin about the *Times* story on Sunday morning. Shilts says Heckler "added a nod to the efforts of the Pasteur Institute" to her statement, and predicted that LAV and HTLV-3 "will prove to be the same." The videotape of Heckler's statement shows that she never spoke those words. Shilts has the degree of genetic variation between ARV and LAV at 6 percent, rather than the actual and more significant distance of 12 percent. He places the isolations of LAV and HTLV-3B seventeen months apart, rather than the actual ten months. Shilts states that the Gallo AIDS test patent was issued "immediately" after the application was filed, rather than thirteen months later. Finally, he maintains, incorrectly, that without a patent of its own the Pasteur "could not market its blood test in the United States." Only FDA approval was necessary before the Pasteur AIDS test went on the American market.

b.R. Riseberg to R. Windom, December 23, 1987. L. Harmison to R. Windom, January 4, 1988. Subpoenaed by Representative John J. Dingell's Subcommittee on Oversight and Investigations, Harmison spent an uncomfortable few hours pleading memory failure to questions about his departure from HHS and the whereabouts of his files, prompting an exasperated Dingell to ask, "Do you remember what your job was? Do you remember picking up your paycheck?"

c.Osler actually said, "In science the credit goes to the man who convinces the world, not to the man to whom the idea first occurs," which didn't bode well for Gallo's claim to have been first to propose that the cause of AIDS was a retrovirus.

d.Nominations for the foundation's board of trustees included King Juan Carlos of Spain, Jonas Salk, Helmut Schmidt, Elizabeth Taylor, the Aga Khan, Giovanni Agnelli, Carlo de Benedetti, Malcolm Forbes, Armand Hammer, Baron Edmond de Rothschild, the Sultan of Brunei — and Robert Maxwell.

e.Crewdson J. "The Great AIDS Quest." *Chicago Tribune*, November 19, 1989. In accordance with the agreement, HHS withheld the first 20 percent of its total royalties and wrote the French and American AIDS foundation a check for the remaining $3.1 million. The check from Pasteur, for $471,105, reflected smaller sales by Genetic Systems, which never had been allowed to make more than a tiny dent in the U.S. market. When the redistribution was complete, HHS and Pasteur each received a refund of $1.36 million, with the remaining $910,432 set aside for the newly established World AIDS Foundation, whose mission was to fund AIDS research in the Third World (J. Mahoney to J. Wyngaarden, February 16, 1988). Vince DeVita claimed 90 percent of the money flowing back to HHS, about $1.2 million a year, for the National Cancer Institute, arguing that research at NCI had made the patent possible (V. DeVita to J. Wyngaarden, May 3, 1988, and J. Wyngaarden to V. DeVita, June 16, 1988).

f.One concerned Lee Ratner's partial sequence of HTLV-1B, the virus initially believed by Gallo to have come from a Houston AIDS patient, but which was later traced to an African leukemia patient (Ratner, L., *et al.* "Nucleotide sequence analysis of a variant human T-cell leukemia virus (HTLV-1b) provirus with a deletion in Px-1." *J. Virol.* 54,3:781, June 1985). When Ratner's HTLV-1B sequence was compared with the HTLV-1 from the Japanese it was a very close match (Seiki, M., *et al.* "Human adult T-cell virus: Complete nucleotide sequence of the provirus genome integrated in leukemia cell DNA." *PNAS* 80:3618, June 1983). Only after Ratner's sequence was in print did the Japanese reexamine their own HTLV sequence and discover an embarrassing, and not inconsequential, error: a single nucleotide, a "C," had been omitted at a critical juncture. Where the published sequence had read AT**CCCC**TC, the corrected sequence read AT**CCCCC**TC. Because it shifted the reading frame, the extra "C" created space for a gene whose absence had been a source of puzzlement (Inoue, J., *et al.* "Nucleotide sequence of the protease-coding region in an infectious DNA of simian retrovirus (STLV) of the HTLV-1 family." *Virology* 150:187–195,

1986). It fell to Abraham Karpas to point out that Ratner's sequence of HTLV-1B, published *before* the Japanese made their correction, also lacked a fifth "C"— and at precisely the same position (Malik, K. T., *et al.* "Molecular cloning and complete nucleotide sequence of an adult t cell leukaemia virus/human T cell leukaemia virus type I (ATLV/HTLV-I) isolate of Caribbean origin: relationship to other members of the ALTV/HTLV-I subgroup." *J. Gen. Virol.* 69:1695, June 1988). Ratner claimed that although the Japanese might have made an error, he, Ratner, had not copied their sequence. The Japanese HTLV-1 might have five Cs at that position, Ratner said, but HTLV-1B had only four.

g.R. Gallo to P. Fischinger, January 10, 1988. Gallo's first complaint concerned Koch's treatment of the December 1983 letter from Gonda to Popovic from which someone — Gallo still denied it had been anyone in his lab — had excised all references to Gonda's micrographs of LAV and, by extension, obscured Popovic's success in growing the French virus. Koch's book, Gallo told Fischinger, "implies that the alterations were made in Dr. Gallo's laboratory in order to cover up the importance of the LAV sent by Montagnier." Gallo's German must have been rusty, because Koch never suggested the Gonda letter had been redacted by Gallo's lab — only that it was "mysterious" that the two incriminating paragraphs were missing: "*In einer dem Institut Pasteur ausgehändigten Kopie dieses Briefes fehlten mysteriöserweise jene zwei kompromittierenden Zeilen*" ("In a copy which was found at the Institut Pasteur, mysteriously, these two revealing lines were missing"). What Gallo described as "Koch's second attack" concerned the letter Gallo sent to several European scientists more than two weeks after Popovic had begun growing LAV, denying that he had ever seen "the virus that Luc Montagnier has described." At the time he mailed the letter, Gallo explained to Fischinger, the statement had been technically correct, because "there was nothing to 'see' in those samples." Koch's "final defamation" involved what Gallo saw as Koch's implication that he had "bullied the Japanese out [of] a rightful claim to the discovery" of HTLV-1. The same opinion was held by others, but Koch was well acquainted with a number of Swedish academics, including several at the Karolinska Institute in Stockholm, whose faculty confers the Nobel Prize in medicine.

h.While Gallo and Koch were still on speaking terms, Koch had asked for copies of electron micrographs of HTLV-1 and HIV to include as illustrations in his book. These Gallo provided, with a note expressing the hope that "they are helpful to you." Koch credited each of the micrographs with a copyright to *Science* magazine, where they had appeared originally. According to Windom, however, the pictures were "the property of the United States government," not *Science,* and therefore "not subject to copyright." Because Koch's book had failed to note this fact, Windom declared Koch and his publisher in violation of Section 43(a) of the Lanham Act, a statute that protects commercial enterprises — but not the federal government — from infringement and other false designations of origin — an utterly preposterous charge, the more so for having come from a senior government official.

i.Five years before, Gallo and Koprowski had reported in *Nature* that victims of multiple sclerosis, the debilitating neurological disease, appeared to be infected with a previously undiscovered strain of HTLV. The news that an "MS virus" had at last been identified, and that it was somehow related to the AIDS virus, prompted a flood of calls from alarmed MS patients who wondered if they were likely to get AIDS ("Link found between MS, virus that causes AIDS." *Los Angeles Times*, November 15, 1985). The cause of MS, which strikes some 10,000 Americans each year, mostly young people, has long been a research priority, and its occurrence within the same families had led some researchers to think it might be caused by a transmissible agent. That the Gallo-Koprowski paper appeared in *Nature* had given it enormous visibility, and *Nature*'s deputy editor, Peter Newmark, remembered trying unsuccessfully to persuade John Maddox to take a pass. "Maddox said, 'If it's by Gallo and Koprowski, we're going to publish it,'" recalled Newmark, who had a doctorate in biology and remembered thinking the paper was classic Gallo: "always looking for the dramatic twist, so he takes a shred of information and blows it up into something it's not." Harold Varmus called the Gallo-Koprowski paper "a joke"; Robin Weiss remembered it as "embarrassing to us all." Newmark's caution proved well-advised; within six months, *Nature* had published two subsequent papers, including one from Abraham Karpas, reporting that nothing resembling HTLV-1 could be detected in central nervous system tissues from MS patients (Karpas, A., *et al.* "Multiple sclerosis: Lack of evidence of the involvement of known human retroviruses in multiple sclerosis." *Nature* 322:177, July 10, 1986; Hauser, S. L., *et al.* "Analysis of human T lymphotropic virus sequences in MS tissue." *Nature* 322:176, July 10, 1986). Koprowski and Gallo replied that the tests used by the other groups weren't as sensitive as their own, and that their detractors had mistakenly been looking for HTLV-1, whereas the virus they had detected was merely an HTLV-1-*like* virus. Even so, labs in Canada and Germany still found it impossible to reproduce the Gallo-Koprowski results (Rice, G. P., *et al.* "Absence of antibody to HTLV-1 and HTLV-3 in sera of Canadian patients with multiple sclerosis and chronic myelopathy." *Ann. Neurol.* 4:533, October 20, 1986; Schneider, J., *et al.* "Multiple sclerosis and human T-cell lymphotropic retroviruses: negative serological results in 135 German patients." *J. Neurol.* 235(2):102, 1987. *Grimaldi et al.* report no evidence of HTLV-1 in MS). It eventually emerged that the familial basis of multiple sclerosis, rather than being infectious, was genetic. People weren't catching MS from siblings or other family members; they were *inheriting* it (Sawcer, S., *et al.* "A genome screen in multiple sclerosis reveals susceptibility loci on chromosome 6p21 and 17a22. *Nature Genetics* 13:464-468, 1996; The Multiple Sclerosis Genetics Group. "A complete genomic screen for multiple sclerosis underscores a role for the major histocompatibility complex." *Nature Genetics* 13:469–471, 1996; Ebers, G. C., *et al.* "A full genome search in multiple sclerosis." *Nature Genetics* 13:472–476, 1996; Farrall, M. "Mapping genetic susceptibility to multiple sclerosis." *Lancet* 348:1674, December 21/28, 1996).

Chapter 16. "Einstein, Freud — I'd Put Him on a List Like That"

[a] According to Popovic's notes for November 9–11, 1983, "HUT-78" was cloned twenty-one times. On November 29, Popovic infected the fourth of these clones, Htu4, with MOV. When Popovic sent MOV to Sarngadharan a week later, he called it "HT/mov." In a September 6, 1985, memo to Peter Fischinger, Popovic claimed it

was the "HT" cell line he had cloned on November 9. "We cannot make a definitive conclusion whether the designated HT cells are identical with the original HUT-78 or not," Popovic told Fischinger.

b.In the summer of 1988, four years after H-9 was published in *Science,* an ATCC official, Rob Hay, confirmed that "We've been trying to get that line, but no one has been willing to give it out to us. We've made inquiries and it hasn't been released to us."

c.S. O'Brien to Director, DCBD, NCI, January 31, 1989. According to O'Brien's manuscript, the record could have been corrected years before. In the summer of 1984, just as Gallo was beginning to pass out H-9 to selected colleagues, another NCI researcher, at Gallo's request, had compared H-9 genetically with HUT-78. At that time, the two cell lines "had been found to be one and the same." O'Brien wrote that, in 1984, "the HLA phenotype of HT, H4 and H9" had been determined to be "identical to HUT-78 (L); namely, HLA-A1, B62, C3, DR4, DQ3 (5)." The fact that the identity of H-9 had been known in 1984 was omitted from the published manuscript.

d.In a 1991 interview with the OSI, O'Brien recalled that "Bob and I did have a conversation about it and he said, 'Look, this is not something worth making a big announcement about, that that's what you do when you go to *Science.* I've got enough trouble with this, so I'm perfectly happy to send this to *AIDS Research.* All the people who need to know will see it and that's fine.'" When one of O'Brien's co-authors, Dean Mann, telephoned *Science* "to see if they were interested in publishing it," Mann recalled that "[t]heir reaction was, 'Well, is it a correction?' I said, 'No, it is not a correction, it is an explanation.' My recollection was [*Science*] told me that, 'Well, then you probably should write it up as an article rather than as a Letter to the Editor.' And I said, 'Well, you know, it really isn't worth all of that, as far as I was concerned.' And it was my impression that she wasn't interested."

e.Alfred Nobel's will created five annual prizes for "those who, during the preceding year, shall have conferred the greatest benefit on mankind" in the fields of physics, chemistry, physiology or medicine, literature, and peace." Because science nowadays is vastly more complex than in Nobel's era, it often takes years, or even decades, for the full importance of work in physics or biology to be understood. Thus, the "preceding year" caveat is frequently ignored, although some prizes are still awarded within a year or two of their underlying discoveries.

f.The Nobel Prizes are awarded by different learned bodies: physics and chemistry by the Royal Swedish Academy of Sciences; physiology or medicine by the Karolinska faculty; literature by the Swedish Academy; and peace by the Norwegian Nobel Committee. The prize for economics, not provided for in Alfred Nobel's will, was established in 1968 by the Bank of Sweden. Although presented by the Royal Swedish Academy of Sciences through the Nobel Foundation, it is properly called the Prize in Economic Sciences in Memory of Alfred Nobel.

^{g.}In 1988, the Nobel committee for medicine included a former winner of the prize, Bengt Samuelsson, and four other Karolinska professors: Sten Orrenius, Jan Wersäll, Tomas Hökfelt, and Hans Wigzell.

^{h.}The Danish scientist, Johannes Fibiger, wasn't alone. The Nobel for 1959 was awarded to an American, Arthur Kornberg, for discovering what Kornberg mistakenly believed to be the enzyme, or polymerase, that DNA uses to copy itself. Kornberg's discovery proved to be another enzyme, used to repair broken DNA; his son, Roger, subsequently discovered the DNA-copying polymerase.

^{i.}Montagnier's portion of the article mentioned Jean-Claude Chermann, Françoise Barré, Jacques Leibowitch, Willy Rozenbaum, and David Klatzmann — but not Françoise Brun or Christine Rouzioux. The French ELISA, wrote Montagnier, had been developed "in collaboration with virologists from the Claude Bernard Hospital."

^{j.}Alizon, M., *et al.* "Molecular cloning of lymphadenopathy-associated virus." *Nature* 312:757, December 20/27, 1984; Hahn, B., *et al.* "Molecular cloning and characterization of the HTLV-3 virus associated with AIDS." *Nature* 312:167, November 8, 1984. Mal Martin had a genome, BRUNL43, which he had fashioned from partial clones of two viruses, LAV-*Bru* and an AIDS virus isolate of his own called NL43. The *Bru* portion also contained the maverick *Hind*III site, indicating that the partial LAV clone Martin used was J-81.

^{k.}G. Myers to R. Gallo, July 3, 1989. "I gave you some tree analyses for the 3B and LAV sequences. We have exhaustively verified these results and I just don't think they are going to change from what is seen. The maximum distance separating any 3B from LAV-1 is 1.6%, but the deadly fact is that the 3B cluster (or "clade") is only 0.05% to 0.44% from the LAV-1 cluster. It is this number that must be compared to the Ratner figure of 0.6% (if that indeed is the distance). Thus you must contend that you 'caught' the sexual partner of BRU in Paris just when said partner returned to New York, or something like that. I don't want to get into scenario-building: rather, I want to apprise you of what you are up against. Again, it is probably good that you ask some other sequence analyst to independently perform this analysis. I don't like being the person to have to tell you this, but I'm happier that the information is in my hands than in the hands of someone else. Up ahead, you'll have reason to think that I have worked against you (I don't think that, but I could understand how you would reasonably think so); this is the strongest argument against your position. . . . I have held it for nearly a year now, hoping for some resolution within the tradition rather than within the press. . . ."

^{l.}The *Chicago Tribune* spent many months attempting to interview Gallo, who in December of 1988 finally agreed, through his then-attorney, former senator Birch Bayh, on the condition that he be given a list of questions in advance (B. Bayh to the author, Dec. 1, 1988). The questions were provided eight days later (the author to

B. Bayh, December 9, 1988). The following day, Bayh informed the *Tribune* that it was no longer "in Dr. Gallo's interest" to submit to an interview.

ᵐ·R. Weiss to R. Gallo, January 23, 1990. To Gallo's question about why he had taken the article to Cold Spring Harbor, Weiss explained that "Eli Reichmann, a virologist and friend at the University of Illinois, sent me the copy of the *Chicago Tribune* article which I brought with me on my trip to Birmingham, Alabama, and CSHL. As people had heard about the *Chicago Tribune* article but not seen it, my copy was of interest. It was photocopied in Birmingham. I think I left it with Beatrice Hahn, who returned it to me at CSHL . . . since several of the participants at Banbury were mentioned in the article, it was naturally a topic of interest and gossip."

Chapter 17. "I Have Probably Talked Too Much"

ᵃ·The *Cell* paper described how the insertion of an alien gene into the immune-system cells of a laboratory mouse resulted in the production of proteins that resembled the products of the inserted gene. It appeared to O'Toole, however, that the proteins in question were being assembled by the mouse's native genes rather than the imported ones, and that the data published by Imanishi-Kari therefore couldn't have been correct.

ᵇ·One of the three panelists, Columbia's Frederick Alt, had published more than a dozen papers with Baltimore. Another, James Darnell of Rockefeller University, had co-authored Baltimore's molecular biology textbook. The third member, Ursula Storb of the University of Chicago, had written Imanishi-Kari a job recommendation.

ᶜ·Other issues to be examined included Gallo's role in the handling of the first Pasteur *Science* paper; the *post-hoc* updating of Gallo's Cold Spring Harbor and Park City presentations and Flossie Wong-Staal's paper from the NCI symposium; the genesis of the references to "LAV" in Sasha Arya's notebooks; the derivation of the Popovic pool; the origin of the mystery virus, MOV; Gallo's claims to have isolated HIV before the French; the labeling of the LAV micrographs as pictures of HTLV-3; and the letter from Gonda to Popovic from which references to LAV had been mysteriously redacted.

ᵈ·Watson and Crick shared the Nobel Prize with Maurice Wilkins of the University of London, whose collaborator, Rosalind Franklin, had produced X-ray photographs of crystalline molecules that revealed the approximate shape of the DNA helix (a feat first accomplished not by Franklin herself but British researcher William Astbury during the Second World War). By the time the prize was awarded Franklin had died an untimely death from cancer at the age of thirty-seven. Nobel Prizes are never awarded posthumously, and the question persists of whether, had she lived, Franklin would have taken Wilkins's place as the third recipient. In his memoir *The Double Helix* (New York: Athenaeum, 1968) Watson acknowledges that "the crux of the matter was whether Rosy's new X-ray pictures would lend any support for a helical DNA structure." But in *The Eighth Day of Creation,* Horace Judson quotes Wilkins as saying that Franklin was "going at it wrong" in not trusting her initial x-radiographs showing what did appear to be a double helix, leaning instead toward the notion that DNA was perhaps *not* helical in form. Judson notes that "Wilkins allowed himself to be led by [Franklin's] assertion" in also concluding, incorrectly, that DNA was not helical.

e. Undated memo from S. Broder to S. Siebert. "The compounds I mentioned in my talk," Gallo wrote Stevens on March 30, 1990, "are in the very earliest stages of drug development. In preclinical animal tests, these compounds appear to be very interesting for further investigation. However, neither I nor anyone else can definitively state what these basic science observations mean for human disease. Perhaps my enthusiasm over these preliminary results carried over into my remarks, and this may possibly have led to some misinterpretation of the data as cited in the article in the *New York Native.* If these misinterpretations have led you or any other patients to harbor premature hopes for a soon-to-be available cure for Kaposi's sarcoma, I am truly sorry."

f. The *Tribune* never made such an allegation, nor could it have, since it had no evidence that deliberate misappropriation had occurred.

g. "The Little Law Firm That Could." *Washington Post,* April 22, 1986. Onek's firm did its share of First Amendment and *pro bono* work. But it had also helped the State of Arkansas write a Supreme Court brief arguing that a prisoner should be executed, and one of its principal clients was the American Psychiatric Association (Onek's wife is a practicing psychiatrist), whose members it defended against allegations of malpractice and patient abuse. Onek had gotten himself in a minor bind the year before, while acting as a special counsel in the case of three attorneys for the Securities and Exchange Commission accused of sexual harassment. After interviewing fifty-one witnesses on tape, Onek had concluded there was insufficient evidence of harassment to punish the three lawyers — then destroyed the interview tapes on which his conclusion was based, saying he feared the tapes might be used as a basis for other harassment investigations. A lawyer for one of the women who claimed to have been harassed thought it looked like a cover-up. "It would seem that they're trying to hide information that would be detrimental to the three," she said ("Law firm destroyed probe tapes." *Washington Post,* March 20, 1989).

h. Among them: that Montagnier had withdrawn his collaboration from Gallo in July 1983 (the following September Montagnier sent Gallo a second shipment of LAV); that Gallo had been first to grow HIV in a permanent cell line (Montagnier began growing LAV in B-cell lines within days of Popovic's infection of T-cell lines with the pool virus); that Gallo had developed "the first workable blood test" for AIDS (the Windom-Robertson letter to Michael Koch's publisher pointed out that the CDC comparisons showed the French ELISA, developed months before Gallo's, was the equivalent of the Gallo test); that the S.N. isolate had been put into culture on September 15, 1983, i.e., *before* the arrival of the September LAV sample (S.N. arrived in Gallo's lab the day *after* the September LAV was delivered); that HTLV-3$_{RF}$ had been grown in a permanent cell line since November of 1983, i.e., at the same time as the pool virus HTLV-3B (in a memo to Gallo dated November 28, 1984, Popovic gives the date of R.F.'s transmission to HUT-78 as December 29, 1983); that the H-9 cell line was created in November 1983 (the date in Popovic's notes is January 19, 1984); that HTLV-3$_{RF}$ had been EM-positive in January 1984 (R.F. was EM-*negative* in January 1984, and not EM positive until October 1984, six months after the *Science* papers were published); that "all our notebooks, letters, and documents were available and scrutinized by Pasteur Institute scientists (all of Popovic's key pages reflecting his success in growing LAV were withheld from the Pasteur lawyers, as were memos from Gallo and Popovic to Peter Fischinger acknowledging Popovic's work with LAV); that the official history "frankly stated in writing that there was no wrong doing" by Gallo's laboratory (the official history contains no such statement); and, finally, that Gerry Myers's evolutionary trees indicated that HTLV-3B and LAV might have been derived from two individuals who had had "very close contacts" with one another (Myers's analysis specifically ruled out the possibility that HTLV-3B and LAV had come from separate individuals).

$^{i.}$Lot number 5102-29-9, February 29, 1988. "I wrote them a threatening letter," recalled Papan Devnani of the Office of Federal Patent Licensing. "I told them that nobody is licensed to sell HIV in H-9 and they should stop selling. What they are doing is illegal."

$^{j.}$Pan-Data was founded in April 1984, at a time when Salahuddin was smarting from his relegation to second author on the "isolations and detections" paper in *Science,* and even more from the attention being paid to Mika Popovic. When the company was incorporated, Salahuddin made himself director of corporate development and his wife, Firoza, chairman of the board. Pan-Data also offered data-processing services, but in Gerry Myers's opinion they were a joke. "The database was starting up," Myers recalled, "and I needed some sequence alignments done. Flossie said, 'Why don't you try Pan-Data?' So I did. I had to go there, and I burst out laughing. I actually had a portable computer that had more memory than anything they had. They were kids who were kind of hackers. When I got back to Los Alamos and looked at the data I thought it was awful." Pan-Data's big break had come in June 1985, when the NIH approved a request, over Gallo's signature, for a Blanket Purchase Agreement allowing any member of his lab to order supplies, reagents, and data-processing services from Pan-Data. As justification for the arrangement, the request stated that Pan-Data was the only source of purified viral proteins and other products that were needed by the lab. But NIH records showed no purchases of such proteins, and the GAO found that for at least a year afterward the company had no laboratory in which such proteins could have been produced. Much of Pan-Data's business with Gallo had involved HBLV, the erstwhile B-lymphotropic virus codiscovered by Salahuddin in 1986, subsequently renamed HHV-6. When the government applied for a patent on a diagnostic blood test for HBLV, Gallo and Salahuddin were among its inventors. The same day the application was filed, Pan-Data asked the Commerce Department for an exclusive license to sell the HBLV test — a sequence of events, Commerce officials told investigators, that suggested an improper use of insider information. No license was ever granted, but Pan-Data continued to sell the HBLV test anyway, its sales spurred by Gallo's promotion of HBLV as a potentially important virus that might cause T-cell disorders, including immune system defects, or even AIDS. One of Pan-Data's largest contracts came from the army's massive program to screen millions of active-duty soldiers and potential recruits for the AIDS virus. By then Pan-Data had acquired a laboratory, and to support its bid for the $600,000 contract the company had provided the army with a copy of its lease. But the GAO found that the lease had been changed to show a monthly rent of $4,125 rather than the $1,625 the company actually paid, and 1,650 square feet of laboratory space rather than the 650 square feet it actually had. "It would certainly appear to be fraud," one of the GAO investigators, Clark Hall, told the Dingell subcommittee. A former Pan-Data employee alleged that scientific equipment, some of it still bearing metal NIH identification tags, had been taken from the Gallo lab and used at the Pan-Data facility. When the GAO attempted to verify the employee's allegation, it discovered that, despite an NIH requirement that all government lab equipment be inventoried annually, no inventory had been conducted of Gallo's lab for more than five years. Some $330,318 worth of equipment assigned to Gallo's lab proved to be unaccounted for, including a pair of $35,000 spectrometers, a $25,000 radioassay analyzer and two chromatographs worth $50,000 apiece. The GAO also was told that during 1985 and 1986, before Pan-Data moved into its first real laboratory, several Pan-Data employees had done the company's work in Gallo's lab. According to NIH records, at least five Pan-Data employees had purchased thousands of dollars' worth of supplies from an NIH "self-service" store and charged them to Gallo's NIH credit card. Another $50,000 worth of supplies had been charged to Gallo by thirty-seven other individuals for whom the NIH had no record of employment.

[k.]R. Gallo to J. Jennings, January 20, 1990. That Gallo had seen the article in advance of its nonpublication is suggested by his comment to Jennings that "The *New Yorker* article is rather good and is about ready to go off [*sic*] by its author."

[l.]A Soviet embassy spokesman in Washington said he had no record or memory of any meeting between Gallo and Mikhail Gorbachev.

[m.]R. Gallo to R. Wachter, June 15, 1990. Although Gallo dictated the letter to the NCI Press Office from Moscow on June 15, it evidently wasn't delivered to Wachter until the 18th, the day Gallo was scheduled to appear. Gallo's advance NIH travel itinerary shows him leaving Washington for Moscow on June 9, three days before the San Francisco conference opened, then departing Moscow for Wilsede, Germany, on June 17, two days before the San Francisco conference closed — a schedule that suggests Gallo never intended to be in San Francisco.

Chapter 18. "Of Course We *Did* Grow LAV"

[a.] *Science* is published by the American Association for the Advancement of Science, a trade and lobbying organization. The official publication of the Academy is the *Proceedings of the National Academy of Science.*

[b.] According to *Science*, Gallo acknowledged that Popovic had achieved "low but continuous" growth of LAV in the Ti7.4 cell line. The article didn't recall that Gallo and Popovic had told *Science* a few years before that all the cell lines Popovic had tried to infect with LAV had been "killed by the virus in two or three weeks," or that Gallo's sworn declaration in the interference had claimed that the growth of LAV had been "only temporary in nature." *Science* also quoted Gallo as asking whether LAV had "inadvertently contaminated our cultures and suddenly dominated the culture by rapid growth?" and then answering his own question. "This is certainly possible," Gallo said, "since LAV was present in the same laboratory where some of our isolates were developed." But Popovic had written in his September 6, 1985, memo to Gallo that "the development of H9/HTLV-3B was almost entirely confined to the tissue culture room 6B03A where no LAV was ever used." The *Science* article also contained several mistakes, including the assertion that Gallo's 1984 *Science* articles had "highlighted data on viruses [named for the patients from whom they came] called C.C., MOV, R.F., M.N. and S.N." Had *Science* checked its own files, it would have discovered that nowhere in the four articles published in May 1984 had Gallo mentioned M.N., C.C. or MOV. (M.N. wasn't reported in print until December 1984, long after the AIDS test was in production. Gallo's single published reference to MOV, which said nothing about its source, occurred in 1985, and C.C. was first reported as an AIDS virus isolate in 1986.)

[c.] LTCB response to OSI question 4c. Despite Gallo's claim in the "official history" that Sarngadharan's "anti-p24 hyperimmune" rabbit antiserum had "proved the 48 isolates belong to the same kind of virus," Gallo acknowledged to OSI that he only had ten confirmed HIV isolates: R.F., B.K., L.S., R.C., S.N., DM82613, T.W. (published in *Science* as W.T.), W7144, HP, and 518083. Moreover, the rabbit antibody used to confirm the isolates was made from the whole AIDS virus, not the much more specific p24 protein.

[d.] W. Blattner to S. Hadley, July 12, 1990. Gallo produced only eight of the ten pool samples. The two missing samples were W.T. (T.W.), whose cells Gallo originally had received from Bart Haynes at Duke, and W.A., sent by Mark Kaplan at North Shore Hospital on Long Island from a patient described as suffering from leukemia, not AIDS.

[e.] M. Martin to S. Hadley, September 21, 1990. In a February 7, 1991, letter to Martin, Montagnier provided "some information about the vial of LAV_{Bru} you received from us on April 12, 1984. The virus stock was prepared at the end of 1983 by Françoise Barré Sinoussi by growing the virus on total peripheral blood lymphocytes stimulated by PHA. The label on the vial is C6TX5. The virus was previous grown on JBB (another cytapheresis) in 1983."

ᶠ·M. Popovic to R. Gallo and P. Fischinger, November 28, 1984;. M. Gonda to M. Popovic, December 15, 1983; January 18, February 13, and March 26, 1984. Gonda made three attempts to photograph virus in R.F.'s cells; the March 26 letter reaffirms his lack of success in the earlier attempts.

ᵍ·McGrath's principal contribution to AIDS research had been the claim that a cucumber extract used in China to induce abortions also inhibited the reproduction of the AIDS virus. Besides being an inventor on the University of California's patent for "Compound Q," as the extract was called, McGrath was on the scientific advisory board of a Bay Area company, Genelabs Technology, that was promoting the extract as a possible AIDS cure. Although the Food and Drug Administration hadn't approved Compound Q, it was being provided to a number of San Francisco–area AIDS patients as an "underground" drug by a local AIDS organization called Project Inform. After some of the patients died, the FDA directed Project Inform to discontinue its "unapproved experimentation" and began an investigation. The founding director of Project Inform, a former Jesuit seminarian named Martin Delaney, protested that patients taking Compound Q had experienced a dramatic increase in their T-4 cells; Arnold Relman, the editor of the *New England Journal of Medicine,* dismissed Delaney's data as "black magic." San Francisco General Hospital, where McGrath had his lab, said that while McGrath had known Compound Q was being tested on patients without FDA approval, he hadn't played any role in organizing the trial. Beyond the fact that Compound Q evidently posed a danger to patients, including the risk of coma, it simply didn't work. When several other researchers, including Jerry Groopman, were unable to replicate McGrath's laboratory results, McGrath explained that they hadn't used the special Teflon-coated culture dishes needed to make the experiments work. But Compound Q soon joined Suramin and dextran sulfate as another failed cure for AIDS.

ʰ·An account of the AL-721 story is contained in Bruce Nussbaum's book *Good Intentions* (New York: Atlantic Monthly Press, 1990).

ⁱ·Federal prosecutors offered Sarin the opportunity to plead guilty to two counts with maximum penalties of only six years in prison. Although such a deal would have avoided the expense of a trial, Sarin reportedly balked when prosecutors insisted that any plea-bargain include some jail time.

ʲ·Gallo testified to knowing that Sarin "had an interest" in D-Pen, but not that Degussa had paid Sarin for testing the drug. Or, Gallo added, "If I knew, I don't remember it today." Sarin had been working on D-Pen with Prakash Chandra in Frankfurt, and NIH travel records showed Gallo had been to Frankfurt for a meeting with Chandra "to discuss drugs which inhibit AIDS." Chandra, who appeared as a witness for the prosecution, testified that "Gallo knew very well about the studies, because Gallo has been to Frankfurt and we have discussed Prem Sarin's data with him." Dale Kelberman, the assistant U.S. attorney who had extracted a guilty plea from Zaki Salahuddin, tried to press Gallo on the question. "Well," Kelberman said, "do you believe as we sit here now, you ever knew anything about any financial arrangement that Dr. Sarin may have with Degussa on behalf of the lab?" But the judge cut Kelberman off, and the question was never answered.

Chapter 19. "If Chance Will Have Me King"

[a.]The night before, Gallo had treated many of the attendees to a Chinese banquet at the Far East Restaurant, about a mile from NIH. According to some of those present, Wong-Staal and Gallo departed about 10:30, with Gallo returning home around eleven o'clock to find that his house had been entered through a basement window. Nothing of value was taken, but Gallo told *Science* he believed "the burglar was there to photograph scientific data and papers," and that "a large white plastic bag that had Daniel Zagury's name on it in inch-high letters had been knocked to the floor and apparently gone through." Gallo described the contents of the bag as "about the vaccine work," and told police he suspected the culprit was the author. The police subsequently established that fingerprints found at the scene were *not* those of the author, who was dining with his family at a Bethesda restaurant when the break-in — if there was a break-in — occurred. The spurious burglary allegation was just one of several proffered by Gallo. According to Simon Wain-Hobson, Gallo claimed the author was not really a reporter for the *Chicago Tribune* but a "detective" who was being paid by Gallo's "enemies." To Victor Zonana, a *Los Angeles Times* reporter who later became a spokesman for HHS Secretary Donna Shalala, Gallo claimed the author was "a dangerous psychotic" — not in itself a criminal offense. Gallo insisted to Maxime Schwartz, the director of the Pasteur Institute, that the author was "secretly being paid by Pasteur"— presumably something of which Schwartz, as director, should have been aware. Joanne Belk, the NIH's Freedom of Information officer, recalled Gallo telling her that the Pasteur had paid the author $100,000. To Gerry Myers, Gallo claimed it was Abraham Karpas to whom the *Chicago Tribune* had paid $100,000, for the sequencing of *Brul20C* — the most ludicrous allegation of all, since Karpas cheerfully provided the sequence for free.

[b.]R. Gallo to Y. Cerisier, December 4, 1990. Within the Pasteur, the original LAV_{Bru} isolate, cultured in T-cells from a researcher named Jean-Baptiste Brunet, was known as JBB-LAV. It was JBB-LAV that had been delivered to Gallo by Montagnier in July 1983, and sent again by Françoise Barré in September 1983, this time accompanied by a second LAV sample designated M2T-/B.

[c.]S. Wain-Hobson to R. Gallo, August 22, 1991; Wong-Staal, F., *et al.* "Different isolates of HTLV-3 and lymphadenopathy [*sic*] virus (LAV) are genetic variants of the same virus." The latter is the unpublished manuscript intended for *The Lancet* in the summer of 1984.

[d.]According to Montagnier's lab notes, IDAV-2 (from Eric Loiseau) was actually isolated first, on May 25, 1983, and IDAV-1 (from Christophe Lailler) second, on June 9, 1983. When they were named IDAV, for "immunodeficiency associated virus," the sequence of isolation was reversed.

ᵉ·"If chance will have me king, why, chance may crown me." *Macbeth,* Act I, Scene III.

ᶠ·M. Schwartz to W. Raub, March 25, 1991. In an April 16, 1991, letter to Suzanne Hadley, Schwartz noted that he was sending OSI one vial of the JBB/LAV previously sent to Gallo on July 17 and September 21, 1983, a second vial of Montagnier's B-LAV, and a third of M2TB/LAV, which "was also sent . . . to Drs. Gallo and Popovic on September 21st, 1983."

ᵍ·Gallo, R. ". . . and his response." *Nature* 351:358, May 30, 1991. Gallo's statement was accompanied by a note from Marv Reitz finally correcting the typographical errors in the sequence of "true Bru" and acknowledging what Gerry Myers and Simon Wain-Hobson had already reported in *Science,* that "our method for computing percentage similarity was considered to have given an 'inflated' impression" of the difference between Bru and 3B (Reitz, M., *et al.* "Gallo's virus sequence." *Nature* 351:358, May 30, 1991).

ʰ·The mother of Claude Rouquier, one of the dead patients, recalled Zagury's principal collaborator, Odille Picard, telling her that Picard planned to fly to Bethesda to discuss her son's death with Gallo. Picard later denied having made such a statement.

ⁱ·Zagury claimed the peptides which formed the cocktail he was using as a "vaccine" had been made in France, even though Gallo had been shipping him quantities of many of the same peptides, including one custom-manufactured for Gallo by the NCI-Frederick laboratory of Takis Papas. Zagury countered that the NCI peptides had been used only in animal experiments, although Zagury hadn't published any animal research. "The real issue," Vince DeVita said later, "was where did Zagury get that material? Because if it came from us it's in violation of the regulations about doing something in another country. We looked into it, we confronted Gallo straight on. We said 'Bob, if you've done this, you've got to tell us because it will be a scandal.' He denied it —'No way, no way.'"

ʲ·"Findings and required actions regarding investigation of noncompliance with HHS regulations for the protection of human research subjects involving the National Institutes of Health intramural research program." Office for Protection from Research Risks, Division of Human Subject Protections, July 3, 1991. Zagury assured OPRR that his research in Zaire hadn't harmed any Zairians, and that the children used in the first set of experiments had suffered no ill effects — although he acknowledged not having seen any of them in years. OPRR hadn't been able to verify Zagury's assurances, the agency said, because Zagury hadn't allowed it to review "the relevant medical and research records in order to obtain independent corroboration of his statements." Nor had the government of Zaire responded to the OPRR's requests for information.

ᵏ·Gallo: April 8, 11, 17, 26, 27; May 10, 16, 25; July 6, 10, 18, 25, 27; August 3, 4; and September 23; December 2, 1990; March 4 and April 12, 1991; Popovic: June 26; December 1, 1990; March 4 and April 10, 1991.

l.Less than a month after the *Tribune* article appeared, Gallo offered to rehire Mika Popovic in his former position. According to Popovic, NIH officials explained that the cloud of suspicion surrounding his research made him no longer welcome (*Mikulas Popovic, M.D., Ph.D. v. United States of America and Suzanne Hadley, Ph.D.* United States District Court for the District of Maryland. Civil Action PJM-96-3106, filed October 2, 1996).

m.**First (11/15/83) & Second (11/22/83) Pools**

W6233: Heterosexual transfusion patient. Original sample received 10/19/83. RT positive 10/20/83. HTLV-1 negative (undated). EM not done. Roche: positive for HIV (multiple viruses) but not HTLV-3B/LAV.

F6367: Jamaican AIDS patient. Original sample received 10/5/83. RT negative 11/15/83, low RT positive 11/14/83. EM negative 12/14/83. No diagnosis. Roche: positive for HIV but not HTLV-3B/LAV.

W6592: Diagnosis unknown. Original sample received 9/14/83. RT negative 11/15/83, RT negative 11/17/83. EM negative 12/14/83. HTLV-1 negative 11/8/83. Roche: Blood sample obtained from patient's physician positive for HIV but not HTLV-3B/LAV.

Third pool (1/2/84)

W7647: Female heroin user. Original sample received 12/23/83. RT negative (undated). HTLV-1 negative (undated). Roche: Gallo declined to provide to OSI; counter sample obtained from submitting physician positive for HIV but not HTLV-3B/LAV.

W7777: AIDS patient. Original sample received 12/22/83. HTLV-1 negative 1/2/84, 1/17/84. RT negative 1/2/84, 1/23/84. EM negative 2/10/84. Roche: positive for HIV but not HTLV-3B/LAV.

W7780: Pre-AIDS patient. Original sample received 12/16/83. HTLV-1 negative 1/2/84. RT negative (undated). EM negative 2/10/84, 3/13/84. Roche: positive for HIV but not HTLV-3B/LAV.

W7644: Hemophiliac. HTLV-1 negative 1/2/84. RT and EM not done. Roche: **negative for HIV.**

W7645: Homosexual. Original sample received 12/12/83. HTLV-1 negative (undated). RT negative 1/9/84, 1/23/84. EM not done. Roche: **negative for HIV.**

W7650: Hemophiliac. Original sample received 12/15/83. RT negative 1/9/84, 1/23/84. HTLV-1 negative 1/17/84, 1/24/84. EM not done. Roche: **negative for HIV.**

W7675: Chronic lymphatic leukemia patient. Original sample received 12/15/83. EM negative 12/16/83. HTLV-1 negative (undated). RT negative (undated). Roche: **negative for HIV.**

[n.]When Tom White tested what purported to be the earliest frozen sample of the pool — Popovic's H-17 clone infected with HTLV-3B on February 29, 1983 — it didn't contain any AIDS virus. Following news reports that he was unable to come up with an archival sample of the Popovic pool, Gallo fired off a letter to *Science* maintaining that his lab had never told OSI the H-17 sample contained any virus. "It would have been more accurate," Gallo said, "to state that we thought H-17 was a sample of the uninfected [HT] clone." However, the label on the vial given to OSI was marked "HTLV-3B/H17." In a January 12, 1992, letter to the OSI, Gallo's administrative assistant, Howard Streicher, contradicted his boss by stating that "[t]he vial was identified as *possibly* containing HTLV-3B from February 1984" [emphasis added]. According to Suzanne Hadley, "The precise label was recorded on the log sheet when I picked up the samples. I am certain the sample was represented as 3B and I took it as such. There would have been no value in analyzing an uninfected sample, since our request was for the earliest 3B culture available." Even though the H-17 clone had been reported as virus-positive in *Science,* Gallo didn't think it mattered that he couldn't produce a remnant of the Popovic pool. "The absence of a 'pool sample' in the freezer in 1991," he told the ORI, "indicates only that the permanent cell line represents a highly selective substrate for growing the HTLV-3B isolate."

[o.]The only report of MOV's existence was a passing reference in a 1985 *Science* article by Flossie Wong-Staal, with a footnote referring the reader to a previously published paper in a different journal. However, the referenced paper contains no reference to MOV. Mentioned in its place is HTLV-3B.

Chapter 20. "I Know I Don't Lie"

[a.]The report would never be made public in this form.

[b.]The original draft of the *Science* paper described virus production as continuing for "more than five months." In the second draft, "five" had been crossed out and replaced by "four." In the fourth draft, "more than four" was crossed out and replaced with "several." In draft eight, "several" had been replaced with "over 5" by Sarngadharan — who, the OSI said, "must have known that the pool experiment did not extend over five months." The papers were submitted to *Science* on March 30, 1984, which meant that if Figure 2A were correct, the virus in question must have begun reproducing in late October 1983 — the same month that Popovic first began growing LAV.

[c.]"Continuous production of HTLV-3," the sentence read, "was obtained after repeated exposure of parental HT cells to concentrated culture fluids harvested from short-term cultures of T cells (grown with TCGF) obtained from patients with AIDS or pre-AIDS. The concentrated fluids were first shown to contain particle-associated RT activity."

ᵈ·The *Lancet* letter stated that HUT-78 had been derived from the T-cells of a patient with Sezary syndrome, which was correct, and HT/H-9 from a patient with Adult T-cell Leukemia; in Popovic's original *Science* paper, the patient from whom HT had come was described as "an adult with lymphoid leukemia," a catch-all that includes Sezary syndrome and ATL. The letter made it sound as if HUT-78 and HT/H-9 had been established from different patients. According to Gallo, he hadn't meant to mislead the *Lancet's* readers into thinking the patient from whom H-9 was established actually had been *afflicted* with adult T-cell leukemia, merely that the H-9 cells fit an "ATL" typology — which, being malignant lymphocytes, they did, as did every other lymphoid cancer.

ᵉ·A few weeks before the four HTLV-3 papers were submitted to *Science,* Gallo assured the editor of *The Lancet* that "no one has been able to work with" the French virus, "and because of the lack of permanent production and characterization it is hard to say they are really 'isolated' in the sense that virologists use this term" (R. Gallo to I. Munro, March 4, 1984). Two months later, Gallo promised Jean-Claude Chermann that "[w]e did not 'mass produce' your virus for characterization. . . . We assumed that was your job" (R. Gallo to J.-C. Chermann, June 15, 1984). To Claudine Escoffier-Lambiotte, Gallo claimed that, at the time the *Science* papers were published, "LAV had not yet been successfully produced in a permanently growing cell line" (July 3, 1985). A month before the Pasteur lawsuit was filed, *Science* had reported that Gallo and Popovic "could not get continuous virus production" with LAV, "so they put the material in the freezer" (Norman, C. "Patent Dispute Divides AIDS Researchers." *Science* 230:610, November 8, 1985). A month after that, Gallo assured the *Wall Street Journal* that "the single [*sic*] LAV sample was too small to be of practical use" (*Wall Street Journal,* December 16, 1985). In April 1986 Gallo told the *New York Times* that "his lab had been able to infect human cells with the virus sample received from France only 'transiently' [and that] further research with the French specimen had not been possible because it failed to infect additional cells" (*New York Times,* April 12, 1986). Gallo also assured *U.S. News & World Report* that it had been "'physically impossible' to grow the particles of virus sent by Montagnier" (*U.S. News & World Report,* January 13, 1986). To Jean Bernard, Gallo had insisted, "We temporarily transmitted [LAV] to human fresh blood T-cells (which soon die) to confirm it was a virus. . . . We did nothing more with this virus which they stated could not be grown in a permanent cell line, which is, of course, exactly what we succeeded in doing with several of our isolates of HTLV-III" (R. Gallo to J. Bernard, February 10, 1986).

ᶠ·"There is no hard evidence," the OSI said, "to disprove Dr. Gallo's claim about the intended meaning of the passage, and the fact is that different interpretations of the passage are possible, including the interpretation that it applies solely to the experiences of the [Institut Pasteur] scientists. . . . There is not sufficient evidence for a finding of scientific misconduct on the part of Dr. Gallo."

g.S. Hadley to R. Lanman, June 4, 1991. Hadley noted that the data tables which "contain entries found in the OSI investigation to be falsified" had been copied verbatim in the application for the patent on the HT and H-9 cell lines. Moreover, the patent application, like the Popovic paper, stated that "the concentrated fluids used to inoculate the 'HT' cell line 'were *first* shown to contain particle associated . . . RT.' This statement is false. Only one sample was first (i.e., before inoculation) shown to be RT-positive. Indeed, several of the constituent samples, when tested later, were found to be RT-negative." As for Gallo's statement under oath that he had an electron micrograph of HTLV-3 in February 1983, Hadley observed that "I am not aware of *any* EM-positive detection *before* 5/83." Gallo's claim to have had between twenty-five and thirty detections 'of this new retrovirus' up to September 1983, was also "not correct." Nor was the assertion that H-9 had been producing the AIDS virus "in large amounts" in November 1983, since the H-9 clone hadn't existed until January 1984. Gallo had maintained under oath that the July LAV shipment had "no detectable virus," but Hadley noted that "Dr. Gonda reported he found lentivirus particles in the culture, in early October 1983." Finally, Gallo's sworn statement that he did "not consider LAV and HTLV-3 to be the same or even substantially the same virus" was "at variance" with Gallo's public statements and his testimony to the OSI. Hadley's memo concluded by noting that the patent applications had been signed by Gallo and Popovic, "who both acknowledged that 'willful false statements may jeopardize the validity of the application or any patent issued thereon.'"

h.When Sharma complained that the admonition was undeserved, there had been a second inquiry in which Healy hadn't been involved. The second inquiry overruled the first, concluding that Sharma was guilty of misconduct in misrepresenting his research. That finding led to a third investigation, which reversed the second finding by concluding that while Sharma had made misleading statements in his grant application, he had not done so with the express intention of deceiving the NIH. Not incidentally, the third panel also concluded that the Cleveland Clinic was under no obligation to return the $1,169,000 awarded to Sharma on the basis of the questioned grant application.

Chapter 21. "Intellectual Recklessness of a High Degree"
a.R. Gallo to L. Montagnier, May 24, 1991. What had begun years before as a day-long picnic for the members of Gallo's laboratory had expanded to include other NIH scientists, then a few university researchers, then many scientists, until the annual invitation list had grown to several hundred. Those with whom Gallo had tangled — Jay Levy, Don Francis, Mal Martin — would never be invited, and the few who dared to decline invitations risked Gallo's wrath. "One year my wife lost a baby," Wolf Prensky recalled, "and I didn't come to the meeting. I got a very tough letter." The attractions included an opportunity for far-flung scientists to meet, and possibly impress, the NCI and NIH higher-ups who dropped by for cocktails or dinner, and who might have something to say about whether their grants got funded. A more immediate attraction was the checks for five hundred or a thousand dollars handed out by Gallo

on the meeting's last day. "It's the only meeting I know of where they paid *you* to go," said one frequent participant. If so, it was money well earned. "You sat there for hours," said another attendee, "listening to talk after talk after talk after talk after talk. The talks would go from nine in the morning till five in the afternoon, when everybody would be exhausted."

ᵇ·To name only two of many: "The first results we obtained with over 1,000 serum specimens showed that between 88 and 100 percent of AIDS patients' sera were positive." In fact, Gallo's ELISA never achieved an accuracy of anything close to 100 percent. Gallo's first HIV serology, his blind testing of the CDC's pedigreed AIDS blood samples, detected AIDS virus antibodies in only 48 percent of AIDS patients. Even Gallo's subsequent data, published in *Science* in May 1984, reported only forty-three of forty-nine AIDS patients' sera positive. On page 158, Gallo writes that "from July 1983 on, we had approval to experiment with LAV particles but not clear permission to publish any results with LAV." But Gallo testified to OSI that "[w]e didn't have to give them co-authorship . . . we had full freedom to do anything we wanted with LAV and publish on our own and solve the problem" (R. Gallo to OSI, May 16, 1990).

ᶜ·Without naming Koch, Gallo asserts that "a major political leader in Bavaria, who was being advised by a country doctor, flirted with the idea of developing camps for HIV-infected people. This doctor had lived in Sweden during the post–World War II years and was a self-proclaimed AIDS expert. . . ." According to Koch, whose anti-Nazi father had been chief prosecutor in Hamburg during the Allied occupation following World War II, no one in the Bavarian government, for whose health ministry Koch served as an adviser on AIDS, ever discussed, or even considered, the idea of "camps for HIV-infected people." Nor, Koch pointed out, would such a thing have been possible, since in Germany all matters of public health are governed by federal German law, not left to the individual states.

ᵈ·On some points Gallo was more conciliatory toward the French. "There were," Gallo conceded, "no doubt many significant differences" between HIV and HTLV-1, a point the Pasteur group had "first argued." Nor was there any doubt that Montagnier "had his own isolate because I knew we had received a bona fide novel retrovirus in 1983 from him"— a sharp departure from Gallo's previous insistence that he didn't know *what* the French had sent him in 1983. After claiming for years that the French had found LAV by following his protocol for isolating HTLV-1, Gallo admitted it had been wrong protocol after all. Perhaps most surprising was Gallo's concession, eight years after writing the Pasteur's *Science* abstract, that in May 1983 LAV had "clearly differed in important ways from what we knew about the HTLV family."

ᵉ·Gallo claimed to have given Chermann the idea of growing LAV in cord blood cells in the spring of 1983 (R. Gallo to OSI, August 3, 1990). But Chermann told OSI Gallo had made the suggestion only "because in HTLV-1 it is better to use cord blood cell [*sic*]"— and that, in any event, it had come after the French had been adding cord blood cells to the Brugière culture for several weeks (J.-C. Chermann to OSI, October 5, 1990).

f.·"On the contrary," Montagnier wrote Gallo, "we sent you again virus samples in September 83 and anti-interferon serum in December 83 at your request, and were eager to receive any news about the use of these reagents in your laboratory." Recounting the 1984 telephone conversation in which he informed Montagnier that HTLV-3B and LAV were "rather close" in their genetic composition, Gallo's book maintains that Montagnier "did not clearly answer" Gallo's suggestion that there had been a contamination in Paris. "This is untrue," retorted Montagnier. "I replied to you that if there were to be a contamination, it had to be one way: 3B contaminated by LAV. This proved later to be real."

g.·The OSI report incorrectly states that "eight of the ten patient-derived samples used to create the HTLV-3B pool had HIV DNA." In fact, four samples, A11, A12, A14, and B6, contained *no* HIV DNA.

h.·The allegation by the Office of Scientific Integrity was that Mika Popovic had improperly assigned a numerical value — 10 percent — to Betsy Read's nonquantitative observation that "very few cells" had been "positive for rabbit antisera." In a May 13, 1992, letter to Bernadine Healy, Read claimed that "very few cells" and "positive for rabbit antisera" were separate statements not meant to be linked, and that "even though there were 'very few cells,' the cells that were on the slide were *positive* with the rabbit poly-clonal anti-sera. . . ."

i.·Present were Fred Richards, Al Gilman, Robert Warner, John Stobo, Mary Jane Osborne, and Judith Areen. Missing were Joe Sambrook of UT-Dallas and Arnie Levine of Princeton, who had submitted his resignation the previous day after informing Bernadine Healy that he had invited the author to lecture his students. Healy's deputy, John Diggs, advised Levine that "I believe you should resign your consultant position with the NIH in order to avoid any perception that your interactions with Mr. Crewdson might bias your advice to the NIH on the Gallo investigation" (J. Diggs to A. Levine, August 30, 1991). Levine advised Diggs that he had withdrawn the informal invitation, which had been tendered over drinks at the Hôtel George V in Paris a few months before, and never formally accepted (A. Levine to J. Diggs, October 11, 1991). Diggs informed Levine that NIH now saw "no basis for concern on your part or ours," and "no reason why you should not continue as a consultant to NIH" (J. Diggs to A. Levine, January 27, 1992). Disgusted with NIH for questioning his integrity in the first place, Levine resigned from the panel anyway.

j.·J. Mason to Director, National Institutes of Health, October 3, 1991. After learning it would be "six to seven more months" before the Sharma case was resolved, Mason concluded that "this length of time is too long for you to be recused from duties involving the OSI. During this period a number of important scientific integrity issues will need to be addressed within the PHS, and I want the benefit of input from the Director, NIH, on these issues."

k.·A third "wise man," Robert Chanock, noted in a March 6, 1992, memo to Healy's executive assistant that "Although Gallo will never be a candidate for an award as the kindest and gentlest scientist, the fairest scientist or the least dissembling scientist, he did develop the first efficient and specific serologic tests for HIV antibodies." Chanock's conclusion, however, is based only on the relative publication dates of blood-test data from the Pasteur and Gallo groups and does not take account of data presented by the French at meetings, *The Lancet*'s six-month delay in publishing the Pasteur's 1983 serology, or the comparative blood testing by the CDC.

[1.]Wrote Korn: "The OSI Report takes the position that Gallo should not be found guilty of scientific misconduct, presumably because he did not personally conduct the experiments nor write the first draft of the paper. Thus, the OSI apparently places Gallo as one removed from Popovic whose own misconduct was judged to be minimal. However, I would take a different position. As the head of the Laboratory, Gallo must assume responsibility for the way it operates. I would not hold him directly responsible if a collaborator falsified or fabricated experimental data. However, as one whose native language is English, as an experienced investigator and author, and as one who must set the 'tone' of the Laboratory, Gallo should be held responsible when he is co-author of a paper that misrepresents and misstates the experimental results that he (Gallo) should have reviewed. Conceivably, Popovic could be a careless investigator and confused by the meaning of English phrases or abbreviations (although I doubt it) but these are specifically Gallo's responsibilities as head of the Laboratory and research team. I have no difficulty in finding Gallo more responsible than Popovic for what has occurred. Specifically, in essentially all 20 of the issues examined Gallo failed in his responsibilities as the head of the Laboratory."

Chapter 22. "It Can't Be the Money"

[a.]Not until July 1985 had heat-treating of blood products begun in Canada, followed a few months later by HIV-antibody testing. During the preceding eight months, according to the *Ottawa Citizen* ("Bad blood's deadly legacy," September 11, 1993), some twenty-eight million units of blood products were distributed in that country. None was recalled, and only 2.5 million units were destroyed. "In retrospect," said a Canadian parliamentary report, "the authorities — including the Canadian Red Cross, the Canadian Blood Committee, Health and Welfare Canada, and the Canadian Hemophilia Society — knew at the time that some of the untreated Factor VIII product remaining on the market was contaminated with the AIDS virus." In mid-1998, at a trial in Tokyo District Court, it emerged that the Japanese government had been aware of the risks posed by untreated blood products a year before it approved their use in 1984. By the time the Japanese government approved the use of heat-treated blood products in 1985, several hundred hemophiliacs had been infected. According to the minutes of the May 6, 1985, meeting of the U.S. Public Health Service Executive Task Force on AIDS, "Manufacturers report that some non-heated AHF [clotting factor] continues to be used though there is no shortage of heated AHF." It was three days after the PHS meeting, on May 9, that Michel Garretta wrote the minister of social affairs of his intention to continue distributing nontreated Factor VIII through July 1985. In May 1997, the four principal American manufacturers of clotting factors — Alpha Therapeutics, Armour Pharmaceuticals, Cutter Laboratories, and Baxter Healthcare — agreed to pay $100,000 to each of more than six thousand HIV-infected hemophiliacs or their survivors, who had charged the companies in a class-action suit with negligence for having failed to begin heat treatment until early 1984. The companies also agreed to reimburse the federal government nearly $12.2 million for payments made by federal health insurance programs. The settlement received almost no attention in the American press.

[b.] A. LeBlanc to R. Netter, February 27, 1985. With a 97 percent accuracy rate, 86 percent of positive samples would be false positives.

[c.] Abbott had planned to supply France and other European countries from a factory in Delkenheim, Germany, which it intended to come on line in May 1995. Because of delays, Delkenheim didn't begin producing test kits until the fall of that year, which meant that any Abbott tests reaching France would have been flown from Abbott's Chicago headquarters, which was unable to make enough tests for the U.S. market.

[d.] R. Gallo to F. Rich, September 27, 1993. The infection of French hemophiliacs was principally due to Michel Garretta's failure to ban the distribution of non-heat-treated Factor VIII. Even if the Abbott test could have been deployed across France beginning in March 1985, given the relatively low incidence of HIV in that country the total number of hemophiliacs and transfusion recipients who might have been spared would almost certainly have numbered between forty and seventy.

[e.] J. Onek to M. Astrue, October 21, 1991. In February 1985 Heckler declared that "only a small number of those with positive test results will go on to develop AIDS." The following month, FDA commissioner Frank Young cautioned that "the public must not leap to the conclusion that a positive test result for antibodies means they have or will get AIDS. That simply is not true."

[f.] Rule 60 of the Federal Rules of Civil Procedure allows for setting aside a judgment or other court-sanctioned agreement if newly discovered evidence comes to light, including evidence of "fraud, misrepresentation, or other misconduct of an adverse party." However, such a motion must be filed within one year of the settlement — a deadline that, for Pasteur, had expired four years earlier.

Chapter 23. "Slander Is the Worst Crime"

[a.] According to *Science and Government Report* (December 1, 1992), Healy's press secretary at first denied that any such meeting had taken place, then confirmed that it had but declined to say when or where it had occurred.

[b.] R. Simon to Federal Bureau of Investigation, March 2, 1992. To the FBI, Healy declared that "the swirl of unauthorized disclosures of confidential information regarding the case of Dr. Robert Gallo has already demonstrably damaged the credibility of the U.S. government's position on patent and other related business matters." Beyond that, the leaks represented "serious breaches of trust and personal integrity." In Healy's opinion, "the damage from this illegal conduct on a range of OSI investigations must be measured as substantial and likely in the millions of dollars" (B. Healy to A. Carroll, March 10, 1992).

c.J. Dingell to W. Barr, January 15, 1992. According to Dingell, HHS officials "may have generated and transmitted" to Justice "false and misleading information about Dr. Gallo's HIV research and HIV blood test" during the patent dispute. Many of the pleadings and other documents filed in that case, Dingell warned, among them Gallo's declaration, appeared to have been flawed by "significant material omissions" or, worse, to have "contained false and misleading information."

d.The ORI corrected several (but not all) of the errors and discrepancies in the OSI's report. The ORI addendum contained at least one glaring error of its own, stating that "between May of 1983 and May of 1984 the Pasteur Institute researchers did not publish any other articles" on LAV. In fact, the Pasteur published a half-dozen articles on various aspects of LAV during this period, notably the April 7, 1984, *Lancet* report of the isolation of LAV from Eric Loiseau.

e.The ORI observed that, "according to Dr. Chermann, in October or November 1983, the French had begun mass-producing LAV, albeit in an EBV transformed lymphoblastoid cell line." It also noted "that the BJAB cell line is a permanent cell line and the French may have grown LAV in this permanent cell line before the *Science* papers were submitted."

f.Despite Popovic's hopes, R.F. never became a player. Of 83,929 scientific articles published on HIV by the end of 1999, only 120 mention HTLV-3$_{RF}$.

g.ORI's professional staff then included thirteen M.D. or Ph.D.-level scientists, all with research backgrounds.

h.Some of those who knew Watson well also thought he was slightly daft. Arnie Levine, who ranked Watson with Einstein as one of the century's two great thinkers, thought Watson's craziness, or apparent craziness, traced to the very young age of twenty-four at which he had done his historic work — thereby condemning Watson, like Jonas Salk, to spend most of his career looking backward. As the *New Republic* wrote in 1990: "One could encounter James Watson for the first time and not immediately think: 'Oh, James Watson — the Nobel Prize–winning scientist who revolutionized biology in 1953 by discovering the structure of DNA.' One could think instead, 'Oh, a deranged person.' Watson's eyes are intense and bugged out yet unfixed; they wander cryptically as he talks, floating from one point in the visual landscape to another and another. His head floats slightly, too, so that altogether he conveys the sort of ethereal detachment that typically signifies either profound inner peace or utter disorientation. And then there's the inappropriate laughter."

i.Watson had fervently disagreed with Healy's plan —"sheer lunacy"— to file patent applications on the human genes as they were discovered, even before anyone had a clue to what function they might perform. Although the patent applications were withdrawn, Watson resigned — effectively forced out, he said later, in a way *Nature* called "discreditable" to the NIH, over a potential conflict of interest involving his ownership of stock in two companies that might someday profit from the genome project. "I had wanted to quit — but not necessarily the way I did," Watson told *Science,* which reported that Healy "roundly" denied having forced Watson to leave the NIH.

Chapter 24. "The Steaks Are Not Done"

[a.]Lusso, P., *et al.* "Human herpesvirus 7 (HHV-7) uses CD4 as a receptor and interferes with HIV infection." Ninth International Conference on AIDS, June 14, 1993. The NCI's six-page news release highlighting Gallo's address in Berlin didn't mention that HHV-7 had been discovered by another NIH researcher, Niza Frenkel.

[b.]"New ways of blocking AIDS virus suggested at conference." *Boston Globe,* June 9, 1993. There never were any human tests. When Gallo tried to publish the data to which he alluded in Berlin, the paper bounced from *Nature* to *Science* to *PNAS,* after which nothing more was heard of an HHV-7 vaccine for AIDS.

[c.]Martin didn't remind Gallo of their conversation in Anthony Fauci's office a few years before, when Martin had characterized Gallo's refusal of the H-9 cells as "obscene." According to Martin, Gallo replied that "I meant it to be obscene. It was to pay you back for mistreating Veffa [one of Gallo's Italian postdocs, Genoveffa Franchini] at Cold Spring Harbor." Gallo confirmed Martin's recollection in a December 5, 1988, memo to the record, admitting that he had refused a reagent to Martin after Martin "abused a few students in my laboratory." Martin denied having "abused" Franchini, recalling instead that he had made uncomplimentary remarks to Franchini about Gallo.

[d.]The trouble arose after Golde gave Gallo another cell line, KG-1, which proved a highly productive source of interferon. After promising in writing to keep KG-1 in his lab and use it only for his own research, Gallo provided the cell line to a former NCI colleague, Sidney Pestka, at Hoffman-LaRoche. When Golde learned his cell line, which was owned by UCLA, had fallen into the hands of a pharmaceutical company, he demanded a meeting with Vince DeVita. "He wanted Dr. DeVita to make some kind of announcement," Gallo testified in a July 1981 deposition in the resulting case, *Hoffman-LaRoche, Inc. v. David W. Golde, et al.* "He wanted to expose this scandal. I remember that conversation pretty well, because I was extremely angry. I said something to that effect on the phone, that if he were in the room I would feel like responding vigorously. I was emotional and abusive. I'll say that for the record. What else could I be? I'm a human being. That's the autonomic nervous system, you know."

[e.]Although the *Bru* results were omitted from Popovic's *Science* paper, the HTLV-3B cultures in that paper were tested in parallel with the rabbit antibody and Frédéric

Brugière's serum. As Gallo admitted to OSI, the correspondence between *Bru* and the rabbit antibody was extremely close, indicating that the French method was just as specific as Gallo's (LTCB response to question 1b). Gallo's claims for the specificity of the rabbit antiserum were also undercut by his own *Science* paper, which reported that "a rabbit antiserum raised against purified HTLV-3 showed some reactivity with antigens of HTLV-2 and, to a lesser extent, with HTLV-1" (Schupbach, J., *et al.* "Serological Analysis of a Subgroup of Human T-Lymphotropic Retroviruses (HTLV-3) Associated with AIDS." *Science* 224:503, May 4, 1984).

[f.]B. Read lab notes, February 15, 1984. Read told the OSI that the designation "S.N./H" referred to a co-culture of the S.N. cord-blood-cell culture with either "HT" or "H4," both of which were HUT-78.

[g.]Following the conclusion of Popovic's appeal, Betsy Read, on the verge of leaving Gallo's lab to pursue a Ph.D. at the University of Maryland, demanded that NCI make her a co-inventor on the blood-test patent and award her an annual $25,000 share of the royalties, a quarter of the sum Gallo and Popovic were receiving. NIH countered by offering Read a one-time $25,000 payment without co-inventorship (R. Lanman to M. Gollin, January 25, 1995).

[h.]In a November 5, 1992, letter to Lang, Gallo wrote that "What you have not perceived in any of your harangues is what I meant by the question 'are you crazy' and the comment 'this is incredible,' which I marked in Popovic's first manuscript."

Chapter 25. "We Did It to Ourselves"

[a.]Bishop's former postdoc, Dominique Stehelin, called the award "unfair and rotten," claiming that he had done the prize-winning work "myself, from A to Z." Robin Weiss thought Peter Vogt should have been the third recipient, or possibly Peter Duesberg. "I don't think they're intellectually as original as the Nobel announcement made them out to be," Weiss said of Bishop and Varmus, "but no one can deny that they did the work. It slightly rankles that in the actual citations it was made out that the concept that the oncogene's retroviruses came from cellular genes was new and surprising. Because several of us proposed precisely this about three or four years before. I was so damn stupid I didn't publish it up front, really. I buried it in a couple of conference symposium findings that were never read. Peter Fischinger at NCI, who I've never thought of as an original thinker, without seeing our paper came out with something very, very similar."

[b.]Another invented scene had Françoise Barré reading Gallo's 1984 articles in *Science* and recognizing — from appearance alone, which would have been impossible — that the picture of "HTLV-3" was really a picture of LAV. A third gaffe saw Francis sharing a late-night snack with Harold Jaffe, played by Charles Martin Smith, in a fictional diner near the CDC — and coming to the realization, as he watches Jaffe play a game of Pac-Man while waiting for his meat loaf, that whatever causes AIDS is "gobbling up" AIDS patients' T-cells. Francis didn't recall having had such a blinding insight into the etiology of AIDS, and the CDC's Paul Feorino pointed out that "there was no place where Harold Jaffe went and had meat loaf, because he doesn't like meat loaf. There was no pinball machine." Nor is there a restaurant anywhere near CDC that serves halfway decent food that late at night.

c. According to White's *Nature* paper, the samples from patients TW, DB, EC, and WA contained no HIV. Notebooks kept by Popovic and Betsy Read showed that none of the three that did contain HIV ever tested positive for reverse transcriptase, indicating that Popovic had been unable to culture the virus in those cells.

d. The affidavit read: "My name is Françoise Barré-Sinoussi, Ph.D. I received my Ph.D. in 1974 from the University of Science, Paris, France. I have been involved in the study of retroviruses at the Pasteur Institute since 1971. From 1980–86 I was an assistant professor from INSERM in the viral oncology unit at the Pasteur Institute in Paris, France. I served three fellowships at the National Institutes of Health in Bethesda, Maryland, between 1973 and 1979, including a collaborative research fellowship in the Laboratory of Tumor Cell Biology at the National Cancer Institute from May to June 1979. I currently am Head of the Retroviruses Biology Unit at the Pasteur Institute in Paris, France. I have first hand knowledge of the following events. At Dr. Gallo's invitation, I attended the 1992 Conference for the Laboratory of Tumor Cell Biology which was held in Bethesda, Maryland, from approximately August 8–15, 1992. During this conference I spoke with Mikulas Popovic. I have known Dr. Popovic for many years. We shared a ride on a van taking participants to another location. Dr. Popovic brought up the OSI findings of scientific misconduct during this ride. Dr. Popovic told me that he was not responsible for the changes in his May 1984 *Science* paper entitled "Detection, Isolation, and Continuous Production of Cytopathic Retroviruses (HTLV-3) from Patients with AIDS and pre-AIDS," that deleted references to LAV. He told me that Dr. Gallo had changed the paper to delete those references and the discussion of LAV. Dr. Popovic stated that he felt it was fortunate that he had saved the drafts of his paper that showed that he tried to give credit to the Pasteur researchers when he wrote the paper. Dr. Popovic told me that he had several viral isolates in 1983. He stated then that he added his isolates to LAV — to try to increase its titer, i.e., to enhance the growth capacity of the virus. Dr. Popovic was describing the "pool" experiment that he had recounted at other times in the past for animal retroviruses. Dr. Popovic stated that he thought that adding additional isolates to LAV would help to increase the growth capacity of the virus. He (as all of us), did not know at that time that there were differences among HIV isolates. He thought that they were like HTLV-1, that means, almost identical. I told Dr. Popovic that he must have thought that LAV would be the isolate that could come through out of the culture infected with such a mixture of viruses because of its adaptation to culture conditions in laboratory *(in vitro)*. I explained to him that a selection for growth capacity was probably established in our lab by passaging the virus several times on primary cultures of human lymphocytes. Dr. Popovic stated that he could not imagine that the virus that resulted from his mixture of viruses would be LAV because he had at least one other virus that also grew well, i.e., R.F. It was clear that Dr. Popovic was highly concerned about this story and I advised him that he had to put the events surrounding the publication of his paper and the problems of the LTCB behind him and get on with his life. I affirm under penalty of perjury of the laws of the United States of America that the foregoing is a true and correct summary of these events. Signed this thirteen [*sic*] day of November, 1993 in Paris, France. Françoise Barré-Sinoussi, Ph.D."

e. In February 1994, Gallo informed Barré that the NIH was considering rehiring Mika Popovic, and that "a clarification of the issue around your conversation with Mika could be very important for him." Gallo urged Barré to respond to a list of questions sent her by a writer for *Science,* Jon Cohen, and to provide "a clarification such as you gave me by phone — either you really do maintain that you are sure *Mika made* a *direct statement* to you that he *deliberately* put LAV (LAI) into the pool (the current interpretation of your statement to ORI or elsewhere); or, you thought that was the meaning of the discussion, based on our having openly acknowledged LAV (LAI) was in the pool (but which occurred as an accidental contamination) and such knowledge, coupled with what you believed was common knowledge (from the Paris press) that he put it in deliberately, caused you to interpret his remarks as you did. This is my understanding of what you said to me by telephone two weeks ago. I look forward to your statement." Barré replied that her "personal belief that LAV has been added to the pool was not caused by the 'Paris press' but, by my intimate knowledge of the events connected with the discovery of the virus from its very beginning." Because she "assumed that LAV had indeed been added to the pool, I mentioned it in the conversation with Mika as an established fact, which was not contradicted by him." Gallo replied that "I understand all your points. When you told me (by phone) about what you thought was well known, I assumed you meant the local propaganda, because I thought you believed it was well known (and acknowledged by Mika) that he stole the virus, i.e. deliberately took LAV, deliberately put it in the pool, and deliberately deceived people. Indeed, this is the current view (as far as I understand things) of ORI and of Suzanne Hadley." The Pasteur lawyers were summoned to sort things out, and Mike Epstein reported that Barré hadn't changed the story she told in the original affidavit. "Her statement," Epstein said, "is 'Dr. Popovic responded by telling me that he mixed LAV with the other viruses to increase the capacity of growth of the virus.' She is saying she doesn't understand why there is any doubt as to what this sentence means. He told her — he, Popovic, told her he was putting LAV into the soup for a specific purpose. She said, 'What I have told everybody is that he gave me the specific reason why he added LAV to the pool.' Which means it was crystal clear that he did it knowingly. Where we're getting hung up is over the word 'deliberate.' He never used the word deliberate, which unfortunately is the question that she answered to Gallo. And she's saying, 'Of course it was deliberate.' If it's accidental, then the phrase 'to increase the capacity of the growth of the virus' makes no sense. The words you have to focus on are 'direct statement.' He never said, 'Françoise, I deliberately did it.' He said, 'Françoise, I put LAV into the pool to increase the capacity of the growth of the virus.' That's a direct statement of deliberateness." At

Epstein's suggestion, Barré swore out a third affidavit that repeated her earlier version of the conversation with Popovic: "My November 13, 1993 Statement states: 'He [Dr. Popovic] stated then that he added his isolates to LAV to try to increase its titer, i.e., to enhance the growth capacity of the virus.' This is a true statement. This sentence reflects my current recollection of my conversation with M. Popovic in August 1992. By this language, it is manifestly clear that Dr. Popovic is stating that he knowingly mixed LAV into the virus pool since he is confirming to me that he did so for the specific reason of increasing the capacity of growth of the virus. During the past few weeks, I have received numerous contacts from Dr. Robert Gallo, both in writing and by telephone, pressuring me to clarify and alter the sentence set forth above from my November 13, 1993 Statement. I believe Dr. Gallo's behavior in this regard is improper. I believe it was improper for Dr. Gallo to try to interfere with the Statements that I gave to the U.S. Department of Health and Human Services and the U.S. Congress. . . . I swear under penalty of perjury pursuant to the laws of the United States of America that the foregoing account is true and correct, to the best of my knowledge and belief." When Peter Stockton saw Gallo's letters to Barré he asked the NIH's legislative liaison, Dotty Tisevich, whether it was true, as Gallo claimed, that the NIH was considering rehiring Popovic. Gallo explained to Tisevich that he had simply been asked by Popovic for a general letter of recommendation, "and it was his understanding Dr. Popovic is applying for several positions at NIH, but he did not know the specifics."

f.Popovic's witnesses included Betsy Read, who had participated in many of the experiments questioned by ORI; his former postdoc, Suzanne Gartner; Jan Svoboda, his elderly mentor from Czechoslovakia; and Gallo.

g."For example," Godek recounted, "they said the ten percent issue 'evidences no intent' because it was in the first draft of the paper. But the fact that the definition for N.D., meaning not done, was put in the seventh draft of the paper — that also 'evidences no intent.' I mean, how the hell do you reconcile those two statements? Another truly amazing one was that we had stipulated that four of the ten samples never had the AIDS virus. Then the Board disregarded the stipulation and said that one of the patients had seroconverted in June 1985 — therefore, seven of the patients had the AIDS virus. What difference does it make if the *patient* had the virus? The *sample* in Dr. Gallo's *freezer* didn't have the virus. It still doesn't, and it never will. Not only did they just totally ignore the stipulation, they actually stuck something into the opinion that's a total joke."

h.According to HHS, the appeals board ruling in the Popovic case also meant that, in order to lead to a finding of misconduct, "a false statement [must] have a material or significant effect on the research conclusions of the paper, and that there be no possibility of honest error." In a November 16, 1993, letter to HHS general counsel Harriet Rabb, Joe Onek declared it "flatly untrue" that the appeals board ever held "that scientific misconduct will not be found unless there is no possibility of an honest error." To the contrary, Onek said, "the Board has consistently reaffirmed that it is employing the 'preponderance of the evidence' standard. Thus, ORI is not required to prove that there is no possibility of honest error; it is only required to prove that the preponderance of the evidence supports a finding of no honest error."

[i.]Wade, N. "The vindication of Robert Gallo." *New York Times Magazine,* December 26, 1993. Wade's column, which he subsequently ceased to write after being replaced as science editor, contained many misstatements. "For years," Wade wrote, "Gallo has been under a thick cloud of suspicion that he stole from French scientists the credit for discovering the AIDS virus. The suspicion has proved groundless. As a Government Appeals Board concluded last month: 'One might anticipate that from all this evidence, after all the sound and fury, there would be at least a residue of palpable wrongdoing. This is not the case.'" But the question of whether *Gallo* "stole credit" from Pasteur hadn't been at issue in the *Popovic* hearing, much less adjudicated by the appeals board. Nor had any of the other accusations against Gallo been heard by the board, since the only evidence concerned the misconduct findings against Popovic, which the board itself considered "vestigial" to the Gallo case. Wade's assertion that Gallo had supplied "biological materials to the laboratory of Luc Montagnier" ignored the fact that, except for the monoclonal antibody to HTLV-1 which allowed the Pasteur to prove that LAV_{Bru} was a new human retrovirus, the flow of "biological materials" was entirely from Paris to Bethesda. Wade's declaration that it was Gallo who "put beyond reasonable dispute that the new virus was the cause of AIDS" ignored the CDC's comparative blood-test data, much less Popovic's acknowledgment to OSI that "we were wrong and Barré-Sinoussi was right." Most puzzling was Wade's insistence that, with the discovery that LAV_{Lai} had accidentally contaminated LAV_{Bru} in Paris, "[t]he only evidence for assuming Gallo had appropriated the French virus promptly evaporated."

Chapter 26. "Dr. Gallo Is No Longer Here"
[a.]In a November 26, 1985, memo to Gallo, Popovic acknowledged that the successful infection of Ti7.4 with LAV had been confirmed by "positive immunofluorescence," on December 14, 1983 — evidently the same experiment overwritten in Betsy Read's notes. Because the memo was withheld from the Pasteur lawyers, the French never knew about the confirmed growth of LAV in two cell lines until the memo surfaced after the 1987 settlement.

[b.]"Throughout the negotiations," the affidavit said, HHS "consistently maintained" that HTLV-3B "was not the same virus that had been earlier discovered by scientists at Pasteur — there were two separate viruses, and their similarities were coincidental." Also, HHS had affirmed that "Dr. Gallo's laboratory was unable to grow, or make any practical use of, the sample viruses sent to Dr. Gallo by Pasteur 'for research purposes only.' The sample viruses were essentially 'dead on arrival.'" In persuading the Pasteur to settle, Epstein said, HHS had assured the French that the government "had diligently performed a complete investigation into the allegations made by Pasteur, and had uncovered the facts that Pasteur would be able to discover through a thorough civil litigation process." Finally, the Pasteur had received an assurance that the government's investigation "had uncovered *no evidence* that was contrary to their factual assertions, or in support of Pasteur's claims that Dr. Gallo's virus *was* the Pasteur virus of which Pasteur had sent him samples in 1983."

c.To OSI, Gallo admitted that, prior to 1984, "there were not, of course . . . any reagents for testing the presence of the AIDS virus" (LTCB Exhibit CC4 to OSI).

d."The relevance of the IP work to that of *Gallo et al.* was affirmed by the PTO examiner when she became aware of it," the memorandum states. "The examiner advised the OIG that, had she been aware of the IP prior art at the time she examined the blood test application of Gallo, she would have suspended prosecution of the Gallo application and declared an interference between the two applicants. An interference was eventually declared, but not until two years after the initial Gallo submission. The IP scientists were eventually named Senior Party in the interference, confirming their priority in submitting a patent application on the HIV antibody blood test. By the time the interference was declared, the Gallo patent had long since been issued."

e.Gallo noted that he had "already publicly acknowledged in 1991, in a letter to *Nature* magazine that we accidental [*sic*] contaminated one of our AIDS virus samples with a virus from the Institut Pasteur. Ironically, the same accidentally [*sic*] contamination occurred earlier at the Institut Pasteur. Though we had many other independent isolates of HIV, at least one of which could have been used for our blood test at the same time, unfortunately the one contaminated by the virus from the Institut Pasteur was the one we selected because it was slightly more productive. Our work in 1983–84 showed how to mass produce the virus for the first time, led to the first reliable blood test for HIV, and was important for showing HIV was the cause of AIDS. I do not believe that there is any truthful, new, substantive information since the 1987 agreement which bears upon the history of our respective scientific contributions. However, I have learned that the sharing of the royalties was actually not 50/50 but markedly favored the U.S. Consequently, I am for a more equitable financial agreement where there is a true roughly 50/50 sharing of royalties. This feeling is intensified by the hope that this will make a permanent end to financial bickering and a return of the lawyers to dealing with lawyers and business and politics and not science; but it is made less enthusiastic by the unprecedented vicious attacks on me and spread of misinformation leading up to this day. During this period I have learned that when politics and financial interests take over, science loses, scientist [*sic*] loose [*sic*], truth often becomes a dispensable commodity, and most important of all, peoples' lives can be lost. Let us once and for all get this behind us and move above our base interests to better goals — let's try to cure AIDS."

f.M. Schwartz to H. Varmus, July 11, 1994. "Further to concluding our discussions regarding the concerns raised by the Institut Pasteur with the United States subsequent to the signing of the March 30, 1987 settlement agreement concerning the Montagnier *et al.* and the Gallo *et al.* patents on the HIV diagnostic test kits and other matters related thereto, by this letter Institut Pasteur confirms that the resolution adopted by the Trustees of the French and American AIDS Foundation (FAAF) regarding the awards of FAAF royalties and the American acknowledgement that U.S. scientists used a French virus when they invented the American HIV test kit brings to a satisfactory conclusion all of the concerns we have raised with you regarding these matters."

Epilogue. "Rather Does the Truth Ennoble All"

[a.]ORI records show that 35 cases were opened in 1993, 38 in 1994, 49 in 1995, 39 in 1996, 26 in 1997, 32 in 1998, and 30 in 1999.

[b.]Gallo chose the name because its initials were a permutation of HIV. But when the head of the Biotechnology Institute advised Gallo she was renaming Gallo's institute the "Center for Human Virology," Gallo demanded that the name be left as it was. "Originally I did not care," Gallo said. "Now I do because it has been openly world-wide written about and discussed as an Institute. We cannot change back to a Center again. We will all look utterly ridiculous. . . . Indeed, we already have symbols: Company is now HVI (Human Virology, Inc.), the virus is HIV, the Institute is the IHV!" (R. Gallo to R. Colwell, August 16, 1995).

[c.]The funding cuts imposed by Bernadine Healy and Sam Broder dropped Gallo's laboratory to fourth place among NIH labs in terms of annual dollars spent, although the bulk of the cutbacks entailed moving the money used to pay Gallo's contract laboratories to another part of the NCI budget. According to *Science* (261:1123, August 27, 1993), the biggest and best-funded NIH lab was that of gene researcher Ron Crystal, with thirty-four doctoral-level employees and a $4.4 million budget, compared to Gallo's nineteen doctoral employees and $2.6 million. The tenth-place NIH lab had a budget of $1.8 million, still larger than almost all university laboratories.

[d.]Although Gallo's paper was scheduled to appear in the December 15, 1995, issue of *Science,* the journal "released" it a week early, to coincide with Reinhard Kurth's publication that same day in *Nature* of his own candidate for the HIV suppression factor, interleukin-16 (Baier, M., *et al.* "Why monkeys don't get AIDS." *Nature* 378(6557):563, 1995). The previous weekend, Gallo and Kurth had appeared at a scientific meeting in Rome, where Kurth apologized for being unable to discuss his interleukin-16 data because of its impending publication. According to the *Washington Post,* the subsequent lifting of the *Science* embargo had been engineered by the public relations firm of Hill & Knowlton. In submitting his paper to *Science,* Gallo instructed that it not be sent to Jay Levy or Reinhard Kurth for review (R. Gallo to B. Jasny, September 6, 1995).

[e.]Gray's departure, said the *Washington Post,* had come "on the heels of a series of staff defections, a sharp fall in revenue and a wave of negative publicity" for the firm, which "has come under heavy criticism for a string of controversial clients it took on in recent years, including the Bank of Credit and Commerce International and Citizens for a Free Kuwait."

ᶠSylvia Lee-Huang, the New York University researcher who first demonstrated the anti-HIV properties of hCG, isolated what she said was the elusive factor — an enzyme, lyzozyme, that was found in the urine of pregnant women and which simply joined forces with hCG to attack the AIDS virus. Several years later, Bruce Patterson of Children's Memorial Hospital in Chicago also claimed to have identified and isolated Gallo's HAF — a protein called leukemia inhibitory factor found normally in the placenta.

ᵍ*Science* 224:497: The "HT" cell line represents a "new immortalized T-cell population . . . derived from an adult with lymphoid leukemia." "The concentrated fluids were first shown to contain particle-associated RT." "Serum from E.T. also contained antibodies to proteins of disrupted HTLV-3 but did not react with cells infected with HTLV-1 or HTLV-2." R.F. RT Activity: 2000 cpm. R.F. Electron microscopy: N.D. (Not Done). S.N. RT Activity: 63,000 cpm. S.N. Electron microscopy: positive. B.K. Electron microscopy: positive. L.S. Electron microscopy: positive. "HTLV-3 has also been isolated in our laboratory from a total of 48 patients by the more conventional methods for isolation of HTLV." "HTLV-3 is related to HTLV-1 and HTLV-2 and, by all criteria, this new virus belongs to the HTLV family of retroviruses." "HTLV-3 and LAV may be different." "LAV . . . has not yet been transmitted to a permanently growing cell line for true isolation and therefore has been difficult to obtain in quantity." *Science* 224:500: "Retroviruses belonging to the HTLV family and collectively designated HTLV-3 were isolated from a total of 48 subjects. . . ." "That these new isolates are members of the HTLV family . . . is indicated by their morphological, biological, and immunological characteristics." "Another HTLV isolate was obtained from the lymph nodes of a patient with lymphadenopathy and at risk for AIDS. This isolate has been difficult to grow in quantities sufficient to permit its characterization." *Science* 224:503: "HTLV-3 is a true member of the HTLV family and . . . is more closely related to HTLV-2 than to HTLV-1." *Science* 224:506: "HTLV-3 . . . has a reverse transcriptase with a molecular weight of about 100,000 . . . however it lacks a band separating at a molecular weight of 19,000 (p19)." The "relatedness" between HTLV-1, HTLV-2, and HTLV-3 has "been confirmed by comparison of nucleotide sequences of the three types of HTLV." "The virus has been isolated from several children with AIDS as well as from their mothers."

DRAMATIS PERSONAE

MARC ALIZON: Molecular biologist at the Institut Pasteur; obtained first molecular clone of French AIDS virus LAV.

SURESH ARYA: Molecular biologist in Gallo's lab who "overinterpreted" genetic similarities between the AIDS virus and HTLV-1 and HTLV-2; references to "LAV" in Arya's notebooks later raised questions about Gallo lab's work with the French virus.

MICHAEL ASTRUE: HHS general counsel; recommended unsuccessfully that HHS pay reparations to the Institut Pasteur for Gallo's use of LAV in development of blood antibody test for HIV.

DAVID BALTIMORE: Molecular biologist, Whitehead Institute, Massachusetts Institute of Technology; codiscoverer, with Howard Temin, of *reverse transcriptase,* for which he was awarded the Nobel Prize.

FRANÇOISE BARRÉ-SINOUSSI: Institut Pasteur virologist; with Luc Montagnier and Jean-Claude Chermann, codiscoverer of the AIDS virus.

LYLE BIVENS: Chief of the Office of Scientific Integrity Review and, later, Office of Research Integrity; reversed Office of Scientific Integrity in finding that Gallo had committed scientific misconduct.

OTIS BOWEN: Succeeded Margaret Heckler as Secretary of Health and Human Services; presided over 1987 settlement with the Institut Pasteur.

EDWARD BRANDT: Assistant HHS secretary for health; pressed Gallo unsuccessfully to say whether Gallo's HTLV-3 was the same kind of virus as Pasteur Institute's LAV.

SAMUEL BRODER: NCI lab chief who succeeded Vincent DeVita as director of NCI; initially compared Gallo to Einstein, later urged him to leave the cancer institute.

FRÉDÉRIC BRUGIÈRE: French AIDS patient; source of first AIDS virus isolate, LAV_{Bru}.

FRANÇOISE BRUN-VÉZINET: Virologist at Claude Bernard Hospital, Paris; with Christine Rouzioux, developed first blood antibody test for the AIDS virus and established LAV as the presumptive cause of AIDS; with François Clavel, codiscoverer of the second AIDS virus, HIV-2.

MARTY BRYANT: Graduate student in Murray Gardner's lab at University of California, Davis; first researcher outside Gallo laboratory to discover genetic identity of Pasteur's LAV and Gallo's HTLV-3B.

CIRILO CABRADILLA: CDC virologist; worked closely with Don Francis in helping the French establish LAV as the cause of AIDS.

CDC: U.S. Centers for Disease Control and Prevention, Atlanta.

CLAUDE CHARDON: French geologist doubly infected with HTLV-1 and HIV from a blood transfusion in Haiti; Chardon's infected T-cells misled Robert Gallo and Mikulas Popovic into suspecting that HTLV-1 might be the cause of AIDS.

JEAN-CLAUDE CHERMANN: Institut Pasteur virologist and chief of lab in which the AIDS virus was discovered.

MARCUS CHRIST: Attorney for Office of Research Integrity; unsuccessfully argued government's case in Mikulas Popovic's appeal of his finding of scientific misconduct.

FRANÇOIS CLAVEL: Institut Pasteur virologist; codiscoverer, with Françoise Brun-Vézinet, of the second AIDS virus HIV-2.

JAMES CURRAN: Chief of the CDC's AIDS epidemiology program; presided over 1984 blood testing competition which established that the Institut Pasteur's LAV and Gallo's HTLV-3 were both the likely cause of AIDS.

RAYMOND DEDONDER: Director of the Institut Pasteur during initial French challenge to Gallo patent on HIV blood test; agreed to settle the case after being assured by Reagan administration that Gallo's HTLV-3B represented an independent discovery and was not Pasteur's LAV by another name.

VINCENT DEVITA: Director, National Cancer Institute.

JOHN DINGELL: Chairman, House Energy and Commerce Committee; angered scientific community with investigations of possible scientific misconduct, including Gallo's AIDS research.

MICHAEL EPSTEIN: New York attorney; with Rob Odle, represented the Institut Pasteur during 1994 settlement.

CLAUDINE ESCOFFIER-LAMBIOTTE: Medical editor of Paris newspaper *Le Monde;* tried unsuccessfully to head off impending Franco-American crisis.

MYRON T. "MAX" ESSEX: Virologist at Harvard School of Public Health whose experiments with HTLV-MA misled Robert Gallo into believing that HTLV-1 might be the cause of AIDS; discoverer of purported second AIDS virus, "HTLV-4," later shown to be a monkey-virus contamination.

FDA: U.S. Food and Drug Administration; agency within HHS responsible for licensing medical devices including blood diagnostic tests.

PAUL FEORINO: CDC virologist; succeeded in growing LAV and isolating LAV-like viruses from the CDC's "transfusion pair," providing crucial epidemiological link between AIDS virus and disease.

ROLLAND FERDINAND: Haitian immigrant who died of AIDS in Philadelphia; source of Gallo AIDS virus HTLV-3$_{RF}$ that provided first clue to the suspicious similarity of HTLV-3B and LAV.

PETER FISCHINGER: Deputy director, NCI; conducted internal investigation purporting to show that Gallo had independently isolated HTLV-3B, proved it was the cause of AIDS and invented the blood antibody test for the AIDS virus.

DONALD FRANCIS: CDC epidemiologist; initially persuaded by Max Essex that HTLV-1 played a role in AIDS, later instrumental in demonstrating that the probable cause of AIDS was Institut Pasteur's LAV.

ROBERT GALLO: Chief of the National Cancer Institute's Laboratory of Tumor Cell Biology.

MURRAY GARDNER: University of California virologist; at Gallo's behest, ordered Marty Bryant not to publish his data showing identity of LAV and HTLV-3B.

ADI GAZDAR: NCI pathologist; established HUT-102 cell line in which Bernard Poiesz and Frank Ruscetti discovered HTLV-1 and HUT-78 cell line in which Mikulas Popovic succeeded in growing the AIDS virus.

STEVEN GODEK: Attorney for Office of Research Integrity; with Marcus Christ, unsuccessfully argued government's case in Mikulas Popovic's appeal of his finding of scientific misconduct.

SUZANNE HADLEY: Deputy director, Office of Scientific Integrity: headed initial investigation which found Popovic, but not Gallo, guilty of scientific misconduct; later assigned to Dingell subcommittee staff, where she produced comprehensive report of "continuing HHS cover-up" of Gallo's claimed discovery of the cause of AIDS.

BEATRICE HAHN: Molecular biologist in Gallo's lab; with partner George Shaw, first determined that HTLV-3$_{RF}$ was genetically distinct from HTLV-3B, raising initial alarms about the similarity of HTLV-3B and LAV.

JULES HALLUM: Director, Office of Scientific Integrity; softened the OSI's report censuring Gallo for having contributed to scientific misconduct by Mikulas Popovic.

BERGE HAMPAR: General manager of NCI's Frederick, Maryland, satellite campus; an attorney as well as a scientist, Hampar attempted to warn other NCI officials that the Reagan administration's defense against the Institut Pasteur was weak.

LOWELL HARMISON: Deputy assistant HHS secretary for health; led American delegation which heard accusations from the Institut Pasteur that Reagan administration had taken credit for French discovery of AIDS virus and blood antibody test.

BERNADINE HEALY: Director, National Institutes of Health; determined "to clear Dr. Gallo's reputation with regard to accusations of misconduct."

MARGARET HECKLER: Secretary of Health and Human Services; announced discovery by "our eminent Dr. Robert Gallo" that HTLV-3 was the cause of AIDS.

HHS: U.S. Department of Health and Human Services; among the scores of agencies under the HHS umbrella are the National Institutes of Health, National Cancer Institute, Centers for Disease Control, and Food and Drug Administration.

YORIO HINUMA: Japanese virologist who established HTLV-1 as the cause of Adult T-cell Leukemia.

ABRAHAM KARPAS: Cambridge University virologist and indefatigable critic of Gallo's research on HTLV-1 and AIDS; first to declare publicly that Gallo's HTLV-3B and Institut Pasteur's LAV had come from the same patient.

DAVID KLATZMANN: French virologist; first to show that the AIDS virus infects T-4 cells, first to identify CD-4 receptor as HIV portal on T-4 cells; established highly productive clone of CEM cell line used for commercial growth of LAV.

V. S. KALYANARAMAN: Virologist in Gallo's laboratory who discovered HTLV-2.

MICHAEL KOCH: Swedish physician who angered Reagan administration with his book questioning aspects of Gallo's research on AIDS.

CHRISTOPHE LAILLER: French student from whom Luc Montagnier isolated the Pasteur's third AIDS virus, LAV_{Lai}.

JACQUES LEIBOWITCH: Paris physician convinced that HTLV-1 was the cause of AIDS; provided Robert Gallo with blood samples from HTLV-1-infected AIDS patients, including Claude Chardon, contributing to Gallo's misperception that AIDS was caused by a close relative of HTLV-1.

JAY LEVY: Virologist at University of California, San Francisco; discoverer of ARV-2, first AIDS virus isolated in the United States.

ERIC LOISEAU: French hemophiliac infected with LAV via clotting factor transfusions; source of second Pasteur AIDS virus isolate LAV_{LOI}.

PAUL LUCIW: Molecular biologist at University of California, Davis; headed team that produced DNA sequence and gene map of Jay Levy's ARV-2, which proved significantly different from the Institut Pasteur's LAV and Robert Gallo's HTLV-3.

JOHN MADDOX: Editor, *Nature* magazine; longtime Gallo supporter, later criticized Gallo for seeking "to diminish the discovery of the virus by Luc Montagnier."

MALCOLM MARTIN: NIH lab chief; first to identify genetic signature shared by Gallo and French AIDS viruses suggesting they had come from the same patient.

JAMES MASON: CDC director and, later, assistant HHS secretary; nearly lost his job after acknowledging to the *New York Times* that the Institut Pasteur had found the cause of AIDS.

IRA MILLSTEIN: Managing partner of the New York City law firm Weil, Gotshal & Manges; represented Institut Pasteur in negotiations resulting in the 1987 settlement with HHS and second settlement in 1994.

ISAO MIYOSHI: Japanese researcher who was first to grow HTLV-1 in a continuous culture.

LUC MONTAGNIER: Institut Pasteur's chief of viral oncology; with Françoise Barré and Jean-Claude Chermann, codiscoverer of the AIDS virus.

DORIS MORGAN: Cell tissue culture expert in Gallo's lab; discoverer of T-Cell Growth Factor, later renamed interleukin-2.

JAMES MULLINS: Virologist at Harvard School of Public Health; discredited purported discoveries by his department chairman, Max Essex, of African green monkey and second AIDS virus HTLV-4.

GERALD MYERS: Scientist at Los Alamos National Laboratory, New Mexico; based on his genetic analysis of HTLV-3 and LAV, warned NIH that Gallo's story about the origin of HTLV-3B constituted a "double fraud."

NCI: U.S. National Cancer Institute, Bethesda, Maryland; site of Robert Gallo's Laboratory of Tumor Cell Biology.

PETER NEWMARK: Deputy editor, *Nature* magazine; regretted his decision not to publish the Institut Pasteur's DNA sequence of LAV.

NIAID: U.S. National Institute of Allergy and Infectious Diseases, Bethesda, Maryland; site of Malcolm Martin's laboratory.

NIH: U.S. National Institutes of Health, Bethesda, Maryland.

ROBERT NOWINSKI: President of Seattle-based Genetic Systems, Inc., which attempted to market Institut Pasteur HIV antibody blood test in the United States.

ROB ODLE: New York attorney with Weil, Gotshal; with Michael Epstein, represented Institut Pasteur during 1994 settlement.

JOSEPH ONEK: Washington, D.C. attorney; represented Robert Gallo during investigations by OSI, OPRR and ORI.

OPRR: Office of Protection from Research Risks; NIH agency charged with ensuring safety of human subjects in experiments by NIH-funded scientists.

ORI: Office of Research Integrity; successor to Office of Scientific Integrity as federal agency responsible for investigating possible scientific misconduct.

OSI: Office of Scientific Integrity; first NIH agency given responsibility for investigating possible scientific misconduct by government-funded researchers; later supplanted by Office of Research Integrity.

BERNARD POIESZ: Postdoc in Gallo's lab; with Frank Ruscetti, codiscoverer of the first human retrovirus HTLV-1.

MIKULAS POPOVIC: Czech virologist working in Robert Gallo's lab; finding of scientific misconduct for alleged falsifications in his landmark *Science* article was overturned on appeal.

WILLIAM RAUB: Acting Director, NIH, who initiated OSI investigation of Gallo and Popovic.

BETSY READ: Mikulas Popovic's principal technician; first to successfully infect continuous T-cell lines with the French AIDS virus LAV.

ERSELL RICHARDSON: Mikulas Popovic's technician; first to recognize that cells from Claude Chardon were infected with HTLV-1.

RONALD ROBERTSON: HHS General Counsel during negotiations leading to the 1987 settlement with the Institut Pasteur; succeeded by Mike Astrue.

CHARLIE ROBINSON: Leukemia patient in whose T-cells Bernard Poiesz and Frank Ruscetti discovered HTLV-1.

FRANK RUSCETTI: Virologist in Gallo's lab; with Bernard Poiesz, codiscoverer of the first human retrovirus HTLV-1.

SYED Z. SALAHUDDIN: Virologist in Gallo's laboratory and codiscoverer of HHV-6; first to raise questions about the source of human T-cell line Gallo and Popovic called "HT" but which proved to be Adi Gazdar's HUT-78.

PREM SARIN: Deputy chief of Gallo's lab who conducted assays for reverse transcriptase which initially misled Mikulas Popovic into concluding that LAV was not the cause of AIDS; later found guilty of embezzling federal funds.

M. G. SARNGADHARAN: Protein chemist employed by Litton Bionetics under contract to Gallo lab; developed the American version of the AIDS blood antibody test using what later proved to be the French virus LAV.

PRISCILLA SCHAFFER: Professor of Medicine, Harvard University; as one of three "outside experts" recruited to participate in OSI investigation of Robert Gallo and Mikulas Popovic, favored finding both Gallo and Popovic guilty of scientific misconduct.

MAXIME SCHWARTZ: Succeeded Raymond Dedonder as director of Institut Pasteur; presided over 1994 settlement in which NIH finally acknowledged that Gallo's HTLV-3B was LAV and ceded $6 million in future blood test royalties to the French.

PETER STOCKTON: Chief investigator for John Dingell's Subcommittee on Oversight and Investigations.

JAMES SWIRE: Attorney with New York law firm of Townley & Updike; chief litigator for Institut Pasteur during first dispute.

HOWARD TEMIN: Nobel Laureate from the University of Wisconsin; codiscoverer, with David Baltimore, of reverse transcriptase.

GEORGE TODARO: NCI cancer virologist; led effort to show that Gallo's purported human cancer virus HL-23 was a monkey-virus contamination; later, as scientific director of Genetic Systems, attempted to market rival Institut Pasteur HIV antibody blood test in the United States.

HAROLD VARMUS: Replaced Bernadine Healy as director of NIH; presided over 1994 settlement with Institut Pasteur, in which NIH acknowledged that Gallo's HTLV-3B was actually Pasteur's LAV_{Lai}.

SIMON WAIN-HOBSON: Molecular biologist at Institut Pasteur; headed team that produced the first DNA sequence and gene map of the AIDS virus.

JAMES WATSON: Codiscoverer, with Francis Crick, of the DNA Double Helix; Nobel Laureate and director, Cold Spring Harbor Laboratory.

ROBIN WEISS: Scientific director, Chester Beatty Laboratories, London, who isolated HL-23V, putative first human cancer virus which proved to be a monkey virus contaminant; later isolated AIDS virus CBL-1 which proved to be contaminant of Pasteur's LAV.

ROBERT WINDOM: Succeeded James Mason as assistant HHS secretary; acknowledged in 1988 that CDC-led blood test comparisons four years earlier had established LAV as the cause of AIDS.

FLOSSIE WONG-STAAL: Gallo's chief molecular biologist; first to determine definitively that Gallo's HTLV-3B and Pasteur's LAV were genetically indistinguishable, though her results were never published.

JAMES WYNGAARDEN: NIH director during 1987 settlement with Institut Pasteur.

DANIEL ZAGURY: University of Paris virologist and Gallo's closest collaborator in France; sanctioned by NIH for unauthorized testing of putative AIDS vaccine in African children and failing to report vaccine-related deaths of adult AIDS patients in Paris.

THOMAS ZUCK: Army Colonel in charge of FDA monitoring of AIDS blood antibody test; critic of efforts by Abbott Laboratories to resolve problems with false positives and negatives produced by company's AIDS test.

GLOSSARY

ADENINE: Main component of one of the four nucleotides from which DNA and RNA are formed, usually abbreviated as the letter "A."

ADULT T-CELL LEUKEMIA: A rare blood-cell cancer in which malignant T-lymphocytes transformed by the human retrovirus HTLV-1 proliferate out of control. ATL is prevalent in southwestern Japan, and to a much lesser degree in Africa and parts of the Caribbean, but is virtually unknown in the rest of the world.

AMINO ACIDS: Organic compounds from which proteins are made. There are twenty known amino acids which have their own three-letter DNA code, known as a codon. For example, the code for the amino acid leucine is the nucleotide string C-T-C. Because there are sixty-four possible arrangements of three nucleotides, many amino acids are designated by more than one codon. DNA is transcribed into "messenger RNA." Through the intervention of "transfer RNA," the appropriate amino acids are assembled and coupled together, producing a protein. There are eight amino acids (valine, leucine, phenylalanine, tryptophan, lysine, isoleucine, methionine, and threonine), which cannot be synthesized by humans and must be obtained from nutritional sources.

ANTIBODY: A protein synthesized by the immune system in response to an invasion by foreign molecules, or antigens, such as viruses. The antibody is specifically "designed" by the immune system to attach itself to the antigen that stimulated the immune system, forming an antigen-antibody complex, and to neutralize the invader. The resulting combination is called an antigen-antibody complex. Antibodies remain present long after the antigen which gave rise to them has disappeared, thereby protecting the host against a future infection. Vaccines induce the artificial formation of protective antibodies by provoking the immune system with non-lethal amounts of viruses or other antigens.

ANTIGEN: Any foreign substance, often a protein, which is capable of stimulating the production of antibodies.

ANTIGEN-ANTIBODY COMPLEX: The structure formed when an antibody adheres to the antigen it has been designed by the immune system to neutralize.

ANTI-INTERFERON: An antibody produced by inoculating a goat, sheep or other animal with interferon, and which neutralizes interferon's natural ability to interfere with virus production. In laboratory experiments, anti-interferon enhances the growth and cultivation of viruses.

ANTISERUM: Blood serum known to contain antibodies to a particular antigen.

ARENAVIRUS: RNA viruses naturally found in rodents and occasionally in humans, and which bear a vague resemblance to retroviruses. The virus that causes Lassa fever is an Arenavirus.

ARV: Aids-Related Virus, Jay Levy's name for the AIDS virus HIV.

ATL: See *Adult T-Cell Leukemia.*

BACTERIA: A single-celled organism, neither animal nor plant, that represents the simplest form of life. Bacteria exist in large numbers; an ounce of soil may contain several hundred million. Some bacteria are helpful, aiding in the breakdown of food to its nutritive elements. Others cause such serious diseases as tuberculosis, diphtheria, typhoid and pneumonia. Bacterial diseases are usually treatable with antibiotics. Because they reproduce very rapidly, certain strains of bacteria, such as *E. coli,* are used as vehicles for DNA cloning.

B-CELL LINE: A collection of B-lymphocytes, or B-cells, that has been transformed into continuously replicating cells, sometimes by exposure to the Epstein-Barr Virus, as was done by Luc Montagnier in creating the continuous B-cell line FR-8.

B-CELL: See *B-lymphocyte.*

B-LYMPHOCYTE: A white blood cell, a principal component of the immune system, also known as a B-cell. The B-lymphocyte originates in the bone marrow — hence the designation "B"— and plays an integral role in the production of antibodies by the immune system. More than one million distinct B-lymphocytes may be produced in each individual, enabling the immune system's defense against over a million different antigens. So-called memory B-cells often remain in the wake of an infection, to confer protection against a future encounter with the same antigen. The concept of persistent immunity is integral to the success of vaccines.

cDNA: See *complimentary DNA.*

CELL CULTURE: Also known as tissue culture; a method of keeping animal, plant or human cells alive in the laboratory after they have been separated from their host organism. The cells are incubated at body temperature in a flask or test tube to which nutrients, such as fetal calf serum, and other life-supporting chemicals have been added. A cell culture provides a vehicle for the reproduction of viruses which infect the particular type of cell being cultured. Thus, a culture of T-4 lymphocytes is necessary for the growth of the AIDS virus HIV.

CELL LINE: A collection of cells of a particular class, usually from the same source.

CELL: The basic building block of all living organisms. The human body contains about a trillion cells, of which there are at least 200 distinct types. In every case, the cell contains a complete copy of the host organism's DNA genome, in the form of chromosomes. Cells reproduce by dividing, a process that begins with the unwinding of the DNA helix to form another, identical helix which becomes the genome of the new cell. Some cells, like the epithelial cells that line the intestines, renew themselves frequently through reproduction. Others, such as endothelial cells of which blood vessels are formed, reproduce only when new vessels are required, such as in the healing of a wound.

CEM: A continuous T-cell line established in 1966 at Children's Hospital in Boston from T-4 lymphocytes of a four-year-old girl with leukemia. It was the C-30 clone of this cell line from David Klatzmann in which the Institut Pasteur grew LAV for the production of its HIV ELISA.

CHROMOSOME: A strand of DNA containing the genetic code for many genes. Chromosomes occur in the form of identical pairs. The fruit fly Drosophila has four pairs of chromosomes. Each human cell contains a full complement of twenty-three chromosome pairs, designated 1 through 22, which collectively hold the genetic code for around 30,000 genes, plus a pair of sex chromosomes designated "X" or "Y" that determine the gender of an offspring.

CLONE: An identical copy, in microbiology usually referring to a genetic copy of DNA, but also applied to a colony of identical cells or antibodies.

CLONING: The process of multiplying fragments of DNA hundreds of thousands of times, usually to facilitate the search for a particular gene or genes. The DNA of interest is fragmented with restriction enzymes, and the fragments inserted into a phage or plasmid, which integrate the fragment into the DNA of bacteria, often *E. coli*. As the bacteria reproduce, they reproduce — clone — the inserted DNA along with their own.

CODON: A group of three sequential nucleotides found initially in DNA and subsequently transcribed into messenger RNA. A "start codon," ATG (adenine, thymine, guanine) signals the beginning of a coding region for a gene. A "stop codon"— TAA, TGA or TAG — marks the end of a gene. In between, each successive codon dictates which amino acid is to be added to the protein chain.

COMPLEMENTARY DNA: Also known as cDNA. A double helical DNA copy of an RNA molecule.

CONTINUOUS CELL LINE: Also called a permanent cell line. A population of cells which has acquired the ability to continue reproducing in a laboratory culture, and thus provide an unending source of identical cells. Such continuous cell lines are particularly useful for culturing cell-killing viruses, because they provide the virus with an unending source of fresh cells to infect. The continuous T-cell lines HUT-102, HUT-78, and CEM were established from the blood cells of patients with T-cell leukemia. In the case of HUT-102 the cells had been transformed, or rendered malignant, by the Adult T-Cell Leukemia Virus HTLV-1. However, not all continuous cell lines consist of transformed cells; for example, there is no evidence of transforming virus in HUT-78 cells, which were taken from a patient with a nonviral form of leukemia. Nonleukemic cells can also be artificially stimulated to reproduce by the addition of various chemical or biological stimulants.

CORE PROTEIN: The protein that forms the core of a virus particle, or virion. The core protein of the AIDS virus is referred to as p24, even though its molecular weight is nearer to 25,000 daltons.

CYTOSINE: Main constituent of one of the four nucleotides of which DNA and RNA are formed, abbreviated as the letter "C."

DALTON: A measure of molecular weight that is used to sort and identify proteins by size. The envelope protein of HIV, gp120, has a molecular weight of 120,000 daltons.

DNA CLONE: DNA clones are produced when a piece of DNA is inserted into the DNA of a bacterial plasmid or phage, which reproduce the inserted DNA as they multiply.

DNA PROBE: A piece of radioactively labeled DNA used in hybridization experiments with other strands of DNA.

DNA SEQUENCE: See *nucleotide sequence*.

DNA VIRUS: A virus whose genome is composed of DNA. Pox viruses, herpesviruses and adenoviruses are DNA viruses.

DNA: Deoxyribonucleic acid, the genetic material which contains the "life code" for all living things. The DNA genome is composed of a very long string of four very small molecules called nucleotides, which contain the nucleosides adenine, cytosine, guanine and thymine. The order in which the nucleotides are arranged determines where genes begin and end, and the structure and function of the proteins for which those genes hold the genetic code. In most organisms except for some viruses, DNA is first transcribed into RNA, which is then used as a template for the construction of proteins.

DOUBLE HELIX: The spiral structure formed by two strands of DNA (primary and complementary) that have paired together. The nucleotide sequences of the two strands are mirror images of one another. When a cell reproduces itself, the strands unwind, each serving as a template for the construction of a new complementary strand. In this way one Double Helix becomes two, with the second helix forming the genome of the new cell.

ELISA: Enzyme-Linked Immunosorbent Assay, a method for detecting the presence of antibodies to a particular antigen, often a virus or viral protein, in blood serum. The antigen in question is used as a "lure" for virus-specific antibodies. For example, the presence of antibodies reactive with HIV indicates an infection with HIV. When blood is exposed to the proteins of the virus, the combination of the viral proteins and their specific antibodies causes a color change that signals the presence of viral antibodies in the blood.

ENVELOPE: The protective fatty membrane that forms the outer shell of many viruses, including the AIDS virus HIV. The HIV envelope is overlaid with a long envelope protein.

ENVELOPE PROTEIN: Known as gp120 in the AIDS virus, so named because it is a glycoprotein with a molecular weight of 120,000 daltons.

ENZYME: A protein, such as reverse transcriptase, that is capable of catalyzing a biochemical reaction. Almost all enzymes are proteins.

EQUINE INFECTIOUS ANEMIA VIRUS: A lentivirus which causes disease in horses; one of the first animal retroviruses to have been discovered.

FACTOR VIII: A clotting substance given to hemophiliacs to enhance the coagulation of their blood.

FELINE LEUKEMIA VIRUS: A retrovirus specific to cats which causes both feline leukemia and immuno-suppression.

GENE MAP: An overlay of a DNA sequence showing the reading frames, or genes, that contain the codons for the manufacture of particular proteins.

GENE: A region of DNA which contains the genetic code for a particular protein and instructions for its transcription. In living things, the primary unit of inheritance. The human genome is believed to contain something like 30,000 genes.

GENETIC CODE: A set of instructions, written in *RNA*, which directs the assembly of proteins.

GENETIC SEQUENCE: See *nucleotide sequence.*

GLYCOPROTEIN: A protein with an attached carbohydrate molecule. Antibodies and hormones are often glycoproteins. The envelope protein of the AIDS virus, gp120, and the transmembrane protein, gp41, are glycoproteins.

GP120: The envelope protein which occurs on the surface of the AIDS virus HIV; a glycoprotein, named gp120 because it has a molecular weight of 120,000 daltons; the largest of the AIDS virus's proteins. Both gp120 and gp41 are the product of a larger protein, gp160.

GP41: The transmembrane protein of the AIDS virus HIV, a glycoprotein, which connects the viral envelope to the viral core. So named because it has a molecular weight of 41,000 daltons, which places it between the virus's core protein and envelope protein in size.

GUANINE: Main component of one of the four nucleotides of which DNA and RNA are formed, abbreviated as the letter "G."

H-9: A continuous human T-cell line established by Mikulas Popovic from a single cell derived from the HUT-78 cell line.

HERPESVIRUS: A class of DNA viruses responsible for herpes simplex and herpes zoster, or chickenpox.

HIV: A retrovirus, the Human Immunodeficiency Virus, that causes AIDS. HIV, a member of the lentivirus family, was originally called LAV by its discoverers at the Pasteur Institute of Paris, and later HTLV-3 by Robert Gallo. The HIV genome consists of some 9,200 nucleotides. By contrast, the human genome has three *billion* nucleotides.

HTLV: Human T-cell Leukemia Virus, of which two distinct strains have been isolated, HTLV-1 and HTLV-2.

HTLV-1: The first known human retrovirus, isolated in 1980 by Bernard Poiesz and Frank Ruscetti.

HTLV-2: The second known human retrovirus, isolated in 1981 by V. S. Kalyanaraman.

HTLV-3: Robert Gallo's name for the AIDS virus; later rejected by scientific colleagues on grounds that the virus was not a member of the "HTLV family."

HTLV-3B: Robert Gallo's prototype AIDS virus, which Mikulas Popovic claimed to have isolated in late 1983 from the pooled cells of ten AIDS patients. HTLV-3B formed the basis of the Gallo laboratory's AIDS research and was used by Abbott Laboratories and other American companies to manufacture the commercial ELISA for AIDS.

HTLV-3$_{RF}$: AIDS virus isolated in December 1983 in Gallo's laboratory by Betsy Read from the T-cells of a Haitian immigrant, Roland Ferdinand, who died of AIDS in Philadelphia.

HTLV-MA: HTLV Membrane Antigen. According to Max Essex, a protein on the surface of HTLV-infected T-cells which served as a "marker" for such infections. Essex assumed, incorrectly, that patients with antibodies to HTLV-MA were infected with HTLV-1. Essex's test for HTLV-MA antibodies proved to be highly unspecific and produced numerous false positive reactions.

HUT-102: A continuous T-cell line established by Adi Gazdar from the transformed cells of Charles Robinson, a patient with T-cell lymphoma. It was from HUT-102 that Bernard Poiesz and Frank Ruscetti first isolated HTLV-1.

HUT-78: A continuous T-cell line established by Adi Gazdar from a patient, L.G., with T-cell lymphoma. Unlike HUT-102, HUT-78 does not contain HTLV-1 or any other transforming virus.

HYBRIDIZATION: Use of a single strand of DNA (or RNA) as a probe to seek out a complementary strand of DNA (or RNA). To permit later detection the probe is labeled in some way, often with a radioactive isotope. The DNA to be analyzed is digested with restriction enzymes separated through a gel by an electric current, then transferred to a filter paper via the Southern Blot. When the filter is placed in a solution with a second strand of DNA, it is possible to measure the degree to which the two strands share similar genetic sequences. The greater the annealing between the two strands, the greater the presumed similarity between the their nucleotide sequences. However, the degree of annealing depends on the conditions under which the experiment is conducted, such as temperature and salinity. Conditions which are too stringent, or not stringent enough, may give misleading results.

HYPERIMMUNE ANTISERUM: Blood serum, usually from a rabbit or other animal which has been inoculated many times with a particular virus or other antigen. The resulting serum, which *contains antibodies* specific to the antigen in question, can be used to test for the presence of that antigen in cell cultures.

IMMUNOFLUORESCENCE ASSAY: A method of testing for antibodies in which an antigen tagged with a fluorescent molecule emits a faint greenish glow upon formation of an antigen-antibody complex.

INTERFERON: A protein produced by the immune system of a human or animal infected by a virus, and which interferes with the ability of the virus to multiply.

INTERLEUKIN-2: A lymphokine secreted by T-4 lymphocytes and discovered by Doris Morgan in 1975. Originally called T-Cell Growth Factor, IL-2 stimulates the growth and production of T-lymphocytes.

ISOLATE: A virologist's term for a virus which has been isolated from an infected cell by transmission to a previously uninfected cell.

JULY LAV: The vial of supernatant containing the LAV_{Bru} virus from Frédéric Brugière, delivered by Luc Montagnier to Robert Gallo's house in July of 1983.

LAV: Lymphadenopathy-Associated Virus, the name first given to the AIDS virus by its discoverers at the Institut Pasteur of Paris.

LAV_{Bru}: AIDS virus strain isolated at the Institut Pasteur of Paris from the patient Frédéric Brugière. Françoise Barré's LAV_{Bru} culture was accidentally contaminated by LAV_{Lai}.

LAV_{Lai}: AIDS virus strain isolated at the Institut Pasteur of Paris from the patient Christophe Lailler. Contaminated Françoise Barré's LAV_{Bru} culture.

LENTIVIRUS: A subfamily of retroviruses, of which the AIDS virus is the only known human virus, so named because they take years to cause disease. Lentiviruses don't cause cancer, but rather immuno-suppressive and central nervous system diseases. Animal lentiviruses include Visna virus, which infects sheep, Equine Infectious Anemia Virus, which infects horses, and caprine arthritis-encephalitis virus, which infects goats.

LEUKEMIA: A cancer of the blood, in which a particular class of blood cell begins to multiply without restraint. The two general classes of leukemias are lymphoid leukemia and myeloid leukemia.

LYMPHADENOPATHY SYNDROME: Precursor of AIDS, and a marker for infection with HIV, in which lymph nodes remain enlarged for a period of weeks or months as the immune system makes its initial response to infection with the virus. Frequently associated with flu-like symptoms such as muscle pain, sore throat, and headache.

LYMPHOCYTE: A class of white blood cells that includes B-cells and T-cells, also known as B-lymphocytes and T-lymphocytes. Lymphocytes are the primary component of the immune system. B-lymphocytes, or B-cells, foster the production of protective antibodies, while T-lymphocytes direct the production of cells, such as macrophages, which attack the invading antigen. An elevated "white blood count" is evidence of the presence of an infection.

LYMPHOID LEUKEMIA: Also known as lymphoma; a cancer of the blood in which lymphocytes, including B-lymphocytes and T-lymphocytes, multiply without restraint.

LYMPHOMA: Blood-cell cancer involving T- or B-lymphocytes.

M2T-/B: AIDS virus preparation which Françoise Barré believed had been made from LAV_{Bru} isolated from Frédéric Brugière, but which actually contained LAV_{Lai} isolated from Christophe Lailler.

MESSENGER RNA: Abbreviated as mRNA, messenger RNA is a genetic copy of a gene in the *DNA* genome used as a template for the synthesis of proteins via ribosomes.

MONOCLONAL ANTIBODY: An antibody produced artificially, in the laboratory, often by inoculating a rabbit or mouse with a specific *virus* or other *antigen*. A single antibody-secreting B-lymphocyte is removed from the animal's spleen and fused with a myeloma cell capable of continuous reproduction. The resulting hybrid cell is grown in culture, producing a large number of identical B-cell clones capable of producing identical antibodies that react specifically with the target antigen.

MOV: Mikulas Popovic's name for the AIDS virus isolate used in the Gallo lab's principal experiments underlying Gallo's announcement that he had discovered the cause of AIDS and developed a blood antibody test for the virus; MOV was eventually shown to be LAV_{Lai} discovered at Institut Pasteur.

MYCOSIS FUNGOIDES: Skin cancer involving malignant T-lymphocytes.

MYELOID CELLS: A class of white blood cells which give rise to macrophages and polynuclear cells. Myeloid leukemia, also known as myeloma, is a cancer of the blood in which myeloid cells multiply without restraint.

NUCLEOTIDE SEQUENCE: The sequential order, reading from left to right, or "upstream to downstream," of the nucleotides adenine, guanine, cytosine and thymine, that form *DNA*, for example: C-A-T-T-G-C-G-A. DNA is "read" in groups of three nucleotides, called *codons*. It is the order in which the nucleotides appear that make a particular piece of DNA unique, much like a sentence in a book.

NUCLEOSIDE: An organic molecule, the basic building block from which DNA and RNA are constructed. There are only five nucleosides: adenine, guanine, cytosine, thymine, and uracil (which replaces thymine in *RNA*). Nucleosides are the main constituent of nucleotides.

ONCOGENE: A gene, often but not always, carried by an oncovirus, which can transform a normal cell into a malignant cell following integration into the cell's own DNA.

ONCOVIRUS: A retrovirus which inserts an oncogene into the DNA of the infected cell. The human oncoviruses HTLV-1 and HTLV-2 have been associated with Adult T-Cell Leukemia and Hairy T-Cell Leukemia, respectively. The Human Papilloma Virus has been associated with some forms of cervical cancer, and the Epstein-Barr virus with Burkitt's Lymphoma in some African children. There are a number of known animal oncoviruses, including Rous Sarcoma Virus, Rauscher Murine Leukemia Virus and Feline Leukemia Virus.

P24: The core protein of the AIDS virus HIV.

PCR: See *polymerase chain reaction.*

PERMANENT CELL LINE: See *continuous cell line.*

PHAGE: A bacteria-infecting virus into which foreign DNA can be inserted as an intermediate step in the process of DNA cloning.

PLASMID: A circle of DNA found in many bacteria which is not part of the bacteria's principal chromosome and which can reproduce independently of that chromosome. Plasmids carry genes which confer resistance to antibiotics. When foreign DNA is inserted into a plasmid, and the plasmid introduced into a strain of plasmid-free bacteria, the growth of the bacteria produces many copies of the inserted DNA.

POLYMERASE CHAIN REACTION: A powerful technique which permits the rapid production of many copies of a particular strand of DNA, making possible the analysis of DNA fragments in samples which have too little DNA to permit other types of analysis, such as a drop of blood at a crime scene. PCR can also identify disease-causing viruses and bacteria with great precision. Essentially, two short strands of DNA, called primers, are used to "fish out" a longer, often much longer, strand of DNA which has nucleotide sequences complementary to both primers at or near its ends. In just a few minutes, many new copies of the longer strand are assembled from free nucleotides. Repeating the procedure doubles the number of copies; it only requires thirty repetitions to amplify the target DNA one billion times.

PROTEIN: A large and intricately folded string of hundreds or thousands of amino acids. Countless proteins of differing sizes, constructions and functions, often joined together in polypeptide chains, are present in all living things.

PROVIRAL DNA: Retroviral *DNA* that has been inserted into the DNA of an infected cell.

RAUSCHER MURINE LEUKEMIA VIRUS: A mouse leukemia retrovirus, in which David Baltimore discovered reverse transcriptase.

READING FRAME: A region of DNA which contains the genetic code, expressed in *codons,* for a particular protein. The beginning and end of the reading frame, which demarcates a gene, are marked by "start" and "stop" codons.

RESTRICTION ENZYME: An enzyme, the product of bacteria, which cleaves a strand of DNA at a particular place in the nucleotide sequence. The normal function of restriction enzymes is to protect against the invasion of foreign DNA. The discovery that restriction enzymes make it possible to cut a complete DNA genome at specific places into fragments of a specific length virtually revolutionized molecular biology. For example, the restriction enzyme *Hind*III always cleaves DNA at the nucleotides A-A-G-C-T-T. *Eco*RI (pronounced "Ecore one"), a product of the bacterium *E. coli,* devours the nucleotides G-A-A-T-T-C. *Bgl*II ("Beagle two"), from the bacterium *Bacillus globigii,* digests only A-G-A-T-C-T. Identical strands of DNA will have restriction sites in exactly the same places, while similar strands will share some sites but not others. Dissimilar strands will have few or even no sites in common. Once the DNA of a particular virus has been "digested," the DNA fragments can be arranged to form a genetic "fingerprint" unique to that virus. This process is often useful in criminal investigations. Restriction mapping was used to prove that bloodstains at the scene of Nicole Simpson's death had come from O. J. Simpson. The restriction enzyme *Hae*III was used by the F.B.I. laboratory in reaching the conclusion that DNA extracted from a semen stain on a navy blue dress once worn by Monica Lewinsky had come from President Clinton.

RESTRICTION MAP: An illustration of the location of various restriction sites at which a particular DNA sequence has been, or would be, cut by a number of different restriction enzymes.

RESTRICTION SITE: The short sequence of nucleotides known to be recognized by a particular restriction enzyme. For example, the DNA sequence A-A-G-C-T-T is referred to as a *Hind*III restriction site, because *Hind*III cleaves that sequence into "A" and "A-G-C-T-T."

RETROVIRUS: An RNA virus consisting of several proteins surrounded by an envelope. At the core are two RNA genomes which include a gene that contains the genetic code for the enzyme reverse transcriptase. After infecting a cell, retroviruses employ reverse transcriptase to copy their RNA into proviral DNA, which is integrated into the DNA at the core of the cell. Cellular enzymes then recopy the proviral DNA into RNA, from which proteins are made and subsequently assembled into new retrovirus particles.

REVERSE TRANSCRIPTASE: The enzyme retroviruses employ to copy their RNA genomes into double stranded DNA. Discovered jointly by Howard Temin and David Baltimore. So named because it reverses the usual transcription process, in which DNA is translated into RNA. The viral DNA is then incorporated into the DNA genome of the infected cell — in the case of HIV, usually a T-4 lymphocyte — where it manufactures new virus particles which escape the cell and go in search of other T-lymphocytes to infect. The detection of reverse transcriptase in a cell culture is evidence of the presence of a replicating retrovirus.

RNA VIRUS: A virus whose genome is made of RNA. All retroviruses, including the AIDS virus HIV, are RNA viruses, but not all RNA viruses are retroviruses. For example, the virus which causes poliomyelitis is an RNA virus, but it is not a retrovirus.

RNA: *Ribonucleic acid.* Much like DNA, except that the nucleotide containing the nucleoside thymine is replaced by uracil. There are various forms of RNA, including transfer RNA and messenger RNA, which play a central role in translating DNA into proteins by assembling chains of amino acids according to the codon instructions contained in the DNA.

ROUS SARCOMA VIRUS: A retrovirus, the first known animal oncovirus, specific to chickens, discovered in 1910 by Peyton Rous. Reverse transcriptase was discovered by Howard Temin in the Rous Sarcoma Virus.

RT: See *reverse transcriptase.*

SEPTEMBER LAV: The preparation of LAV shipped to Gallo's lab by Françoise Barré in September of 1983. Although Barré believed the virus in question had come from Frédéric Brugière, subsequent analysis showed it had come from another patient, Christophe Lailler.

SERUM: Blood plasma from which the blood clotting factors, such as *Factor VIII,* have been removed.

SEZARY'S SYNDROME: A T-cell cancer analogous to mycosis fungoides.

SOUTHERN BLOT: A technique, invented by Oxford University's Edward Southern, in which different-sized fragments of DNA that have been cut by restriction enzymes are sorted by size through a slab of gel by the application of an electrical current. Because DNA has a negative charge, the DNA will be attracted by the positive electrode at one end of the gel. Smaller fragments move more quickly than larger ones, and so end up closer to the positive terminus. The DNA fragments, separated by size, are blotted from the surface of the gel with a nitrocellulose filter paper, then identified with radioactively labeled DNA probes which hybridize to the DNA fragments of interest. The resulting fragment pattern is often referred to as a DNA fingerprint.

SUPERNATANT: The fluid produced when a test tube containing virus-infected cells is placed in a centrifuge. The supernatant, which contains virus but no cells, is drawn off as a liquid after the cells have collected at the bottom of the tube.

T-4 CELL: Also called T-4 lymphocyte, the T-4 cell is a principal target of infection by the AIDS virus. T-4-lymphocytes, produced in the presence of an antigen, activate antibody production by B-lymphocytes. The gradual loss of T-4 lymphocytes in patients with AIDS hampers their immune response and leads to a variety of infections.

T-8 CELL: Also called T-8 lymphocyte, or "killer T-cell," the T-8 cell plays a key role in attacking and neutralizing infected cells.

T-CELL GROWTH FACTOR: See *Interleukin-2*.

T-CELL LINE: A culture of continuously replicating T-cells taken from a patient with leukemia, or transformed in the laboratory by exposure to a leukemia-causing virus.

T-CELL LYMPHOMA: A cancer of the blood in which T-lymphocytes have become malignant.

T-CELL: See *T-lymphocyte*.

THYMINE: Main component of one of the four nucleotides of which *DNA* is formed, abbreviated as the letter "T." Thymine is replaced by *uracil* in *RNA*.

TISSUE CULTURE: See *cell culture*.

T-LYMPHOCYTE: A white blood cell, an essential component of the immune system, which originates in the bone marrow but completes its development in the thymus — hence, the designation "T." With *B-lymphocytes,* T-lymphocytes play a key role in determining the immune response. When presented with an antigen, T-lymphocytes divide and produce new "killer T-cells" specifically intended to seek out and neutralize the target antigen, as well as *T-4 lymphocytes* which activate B-lymphocytes, and *T-8 lymphocytes* which turn off B-lymphocyte activation once the antigen has been disposed of.

TRANSFER RNA: A form of *RNA* whose function is to assemble *amino acids* into *proteins* according to the sequence dictated by *messenger RNA*.

TRANSFORMATION: The inducement of normal cells, sometimes by a virus, to become malignant. Normal B-cells can be transformed into malignant B-cells via exposure to the Epstein-Barr Virus. Normal T-cells can be transformed into malignant T-cells via infection with HTLV-1.

URACIL: One of the four nucleosides of which *RNA* is formed, abbreviated as the letter "U." Uracil is replaced by *thymine* in *DNA*.

VACCINE: A preparation containing *antigens,* generally from a *virus* that has been killed, weakened or genetically altered, and is incapable of causing disease. The presence of the viral antigens provokes an immune response that results in the production of viral antibodies, which confer long-lasting immunity against a future infection with the particular virus.

VIRION: A mature virus particle.

VIRUS: A submicroscopic infectious agent consisting of structural and functional proteins and a core nucleus that contains the genome of the virus, written in either DNA or RNA. Virally induced diseases include the common cold, influenza, polio, smallpox, measles and yellow fever. In the more complex animal viruses, and in the AIDS virus HIV, the genome is protected by a protein envelope. The virus must infect a host cell before the viral genes can be transcribed and new viral proteins assembled.

VISNA VIRUS: An *RNA virus,* which is both a retrovirus and lentivirus, specific to sheep.

WESTERN BLOT: A relative of the Southern Blot, in which proteins (rather than fragments of DNA) are placed at one end of a thin slab of gel and pulled through the gel by an electric current. Because smaller proteins move faster than larger ones the proteins are eventually separated by size and weight, then blotted onto a sheet of filter paper where they can be stained or exposed to antibodies tagged with a fluorescent protein or radioactive isotope. The positions of the proteins to which the antibodies adhere, and therefore their relative sizes and weights, show up as bands of light or smudges on a piece of X-ray film. In the simplified Western Blot used for HIV testing, the proteins of the AIDS virus are laid out from largest to smallest on a strip of film, which is exposed to the blood sample to be tested. HIV antibodies in the sample will adhere to the proteins for which they are specific — anti-gp120, for example, will bind only to the HIV envelope protein gp120. Anti-p24 will bind to the core protein, p24. An enzyme is added which binds to the antibodies, followed by a chemical which changes color when it comes in contact with the protein-antibody-enzyme complex. The presence of antibodies is indicated by shaded bands on the film strip which correspond to particular HIV proteins. The presence of antibodies to three of the nine major HIV proteins is generally considered conclusive evidence of infection with HIV. Because the Western Blot uses the constituent proteins of HIV rather than the whole virus, as in the HIV ELISA, it is far less likely to give a false-positive response by reacting with non-HIV antibodies.

INDEX

Aaronson, Stu, 31, 210, 480

Abbott Laboratories
  AIDS blood tests' accuracy and, 254–55, 256, 257, 280–81
  AIDS blood tests' competition, 220, 288
  AIDS blood tests' development, 146–48, 164, 185, 186–87
  AIDS blood tests' false negatives and, 250, 251, 252–53, 255, 256, 279, 448, 528, 574–75nn. b, c
  AIDS blood tests' false positives and, 187, 189, 219, 228, 229, 249–50, 251, 255, 280, 447, 528
  AIDS blood tests' licenses, 226
  AIDS blood tests' profits and, 219
  Food and Drug Administration and, 148, 219, 229, 251–52, 255, 279–80, 281–82, 291, 447, 448–49, 528, 575n. d
  in France, 446–49
  patent royalties and, 202, 223

ABC News, 442–43, 450, 451

Ablashi, Dharam, 324-25

actinomycin B, 6

Adamson, Richard, 350-51, 352, 355, 424, 515, 532

Adenine, defined, 629

Adult T-Cell Leukemia
  cause of, 28
  defined, 629
  DNA and, 34–35, 544n. l
  HTLV and, 29, 31, 32, 34, 35, 36, 79–80, 542–43n. g

Poiesz and, 26
  retroviruses and, 29

Africa, 51, 66, 77, 99, 187, 231–33, 235, 306, 325, 406

AIDS (acquired immune deficiency syndrome)
  asymptomatic carrier state and, 117
  early cases of, 13
  epidemiology of, 163, 563–64n. j
  Gallo and, 39, 43, 44, 52, 57, 59–60, 62–63, 76, 95–97, 105–07, 548n. q
  Haitian community and, 43, 51, 62, 548n. r
  history of epidemic, 311
  history of research on, 289, 293–97
  HTLV and, 38–43, 51–54, 58–59, 61, 62–63, 66, 68–70, 72–77, 81–83, 91, 94
  HTLV-1 and, 85, 105, 122, 144, 173–74
  HTLV-3 and, 112, 130, 135, 137, 138
  Institut Pasteur and, 58, 60, 90, 101, 106–07, 153, 447
  LAV and, 65, 71, 81–82, 101, 102, 103–04, 107–08, 130, 133, 153
  Levine and, 38–39
  rise in diagnosis of, 58
  T-lymphocytes and, 50

AIDS blood test patents
  CDC blood-test data and, 322, 436
  Chicago Tribune article and, 357
  Dingell and, 430
  Gallo and, 205–08, 294, 297, 301, 309, 321, 371, 428, 429, 432–33, 456, 462–63, 506, 517, 519, 539, 557n. k, 605n. g, 610n. c

AIDS blood test patents (*cont.*)
  Hadley and, 419–20, 434, 605n. g
  Health and Human Services Department
    and, 128, 224, 237–38, 260, 284–85,
    289–90, 294–95, 309, 317, 444, 454–56,
    519, 520, 585n. d, 589n. e
  Health and Human Services/Institut Pas-
    teur 1987 settlement and, 300–303, 322,
    357, 430, 434, 435, 444, 453, 454, 455,
    456–57, 509, 511, 523, 616–17n. b
  Health and Human Services/Institut Pas-
    teur 1994 settlement and, 521–24, 525
  Institut Pasteur and, 191–93, 196–97,
    200–203, 211–12, 224, 227, 236–37, 254,
    278, 282–89, 294, 294–95, 310, 317–18,
    454, 458, 523, 582–83n. b, 589n. e
  Institut Pasteur's interference claim, 222,
    243, 244, 246, 282, 372, 517, 617n. d
  Justice Department and, 260, 283–84, 287,
    371, 419, 431, 433, 462–63, 478, 610n. c
  LAV and, 404
  Office of Scientific Integrity and, 354, 357,
    422, 430, 457
  Research Integrity Adjudication Panel and,
    502, 503–04
  royalties and, 202, 223, 249, 294, 310, 317,
    409, 435, 444, 449, 453, 454–55, 464,
    510, 511–12, 514, 517, 518, 520–23, 535
  Wain-Hobson and, 401, 402
AIDS blood tests
  blood supply and, 146, 186, 187, 446–47
  CDC and, 150, 176, 189, 284, 583n. c
  Essex and, 145
  Food and Drug Administration and, 147,
    148, 185, 186
  Gallo and, 120–21, 123, 128, 135, 140, 141,
    146, 148, 156, 164, 166, 178, 191,
    192–93, 205, 224–25, 257, 278, 283–85,
    293, 324, 333, 337, 343, 379, 381, 499,
    506, 518
  Health and Human Services Department
    and, 146–48, 189
  Heckler and, 185–87
  Institut Pasteur and, 128, 133, 137, 176,
    191–93, 196–98, 201, 207, 209, 225, 226,
    227, 230, 237, 246, 249, 284–85, 288,
    290, 343, 447–49, 472, 518, 522,
    568–69n. d
  profits from, 219
  Sarngadharan and, 128, 193, 557n. k
  Weiss and, 188–89
AIDS Discoverers' Club, 327–28
AIDS Research and Human Retroviruses, 76,
  334, 534

AIDS — Vom Molekul zur Pandemie (Koch),
  319–22
AL-721, Sarin and, 390
Albert Lasker Clinical Medical Research
  Award, 36–37, 276–77, 337, 489
Alizon, Marc, 116–17, 168, 169, 247–48, 309,
  328–29, 330, 339, 340
Allain, Jean-Pierre, 446, 447
Altman, Lawrence K., 129–31, 132, 133, 142,
  246, 430
American Cancer Society, 10
American Red Cross
  Abbott Laboratories and, 291–92
  AIDS blood tests and, 285, 448
  AIDS blood tests competition, 219–20, 249
  AIDS blood tests development and, 185,
    186
  AIDS blood tests' false negatives and, 253,
    255–56, 279, 280, 281
  AIDS blood tests' false positives and, 189,
    190, 219
  Gallo AIDS test and, 293, 294
  Genetic Systems and, 190, 226, 255,
    256–57, 280, 281, 282, 291–92
  Healy and, 527–28
  Institut Pasteur and, 290
American Tissue Type Culture, 273
American Type Culture Collection, 333, 335
Amersham Laboratories, 189
amino acids, defined, 629
And the Band Played On (HBO movie),
  489–91, 530
And the Band Played On (Shilts), 311, 489,
  587–88n. a
Anderson, Jack, 206
Angier, Natalie, 370
Anglia, Max, 265
Annals of Virology, 117
antibodies, defined, 629–30
antigen-antibody complex, defined, 630
antigens, defined, 630
anti-interferon, defined, 630
antiserum, defined, 630
Areen, Judith, 358, 359, 383
arenavirus, 98, 143, 548n. n, 630
Armand Hammer Cancer Research Award,
  177
Arthur, Larry, 120, 148
ARV (AIDS-Related Virus), 143, 157–58,
  166–67, 173, 178–79, 250, 561–62n. t,
  630
ARV-2, 236, 304, 305
Arya, Sasha, 266, 267, 277, 370, 515
Ascher, Mike, 250–55, 279

Ashwell, Gilbert, 440
Associated Press, 131–32, 422
Astrue, Michael, 431, 451–52, 453, 455, 456, 459, 510, 512
ATL. *See* Adult T-Cell Leukemia
ATLV, 31–35, 70, 75, 545n. n
AZT, 331–32, 479

bacteria, defined, 630
Baltimore, David
    AIDS blood test patents and, 290
    Dingell and, 347, 348–50, 390
    Gallo and, 31, 300, 314–15
    HTLV and, 27, 28
    Montagnier and, 300
    mouse leukemia virus and, 15, 60
    National Academy of Sciences and, 353
    Nobel Prize for physiology or medicine and, 9, 37
    Office of Research Integrity and, 529
    reverse transcriptase and, 8–9, 11, 15, 302
Baltimore Sun, 154, 375, 405, 534
Barin, Francis, 233
Barré-Sinoussi, Françoise
    AIDS and, 65
    AIDS blood test and, 192
    AIDS blood test patent and, 294, 309
    AIDS Discoverers' Club and, 327
    Brugière and, 54–55, 56, 57, 61
    Chermann and, 48, 50, 395
    Gallo and, 48, 49, 60, 61, 68, 91, 109, 139, 143–44, 155, 193, 344, 394, 397, 520, 558n. a
    Japan Prize nomination and, 159
    lab contamination and, 399–400
    LAV and, 76, 82, 85, 89, 91, 93, 152, 162, 163, 213
    Martin and, 60–61
    Montagnier and, 46, 50, 117, 328
    Nobel Prize for AIDS, rumors and, 326, 327
    Office of Research Integrity and, 495, 499–500, 613–15nn. d, e
    Office of Scientific Integrity investigation and, 408
    Popovic and, 83, 495–96, 499, 513, 525, 613–15nn. d, e
    records of, 206
    retroviruses and, 55
    reverse transcriptase and, 48, 49–50, 55
    Wain-Hobson and, 395, 397, 400, 401
    Weiss and, 531
Barr, Tony, 26
Barzach, Michèle, 249, 290–91, 318
Baxter-Travenol, 146, 147

Bazell, Robert, 479
B-cell lines
    defined, 630
    HBLV and, 324
    LAV and, 102–03, 110, 128, 157, 161, 162, 413
Becton Dickinson, 146, 147
Belk, Joanne, 260–61, 263, 338, 489
Bennett, Richard D., 462–63
Berger, Ed, 535
Bernard, Jean, 197, 198, 237, 571n. h
Berneman, Danielle, 68, 86, 202, 248–49
Berns, Kenneth, 388, 389, 410, 412, 414, 422, 435, 481, 483
Betke, Todd, 485–86
Biberfeld, Peter, 450
Bieker, Terry, 291
Biotech Research Laboratories, 146, 147, 261, 266, 267
Bishop, J. Michael, 27, 36, 36–37, 60, 489, 545–46n. q
Bivens, Lyle, 464–68, 485, 487, 494, 500, 504–05, 515, 529
BJAB, 103
Black, James, 338
Black, Paul, 11
Blattner, Bill, 480
Blayney, Doug, 39, 52, 85, 92
Bliley, Thomas, 527
Blomberg, Jonas, 337
blood supply
    AIDS blood tests and, 146, 186, 187, 219, 227, 228, 229, 252, 254, 285, 326, 446–47
    American Red Cross and, 256, 280–81, 448, 575n. e
    Food and Drug Administration and, 446
    in France, 445–46, 473
    heat-treating of blood, 445–46, 608–09n. a
    Nowinski and, 280–81
B-lymphocytes, defined, 22, 630
Bodmer, Walter, 126, 184
Bok, Derek, 309
Bolognesi, Dani, 68, 76, 180, 184, 202, 215, 299, 336, 393, 405
Boston Globe, 80, 154, 240, 311, 351, 353, 405, 537
Boutte, Otto, 292
Bowen, Otis T., 288, 290–91, 297, 301
Brandt, Ed
    AIDS vaccine and, 138
    CDC and, 128–29, 130, 151
    Gallo and, 113, 155, 163, 506
    Haddow and, 133
    Heckler and, 135

Brandt, Ed (*cont.*)
  HTLV-3 and, 110, 123, 126–27, 163, 555n. d
  Institut Pasteur and, 101, 140
  LAV and, 165
  Mason as replacement for, 208–09
  Office of Research Integrity and, 495
Breitman, Ted, 11, 37, 51
Brenner, Sydney, 5
Breuning, Stephen, 347
Broder, Samuel
  Gallo and, 271, 331, 357–58, 359, 423–24, 425, 480, 514, 515–16, 532
  Gazdar and, 335
  Hadley and, 513, 514–16
  Montagnier and, 170
  National Academy of Sciences panel and, 353
  Stevens and, 355
  Varmus and, 531–32
Brugière, Frédéric
  AIDS and, 65
  AIDS blood test and, 282
  Barré-Sinoussi and, 54–55, 56, 57, 61
  Brun-Vézinet, and, 42, 44, 47
  death of, 330
  ELISA and, 66
  Gallo and, 180, 214, 237
  HTLV and, 54–55, 56, 60, 548n. n
  HTLV-3 and, 124
  LAV and, 86, 89, 93, 142, 293, 402
  Montagnier and, 54, 55–56, 68, 69, 164, 243
  Popovic and, 84, 484
  provenance of virus, 53, 55–56
  Read and, 283
Brunet, Jean-Baptiste, 397
Brun-Vézinet, Françoise
  AIDS and, 43–44, 65–66
  AIDS blood test patent and, 294, 309
  AIDS research history and, 296
  Brugière and, 42, 44, 47
  ELISA and, 66–67, 76, 80, 85, 86, 98, 103, 104, 106, 157
  LAV-2 and, 232
  LAV-2$_{FG}$ and, 308
  LAV and, 102, 157
  Leibowitch and, 52
  Montagnier and, 47
  Science and, 55
Bru virus. *See* LAV$_{Bru}$
Bryant, Marty, 166–68, 180, 402, 506
Buc, Nancy, 222–24, 238, 240, 261, 264, 265
Buck, Gerald, 54

Bundren, Bill, 127–28, 134, 203
Burkitt's Lymphoma, 26
Burney, Arsène, 170
Burroughs Wellcome, 189, 517
Burt, Cyril, 347
Bush, George H., 306, 452, 458–59, 510–11
Bush administration, 346, 404, 449, 454, 459
Business Week, 535
Butler, Declan, 370
Byrnes, Tom, 243, 258, 286

C-30 cell line, 190–91
Cabradilla, Cirilo, 40, 61, 73, 74, 100, 107, 128, 171, 172
CAF, 535
Cambridge BioScience, 53–54, 58, 146, 250
Cancer Act of 1971, 10
Cancer Research, 175
cancer vaccine, 10
Capote, Truman, 311
Casey, Connie, 489
CBL-1, 189, 517
CD-4, 190–91, 479
CDC (Centers for Disease Control and Prevention)
  AIDS and, 39, 73, 76, 105–07
  AIDS blood test and, 150, 176, 189, 283, 284, 286, 287, 322, 343, 436, 583n. c
  AIDS Task Force and, 68
  Barré-Sinoussi and, 61
  Chermann and, 100–101
  Gallo and, 73–74, 101, 105–07, 112–13, 118, 119, 129, 133, 137, 138, 151, 153, 154, 284, 322, 343, 554–55n. p
  HTLV-2 and, 163
  HTLV-3B and, 150, 151, 155–56, 165
  Institut Pasteur and, 102, 104, 105–07, 112–13, 128, 129, 131, 133, 153, 206, 284, 322, 343
  LAV and, 165, 209
  transfusion pair and, 157, 209, 213–14
cDNA. *See* complementary DNA
Cell
  Baltimore and, 347, 348
  Martin and, 181
  Wain-Hobson and, 171–72, 173, 174, 175, 394, 398, 400–401
cell culture, defined, 630–31
cell lines
  AIDS blood test and, 146
  defined, 631
  Gazdar and, 24
  LAV and, 142, 143
  Miyoshi and, 30

National Institutes of Health policy and, 148, 559n. g
cells, defined, 631
CEM
  AIDS blood tests and, 230, 251
  defined, 631
  Klatzmann and, 190
  Montagnier and, 567–68n. k
  Volsky and, 376–77
  Weiss and, 127, 128
  Zagury and, 88
Centers for Disease Control. *See* CDC (Centers for Disease Control and Prevention)
Centocor, 170
Cetus, 146, 147
Chabner, Bruce, 532
Chafin, Bruce, 390, 427, 462, 512, 519
Chandra, Prakash, 295
Chanock, Robert, 440, 607–08n. k
Chardon, Claude
  electron micrograph of virus, 70, 287
  Gallo and, 70–71, 242, 243–44
  $HTLV_{CR}$ and, 92
  Leibowitch and, 51–52
  Modigliani and, 51, 53
  Popovic and, 83, 85, 364
Charleston Post & Courier, 516
Charrow, Robert, 297, 358
Chase, Marilyn, 271
chemokines, 535, 537
Chen, Irvin, 482
Chermann, Jean-Claude
  AIDS and, 60, 63, 65
  AIDS blood test and, 192, 284
  AIDS blood test patent and, 294, 302, 309
  AIDS Discoverers' Club and, 327–28
  AIDS research history and, 296–97
  Barré-Sinoussi and, 48, 50, 395
  Brugière and, 56
  Brun-Vézinet and, 47
  CDC and, 209
  ELISA and, 105
  Francis and, 100, 105, 112, 153
  Gallo and, 87, 95, 109, 112, 118, 119, 125, 139, 144, 155, 193, 198–99, 210, 270, 285, 343, 344, 361, 393, 394, 395, 429, 568n. n, 606n. e
  Gottlieb and, 97, 99, 149
  HTLV-3B and, 152, 156, 175–76
  Klatzmann and, 62
  LAV and, 76, 88, 98–100, 101, 130, 132, 152, 163, 175–76, 216
  LAV_{Bru} and, 395
  Montagnier and, 46, 47–48, 117, 274, 394

Nobel Prize for AIDS rumors and, 326, 327
Office of Research Integrity and, 495, 499
Office of Scientific Integrity investigation and, 408
peptide research of, 531
Popovic and, 99–100, 164
Reitz and, 402
retroviruses and, 43, 55
Rouzioux and, 67
Science and, 55
Weiss and, 153
Chicago Tribune, 342–45, 350–52, 355–57, 407, 451, 468, 525, 532
Chirac, Jacques, 300, 301, 302, 305, 430, 445
Chiron, 146, 147, 166
Christ, Marcus, 476–77, 478, 484–87, 492, 494–95, 499, 500–501, 504
chromosomes, defined, 631
Citation Index, 322
C-LAV, 189
Clavel, François, 231–35, 308, 309, 329, 330
Cleveland Plain Dealer, 427
Clinton, Hillary, 532
Clinton, William Jefferson, 458, 459, 488
Clinton administration, 474, 511–12
clones, defined, 631
cloning, defined, 631
CNN, 451
CNTS scandal, 445–50
codon, defined, 631–32
Cold Spring Harbor Agreement, 179
Cole, Stuart, 169
Commerce, U.S. Department of, 189, 200, 254
complementary DNA, defined, 632
Comptes Rendus, 234
Connor, Steve, 297–99, 370
continuous cell line, defined, 632
Contracts Dispute Act, 258
Coppola, Francis Ford, 526
core protein, defined, 632
Cousins, Norman, 329
Crick, Francis, DNA structure and, 4–5, 6, 302, 594–95n. d
Crosby, Kandra Kae, 282
Crosby, Michael, 282
Crowell and Moring, 432
Crozemarie, Jacques, 87
Culliton, Barbara, 369–71, 372, 401, 536
Cure, The (Coppola and Johnston), 526
Curien, Hubert, 435
Curran, James
  AIDS and, 106–07, 109
  AIDS Task Force and, 68
  And the Band Played On, 491

Curran, James (*cont.*)
 Chermann and, 100–101, 491
 deVita and, 128
 ELISA and, 106
 Francis and, 287
 Gallo and, 108, 129, 130, 138, 143, 154, 184–85
 Harmison and, 209
 Heckler and, 136
 HTLV and, 73
 LAV and, 69, 108, 130
 Mullins and, 74
Current Contents, 322
Curt, Gregory, 375
Cushman, Darby & Cushman, 287
cyclosporin, 96
cytosine, defined, 632

Daily Telegraph, 188
Dalgleish, Angus, 188
dalton, defined, 632
D'Angelo, Mario, 218–19
Daniel, Muthiah, 308
Danos, Olivier, 169
Darsee, John, 347
Dauguet, Charles, Brugière and, 48–49
Dean, John W., III, 221
Dedonder, Raymond
 AIDS blood test patent and, 200–201, 221, 302–03, 317, 318, 455
 Connor and, 299
 Food and Drug Administration and, 227
 French and American AIDS Foundation and, 454, 522
 Haddow and, 208, 212
 retirement of, 401
 Schwartz and, 521
 Swire and, 238
Dee, Lynda, 533
Defense, U.S. Department of, 431
Deinhardt, Fritz, 122, 319, 479
Delbrück, Max, 5
Dennis, Beverly, 521
Desrosiers, Ron, 233, 308
DeVita, Vincent
 AIDS and, 39, 58
 AIDS blood test and, 147
 AIDS textbook of, 241
 Brandt and, 128–29
 Essex and, 276
 Fischinger and, 203, 207, 208, 330
 FOCMA and, 41
 Gallo and, 20, 31–32, 59–60, 96, 110, 113, 149, 155, 160, 193–94, 216, 241–42, 260, 314–15, 316, 480

H-9 and, 333–34
Harmison and, 230
Heckler and, 135
HTLV-3 and, 126, 163
Kaplan and, 27
Lasker Prize and, 37
Memorial Sloan-Kettering Cancer Center and, 331
National Cancer Institute and, 145–46
Dextran sulfate, 331, 534
Diagnostics Pasteur, 458
Dingell, John D.
 AIDS blood test patents and, 430, 431
 Baltimore and, 347–49, 382
 Gallo and, 362–63, 460, 491–92, 506, 513, 515, 526
 Hadley and, 434, 461, 472
 Healy and, 423, 425–26, 439–40, 459–60, 462, 474, 527, 610n. c
 loss of chair of Committee on Energy and Commerce, 526
 Office of Research Integrity and, 472, 476
 Office of Scientific Integrity and, 460–62, 465
 Office of Scientific Integrity Review and, 464
 Rabb and, 519
 Raub and, 350–51, 352, 353, 362–63, 391–92, 468
 Read and, 509
 Reagan administration and, 346
 Sarin and, 391
 Schwartz and, 510
 Varmus and, 512
 Watson and, 473
Dingell Report, 526–27
Discover, 342
DNA
 Adult T-Cell Leukemia and, 34–35
 AIDS and, 41
 defined, 632–33
 HTLV-3B and, 156
 LAV and, 156
 Montagnier and, 585n. a
 polymerase chain reaction and, 374
 structure of, 4–5
DNA clones, defined, 632
DNA probes
 CDC and, 73, 74
 defined, 632
 HTLV and, 59
DNA sequence. *See* nucleotide sequences
DNA virus, defined, 632
Donaldson, Sam, 442–43, 450, 451
double helix, defined, 633
Dowdle, Walter, 101, 129, 151

D-penicillamine, 390–91, 600n. j
Duesberg, Peter, 324
Dufoix, Georgina, 446, 449
Dulbecco, Renato, 5, 6, 290
DuPont, 147, 170, 255, 291

Eastment, Tina, 25
Economist, The, 451
Edlinger, Ewald, 69
Edsall, John, 527
Edwards, James, 517
Einstein, Albert, 96
Eisen, Harvey, 116, 336
Electronucleonics, 146, 147, 186, 227, 254,
   266, 267, 287, 362
Electrostatic Detection Apparatus, 506–10
Elion, Gertrude, 338
ELISA
   AIDS blood tests and, 185
   Brun-Vézinet and, 66–67, 76, 80, 81, 85,
      157
   commercial production of, 118, 120, 189
   defined, 633
   Gallo and, 108, 117, 120, 136, 146, 176,
      208, 250, 283–84, 352
   HTLV-3B and, 148
   Institut Pasteur and, 86, 117, 146, 176, 204,
      216
   LAV and, 66–67, 76, 102, 106, 107–08, 117,
      133
   patent on, 85, 86, 551–52n. n
   Sarngadharan and, 104–08, 112, 264
Enders, John, 32, 503, 584–85n. k
Engler, Seymour, 265, 266
envelope, defined, 633
envelope protein, defined, 633
Environmental Protection Agency, 431
enzymes, defined, 633
Epstein, Mike, 455–56, 518, 520–22
Epstein, Yvonne, 26
Epstein-Barr virus, 26, 29, 325
Equine Infectious Anemia Virus, 69, 81,
   93–94, 98, 117, 210, 585n. a, 633
Ernberg, Ingemar, 325
Escoffier, August, 195
Escoffier, Jean-Bernard, 195
Escoffier-Lambiotte, Claudine, 87–88, 194–99,
   246, 318, 327
ESP-1, 14–15
Essex, Myron T. "Max"
   Abbott blood test and, 250
   AIDS and, 68, 76, 77–78, 97
   AIDS blood test and, 145
   Albert Lasker Clinical Medical Research
      Award and, 276

Cambridge BioScience and, 53–54, 146
CDC and, 73, 100
FOCMA and, 40–41, 97, 145
Francis and, 72, 74
Gallo and, 53–54, 55, 58, 79, 136, 145, 336
HIV-2 and, 293
HTLV-1 and, 40, 145
HTLV-3B and, 151
HTLV-4 and, 233, 234, 235, 236, 276,
   308–09
HTLV-MA and, 40, 41, 42, 52, 53–54, 58,
   59, 67, 77, 80, 90, 92, 100, 136, 145, 247
Martin and, 215
monkey AIDS virus and, 232–33, 307, 308,
   586n. h
Office of Research Integrity and, 478
Purtilo and, 76
Retroviridae Study Group and, 179
ethics
   Gallo and, 209, 248, 407, 520, 535, 540
   Hadley and, 528
   in science, 158, 197, 198, 347–48
   Zagury and, 406–07

Fabius, Laurent, 445, 446, 449
Factor VIII, defined, 633
Falkow, Stanley, 358, 412
Farber, Sidney, 15
Farr, Bart, 358
Fauci, Anthony, 215, 254, 480
Federal Bureau of Investigation, 461–62
Federal Technology Transfer Act, 278
Feline leukemia virus, 54, 62, 633
Feorino, Paul, 100, 107, 213–14, 217
Ferdinand, Roland, 121, 160
Ferris, Tom, 192
Financial Times, 525
Finch, Julie, 263
Finnegan & Henderson, 284
Fischinger, Peter
   AIDS blood test patents and, 123, 430, 455
   AIDS blood tests and, 192, 193, 205
   Connor and, 297, 298
   Deinhardt and, 319
   DeVita and, 203, 207, 208, 330
   Gallo and, 54, 155, 160, 202, 203, 204,
      205–08, 210, 212, 215, 216–17, 237, 244,
      259, 260, 261, 266, 285, 350, 371, 415,
      425, 503, 532, 573n. u
   Gardner and, 167
   Hampar and, 84
   Heckler and, 135
   HTLV-3B and, 148–49, 162–63, 165, 559n. i
   Institut Pasteur and, 200, 201, 202,
      568–69n. d

Fischinger, Peter (*cont.*)
  Koch and, 320
  Popovic and, 388
FOCMA (feline oncornavirus membrane antigen), 40–41, 97, 145
Food and Drug Administration
  Abbott Laboratories and, 148, 219, 229, 251–52, 255, 279–80, 281–82, 291, 447, 448–49, 527–28, 575n. d
  AIDS blood tests and, 147, 148, 185, 186, 191
  AZT and, 332
  blood supply and, 446
  Dingell and, 431
  Genetic Systems and, 220, 223, 226, 227, 252
  herpesvirus and, 69
  Institut Pasteur and, 290
  vaccines and, 405
Forbes, 539
Ford, Cecilia Sparks, 481, 487
Foundation for Advanced Education in the Sciences, 391
Fradellizi, Didier, 47
Francis, Donald
  AIDS and, 73
  AIDS Task Force and, 68
  Amersham Laboratories and, 189
  And the Band Played On, 490
  Barré-Sinoussi and, 61
  CDC blood-test data and, 436
  Chermann and, 100, 105, 113, 153
  Curran and, 287
  DeVita and, 128
  Donaldson and, 443
  ELISA and, 105–06, 176
  Essex and, 72
  Gallo and, 74, 108, 113, 118–19, 130, 154, 183, 312–13, 443, 479
  Genentech and, 529
  Harmison and, 209
  HTLV and, 39, 61, 100, 546–47n. d
  Institut Pasteur and, 102
  LAV and, 108, 130, 153
  Martin and, 378
  Montagnier and, 81, 104, 117, 129, 443, 583n. c
  Office of Research Integrity and, 495
  Office of Scientific Integrity investigation, 408
  Popovic and, 164
  Salk and, 288, 295
  Shilts and, 311, 313
  Swire and, 294
  vaccines and, 479, 529

Frank, Barney, 222
Frankel, Max, 444
Franklin, Rosalind, 354, 531, 594–95n. d
Freedom of Information Act, 259–63, 265, 266, 294, 297, 378, 453
French and American AIDS Foundation, 454, 514, 518–19, 521–24, 617–18n. f

Gairdner Prize, 313
Gallagher, Robert, 16–18, 20, 21, 22, 24, 25, 27, 541–42n. b
Gallin, John, 441
Gallo, Judith, 15
Gallo, Mary Jane, 177, 194
Gallo, Robert Charles
  AIDS and, 39, 43, 44, 52, 57, 59–60, 62–63, 76, 85, 95–97, 105–07, 122, 187–88, 548n. q
  AIDS blood test and, 120–21, 140, 146, 148, 156, 178, 191, 192–93, 205, 224–25, 257, 278, 283–85, 293, 318, 324, 333, 337, 352, 379, 381, 499, 506
  AIDS blood test patent and, 294, 301, 309, 321, 428, 429, 432–33, 456, 462–63, 520, 605n. g, 610n. c
  AIDS Research and, 76
  And the Band Played On, 490–91
  awards of, 158
  Barré-Sinoussi and, 48, 49, 60, 61, 91, 109, 143–44, 193, 344, 397, 520, 558n. a
  Bolognesi and, 68
  Broder and, 332
  Buc and, 222
  Cambridge BioScience and, 53–54, 58
  CDC and, 73–75, 101, 105–07, 112–13, 118, 119, 129, 138, 151, 153, 154, 554–55n. p
  CEM and, 230
  Chermann and, 87, 95, 98, 109, 112, 118, 119, 125, 139, 144, 154–55, 193, 198–99, 210, 270, 285, 344, 361, 393, 394, 429, 568n. n, 606n. e
  CNTS scandal and, 449, 450
  Connor and, 297–99
  determination of, 15, 31
  DeVita and, 20, 31–32, 59–60, 96, 110, 113, 149, 155, 160, 193–94, 216, 241–42, 260, 314–15, 316, 480
  Dingell and, 350, 431–32, 491–92, 513, 515, 526, 527
  Donaldson and, 442–43, 450, 451
  Escoffier-Lambiotte and, 196–99, 246
  Essex and, 308
  Fischinger and, 54, 155, 160, 202, 203, 205–08, 210, 212, 215, 216–17, 237, 244,

259, 260, 261, 266, 285, 350, 371, 415, 425, 503, 532, 573n. u
FOCMA and, 41, 312
Francis and, 74, 108, 112–13, 118–19, 130, 154, 183, 312–13, 443, 479
French and American AIDS Foundation and, 454, 455, 456, 522, 617–18n. f
growth factor and, 16
Heckler and, 134, 135, 136, 141, 557n. n
Henle and, 75
HIV-3 and, 306
HIV and, 236
HL-23 and, 20, 21, 316, 336
HL-23V and, 19
HTLV and, 14, 26–36, 49, 51, 59, 64, 66, 68, 71, 77–80, 82–83, 87, 90, 92, 96, 99, 160, 298, 542–43n. g, 543n. i, 543–44nn. k, l, 549–51n. f, 551n. i
HTLV-1 and, 85, 97, 105, 114, 123, 132, 142, 144, 145, 155, 159, 213, 215, 243–44, 247, 260, 263, 269, 283, 286, 314, 321, 585n. a
HTLV-2 and, 39, 80, 114, 116, 123, 124, 139, 155, 159, 215, 269
HTLV-3 and, 109, 114–15, 116, 122, 123, 130, 132, 138–39, 142, 144–45, 155, 164, 170, 178–80, 215–16, 236, 244–45, 247, 285, 297, 314, 433, 558n. b
HTLV-3B and, 148–50, 153, 173, 193, 200, 261, 272, 275, 361, 393, 469, 476, 498, 564–65n. m, 565–66n. s
HTLV-3$_{RF}$ and, 160–62, 166, 181, 217, 260, 272–73, 275, 562n. c, 563n. g
HUT-78 and, 416, 604n. d
HUT-102 and, 24–25
Institute of Human Virology, 532–33, 535–37, 618n. b
Institut Pasteur and, 112, 137, 140, 154–55, 183, 184–85, 195, 200, 211, 226, 258, 277–78, 287, 297, 361, 371, 444, 452
Japan Prize and, 159, 160
Kaposi's sarcoma and, 354–55, 595n. e
Karpas and, 32–34, 64, 79, 183, 218, 247, 268, 319, 320, 332, 340, 367, 489, 505
Koch and, 319–21, 590nn. g, h
Koprowski and, 323, 590–91n. i
lab's contamination, 19–20, 320, 352, 356, 357, 376, 402, 492
Lasker Prize and, 37
LAV and, 68–69, 81, 84, 91–92, 128, 131, 140, 143, 169, 178, 193, 196, 224, 235, 237, 241, 257, 269–70, 275, 285, 286, 290, 321, 345, 352, 356, 371, 380, 381,

390, 418, 432–33, 468–70, 570–71n. g, h, i, 581–82n. l, 598n. b, 604n. e
Leibowitch and, 49, 50–51, 52
Levine and, 38–39
memoirs of, 428–29, 446, 606nn. b, c
Morgan and, 20–21, 22, 23
MOV and, 104
National Academy of Science panel and, 373, 438, 451
New Jersey Pair and, 304, 586n. f
Nobel Prize for AIDS, rumors and, 326, 536
Nobel Prize aspirations, 336, 337, 338, 368
notebooks of, 355, 369, 378
Office of Research Integrity and, 467–72, 475–81, 492–95, 505, 509, 515, 610n. d
Office of Scientific Integrity and, 351–52, 358, 359, 360, 361, 369, 408, 410, 414–25, 428, 435, 438, 451, 453, 460, 463, 506, 595–96n. h, 604n. f
Pan-Data Systems and, 362
patent royalties and, 310, 333, 335, 510, 517, 533
Popovic and, 110–11, 114, 136, 180, 212, 248, 286, 294, 360, 388, 393, 411, 467, 485, 493, 533
Redfern and, 122, 125, 126, 556n. f
Research Integrity Adjudications Panel and, 475
retirement from National Institutes of Health, 532–33, 539
Retroviridae Study Group and, 179–80
retroviruses and, 24, 25, 27, 31, 57
reverse transcriptase and, 11, 14, 16, 541–42n. b
Salk and, 288, 293, 295
Sattaur and, 182–85
Shilts and, 311–12, 367, 443
Swire and, 259–60
Todaro and, 19, 31–32, 156, 160, 324, 337
Varner and, 217–18
Wain-Hobson and, 171
Zagury and, 393, 405–08, 428, 449, 514, 600n. a
Gallochat, Alain, 317, 454, 455, 521
Gallo/Montagnier relationship
  AIDS blood test award and, 384
  AIDS blood test patents and, 429–30
  Chermann and, 198
  Chicago Tribune article, 343, 344, 345
  correspondence of, 206
  D'Angelo and, 218
  Essex and, 234
  Gallo's memoirs and, 428–29, 607n. f
  history of HIV and, 289, 295–97

Gallo/Montagnier relationship (*cont.*)
  HTLV and, 551n. h
  HTLV probes and, 49, 53
  HTLV-3/LAV comparison and, 109–10, 115, 118, 139, 142, 155, 162, 175–76, 193, 248–49, 271–76, 284, 563n. g, 583n. c
  Institut Pasteur's *Science* article and, 344
  isolates and, 113
  lab contamination and, 492, 563n. g
  LAV and, 64, 81–83, 87–89, 94, 115–16, 127, 143, 154, 235–36, 357, 380, 404, 418, 548–49n. s, 549n. b
  LAV_{Bru} and, 395
  Maddox and, 530
  Montagnier's *Science* paper and, 55, 56–57, 548n. o
  Noble Prize rumors and, 337–38, 537
  Office of Research Integrity and, 471, 495
  San Francisco Examiner and, 366
  Temin and, 377
  Varmus and, 179
Gardner, Murray
  Abbott's blood test and, 250
  AIDS blood tests and, 189, 254
  ARV and, 166, 169
  Chermann and, 99
  FOCMA and, 41, 97
  Gallo and, 115, 116, 120, 149–50, 167
  HTLV-3B and, 166, 169, 308
  LAV and, 166, 168, 169, 308, 397, 402–03
  Montagnier and, 117, 118
  retroviruses and, 80
  Swire and, 294
Garretta, Michel, 445–46
Gazdar, Adi
  Gallo and, 333, 334–35
  HTLV and, 28, 36
  HUT-78 and, 90, 416
  Minna and, 25
  Office of Scientific Integrity and, 416–17
  Popovic and, 332, 333, 334
  Robinson and, 24
Gelmann, Ed, 41–42, 49, 52, 53, 85, 585n. a
GEM-91, 534
gene maps, defined, 633
Genentech, 173, 294, 529, 538
General Accounting Office, 362, 390, 391–92
General Motors Cancer Research Award, 85, 158
genes, defined, 633
genetic codes, defined, 633
genetic sequence. *See* nucleotide sequences
Genetic Systems
  AIDS blood test patent and, 284, 289

AIDS blood tests' accuracy, 229–30, 252, 254
AIDS blood tests supply, 251
American Red Cross and, 190, 226, 255, 256–57, 280, 281, 282, 291–92
Food and Drug Administration and, 220, 223, 226, 227, 252
Todaro and, 156–57
Germany, 189–90
Gilden, Ray, 240, 242
Gillespie, Dave, 15, 19
Gilman, Alfred, 358, 373, 412, 437, 438–39, 495, 526
Gilot, Françoise, 287
Glauser, Michel, 114
Glendening, Parris, 532–33
Global AIDS News, 472
glycoprotein, defined, 634
Godek, Steve, 478, 481–84, 494, 502–04, 615n. g
Golde, David, 482, 538, 611n. d
Gomez, Fernando, 307
Gonda, Matthew
  Gallo and, 320, 482
  Gallo inquiry and, 370
  HTLV-3 and, 123
  $HTLV-3_{RF}$, 121, 388
  LAV and, 70, 84, 91–92, 93, 237, 238, 239, 241, 298, 571n. i, 572n. k, 577n. l
  Montagnier and, 69
  Popovic and, 124, 207, 224, 238–39, 240, 264, 265, 298, 343, 508, 577–78n. m, 581–82n. l
  Swire and, 238–40, 259, 294, 571–72n. j
Good, Robert, 75
Gorbachev, Mikhail, 368
Gore, Al, 459
Gottlieb, Michael
  acquired T-cell defect and, 13
  AIDS and, 42, 539
  AIDS Discoverers' Club and, 327
  Chermann, 97, 99, 149
  Gallo and, 144
  HTLV-3B and, 149
  LAV_{Bru} and, 63
  Montagnier and, 329
  Nobel Prize for AIDS rumors and, 326
Gottlieb, Robert, 367
gp41
  AIDS blood tests and, 255, 279, 280, 281, 292, 582–83n. b
  defined, 634
gp120, defined, 634
Gray, L. Patrick, III, 221

Gray, Robert K., 358, 536, 618–19n. e
Great Britain, 188
Greenspun, Julian, 362
Griffuel Prize, 87
Grinstead, Darrel, 222
Groopman, Jerome, 95, 97, 149, 163, 563–64n. j
Gros, François, 197, 198, 448, 449
Gross, Ludwik, 174–75, 323, 353, 358
Gruest, Jacqueline, 56, 63, 397, 548–49n. s
guanine, defined, 634
Guétard, Denise, 232
Guroff, Marjorie
    AIDS and, 85, 109, 145
    ELISA and, 66, 92
    HTLV and, 29, 40, 52, 70, 77, 96, 105,
        542–43n. g
    Montagnier and, 551n. h
Gutterman, Jordan, 51

H-9
    AIDS blood tests and, 147, 149, 332, 448,
        604–05n. g
    AIDS blood tests' false positives and,
        189–90, 192, 229
    defined, 634
    DeVita and, 333–34
    Fischinger and, 149
    Gallo and, 148, 149, 150, 251, 293, 314,
        333, 334, 416, 438, 469, 476, 480, 493,
        604n. d, 611n. c
    HTLV-3$_{RF}$ and, 161, 181
    Institut Pasteur and, 152
    LAV and, 257
    Levy and, 150
    Pan-Data Systems and, 362
    patents for, 149
    Popovic and, 105, 110–11, 124, 202, 208,
        217, 259, 266, 332, 382, 409, 416, 503
Haddow, C. McLain, 133, 134, 208, 212, 220,
    443–44
Hadley, Suzanne
    AIDS blood test patents and, 419–20, 431,
        434, 526, 605n. g
    And the Band Played On, 489–90
    Bivens and, 485
    Dingell and, 434, 461, 472
    ethics and, 528
    Gallo and, 351–52, 355, 358, 360, 369, 375,
        379–80, 393, 411–12, 419, 425, 433–34,
        463, 467, 472, 492, 509, 514, 515, 516, 520
    Gallo report and, 437, 464–65
    Hallum and, 372, 408–09, 420–21, 461
    Healy and, 420–22, 426–27, 435, 460,
        461–62

interviews of, 408
Justice Department and, 357
Martin and, 377
Montagnier and, 400
National Academy of Sciences panel and,
    359, 379, 413
Odle and, 431
Office of the Inspector General and, 433
Office of Research Integrity and, 476–78
Onek and, 432–33
Popovic and, 363, 364, 365, 375, 386, 389,
    410, 411–13, 420, 483, 496, 502, 503–04,
    506–07, 517–18, 533
Rabb and, 511
Raub and, 353, 381, 413, 414
Varmus and, 512
HAF, 537–38
Haguenau, Françoise, 87
Hahn, Beatrice
    Gallo and, 360
    HIV and, 339
    HTLV-3B and, 161, 168, 181, 213, 223,
        338–39, 340, 565n. p
    HTLV-4 and, 308
    LAV and, 93, 161, 277, 552–53n. w
    MOV and, 413
    Myers and, 338
    patent royalties and, 278
    restriction mapping and, 92
Hahn, Otto, 326
Haitian community, 43, 51, 62, 66, 69, 548n. r
Hallum, Jules
    Francis and, 436
    Gallo and, 411, 414, 435, 460–61
    Gallo report and, 464
    Hadley and, 372, 408–09, 420–21, 461
    Healy and, 427, 440
    Martin and, 377
    Myers and, 372, 373
    Office of Research Integrity and, 466
    Popovic and, 386, 388
HALV (human AIDS/lymphotropic virus), 179
Hampar, Berge
    AIDS blood test patent and, 301–02
    Fischinger and, 84
    Gallo and, 151, 242, 245, 371, 382
    Institut Pasteur and, 200, 203–05
    LAV and, 240, 571–72n. j
    Martin and, 378
    Office of Scientific Integrity and, 382, 416
    patent royalties and, 278
    Swire and, 271, 579–80n. d
Hanafusa, Hidesaburo, 7–9
Harada, Shinji, 75

Harmison, Lowell
AIDS blood test patents and, 430, 455
AIDS blood tests and, 147, 185, 188–89, 192, 193, 205
Berneman and, 249
CDC and, 209, 287
Fischinger and, 207, 212, 216, 568–69n. d
Gallo and, 223, 230, 260, 425
Genetic Systems and, 156
Health and Human Service Department leadership and, 222
HTLV-3B and, 148–49, 559n. i
Institut Pasteur and, 200, 201, 202
Martin and, 212, 214, 215
Mason and, 220
Maxwell and, 315
Montagnier and, 271
resignation of, 316, 589n. b
Zuck and, 230
Harriman, Pamela, 459
Haseltine, Florence, 474
Haseltine, William
Chermann and, 97–98
Essex and, 53–54, 68
Francis and, 153–54
Gallo and, 84, 360
H-9 and, 149
HTLV-3B and, 170, 565–66n. s
Martin and, 215
Sattaur and, 182
Wain-Hobson and, 171
Hausen, Harald zur, 122
HBLV, 324–25, 362
hCG, 537–38
Health and Human Services, U.S. Department of. *See also* Office of the Inspector General (HHS); Office of Research Integrity; Research Integrity Adjudications Panel
AIDS and, 123, 141
AIDS blood tests and, 146–48, 189, 192
AIDS blood tests patents and, 128, 224, 237–38, 260, 284–85, 289–90, 294–95, 309, 317, 444, 454–56, 519, 520, 585n. d, 589n. e
Buc and, 240
Connor and, 299
Dingell and, 431, 434–35
Dingell Report and, 526
Fischinger report and, 208, 212
Gallo and, 123, 286, 287, 350, 357, 358, 423
Gallo report and, 436
Genetic Systems and, 229–30
Institut Pasteur and, 101, 200, 201, 202, 208, 221, 223, 224, 249, 282

Koch and, 321–22
Myers and, 340
Office of Scientific Integrity and, 460
Onek and, 412
regulations of, 348
Regulations for the Protection of Human Subjects, 405
Salk and, 288–89
Swire and, 261, 262, 265, 579–80n. d
Healy, Bernadine
and American Red Cross, 527–28
Dingell and, 423, 425–26, 439–40, 459–60, 462, 474, 527, 609–10n. b
French and American AIDS Foundation and, 454, 455, 456, 522
Gallo and, 405, 408, 423–24, 425, 440–41, 451–52, 453, 460, 480
Gallo report and, 436–38, 464, 465
Hadley and, 420–22, 426–27, 435, 460, 461–62
Institute of Human Virology and, 536
National Academy of Sciences panel and, 437, 438–40, 441
as National Institute of Health director, 404–05, 439–40, 459, 466, 474, 488, 489
Office of Research Integrity and, 468
Office of Scientific Integrity Review and, 465
Sharma and, 425–27, 494
Watson and, 473
Heckler, Margaret
AIDS blood tests and, 147, 185–87, 219, 449–50
as ambassador to Ireland, 221–22
Institut Pasteur and, 101, 134, 136, 154, 200, 208
news conference announcing Gallo's results, 126–27, 128–29, 130, 133, 134–36, 141, 143, 146, 149, 153, 154, 160, 181, 275, 286, 334, 558n. n
Henle, Werner, 75
Henry Kaplan Memorial Lecture, 158
hepatitis B, 73, 102, 146, 250
hepatitis viruses, 65
herpesvirus, 26, 65, 69, 325, 634
Hervé, Edmond, 446, 449
HHH. *See* Health and Human Services, U.S. Department of
HHV-6, 325, 533
HHV-7, 479
Hill, Fergal, 341
Hilts, Phillip, 523
Hinuma, Yorio
ATLV and, 75, 585n. a
Epstein-Barr virus and, 29

Gallo and, 60, 79
Harada and, 75
HTLV and, 35, 36
Karpas and, 34, 60, 75
retroviruses and, 30–31, 543n. h
Hitchings, George, 338
HIV (Human Immunodeficiency Virus)
Abbott blood test and, 250
defined, 634
Gallo and, 356
history of discovery, 342
Koch and, 320
Read and, 508
Varmus and, 236
HIV-1, 236
HIV-2, 236, 293, 308, 309
HIV-2$_{NIH-Z}$, 308, 587n. k
HIV-3, 306
HIVAC, 405
HIV Sequence Database, 303–06, 341, 393
HL-23
DeVita and, 31
Gallagher and, 16, 17–18, 21, 27
Gallo and, 20, 21, 316, 336
Kaplan and, 27
Ruscetti and, 22
HL-23V, 18, 19
Ho, David, 536
Hodgkin's disease, 27
Hoffman–La Roche, 374
Homburg Degussa Pharma, 390–91
Homosexuality
acquired T-cell defect and, 13–14
AIDS and, 43, 51, 52, 58, 60, 76
HTLV and, 39, 42, 53
Hovanessian, Ara, 46
Hoxie, James, 111, 121, 181–82
HSB-2, 88
HTLV (Human T-cell Leukemia Virus)
AIDS and, 38–43, 51–54, 58–59, 61, 62–63,
66, 68–70, 72–77, 81–83, 91, 94
ATLV and, 31–35, 70
defined, 634
ELISA and, 66
Gallo and, 14, 26–36, 49, 51, 59, 64, 66,
68, 71, 77–80, 82–83, 87, 90, 92, 96, 99,
160, 298, 542–43n. g, 543n. i, 543–44nn.
k, l, 549–51n. f, 551n. i
Guroff and, 29, 542n. g
Karpas and, 34, 543–44n. k
mycosis fungoides and, 28, 542n. e
Poiesz and, 26–29, 31, 32, 35, 37, 64, 80, 82,
333, 542n. d, 543–44nn. k, l
transmission of, 39, 62

HTLV-1
Adult T-Cell Leukemia as, 79–80
AIDS and, 85, 105, 122, 144, 145, 173–74
defined, 634
ELISA and, 104
Essex and, 40
Gallo and, 85, 97, 105, 114, 123, 132, 139,
142, 144, 145, 155, 159, 213, 215,
243–44, 247, 263, 314, 321, 585n. a
HTLV-3 and, 163, 164, 171, 173, 178
Institut Pasteur and, 139
isolates of, 161
LAV and, 113, 139, 144, 171, 269, 565n. q
Pan-Data Systems and, 362
Popovic and, 71, 84
Robinson and, 124, 164
Schupbach and, 383
HTLV-1B, 93, 552n. u, 589–90n. f
HTLV-2
AIDS and, 173–74
defined, 634
ELISA and, 104
Gallo and, 39, 80, 114, 116, 123, 124, 139,
155, 159, 215
and hairy cell leukemia, 546n. b
HTLV-3 and, 164
Institut Pasteur and, 139
Kalyanaraman and, 324
LAV and, 113, 163, 269
Pan-Data Systems and, 362
Popovic and, 124
Schupbach and, 383
HTLV-3
AIDS and, 112, 130, 135, 137, 138, 179
AIDS blood test and, 147, 149, 227
defined, 634
DeVita and, 193
ELISA and, 120–21
Gallo and, 109, 114–15, 116, 122, 123, 130,
132, 138–39, 142, 144–45, 155, 178–80,
215–16, 236, 244–45, 247, 285, 293, 297,
314, 433, 558n. b
HTLV-1 and, 163, 164, 171, 173, 178
LAV and, 110, 111, 112, 113–14, 115, 116,
118, 129, 132, 133, 138, 140, 142, 146,
150, 151, 152, 156, 204, 206, 237–38,
249, 257, 284, 286, 298, 583n. c
Montagnier and, 70
MOV and, 109
Redfern and, 122, 125–26
Salahuddin and, 112, 123–24
Schupbach and, 383
HTLV-3B
AIDS blood tests and, 120–21, 147–50, 284

HTLV-3B (*cont.*)
  Arthur and, 120
  cloning of, 168, 565n. p
  defined, 634
  DNA and, 166–67, 170
  Fischinger and, 149
  Gallo and, 148–50, 153, 164, 200, 261, 272,
    275, 361, 393, 469, 476, 498
  Gallo inquiry and, 370
  Hahn and, 181, 213, 223, 338–39
  HTLV-3$_{RF}$ and, 161
  LAV and, 151, 152, 155–56, 161, 162–63,
    165–66, 173, 175–76, 180–81, 193, 196,
    200, 207, 208, 210–14, 223, 238, 267,
    274–75, 277, 285, 286, 290, 298–99,
    305–06, 309, 318, 320, 338–39, 341–43,
    356, 372, 376, 402, 421, 563n. g, 565–66n. s
  LAV$_{Bru}$ and, 342, 345, 350, 375, 394, 400
  LAV$_{Lai}$ and, 399, 403, 436, 491
  MOV and, 416
  naming of, 236
  Office of Scientific Inquiry and, 377, 379
  pictures of, 241
  polymerase chain reaction and, 374
  Popovic and, 120–21, 164–65, 180, 207, 259,
    265, 364, 387, 409, 415, 566n. a
HTLV-3$_{MN}$, Myers and, 304
HTLV-3$_{RF}$
  defined, 634
  ELISA and, 120–21
  Gallo and, 160–62, 166, 181, 217, 260,
    272–73, 275, 372, 562n. c
  Hadley and, 375
  Myers and, 304, 305
  Popovic and, 148, 181, 387–88, 496, 498–99,
    567n. b
HTLV-4
  Essex and, 233, 234, 235, 236, 276, 308–09
  Gallo and, 307–08
  Hahn and, 308
  Mullins and, 307, 586–87n. i
HTLV$_{CR}$
  Chardon and, 93
  electron micrographs of, 124
  Gelmann and, 41
  Popovic and, 70, 77
HTLV-MA
  defined, 634–35
  Essex and, 40, 41, 42, 52, 53–54, 58, 59, 67,
    77, 80, 90, 92, 100, 136, 145, 247
Hudson, Rock, 193
Human T-cell Leukemia Virus. *See* HTLV
  (Human T-cell Leukemia Virus)
HUT-78
  defined, 635

Gallo inquiry/investigation and, 370, 419
Gazdar and, 24, 332, 334, 335
H-9 and, 333–35, 343, 416, 493, 592n. c
LAV and, 121, 155, 237, 264, 269, 576n. j
Levy and, 150
Popovic and, 88, 89, 90, 104–05, 128, 212,
  223, 264, 266, 416, 591–92n. a
HUT-102
  defined, 635
  Essex and, 40
  Gazdar and, 24, 333
  Ruscetti and, 24–25, 333
Hyatt, Howard, 424
hybridization, defined, 635
hydroxyurea, 534
hyperimmune antiserum, defined, 635

IDAV (immune deficiency associated virus),
  65
IDAV-1, 397, 399
IDAV-2, 397, 399
Imanishi-Kari, Thereza, 348, 351, 529
IMClone, 538
immunofluorescence assay, defined, 635
In Cold Blood (Capote), 311
INSERM, 76, 531
Institute for Scientific Information, 322–23
Institut Pasteur
  AIDS and, 58, 60, 90, 101, 106–07, 153, 447
  AIDS blood test and, 128, 133, 137, 176,
    191–93, 196–98, 207, 209, 227, 230, 237,
    246, 249, 284–85, 288, 290, 447–49, 472,
    568–69n. d
  AIDS blood test patent and, 191–93,
    294–95, 310, 317–18, 454, 458, 589n. e
  AIDS postage stamp and, 513
  CDC and, 102, 104, 105–07, 112–13, 128,
    129, 153, 322
  ELISA and, 86, 117, 146, 190, 204, 220
  Escoffier-Lambiotte and, 195
  Gallo and, 112, 137, 140, 154–55, 183,
    184–85, 195, 200, 208, 211, 226, 258,
    277–78, 287, 297, 361, 371, 444, 452
  Gallo's memoirs and, 429, 606n. d
  Gardner and, 167
  Genetic Systems and, 157
  Health and Human Services and, 200, 201,
    202, 208, 221, 223, 224, 249, 282
  history of, 45
  HIV-2 and, 309
  HTLV-3B and, 152, 165
  Hudson and, 193
  Japan Prize and, 159
  LAV and, 68, 76, 81–82, 111, 112, 128, 131,
    224, 257–58, 498, 557nn. k, l

LAV-2 and, 234, 308
LAV$_{Bru}$ and, 378, 393
Martin and, 378
National Cancer Institute and, 137
interferon
    defined, 635
    Montagnier and, 46–47, 49, 585n. a
Interleukin-2
    defined, 635
    Gallo and, 23, 29, 49, 195, 585n. a
    Gazdar and, 24
    Institut Pasteur and, 139, 143
    Montagnier and, 47
    Pan-Data Systems and, 362
Irish Times, 539
isolates
    defined, 635
    Gallo and, 107, 112, 118, 126, 138, 140,
        142, 148, 161, 181, 184–85, 196, 201,
        215, 243, 275, 286, 293, 302, 343, 344,
        371, 379, 381–82, 404, 415, 471, 554n. m,
        562n. c, 572–73n. o, 584n. g, 598n. c
    Institut Pasteur and, 396
    Montagnier and, 164, 453
    names of, 236
    Popovic and, 161, 164, 184, 207, 247–48,
        364, 372, 381, 382, 569n. e
    Weiss and, 189
Italian-American Foundation, 158
Ito, Yohei, 29, 59, 77, 79

Jacob, François, 5, 45, 198, 327
Jacobsen, Leon, 323–24, 336–37
JAMA, 62, 75, 318
Jamison, Kay, 473
Japan Prize, 158–59
Jaruzelski, Janina, 512
Jay, Peter, 315–16
Jenner, Edward, 406
Johnson, Corky, 206
Johnston, Diane, 526
Josephs, Steve, 325
Journal of Human Virology, 537
Journal of Virology, 360
July LAV
    defined, 635
    Gallo and, 397
    HTLV-3B and, 394
    Popovic and, 89, 207, 211, 248
Justice, U.S. Department of
    AIDS blood test patent and, 260, 283–84,
        287, 371, 419, 431, 433, 462–63, 478,
        610n. c
    Hadley and, 357
    Office of Research Integrity and, 477–78

Kalyanaraman, V. S., 183–84, 216, 248, 324,
    408, 482, 497, 569–70n. j
Kanki, Phyllis, 235, 308–09
Kaplan, Henry, 27, 28
Kaposi's sarcoma, 354–55, 533–34, 537, 538
Karolinska Institute, 335–36, 537
Karpas, Abraham
    AIDS blood test patent and, 303, 525
    AIDS blood tests and, 189, 340
    Gallo and, 32–34, 64, 79, 183, 218, 247,
        268, 298, 319, 320, 332, 340, 367, 368,
        489, 505
    Hinuma and, 34, 60, 75
    HTLV and, 34, 543–44n. k
    HTLV-1 and, 174
    Karpas 707H and, 531
    LAV and, 340–41, 342
    Sattaur and, 183, 184
    Weiss and, 33, 247, 574n. a
Kelberman, Dale, 376, 509–10
Kennedy, Edward, 316
Kenwood, Michael, 297
Kessler, David, 460
Klatzmann, David
    AIDS and, 43, 62
    CD-4 as AIDS virus receptor and, 190–91
    Chermann and, 119
    Columbia University and, 330
    LAV and, 71, 80
    Nature and, 71–72, 78, 79, 171
    reverse transcriptase and, 63
    T-4 cells and, 144–45, 157
Klausner, Richard, 440, 441, 532
Klein, George, 63, 368
Klein, Joel, 358
Klug, Aaron, 33
Koch, Michael, 319–22, 326, 368, 429, 590nn.
    g, h, 606n. c
Koprowski, Hilary, 323, 353, 358, 405,
    590–91n. i
Korn, Edward, 440, 441, 608n. l
Koshland, Daniel, 401–02
Kramer, Larry, 354
Kulstad, Ruth, 53, 57, 123, 124, 548n. o
Kurth, Reinhard, 336
Kusserow, Richard, 461–62

Lailler, Christophe
    Berneman and, 86
    biopsy of, 399
    Chermann and, 61
    HTLV-3B and, 412
    IDAV and, 65
    IDAV-1 and, 397
    infection of, 398

Lailler, Christophe (*cont.*)
  Institut Pasteur and, 164
  Montagnier and, 69
  Popovic pool and, 402
Lailler, Sophie, 398
Lancet, The
  Abbott Laboratories and, 448
  Chermann and, 175–76
  ELISA and, 98, 117, 128, 157–58
  Essex and, 232–33
  Gallo and, 109, 350, 407, 416, 604nn. d, e
  Guroff-Blayney and, 92, 109, 145
  Institut Pasteur and, 117, 125, 138
  Modigliani and, 53
  Weiss and, 188
  Wong-Staal and, 166
  Zagury and, 407
Lang, Serge, 439, 486
Lange, Michael, 39, 99
Lanman, Robert, 351, 375, 419–20
Lasker Prize, 36–37
LAV (lymphadenopathy-associated virus)
  AIDS and, 65, 71, 81–82, 101, 102, 103–04,
    107–08, 130, 133, 153
  AIDS blood test and, 284
  ARV and, 173
  Barré-Sinoussi and, 76, 82, 85, 88, 89, 91,
    93, 152, 162, 163, 213
  B-cell lines and, 102–03, 110, 157, 161, 162
  Chermann and, 76, 88, 98–100, 101, 130,
    132, 216
  Clavel and, 231–32
  cloning of, 102, 116–17, 168–69, 554n. j
  defined, 636
  DNA and, 166–67, 168, 169, 170
  electron micrographs of, 286
  ELISA and, 66–67, 76, 102, 104, 106,
    107–08, 117, 128
  Equine Infectious Anemia Virus, 81,
    93–94, 98, 117, 210, 585n. a
  Gallo and, 68–69, 81, 84, 91–92, 109, 128,
    131, 140, 143, 169, 178, 193, 196, 224,
    235, 237, 241, 257, 269–70, 275, 321,
    345, 381, 432–33, 468–70, 570–71nn. g,
    h, i, 581–82n. l
  Gonda and, 70, 84, 92, 94, 237, 238, 239,
    241, 298, 571n. i, 572n. k, 577n. l
  HTLV-1 and, 113, 139, 144, 171, 269,
    565n. q
  HTLV-2 and, 113, 163, 269
  HTLV-3 and, 110, 111, 112, 113–14, 115,
    116, 118, 129, 132, 133, 138, 140, 142,
    146, 150, 151, 152, 156, 204, 206,
    237–38, 249, 257, 284, 286, 298, 583n. c

  HTLV-3B and, 151, 152, 155–56, 161,
    162–63, 165–66, 173, 175–76, 180–81,
    193, 196, 200, 207, 208, 210–14, 223,
    238, 267, 274–75, 277, 285, 286, 287,
    290, 298–99, 305–06, 309, 318, 320,
    338–39, 341–43, 356, 372, 376, 402, 421,
    563n. g, 565–66n. s
  Institut Pasteur and, 68, 76, 81–82, 111, 112,
    128, 131, 227, 257–58, 557nn. k, l
  lentiviruses and, 69, 84, 98, 117, 163, 210
  Montagnier and, 68, 69, 71, 78, 80–81, 87,
    93, 127, 128, 144, 207, 225, 227, 236,
    237, 283, 321, 549n. b
  Nature and, 71–72, 78
  Office of Scientific Integrity and, 377
  patenting of, 68, 86
  polymerase chain reaction and, 374
  Popovic and, 83–85, 88–90, 92, 94, 96, 110,
    111, 113–14, 118, 138, 161–62, 202, 206,
    207, 208, 211, 217, 224, 237, 248, 257,
    260–66, 270, 277, 318, 343, 365, 372,
    376, 381, 387, 389, 410, 415, 417, 469,
    496, 508–09, 554n. n, 576n. i, 577n. l,
    581–82n. l
  Stevenson and, 360
  Weiss and, 127
  White and, 413
LAV-1, 394
LAV-2, 2_{FG}, 32–35, 236
LAV-2FG, 307–08, 587n. k
LAV$_{Bru}$
  AIDS and, 62
  Barré-Sinoussi and, 60, 61, 328
  defined, 635
  Gallo and, 394, 400
  HTLV and, 63, 548–49n. s
  HTLV-3B and, 342, 345, 350, 375, 394, 400
  Institut Pasteur and, 378, 393
  naming of, 236
  picture of, 244
  Wain-Hobson and, 397–98
  White and, 413
LAV$_{Lai}$
  defined, 636
  HTLV-3B and, 399, 403, 436, 491
  Rozenbaum and, 398
  virulence of, 61, 65
  Weiss and, 517
  White and, 413
LAV/*Rab*, 93
Lee, Helen, 446
Lee, Phil, 521, 522
Leibowitch, Jacques
  Abbott Laboratories and, 447, 448

AIDS and, 43, 51–52
Gallo and, 49, 50–51, 52, 243, 446, 450
HTLV and, 88
Nobel Prize for AIDS rumors and, 326–27
Le Monde, 194–95, 196, 204, 246, 357, 402, 428, 430, 525
lentiviruses
  chimpanzee lentivirus, 309
  defined, 636
  Equine Infectious Anemia Virus and, 69, 210
  Gonda and, 224, 264
  LAV and, 69, 84, 92, 98, 117, 163, 210
  Levy and, 91
Le Pen, Jean-Marie, 445
leukemia, 14, 15, 58, 59, 636
Levine, Arnold, 358, 374, 379, 489
Levine, Arthur, 38–39, 440, 441
Levy, Jay
  AIDS Discoverers' Club and, 327
  ARV and, 143, 158, 166, 561–62n. t
  Ascher and, 250
  Gallo and, 99, 109, 143, 150, 296, 324, 360, 368, 480, 506, 535
  Gardner and, 167
  lack of recognition for, 158, 159
  LAV and, 90–91
  Maddox and, 296
  Martin and, 167, 169
  news conference announcing Gallo's results, 142–43
  Retroviridae Study Group and, 179
Lewin, Benjamin, 172
Liberation, 343, 357
Lipsey, Charles E., 284–85, 318
Litton Bionetics, 104, 146, 254, 264, 266
Loiseau, Eric, 61, 65, 69, 86, 117, 125, 164, 397, 399
Loi virus, 61
Loop, Floyd, 405
Los Alamos National Laboratory, 303
Los Angeles Times, 237, 300, 525
Luciw, Paul, 166, 171, 173, 248, 326, 332, 360, 366, 368
Lundberg, George, 75
Luria, Salvador, 290
Lwoff, André, 45, 79, 287, 327
lymphadenopathy, 44, 67. *See also* LAV (lymphadenopathy-associated virus)
lymphadenopathy syndrome, defined, 636
lymphocytes, defined, 636
lymphoid leukemia, defined, 636
lymphoma
  defined, 636

ESP-1 and, 14
HTLV and, 52

M2T-/B, defined, 636
McGinnis, J. Michael, 466, 467, 468
McGrath, Mike, 389, 410, 412, 414, 435, 481, 599n. g
McLaughlin, Loretta, 154
Maddox, John Royden
  Chicago Tribune article and, 345, 355–56
  Connor and, 298
  French judicial system and, 446
  Gallo and, 210, 268–75, 296, 355–56, 381, 400, 530
  Karpas and, 247, 268–69, 332, 340
  Montagnier and, 174, 269, 273, 296, 401
  Nature and, 72, 78–79
  Office of Scientific Inquiry and, 380
  Temin and, 8
Maharaj Ji, 15
Mankiewicz, Frank, 358
Manley, Ken, 9
Mann, Dean, 416
Mann, Jonathan, 326
Markham, Phil, 145
Marks, Paul, 160
Martin, Malcolm
  Barré-Sinoussi and, 60
  Clavel and, 330
  Fischinger and, 216
  Gallo and, 131–33, 214–15, 341, 361, 376, 470–71, 479, 480, 532, 611n. c
  HTLV-3B and, 181, 212–14
  Institut Pasteur and, 378
  LAV and, 150, 162, 168–69, 212–14, 217, 378, 397, 413
  Levy and, 167, 169
  Myers and, 305–06, 340, 341, 342, 377
  Office of Research Integrity and, 479–80, 483, 495, 501–02
  Office of Scientific Integrity and, 377–78, 382, 416
Mason, James
  Altmann and, 129–31, 132, 133
  Dedonder and, 220
  French and American AIDS Foundation and, 454, 455, 456
  Gallo and, 358, 430
  Gallo report and, 464
  H-9 and, 151, 494
  Health and Human Services Department and, 222
  Healy and, 441
  Heckler and, 134, 136, 137, 141

Mason, James (*cont.*)
  Institut Pasteur and, 101, 106, 134, 141, 208–09, 212
  Office of Research Integrity and, 468
  Office of Scientific Integrity and, 466
Material Information Disclosure, 284
Mathias, Charles McC., Jr., 288
Maxwell, Robert, 315–17
Maxwell Institute for AIDS Research, 315–16
Meitner, Lise, 326
Mendel, Steve, 316
Merow, James F., 257–59, 261, 286, 294
messenger RNA, defined, 636
Meyers, Gerald, J61 and, 396
MFA, Stevenson and, 360–61
Mildvan, Donna, 99
Millian, Hector, 366, 375, 413
Millstein, Ira, 221, 222, 291, 294, 301, 318, 456–57
Milstein, Cesar, 531
Minna, John, 25, 335
Mir, 231–32, 232, 233, 234
Mishkin, Barbara, 387, 389, 409, 410, 477, 481–83
Mitterand, François, 197
Miyoshi, Isao, 29–30, 30, 31, 32, 70, 79, 585n. a
Mizutani, Satoshi, 6–7, 8, 9
Modigliani, Robert, 51, 53
Molecular biology, 4, 5, 6, 33, 45
Moley, Kevin, 451
monoclonal antibodies, defined, 636
Monod, Jacques, 45, 46
Montagnier, Luc. *See also* Gallo/Montagnier relationship
  AIDS and, 60, 62, 65, 76–77, 118, 173, 531
  AIDS blood test and, 192, 283, 318, 449–50
  AIDS blood test patent and, 294, 309
  AIDS Task Force and, 68
  AIDS vaccine and, 138
  And the Band Played On, 490
  background of, 45–46
  Barré-Sinoussi and, 46, 50
  Brugière and, 54, 55–56, 68, 69, 164, 243
  Brun-Vézinet and, 66
  CEM and, 567–68n. k
  Chermann and, 46, 47–48, 274, 394
  Clavel and, 231–32
  Connor and, 298
  ELISA and, 76, 103–04, 118
  Francis and, 81, 104, 117, 129, 443, 583n. c
  French and American AIDS Foundation and, 454, 522
  Gairdner Prize and, 313
  HIV-3 and, 306
  HTLV-3B and, 152–53, 156, 170, 339
  Institut Pasteur and, 45
  Japan Prize and, 159
  Koch and, 319
  Lasker Foundation and, 276
  LAV and, 68, 69, 71, 78, 79, 80–81, 87, 93, 127, 128, 144, 156, 163, 207, 225, 227, 236, 237, 283, 321, 339, 549n. b
  LAV-2 and, 234, 328
  Maddox and, 174, 269, 356, 401
  mycoplasma, 366
  Newmark and, 174, 210
  Nobel Prize for AIDS, rumors and, 326, 327, 537
  Nobel Prize aspirations, 337
  Office of Research Integrity and, 499
  Office of Scientific Integrity investigation and, 408
  Popovic and, 70, 71, 83, 88, 94, 104, 428
  records of, 206
  respect for, 177–78, 193, 453
  Retroviridae Study Group and, 179
  retroviruses and, 43–44, 55
  Salk and, 293, 295
  Sattaur and, 183
  Swire and, 294
  Tiollais and, 102
  Volsky and, 376–77
  Wain-Hobson and, 329, 400, 401
  Weiss and, 142, 151
Montagnier, Marcel, 471
Moore, John, 500, 538
Morbidity and Mortality Weekly Report, 42, 216
Morgan, Doris, 20–23
Morgan, Howard, 374
Moss, Bernard, 406
MOV
  AIDS and, 107
  CDC and, 106, 108
  defined, 636
  Gallo and, 241
  Gallo inquiry and, 370
  Hadley and, 375
  HTLV-3B and, 416
  LAV and, 277, 372, 375, 389, 413, 464–65
  Popovic and, 104, 181, 264, 265, 266, 267, 283, 361, 365–66, 389, 413, 470, 485, 553n. h, 603n. o
  Sarngadharan and, 104–05, 106, 264, 265, 365, 413, 553n. h
MT-1, Miyoshi and, 30
MT-2, 30, 40

Mullins, James, 41, 53, 74, 149, 307, 360, 393
Mullis, Kary, 374
Multiple sclerosis, 323, 590–91n. i
Munro, Ian, 109
Murphy, Fred, 133, 151, 156, 210, 221
Murrow, Edward R., 86
mycosis fungoides
   defined, 637
   HTLV and, 28, 29, 31, 542n. e
   Karpas and, 34
   retroviruses and, 25
   Robinson and, 23–24, 26, 28, 31, 543n. j
myeloid cells, defined, 637
Myers, Gerald
   Gallo and, 338–42, 360, 396, 436, 593n. k
   Hallum and, 372, 373
   HIV Sequence Database and, 303–06
   HTLV-3B and, 338–40, 396
   Karpas and, 341
   Martin and, 305–06, 340, 341, 342, 377
   New Jersey pair and, 376
   Reitz and, 393
   Temin and, 403
   White and, 491

National Academy of Sciences
   Gallo and, 160, 323, 439, 562n. a
   Gallo inquiry/investigation and, 353, 358, 370, 373–74, 377, 379, 383, 412–13, 437–40, 451, 607n. i
National Cancer Advisory Board, 10, 126, 450–52
National Cancer Institute
   AIDS and, 38, 58, 76, 141
   AIDS blood test patent and, 318
   AIDS Task Force and, 67–68, 70
   CDC and, 73, 74
   FOCMA and, 40–41
   Hinuma and, 30
   HTLV and, 36
   HTLV-3 and, 126, 145
   Institut Pasteur and, 137
   Japan Prize and, 159
   LAV and, 93–94
   War on Cancer and, 10, 20, 532
National Institutes of Health. *See also* Office of Scientific Integrity
   AIDS and, 141
   AIDS blood test patent and, 123, 128, 133, 134, 135, 287, 557n. l
   AIDS blood tests and, 254
   Baltimore and, 348
   Dingell and, 347, 349, 431, 434–35
   Institut Pasteur and, 200, 249

National Cancer Institute and, 10
   rival groups of, 20
Nature
   AIDS and, 58, 79
   AIDS blood test patents and, 453
   AIDS research chronology, 296–97
   Allain and, 446
   Baltimore and, 8, 9, 300
   Connor and, 297–98
   Daniel and, 308
   DNA structure and, 4–5, 6
   Essex and, 308–09, 339
   Gallo and, 142, 193, 210, 242–44, 245, 246, 263, 275, 286, 356, 364, 371, 394, 395, 397, 403–04, 511, 531, 534, 537, 601n. g
   HL-23V and, 18, 19
   HTLV and, 32
   HTLV-3B and, 153, 170, 172–73
   Klatzmann and, 71–72, 78, 79, 171
   LAV and, 71–72, 78, 153
   Meyers and, 377
   Montagnier and, 55, 269
   MT-2 and, 31
   Mullins and, 307
   peer review process and, 7
   Popovic and, 70
   Temin and, 8
   Varmus and, 518
   Wain-Hobson and, 172, 174
   Weiss and, 531
   White and, 491–92
   Wong-Staal and, 179
Netter, Robert, 447
New England Journal of Medicine, 67, 371, 390
New Jersey Pair, 304, 305, 376, 586n. f
Newman, Don, 317, 318
Newmark, Peter, 78–79, 82, 171–74, 210, 269–70, 272, 274, 340
New Scientist, 125, 126, 182–84, 297–99, 340, 556n. f
Newsweek, 9, 58, 300–301, 357, 403, 535, 537
New Yorker, The, 367, 445
New York Times
   AIDS blood test patents and, 525
   Dingell and, 346
   ESP-1 and, 14
   Gallo and, 122, 160, 178, 225, 316, 380, 428, 505, 534, 562n. b
   Haddow and, 444
   HIV-3 and, 306
   LAV and, 132
   Mason and, 129–31, 132, 133
   Onek and, 444–45

New York Times (cont.)
  Pasteur v. Gallo and, 246
  reverse transcriptase and, 9
  science journalists of, 370
  Shilts and, 311
  Swire and, 238
Nixon, Richard, 10, 120, 431, 453
Nobel Prize for physiology or medicine
  AIDS and, 325–26
  Baltimore and, 9, 37
  Black and, 338
  Crick and Watson and, 5
  Elion and, 338
  Gilman and, 526
  Hitchings and, 338
  Monod and, 45
  Rous and, 4
  Temin and, 6, 9, 37
Nobel Prizes, selection process of, 335–37,
  592nn. e, f
Norman, Colin, 210–11, 370
Norwood, William "Pete," 253
Nouvel Observateur, 467
Nowinski, Robert
  AIDS blood test and, 190, 227, 251
  AIDS blood test patents and, 200, 201,
    204–05
  blood supply and, 280–81
  Genetic Systems and, 156–57
  Martin and, 378
  Saah and, 256
  VaxGen and, 530
nucleosides, defined, 637
nucleotides, defined, 637
nucleotide sequences
  of ARV, 171, 173, 180
  defined, 637
  of HTLB-3B, 170, 172, 173, 175, 177, 178,
    180, 193, 271, 293–94, 360, 381, 403,
    421, 565–66n. s, 570n. k
  of LAV, 169–70, 172, 173, 175, 177, 178,
    180, 193, 271, 293–94, 341, 360, 381,
    421, 565–66n. s, 570n. k
  of LAV$_{Bru}$, 403
  of MFA, 360
  Myers and, 303–04
  of New Jersey Pair, 304, 586n. f
Nussbaum, Bruce, 384–86

O'Brien, Steve, 334
Observer, 188
O'Connor, Nancy, 476–77, 495, 499
Odle, Robert, 430–31, 454–56, 458, 485, 511,
  518–21

Office of the Inspector General (HHS), 433,
  517, 518, 523
Office of Protection from Research Risks,
  405–08, 409, 423, 601n. j
Office of Research Integrity
  creation of, 466, 475
  Gallo and, 467–72, 475–81, 492–95, 504–05,
    509, 515, 610n. d
  Imanishi-Kari and, 529
  Popovic and, 470, 478, 481–87, 501–05
  Sharma and, 474
Office of Scientific Integrity
  AIDS blood test patents and, 419, 430, 457,
    605n. g
  Dingell and, 460–62
  Gallo and, 351–52, 358, 359, 360, 361, 369,
    408, 410, 414–25, 428, 435, 438, 451,
    453, 460, 463, 478, 494, 506, 514,
    595–96n. h, 604n. f
  Gallo inquiry upgrade to investigation, 379
  Gallo investigation team, 384
  Gallo report, 436–38, 440–41, 460, 464,
    465–66, 608n. l
  Gallo's isolates and, 371, 373
  Imanishi-Kari and, 351
  National Institute of Health's review of, 425
  Popovic and, 352, 363–65, 374, 376,
    386–90, 408, 409–13, 414, 415–16, 420,
    422, 435, 438, 460, 487, 497–98, 501,
    528, 607n. h
  Popovic's pool samples and, 375, 413,
    602–03n. m
  scientific misconduct and, 349
  Sharma and, 426
Office of Scientific Integrity Review, 464
oncogenes, defined, 637
oncoviruses, defined, 637
Onek, Joseph
  AIDS blood tests and, 447
  CNTS scandal and, 449, 450
  Dingell and, 383, 527
  Francis and, 443
  French and American AIDS Foundation
    and, 522
  as Gallo's attorney, 358, 432, 440, 452–53
  Gallo's notebooks and, 355
  Hadley and, 380
  HTLV-3B and, 393, 394
  Imanishi-Kari and, 529
  LAV and, 469
  McGrath and, 481
  Martin's notebooks and, 378
  New York Times and, 444–45
  Office of Inspector General and, 517

Office of Research Integrity and, 468, 475, 477, 478, 480
  Raub and, 381
  Sharma and, 494
Onek, Klein and Farr, 358, 432, 595n. g
Organon, 147
Orth, Gerard, 178
Osborne, Mary Jane, 358, 359
OSI. *See* Office of Scientific Integrity
Osler, William, 317
O'Toole, Margot, 348–49

p24
  Abbott Laboratories and, 292
  AIDS blood tests' false negatives and, 250–51, 254, 255, 256, 279
  defined, 637
  Institut Pasteur's test and, 251, 292, 582–83n. b
Palca, Joe, 269, 271
Pan-Data Systems, 362–63, 375–76, 390, 391, 596–97n. j
Parkman, Paul, 352, 366
Parks, Wade, 68, 69
Parrish, Debbie, 476–77
Pascal, Oscar, 464–65, 468, 529
Pasteur v. Gallo, 346
Patarca, Roberto, 173
Paul Ehrlich Prize, 536
Paulucci, Jeno, 158
PCR. *See* polymerase chain reaction
peer review process, 7
Peetoom, France, 281
People, 177, 178, 451
"peptide cocktail" vaccine, 407–08, 601n. i
permanent cell line. *See* continuous cell line
Perot, Ross, 459
Perutz, Max, 33
PHA, Morgan and, 21
phage, defined, 637
Philadelphia Inquirer, 58–59, 77–78
Picasso, Paloma, 329
Pierce, Fred, 125
Piot, Peter, 103, 105, 157, 296, 472
plasmid, defined, 637
PNAS. *See Proceedings of the National Academy of Sciences*
Pneumocystis carinii, 13, 58, 62, 539
Poiesz, Bernie
  HTLV and, 26–29, 31, 32, 35, 37, 64, 80, 82, 164, 333, 541–42n. d, 543–44nn. k, l
  HUT-102 and, 24–25, 333
  LAV and, 82
  Miyoshi and, 30

mycosis fungoides and, 24
  Office of Research Integrity and, 495
  Popovic and, 88
  reverse transcriptase and, 24
  Ruscetti and, 23
polymerase chain reaction
  defined, 637–38
  Hoffman–La Roche and, 374
  White and, 413
Popovic, Mikulas
  AIDS blood test and, 193, 274, 283, 482
  AIDS blood test patent and, 294, 301, 309, 335, 605n. g
  AIDS receptor problem and, 191
  Alizon and, 247
  Barré-Sinoussi and, 83, 495–96, 499, 513, 525, 613–15nn. d, e
  Chermann and, 99–100
  Gallo and, 110–11, 114, 136, 180, 212, 248, 286, 294, 360, 388, 393, 411, 467, 485, 493, 533
  Gonda and, 91–92, 124, 207, 224, 238–39, 240, 264, 265, 298, 343, 508, 577–78n. m, 581–82n. l
  H-9 and, 105, 110–11, 124, 202, 208, 217, 259, 266, 332, 333, 409, 503
  HTLV and, 32, 35, 42, 53, 77, 83
  HTLV-3 and, 142, 148
  HTLV-3B and, 120–21, 164–65, 180, 207, 265, 305, 339, 342, 343, 364, 387, 409, 415, 566n. a
  HTLV-3$_{RF}$ and, 161, 181, 496, 498–99, 567n. b
  HUT-78 and, 88, 89, 104–05, 128, 212, 223, 264, 266, 333, 416, 591–92n. a
  Kalyanarman and, 184
  Kulstad and, 123
  LAV and, 83–85, 88–89, 92, 94, 96, 110, 111, 113–14, 115, 118, 138, 155, 161–62, 202, 206, 207, 208, 211, 217, 223, 224, 237, 248, 257, 260–66, 270, 277, 318, 343, 344, 352, 365, 372, 376, 380, 381, 387, 389–90, 410, 415, 417, 469, 496, 508–09, 554n. n, 576n. i, 577n. l, 581–82n. l
  LAV$_{Bru}$ and, 394
  Maddox and, 274
  Montagnier and, 70, 71, 83, 88, 94, 104, 109, 411
  MOV and, 104, 181, 264, 265, 266, 267, 283, 361, 365–66, 389, 413, 470, 485, 553n. h, 603n. o
  National Academy of Science panel and, 373
  New Mexico State University and, 330–31, 363

Popovic, Mikulas (*cont.*)
  Nobel Prize for AIDS, rumors and, 326
  Office of Research Integrity and, 470, 478,
    481–87, 501–04
  Office of Scientific Integrity and, 352,
    363–65, 376, 386–90, 409–13, 414,
    415–16, 420, 422, 435, 438, 460, 487,
    497–98, 501, 528, 607n. h
  patent royalties and, 333, 335, 409, 510
  pool samples of, 375, 413, 415–16, 435,
    470, 483, 484, 491, 496, 497, 499,
    602–03nn. m, n
  records of, 206–07, 222–24, 259–62,
    364–65, 373, 374, 379, 389, 417, 425,
    434, 470, 506–08, 526
  Research Integrity Adjudications Panel
    and, 475
  reverse transcriptase and, 82
  Salahuddin and, 124
  Swire and, 294
  T-cell line and, 105–06, 110–11
  Temina and, 451
Praxis Pharmaceuticals, 390
Premio Internazionale Tevere Roma, 215
Prensky, Wolf, 41
Priori, Elizabeth S., 14–15
*Proceedings of the National Academy of
  Sciences*
  Gallo and, 514, 515, 534, 537
  HTLV and, 27, 28, 542n. d
  Montagnier and, 79
  Purtilo and, 75
  retroviruses and, 30–31
protease inhibitors, 536, 538
proteins, defined, 638
proviral DNA, defined, 638
Public Health Service, 209, 230, 330, 421, 423
Public Health Service Executive Task Force,
  186
Purtilo, David, 75–76

Rabb, Harriet
  Institut Pasteur and, 511, 518–20
  Varmus and, 512, 519, 521
Radioimmuno precipitation assay, 107
Ralbovsky, Donald M., 380
Ratner, Lee, 165, 170, 173, 304, 306, 344, 398,
  506, 589–90n. f
Raub, William
  AIDS blood test patents and, 419
  Chicago Tribune article, 352
  Connor and, 297
  Dingell and, 350–51, 353, 362–63, 391–92,
    468

  Gallo and, 358, 411
  Gallo inquiry upgraded to investigation, 379
  Gallo's isolates and, 381–82
  Hadley and, 355, 413, 414
  Hallum and, 372
  National Academy of Sciences panel and,
    359, 373–74, 379, 412, 437
  Office of Scientific Integrity and, 351,
    420–21, 422, 472
  replacement of, 404
  Schwartz and, 400
Rauscher Murine leukemia virus, defined,
  638
Read, Betsy
  Gallo and, 136, 216, 482
  HLTV3$_{RF}$ and, 121, 161
  HUT-78 and, 397
  lab sabotaged, 100
  LAV and, 89, 90, 165, 263–64, 270, 283,
    397, 581–82n. l
  MOV and, 365
  Office of Scientific Integrity and, 352, 435,
    607n. h
  Popovic and, 417, 484–85
  records of, 259, 262, 506–09, 526
  Swire and, 294
reading frames, defined, 638
Reagan, Ronald
  AIDS blood test and, 188
  AIDS blood test patent and, 290, 300, 301,
    305, 430
  Federal Technology Transfer Act and,
    278
  Heckler and, 101, 222
Reagan administration
  AIDS blood test and, 141, 146, 186
  AIDS blood test patent and, 200, 283–84,
    288, 318, 444
  Dedonder and, 299
  Dingell and, 346
  Genetic Systems and, 227
  Institut Pasteur and, 257
Redfern, Martin, 122, 125–26, 556n. f
Rehm, Diane, 384, 386
Reitz, Marvin, 393, 396, 402, 549n. t, 549–51n. f
Remnick, David, 310
Research Integrity Adjudications Panel
  appeals process of, 475
  Gallo and, 492–95
  Popovic and, 481–87, 499–505, 512, 517–18,
    615–16nn. g, h
restriction enzymes, defined, 638
restriction maps
  Bryant and, 166–67

defined, 638
  Feorino and, 214
  Hahn and, 93, 168
restriction sites, defined, 638
Retroviridae Study Group, 179–80
retroviruses
  Barré-Sinoussi and, 49
  cell-surface marker for, 40
  Chermann and, 43, 55
  defined, 639
  Gallo and, 24, 25, 27, 31, 57
  Gardner and, 80
  Hinuma and, 30–31, 543n. h
  Montagnier and, 43–44, 55
  Mullins and, 74
  reverse transcriptase and, 9–10, 15–16, 47, 48
  similarity of, 161
  vaccines and, 138
reverse transcriptase
  Barré-Sinoussi and, 48, 49–50, 55
  defined, 639
  Gallo and, 11, 14, 51, 541–42n. b, 585n. a
  Klatzmann and, 63
  LAV and, 83, 117, 127
  Poiesz and, 24
  retroviruses and, 9–10, 15–16, 47, 48
  Ruscetti and, 24
  Salahuddin and, 71
  Spiegelman and, 7, 585n. a
  Temin and, 7–8, 9, 450
Rhesus macaque virus, 61, 307, 308
Rhoades, Larry, 464–65
Richards, Fred, 412, 437, 439, 440, 495, 502, 503
Richardson, Ersell
  AIDS and, 70, 77
  Hahn and, 93
  MOV and, 365
  Office of Scientific Integrity and, 352
  Popovic and, 388
  records of, 259, 262
  Swire and, 294
Riseberg, Dick, 522
RNA (Ribonucleic acid)
  defined, 639
  genetic codes and, 5, 6
  oncoviruses and, 4
RNA viruses
  defined, 639
  Temin and, 6, 7
Roberts, John, 203–05
Roberts, Seth, 367, 368
Robertson, Ron, 291, 294, 317, 321–22

Robinson, Charles
  HTLV-1 and, 124, 164
  HTLV$_{CR}$ and, 41
  mycosis fungoides and, 23–24, 26, 28, 31, 543n. j
  Poiesz and Ruscetti's work and, 23–24, 25, 28, 64, 164, 543–44n. k
  restriction maps and, 92
Roche Diagnostic Systems, 374
Rod, 232
Rous, Francis Peyton, discovery of oncovirus, 4
Rous Sarcoma Virus, 6, 8, 36, 545–46n. q, 639
Rouzioux, Christine, 66–67, 80, 86, 98, 103, 105, 157, 309
Rowland, Bernard, 191, 192–93
Rozenbaum, Willy
  AIDS and, 42–45
  Brugière and, 42, 330
  Lailler and, 398
  Leibowitch and, 52
  Montagnier and, 44
  Science and, 55
RSV. *See* Rous Sarcoma Virus
RT. *See* reverse transcriptase
Ruscetti, Frank
  Gallo and, 25, 30, 37, 79
  H-9 and, 332
  HTLV and, 27–29, 32, 35, 64, 164, 333
  HUT-78 and, 334, 335
  HUT-102 and, 24–25, 333
  Interleukin-2 and, 24
  Morgan and, 22–23
  Poiesz and, 23, 26
Ruscetti, Sandy, 41
Russell, Cristine, 139

Saah, Al, 253–56, 257
Sabin, Albert, 32, 288, 584–85n. k
SAIDS, 114
Salahuddin, Zaki
  AIDS and, 71, 85, 163, 563–64n. j
  Bennett and, 463
  Gallo and, 112, 123, 241, 376, 391, 514
  Gallo's memoirs and, 429
  Gonda and, 239, 240
  growth factor and, 16–17
  H-9 and, 332
  HBLV and, 324, 325
  HTLV-3 and, 112, 123–24, 382–83
  Office of Scientific Integrity investigation and, 408, 423
  Pan-Data Systems and, 362, 363, 375–76, 390, 596–97n. j
  Popovic and, 89, 111

Salahuddin, Zaki (*cont.*)
  retroviruses and, 24
  Swire and, 294
  Wong-Staal and, 194
Salk, Jonas, 86, 287–89, 293–95, 313, 329, 455, 479
Sambrook, Joseph, 358
Sanders, Kingsley, 46
Sandler, Gerry, 255–56, 280–81, 292
San Francisco Chronicle, 311, 367
San Francisco Examiner, 366, 369
Sanger, Fred, 34, 544n. m
SANOFI, 458
Sarin, Prem
  AIDS blood tests and, 251
  Bennett and, 463
  Homburg Degussa Pharma and, 390–91, 599–600nn. i, j
  HTLV-3 and, 129
  Kulstad and, 123
  LAV and, 83
  Office of Scientific Inquiry investigation and, 408, 423
  Stockton and, 390
  Swire and, 294
Sarngadharan, M. G.
  AIDS blood test patent and, 128, 193, 283, 287, 289, 294, 301, 309, 557n. l, 582n. q
  ELISA testing and, 108, 112, 146, 264, 383, 482, 514–15, 553–54n. i
  Gallo and, 107, 152
  HTLV-3B and, 156, 162, 165, 176, 397, 415
  Institut Pasteur and, 140, 151–53
  Karpas and, 247
  Kulstad and, 123
  MOV and, 104–05, 106, 264, 265, 365, 413, 484, 553n. h
  Nobel Prize for AIDS and, 326
  Office of Scientific Integrity investigation and, 410, 435
  Swire and, 294
Sattaur, Omar, 125, 182–85, 297, 299, 370, 497
Schaffer, Priscilla
  Dingell and, 435
  Gallo and, 410
  Hadley and, 412, 414
  Office of Research Integrity and, 481–82, 484, 485, 487, 495, 502
  Popovic and, 388
  Raub and, 422
  scientific misconduct commission and, 529
Schmitt, Victor, 291–92

Schneider, Johanna, 488
Schroeder, Patricia, 474
Schuler, Jack, 147–48, 186
Schupbach, Jorg, 112, 123, 124, 237, 383
Schwartz, Maxime
  AIDS blood test patents and, 458, 517, 520
  Dingell and, 510
  French and American AIDS Foundation and, 454, 455–56, 522
  Gallo and, 429–30
  as Institut Pasteur's director, 394, 401
  Montagnier and, 450
  Raub and, 400
  Varmus and, 511–14, 518, 520–21, 525
Science
  AIDS blood tests and, 147
  Clavel and, 233–34
  Essex and, 233
  Gallo and, 17, 35, 53, 55–59, 71, 75, 107, 110–13, 118, 121–29, 132, 134, 139–40, 141, 142, 144, 149, 152, 161, 164, 181–82, 210, 216, 237, 242, 244, 262–64, 323, 332, 344, 345, 353, 371, 373, 382–83, 415, 465, 468, 477, 486, 492, 503, 514, 535, 539, 540, 570–71n. g, 603n. b, 618n. d
  Gallo inquiry and, 369–70, 598n. b
  HTLB-3B and, 372
  Institut Pasteur and, 55, 56–57, 58, 78, 82, 90, 91, 98, 99, 102, 115, 129, 157, 164, 202, 205, 243, 244, 284, 285, 343, 344, 492–93, 518, 545n. o
  Levy and, 143, 158
  Luciw and, 171, 173
  Martin and, 213, 214, 396
  Myers and, 396
  Nature compared to, 72
  O'Brien and, 334, 335, 592n. d
  Popovic and, 363, 364, 379, 382, 387–90, 409, 410–12, 417–18, 419, 420, 428, 430, 434, 435, 438, 439, 469, 481, 485–86, 493, 496, 498, 508, 539, 540
  Saah and, 254
  T-Cell Growth Factor and, 23
  Wain-Hobson and, 401–02, 412, 531
Science & Government Report, 440, 459, 506
Science Digest, 154
Scientific American, 287, 337–38, 340, 371
Scolnick, Ed, 323
Second Triennial Rameshwardas Birla International Award, 158
Secret Service, 506–08, 526
Securities and Exchange Commission, 431
Selzer, Andrea, 505

September LAV
  defined, 639
  Gallo and, 397
  HTLV-3B and, 394
  Popovic and, 207, 211, 217, 222, 248, 258
  Wong-Staal and, 165–66
Seragen, 146
Sergent, François, 343, 344
Serums, defined, 639
Seytre, Bernard, 446–47, 448
Sezary's syndrome, 24, 25, 29, 31, 34, 417, 542n. e, 639
Sharma, Rameshwar K., 425–26, 474, 494, 605n. h
Shaw, George, 161, 277, 338, 339, 413
Shearer, Gene, 69
Shilts, Randy, 311, 313, 367, 443, 489–90, 587–88n. a
Sidote, Marijane, 229, 279, 281
Siegenthaler, Walter, 115
Sliski, Ann, 276
SLWDQ, 534
SmithKline Beecham, 114
Sodroski, Joseph, 482, 502
Sonigo, Pierre, 116–17, 169
Sonnabend, Joseph, 76
Southern Blot, defined, 639–40
Spiegelman, Sol, 7, 15, 18, 585n. a
SP-PG, 533–34
Spy, 367–68
ST1571, 538
Staal, Steve, 158, 194
Stent, Gunther, 5
Stevens, Jerry, 354, 595n. e
Stevenson, Mario, 360–61, 376, 377
STLV-3A$_{GM}$, 307, 308, 586–87n. i
STLV-3$_{MAC}$, 233, 307, 308, 309, 586–87nn. h, i
Stobo, John, 358
Stockton, Peter D. H.
  AIDS blood test patents and, 463–64
  Baltimore and, 390
  Bennett and, 462–63
  Gallo and, 392, 409–10, 466–67
  Hadley and, 426, 461
  Institut Pasteur and, 511
  Odle and, 430
  Office of the Inspector General and, 433
  Office of Scientific Integrity Review and, 465, 468
  Onek and, 383
  retirement of, 528
  Varmus and, 512
  Watson and, 473
Streicher, Howard, 261, 322, 354–55, 355, 380

Stuntz, Reid, 510–11, 512
Sugen, 538
Sullivan, Louis W., 449, 451, 455, 456
supernatant, defined, 640
Supreme Court, U.S., 85–86
Suramin, 331
Svoboda, Jan, 70
Swire, James B.
  AIDS blood test patents and, 224, 458
  contract for noncommercial use and, 258–59
  Dean and, 221
  Freedom of Information Act, 259–63, 265, 266, 294, 297
  Gallo and, 286–87, 294, 369, 453
  Gonda and, 238–40, 259, 294, 571–72n. j
  Hampar and, 271, 579–80n. d
  LAV and, 247, 258, 264–65, 577n. l
  legal bills and, 318
  Martin and, 378
  MOV and, 416
  Office of Research Integrity and, 477
  Popovic and, 374
  Reagan administration and, 299–300
  Wood and, 580–81n. e
Szybalski, Waclaw, 8

T-4 cells
  defined, 640
  ELISA and, 67
  HIV and, 538
  Klatzmann, 144–45, 190
  LAV and, 71, 80
  LAV$_{Bru}$ and, 62
  Popovic and, 88
T-8 cell, defined, 640
T-cell growth factor. *See* Interleukin-2
T-cell line
  defined, 640
  Popovic and, 105–06, 110–11
T-cell lymphomas
  defined, 640
  HTLV and, 28, 542n. e
T-cells. *See* T-lymphocytes
Tedder, Richard, 325
Teich, Natalie, 18, 19
Temin, Howard
  AIDS blood test patents and, 290
  Gallo and, 314, 342, 450–52, 471
  HTLV-3B and, 377, 394, 395, 403
  Nobel Prize for physiology or medicine and, 6, 9, 37
  oncoviruses and, 4
  Retroviridae Study Group and, 179

Temin, Howard (*cont.*)
  reverse transcriptase and, 7–9, 302
  RNA viruses and, 5–6
  War on Cancer and, 10
Tenth International Cancer Congress, Temin
  and, 7
Thé, Guy de
  Adult T-cell Leukemia and, 28
  Chermann and, 87
  Gallo and, 468
  Guroff and, 29, 542–43n. g
  Hinuma and, 30
  Montagnier and, 68, 81
thymine, defined, 640
Ti7.4, 269, 370, 397, 402
Time
  Gallo and, 14, 141, 206, 277–78, 453, 471
  Ho and, 536
  Institut Pasteur and, 141–42, 277–78, 282
  Montagnier and, 453
  Popovic and, 409
Times, The, 72
Ting, Bob, 146
Tiollais, Pierre, 102, 116
tissue culture. *See* cell culture
T-lymphocytes
  AIDS and, 44
  defined, 640
  Morgan and, 22, 23
  Pneumocystis carinii and, 13
Todaro, George
  ESP-1 and, 15
  Fischinger and, 202–03
  Gallo and, 156, 160, 324, 337
  Gallo compared to, 19, 31–32
  Gallo's lab contamination, 20, 205
  HL-23V and, 18
  HTLV and, 31
  HTLV-3 and, 156
  HTLV-3B and, 169
  lab of, 18
  LAV micrographs and, 571–72n. j
  Martin and, 181, 378
  Montagnier and, 156–57
  mouse leukemia virus and, 15, 60
  National Academy of Sciences and, 323, 353
  National Cancer Institute and, 205
  reverse transcriptase and, 14
  Swire and, 238, 267
  Wong-Staal and, 331
Tomasulo, Peter, 256
Touched with Fire (Jamison), 473
Townley & Updike, 221

Townsend and Townsend, 191
Tramont, Edmund, 352–53
transfer RNA, defined, 640
transformation, defined, 640
Transportation, U.S. Department of, 431
Tristem, Mike, 341

United Press International, 369, 370
United States Patent and Trademark Office, 128, 134, 191–92, 282, 284, 294, 309, 459
uracil, defined, 640
USA Today, 451
U.S. News & World Report, 346

vaccines
  Brandt and, 138
  cancer vaccine and, 10
  defined, 641
  Francis and, 479, 529
  Gallo and, 177, 405–07, 479, 514
  Heckler and, 135
  HIV Sequence Database and, 304, 305
  HTLV-3B, 148
  polio vaccine and, 304
  Salk and, 288, 479, 584–85n. k
  Zagury and, 405–07, 514
vaccinia virus, 406–07
van der Loo, Elizabeth, 25, 35–36
Van Horn, Charlie, 191
Varmus, Harold
  AIDS blood test patents and, 514
  animal cancer viruses and, 60
  French and American AIDS Foundation and, 522–24
  Gallo and, 236, 489, 513, 516, 535
  Memorial Sloan-Kettering Cancer Center, 530
  National Academy of Sciences, 323, 324, 353
  as National Institutes of Health director, 488–89, 530
  Popovic and, 513
  Rabb and, 512, 519, 521
  Retroviridae Study Group and, 179–80
  Rous Sarcoma Virus and, 36–37, 545–46n. q
  Schwartz and, 511–14, 518, 520–21, 525
Varner, Oliver, 217–18
VaxGen, 529–30
virion, defined, 641
viruses, defined, 3, 641
Virus Hunting (Gallo), 429
visna virus, defined, 641
Vogt, Cornell, 374–75
Volsky, David, 376

Wade, Nicholas, 505, 616n. i
Wagner, Robert, 358
Wain-Hobson, Simon
    Barré-Sinoussi and, 395, 397, 400, 401
    chimpanzee lentivirus and, 309
    Gallo and, 273–74, 334, 360, 396
    HTLV-3B and, 394, 403, 412
    HTLV-4 and, 339
    IDAV-2 and, 399
    Institut Pasteur and, 397
    Koch and, 319
    LAV and, 116–17, 168, 169, 170, 171, 174, 175, 331, 340–41, 565n. q
    LAV_{Bru} and, 394
    Maddox and, 530
    Montagnier and, 329, 400, 401, 471
    Tiollais and, 102
    White and, 491
Waksal, Sam, 336
Wall Street Journal, 125, 126, 157, 204, 224, 300, 315, 390, 404
War on Cancer, 10, 20, 120
Warner-Lambert, 146, 147
Washington Post
    AIDS blood test patents and, 300
    AIDS blood tests' false negatives and, 254, 255
    And the Band Played On, 489
    Broder and, 332
    Essex and, 234
    Gallo and, 17, 122, 125, 126, 136, 139, 226, 236–37, 276, 313–14, 337, 355, 357, 360, 362, 394–95, 436, 453, 539
    Gallo/Montagnier relationship and, 471
    Haseltine and, 173
    Healy and, 441, 528
    HTLV and, 182
    Onek, Klein and Farr and, 358
Washington Times, 404
Watkins, Clyde, 435, 461
Watson, James
    DNA structure and, 4–5, 6, 302, 594–95n. d
    Gallo and, 353–54, 467, 472–73
    Healy and, 473, 610–11n. i
    National Academy of Sciences and, 353, 358
    reputation of, 473, 610n. h
    Schwartz and, 401
    War on Cancer and, 10
Watt, James, 86
Webb, Dennis, 282
Weil, Gotshal & Manges, 221
Weinberg, Myron, 262, 263, 266, 374, 580–81n. e
Weinberg, Robert, 489

Weiser, Gerard, 193, 202, 205
Weiss, Robin
    AIDS blood test and, 188–89, 190, 517
    AIDS receptor problem and, 191
    CEM and, 230, 570n. c
    Gallo and, 18, 64, 127, 142, 181, 236, 344–45, 360, 556n. g, 558n. b, 560n. m, 594n. m
    HL-23V and, 19–20
    HTLV and, 35–36
    HTLV-3 and, 127
    HTLV-3B, 148, 149, 151, 165
    Japan Prize and, 159
    Karpas and, 33, 247, 531, 574n. a
    LAV and, 82, 127, 128, 165
    Nobel Prize for AIDS rumors and, 326
    Retroviridae Study Group and, 179
    Sattaur and, 184
Western Blot
    AIDS blood tests and, 185, 189, 190, 219, 229, 252, 253, 255, 279, 280
    Ascher and, 250
    defined, 641
    HTLV-4 and, 235
    Institut Pasteur's AIDS blood test and, 230
White, Tom, 413, 416, 421, 483, 485, 497, 603n. n
Wigzell, Hans, 337, 368, 537
Wilson, Dennis, 512
Windom, Robert, 317, 319, 321–22, 590n. h
Wong-Staal, Flossie
    Arya and, 277
    career of, 331
    Gallo and, 194, 275, 341–42, 359, 492
    HALV and, 179
    Haseltine and, 149
    HTLV-1B and, 93
    HTLV-3B and, 168, 170, 175, 176, 180, 223, 274, 397, 434, 492, 564–65n. m, 566n. v
    Montagnier and, 273
    September LAV and, 165–66
Wood, Tom, 580–81n. e
Woods, Andrea, 25, 26, 37, 52
World AIDS Foundation, 318
World Health Organization, 93, 406
Wyngaarden, James
    Baltimore and, 348
    DeVita and, 331
    Dingell and, 350
    Fischinger and, 149
    Gallo and, 127, 155, 160, 198, 216, 276, 316, 353
    H-9 and, 151
    Heckler news conference and, 135

Wyngaarden, James (*cont.*)
  Institute of Human Virology and, 536
  Institut Pasteur and, 249
  Karpas and, 218, 340
  successor of, 404
  Weiss and, 128

Yang, Sue, 541–42n. b
Young, Frank, 227

Zagury, Daniel
  Broder and, 514

  Chermann and, 88, 198
  Escoffier-Lambiotte and, 196, 197
  Gallo and, 393, 405–08, 428, 449, 514, 600n. a
  Gomez and, 308
  HTLV-3B and, 149
  Morgan and, 23
  Office of Protection from Research Risks and, 408, 601n. j
Zagury, Jean-François, 534
Zeigler, John, AIDS and, 38
Zonana, Victor, 521
Zuck, Tom, 228–30, 251–52, 279, 281–82